Acta Neurochirurgica Supplement 121

Series Editor
H.-J. Steiger

For further volumes:
http://www.springer.com/series/4

Richard L. Applegate • Gang Chen • Hua Feng
John H. Zhang
Editors

Brain Edema XVI

Translate Basic Science into Clinical Practice

Springer

Editors
Richard L. Applegate
Department of Anesthesiology
Loma Linda University School of Medicine
Loma Linda
California
USA

Gang Chen
Department of Neurosurgery
Soochow University The First
Affiliated Hospital
Suzhou
Jiangsu
China

Hua Feng
Department of Neurosurgery
Third Military Medical University Southwest
Hospital
Chongqing
China

John H. Zhang
Departments of Anesthesiology
Physiology and Neurosurgery
Loma Linda University School of Medicine
Loma Linda
California
USA

ISSN 0065-1419
ISBN 978-3-319-18496-8 ISBN 978-3-319-18497-5 (eBook)
DOI 10.1007/978-3-319-18497-5

Library of Congress Control Number: 2015949156

Springer Cham Heidelberg New York Dordrecht London

Printed on acid-free and chlorine-free bleached paper

Springer is part of Springer Science+Business Media (www.springer.com)

Foreword

This book constitutes the proceedings of the 16th International Conference on Brain Edema and Cellular Injury and the 3rd Symposium on Preconditioning for Neurological Disorders, which was held at the Hyatt Regency, Huntington Beach, California, on September 27–30, 2014.

The symposium hosted an impressive group of basic scientists and clinicians from North America, Europe, and Asia.

Sixty-five abstracts were presented over 3 days in three sessions:

Session I	Brain Edema and Ion Channels
Session II	What Is New in Neural ICU and Edema Management
Session III	Experimental Edema Treatment

This symposium was given generous support by:

Platinum Sponsor	Integra
Gold Sponsor	Sechrist

Awards were presented for the best, well-written abstract in each session:

Poster Awards	Group 1	Devin McBride, PhD
	Group 2	Elga Esposito, PhD
	Group 3	Xian-Hua Chen, PhD
	Group 4	Meghan McClure, MD
Oral Awards	Clinical	Keven Sheth, MD
		Changhong Ren, MD, PhD
	Basic Science	Hua Su, MD, PhD
		Rafaella Gesuete, PhD

There were two keynote speakers and three presidential lecturers:

Keynote Speakers	Jun Chen, MD, Professor of Neurology and Pharmacology, University of Pittsburgh
Keynote Speaker	Paul Vespa, Professor of Neurology, UCLA
Presidential Lecture	Miguel Perez-Pinzon, PhD, Professor of Neurology/Neuroscience, Director of the Cerebral Vascular Disease Research Center, Vice-Chair for Basic Science of Neurology, Basic Science Division
Presidential Lecture	Guohua Xi, MD, Professor of Neurosurgery Richard C. Schneider Research Professor, Neurosurgery Associate Director, Crosby Neurosurgical Laboratories
Presidential Lecture	Takeshi Maeda presented for Yoichi Katayama, MD, Chairman and Professor Department of Neurological Surgery, Nihon University School of Medicine

CA, USA Robert D. Martin, MD

Preface

The 16th International Conference on Brain Edema and Cellular Injury and the 3rd Symposium on Preconditioning for Neurological Disorders were successfully held in Huntington Beach, California, from September 27 to 30, 2014. Basic scientists and physician scientists from all over the world attended and discussed mechanisms and treatments for brain edema, as well as preconditioning-induced brain protection. This volume contains more than 60 papers from internationally recognized experts.

Brain edema, an increase in brain water content, can result in increased tissue volume and increased intracranial pressure. Brain edema is a feature of many different neurological disorders and this was reflected by the range of presentations at the meeting, from neonatal hypoxia/ischemia and hemorrhage to adult cerebral ischemia, hemorrhage, and traumatic brain injury. Brain edema is a major determinant of disease/injury outcome.

In 1967, Dr. Klatzo divided brain edema into two basic types, vasogenic and cytotoxic edema. Vasogenic edema results from increased blood-brain barrier permeability, whereas cytotoxic edema is caused by parenchymal cell dysfunction. This classification is still commonly used, and this symposium had a range of papers on altered blood-brain barrier function as well as the mechanisms of parenchymal cell dysfunction in multiple disease states. Although it is important to understand the mechanisms underlying brain edema formation, it is also vitally important to translate that information into therapies for treating edema. The treatment of brain edema has not significantly advanced in decades. The current meeting presented several innovative approaches to treat edema experimentally, but it also presented new data on the current clinical trial on glyburide in ischemic stroke.

Magnetic resonance imaging has advanced significantly over the last decade and can be used to differentiate vasogenic edema from cytotoxic brain edema. Fluid-attenuated inversion recovery (FLAIR) is often performed to detect vasogenic edema, and diffusion-weighted imaging can identify cytotoxic edema. We believe that magnetic resonance imaging and other imaging techniques will be used even more extensively in brain edema studies in the next decade.

Experimental studies suggest that brain edema caused by neurosurgical procedures is preventable. It is well known that neuroprotection is a major neurosurgical issue where procedures may result in edema, hemorrhage, and/or ischemia. Preconditioning-induced brain tolerance refers to an endogenous mechanism for brain protection against different kinds of brain injuries. Preconditioning has been used for heart and brain surgery and is a clinical reality now. In the brain, ischemic preconditioning has been used during clipping of cerebral aneurysm and attenuates tissue hypoxia during aneurysm clipping. Future studies are needed to develop noninvasive preconditioning methods to reduce brain edema and brain injury.

MI, USA	Guohua Xi
MI, USA	Richard F. Keep

Contents

General Section

The Evolution of the Clinical Use of Osmotic Therapy in the Treatment of Cerebral Edema

Michael N. Diringer

Introduction

For decades, one of the primary medical interventions to treat cerebral edema has been the administration of hyperosmolar solutions. The agents used, how they are administered, and the therapeutic targets have evolved considerably over the last century. A review of the process highlights lessons learned, provides insight into current practice, and raises important questions.

Weed and McKibbens [1] were the first to report the ability of hyperosmolar solutions to shrink nervous tissue in 1919. They noted that infusion of a 30 % saline solution produced a marked decrease in brain volume, whereas free water administration resulted in brain swelling. In that same year, Hayden [2] reported a similar effect with 25 % glucose solutions. This was followed by Fay's [3] description of "the treatment of cerebral trauma, by methods of dehydration." Fay initially administered oral hypertonic saline solutions, but because of poor patient tolerance, he switched to intravenous boluses of 15–35 % sodium and magnesium chloride solutions.

Over the next half century, various compounds were investigated, including 50 % glucose, 50 % sucrose, 25 % sodium chloride, 25 % urea, 50 % magnesium sulfate, glycerol, concentrated albumin, and concentrated plasma. Their use was tempered by the caveat that "most of these dehydrating agents have only a temporary effect, which may be followed by a 'rebound phenomenon' during which the intracranial pressure may exceed that which existed before they were administered" [4]. Because of these concerns, osmotic agents were rarely used to treat cerebral edema after the mid-1930s.

M.N. Diringer, MD
Neurocritical Care Division, Department of Neurology, Washington University, Campus Box 8111, 660 S Euclid Ave, St Louis, MO 63110, USA
e-mail: diringerm@wustl.edu

After the introduction of intracranial pressure monitoring (ICP) monitoring to the management of head injury in the1960s, there was a resurgence of interest in the use of osmotic agents. At the same time, mannitol was added to the list of potential osmotic agents [5, 6]. Although initially administered as continuous infusion, the practice of using of intermittent bolus administration evolved rapidly. Mannitol quickly became one of the primary osmotic agents used to treat cerebral edema, primarily because it did not cross the cell membrane, like urea, and was not metabolized, like other sugar solutions. Over time, other concerns about mannitol were noted, including its marked diuretic effect leading to hypovolemia, its association with renal failure, and the identification of "mannitol-resistant" patients.

Hypertonic saline has gained favor because it does not appear to be burdened with these side effects. It has challenged mannitol's position as the preferred osmotic agent [7]. Debates in the literature lay out arguments for and against its use [8, 9]. Additionally, its use has transitioned from administration as a bolus to use as a continuous infusion. This has shifted management to slowly increasing osmolality to a stable high value rather than intermittently and sharply raising osmolality followed by a return to normal levels.

Currently, osmotic therapy is routinely used to treat cerebral edema in a wide range of conditions. Numerous retrospective and prospective series confirm that, in most conditions, a bolus of mannitol or hypertonic saline will lower intracranial pressure, usually to a similar degree. What remains unstudied and poorly understood is the impact of repeated dosing, appropriate fluid management during osmotic therapy, and how to guide therapy. In addition, controversy persists regarding whether osmotic agents act only on normal brain, whether they lose efficacy over time, and whether they leak into the brain. No appropriately designed and powered studies have assessed the impact of osmotic therapy on outcome.

R.L. Applegate et al. (eds.), *Brain Edema XVI: Translate Basic Science into Clinical Practice*, Acta Neurochirurgica Supplement, Vol. 121,
DOI 10.1007/978-3-319-18497-5_1, © Springer International Publishing Switzerland 2016

Physiology of Osmotic Agents

Osmotic Effects

Intravenous administration of a hypertonic solution that is impervious to the cell membrane creates osmotic disequilibrium between the intracellular and extracellular compartments. Water moves rapidly into the extracellular compartment to restore equilibrium. This net shift of water out of the intracellular space results in cell shrinkage.

In the brain, the distribution of osmotic agents is further governed by the blood-brain barrier (BBB), which limits entry of most osmotic agents into the extravascular extracellular space of the central nervous system. The osmotic reflection coefficient indicates the degree to which a solute crosses the BBB; 0 indicating free passage and 1 complete exclusion. Mannitol and sodium are highly excluded by the BBB; the osmotic reflection coefficient for mannitol is 0.9 and that for sodium approaches 1. Yet, in disease states, the integrity of the BBB is often impaired, increasing permeability to solutes as well as increasing hydraulic conductivity.

Hydraulic conductivity (the ease with which water can pass through a membrane) of brain capillaries must also be considered [10, 11]. A family of aquaporin receptors has been identified that appears to play a key role in hydraulic conductivity across the BBB [12]. Changes in permeability of the channels determine the magnitude of the response to osmotic stimuli [13]. Movement of water across the BBB is driven by Starling forces; hydrostatic pressure and osmotic pressure act in opposite directions across the capillary wall, with hydrostatic forces driving fluid out and osmotic pressures pulling it back. The net flux is determined by membrane permeability to solutes (osmotic agents) and solvent (water). The net result of all these factors is described by the tonicity or osmotic effectiveness of a solution, which depends on both the osmotic gradient created and the osmotic reflection coefficient of the membrane for that solute.

Brain Adaptation to the Hyperosmolar State

The beneficial effects of osmotic agents are thought to be the result of their ability to shrink the brain; a single dose of mannitol acutely reduces brain volume by 6–8 % in patients with large stroke and cerebral edema [14]. As this fluid comes from the intracellular compartment, cells shrink, initiating a series of responses targeted at restoring cell size to normal. This process acts in several ways to increase the absolute number of intracellular osmotically active particles to counteract the dehydrating influence of hyperosmolar plasma. Over a few hours, the intracellular content of electrolytes rises, followed by a slower accumulation of organic [15] and idiogenic osmoles [16], which draw water back into the cell. The net effect is restoration of cell size with maintenance of the hyperosmolar state.

This response limits the impact on brain volume that can be achieved when the brain is exposed to a sustained hyperosmolar state. The beneficial reduction in brain volume is lost over time as intracellular osmoles rise. Over 24–48 h, a state is reached where both intracellular and extracellular compartments are hyperosmolar, but cell size has returned to baseline and the reduction in brain volume has been lost. This creates a high risk of rebound edema if osmolality is lowered too quickly. Overly rapid correction that outpaces the dissipation of the accumulated osmoles can have disastrous consequences [17].

Non-osmotic Effects

Administration of any hypertonic solution produces a shift of water into the extracellular (and, thus, intravascular) compartments, increasing blood volume. This leads to hemodilution, increased cardiac output, and increased blood pressure. If the osmotic agent is mannitol, a marked diuresis soon follows, which can lead to hypovolemia and hypotension. Because hypertonic saline is not a diuretic it produces sustained volume expansion, giving it a distinct advantage over mannitol in the setting of hypovolemia.

Mannitol and hypertonic saline also lower blood viscosity. This occurs, in part, as a result of hemodilution but also by decreasing the reducing mechanical resistance of red blood cells, shrinking them, and increasing their deformity [18].

Mannitol and Hypertonic Saline

For decades, mannitol was the osmotic agent of choice in the United States. However, to address some of the possible complications associated with its use, there was renewed interest in hypertonic saline in the late 1980s [19, 20]. The first reports used hypertonic saline to treat "mannitol refractory" patients. Additionally, because, unlike mannitol, hypertonic saline does not have a diuretic effect, it can be advantageous in situations where hypovolemia is a concern, such as in trauma and subarachnoid hemorrhage.

A meta-analysis of randomized clinical trials was performed to determine whether hypertonic saline is superior to mannitol for the treatment of elevated ICP [21]. The selection criteria included only trials that directly compared equiosmolar doses of hypertonic sodium and mannitol in patients undergoing ICP monitoring. The outcome was based on the ICP response for each dose and did not address repeated doses or patient outcome. Five trials with a total of 112 patients and 184 episodes of elevated ICP were analyzed. Overall, the relative risk of ICP control slightly favored hypertonic saline (1.16; 95 % confidence interval [CI] 1.00–1.33), but the difference in ICP was only 2.0 mmHg (95 % CI: 1.6–5.7), a clinically inconsequential difference. Despite this small difference, the authors concluded that hypertonic saline was more effective and may be superior to the current standard of care.

Another meta-analysis included 36 articles, 10 prospective randomized controlled trials (RCTs), 1 prospective and nonrandomized trial, 15 prospective observational trials, and 10 retrospective studies [22]. The analysis was hampered by low patient numbers, few RCTs, and inconsistent methods among studies. Nevertheless, the authors concluded that a greater part of the data suggested that hypertonic saline was more effective in reducing episodes of elevated ICP.

Hypertonic Saline Infusions

The use of continuous infusions of mildly hypertonic solutions has been introduced as a means of treating or preventing cerebral edema. Solutions of 1.5 % up to 7.5 % sodium chloride or sodium chloride/acetate are infused with the goal of reaching a target sodium concentration. To date, the rationale for this approach has not been clearly elucidated and little is known about its impact. A prospective, randomized controlled trial of fluid management in 32 children with severe head injury compared Lactated Ringer's, a hypotonic solution (273 mOsm/l) to hypertonic saline (598 mOsm/l) [23]. In this small study, ICP and cerebral perfusion pressure (CPP) did not differ between groups; those in the hypertonic saline group required fewer interventions ($P<0.02$) and had shorter ICU length of stay.

Another study retrospectively reviewed the use of early hypertonic saline infusion in a cohort of patients with cerebral edema associated with cerebrovascular disease [24]. A heterogeneous group of 100 patients was treated with continuous infusion of 3 % saline, the rate of which was adjusted until a targeted plasma sodium level of 145–155 mmol/l and an osmolality level of 310–320 mOsm/kg were reached. Compared with historical controls, those treated with hypertonic saline had fewer episodes of critically elevated ICP and lower in-hospital mortality. However, when each clinical entity (ischemic stroke, intracerebral hemorrhage, and subarachnoid hemorrhage) was considered separately, no impact on ICP or mortality was seen.

A continuous 3 % saline infusion was used in 26 patients with spontaneous lobar intracerebral hemorrhage, with a goal serum sodium concentration of 145–155 mmol/l and osmolality of 310–320 mOsm/kg [25]. When compared with historical controls, episodes of elevated ICP or new anisocoria were less frequent in those receiving hypertonic saline. In-hospital mortality was 3 (11.5 %) in the hypertonic saline group and 16 (25 %) in the control group.

The use of continuous controlled infusions of hypertonic saline has been reported in refractory intracranial hypertension [26]. A single-center retrospective study of 50 patients with severe head injury used infusions of 20 % saline to reach a target sodium concentration. Over 8 days of use, ICP decreased and CPP increased. No ICP rebound was reported after stopping the infusion.

Conclusion

Equi-osmolar boluses of mannitol and hypertonic saline act in the same way to create an osmotic gradient and reduce brain water and lower ICP. Data regarding the equivalence of mannitol and hypertonic saline for ICP control after a single dose are conflicting and of low quality. The meta-analysis that favored hypertonic saline for ICP control found the difference in ICP was only 2.0 mmHg, a difference of questionable clinical significance. In addition, the ICP response to a single bolus does not necessarily translate into improved outcome; it is important to consider that many other interventions that have had a greater impact on ICP have failed to improve outcome. The relationship between ICP control and outcome has been further challenged by the results of a large international randomized trial treating patients with severe head injury, with and without ICP monitoring, which failed to show any benefit of ICP monitoring [27].

The case for using continuous infusion of hypertonic saline is weak. The rationale is inconsistent with our understanding of the mechanism of action of osmotic agents. Minimal osmotic disequilibrium is created when a continuous infusion is used. The creation of a sustained hyper-osmolar state by continuous hypertonic saline infusion drives the brain's compensatory creation of intracellular osmoles to return cell size to normal. In addition, continuous infusions maintain a concentration gradient favoring movement of solutes into the brain, especially when the BBB may be damaged.

The clinical studies to date do not provide clear evidence of benefit. The only randomized trial was extremely small and compared hypertonic saline to a relatively hypotonic fluid. The retrospective studies suffer from selection bias and used historical controls. At present, the data do not support the use of continuous infusions of hypertonic solution to treat cerebral edema.

Disclosure The author has no relevant disclosures.

References

1. Weed LH, McKibbens PR (1919) Experimental alterations of brain bulk. Am J Physiol 48:512–530
2. Haden RL (1919) Therapeutic application of the alteration of brain volume. JAMA 73:983–984
3. Fay T (1935) The treatment of acute and chronic cases of cerebral trauma by methods of dehydration. Ann Surg 101(1):76–132
4. Pudenz RH, Todd EM, Shelden CH. Head injuries in infants and young children. Calif Med. 1961;94:66–71. PubMed PMID: 13738386; PubMed Central PMCID: PMC1575445
5. Shenkin HA, Goluboff B, Haft H (1962) The use of mannitol for the reduction of intracranial pressure in intracranial surgery. J Neurosurg 19:897–901
6. Wise BL, Chater N (1961) Use of hypertonic mannitol solutions to lower cerebrospinal fluid pressure and decrease brain bulk in man. Surg Forum 12:398–399
7. Marko NF (2012) Hypertonic saline, not mannitol, should be considered gold-standard medical therapy for intracranial hypertension. Crit Care (London, England) 16(1):113
8. Grape S, Ravussin P (2012) PRO: osmotherapy for the treatment of acute intracranial hypertension. J Neurosurg Anesthesiol 24(4):402–406
9. Grande PO, Romner B (2012) Osmotherapy in brain edema: a questionable therapy. J Neurosurg Anesthesiol 24(4):407–412
10. Rosenberg GA, Kyner WT, Fenstermacher JD, Patlak CS (1986) Effect of vasopressin on ependymal and capillary permeability to tritiated water in cat. Am J Physiol 251(3 Pt 2):F485–F489
11. Olson JE, Banks M, Dimlich RV, Evers J (1997) Blood-brain barrier water permeability and brain osmolyte content during edema development. Acad Emerg Med 4(7):662–673
12. Badaut J, Ashwal S, Obenaus A (2011) Aquaporins in cerebrovascular disease: a target for treatment of brain edema? Cerebrovasc Dis (Basel, Switzerland) 31(6):521–531
13. Zelenina M (2010) Regulation of brain aquaporins. Neurochem Int 57(4):468–488
14. Manno EM, Adams RE, Derdeyn CP, Powers WJ, Diringer MN (1999) The effects of mannitol on cerebral edema after large hemispheric cerebral infarct. Neurology 52:583–587
15. Adrogue HJ, Madias NE (2000) Hypernatremia. N Engl J Med 342(20):1493–1499
16. McManus ML, Churchwell KB, Strange K (1995) Regulation of cell volume in health and disease. N Engl J Med 333(19):1260–1266
17. Go KG (1991) The fluid environment of the central nervous system. In: Cerebral pathophysiology. Elsevier, New York
18. Burke AM, Quest DO, Chien S, Cerri C (1981) The effects of mannitol on blood viscosity. J Neurosurg 55(4):550–553
19. Worthley LI, Cooper DJ, Jones N (1988) Treatment of resistant intracranial hypertension with hypertonic saline. Report of two cases. J Neurosurg 68(3):478–481
20. Prough DS, Kramer GC, Uchida T, Stephenson RT, Hellmich HL, Dewitt DS (2006) Effects of hypertonic arginine on cerebral blood flow and intracranial pressure after traumatic brain injury combined with hemorrhagic hypotension. Shock 26(3):290–295
21. Kamel H, Navi BB, Nakagawa K, Hemphill JC 3rd, Ko NU (2011) Hypertonic saline versus mannitol for the treatment of elevated intracranial pressure: a meta-analysis of randomized clinical trials. Crit Care Med 39(3):554–559
22. Mortazavi MM, Romeo AK, Deep A, Griessenauer CJ, Shoja MM, Tubbs RS, Fisher W (2012) Hypertonic saline for treating raised intracranial pressure: literature review with meta-analysis. J Neurosurg 116(1):210–221
23. Simma B, Burger R, Falk M, Sacher P, Fanconi S (1998) A prospective, randomized, and controlled study of fluid management in children with severe head injury: lactated Ringer's solution versus hypertonic saline. Crit Care Med 26(7):1265–1270
24. Hauer EM, Stark D, Staykov D, Steigleder T, Schwab S, Bardutzky J (2011) Early continuous hypertonic saline infusion in patients with severe cerebrovascular disease. Crit Care Med 39(7):1766–1772
25. Wagner I, Hauer EM, Staykov D, Volbers B, Dorfler A, Schwab S, Bardutzky J (2011) Effects of continuous hypertonic saline infusion on perihemorrhagic edema evolution. Stroke J Cereb Circ 42(6):1540–1545
26. Roquilly A, Mahe PJ, Latte DD, Loutrel O, Champin P, Di Falco C, Courbe A, Buffenoir K, Hamel O, Lejus C et al (2011) Continuous controlled-infusion of hypertonic saline solution in traumatic brain-injured patients: a 9-year retrospective study. Crit Care (London, England) 15(5):R260
27. Chesnut RM, Temkin N, Carney N, Dikmen S, Rondina C, Videtta W, Petroni G, Lujan S, Pridgeon J, Barber J, Machamer J, Chaddock K, Celix JM, Cherner M, Hendrix T; Global Neurotrauma Research Group (2012) A trial of intracranial-pressure monitoring in traumatic brain injury. N Engl J Med 27;367(26):2471–2481. doi: 10.1056/NEJMoa1207363. Epub 2012;12. Erratum in: N Engl J Med. 2013 19;369(25):2465. PubMed PMID: 23234472; PubMed Central PMCID: PMC3565432

Transcranial Near-Infrared Laser Therapy for Stroke: How to Recover from Futility in the NEST-3 Clinical Trial

Paul A. Lapchak and Paul D. Boitano

Introduction: Laser Light Mechanisms

Noninvasive transcranial near-infrared laser therapy (NILT) using near-infrared light at a wavelength of 800–820 nm may stimulate mitochondrial function, thereby increasing cellular energy production. This mechanism may be important in NILT-induced neuroprotection and repair, because there is evidence suggesting that the primary mitochondrial chromophore for NILT is cytochrome c oxidase (COX) [4–6, 11]. COX is a terminal enzyme in cellular respiration, located in the inner side of the mitochondrial membrane. Stimulated COX activity regulates cellular bioenergetics by delivering protons across the inner membrane and drives the formation of adenosine triphosphate (ATP) by oxidative phosphorylation. In addition to leading to increased mitochondrial ATP formation, photobiostimulation may also initiate secondary cell-signaling pathways [10, 20], protect against neuronal degeneration by inhibiting apoptosis [26], induce neurogenesis [30], and enhance the production of endogenous neurotrophic factors, which may allow for remodeling of cellular compartments after injury or long-term neurodegeneration [25].

NILT is touted as a novel form of acute neuroprotection that attenuates and reverses many forms of insult in animal models of acute and chronic neurodegenerative diseases [1, 3, 8, 10, 14, 16, 28]. Certainly, there is extensive and convincing preclinical and translational data to support this claim. Of importance to the treatment of acute ischemic stroke (AIS) is the observation that NILT can increase cerebral blood flow (CBF) and possibly attenuate motor function and other diverse clinical deficits [35]. One study demonstrated that there was a correlation between NILT-induced changes in nitric oxide synthase (NOS), nitric oxide (NO), and CBF using power densities in the range of 0.8–3.2 W/cm^2 (these densities are in excess of those used in translational stroke studies and NEST-clinical trials) [35].

Laser-Induced Neuroprotection In Vivo

NILT has been tested in preclinical stroke models in two different species, the rat middle cerebral artery occlusion (MCAO) model and the rabbit small clot embolic stroke model (RSCEM), with slightly different results. The first landmark studies to provide evidence of NILT efficacy resulted from RSCEM studies [22]. It is generally thought that the RSCEM has multiple advantages over most other stroke models used in preclinical or translational research. First, the model uses non-autologous blood clots for embolization, and embolization is performed in the absence of anesthetics. Second, because of the use of quantal analysis, the model includes a heterogeneous population of stroke subjects and the primary endpoint is a well-defined, clinically relevant behavioral measure [15, 34]. Because AIS is usually characterized by motor function deficits, among others (e.g., somatosensory, linguistic (or aphasia), and visual-spatial/attentional (or neglect) deficits), which are the main clinical functions scored on the National Institutes of Health Stroke Scale (NIHSS) and the modified Rankin Scale (mRS), similar clinically translatable endpoints should be used in translational studies [27].

NILT has been shown to be efficacious as a method to reduce or attenuate behavioral deficits in the RSCEM using continuous wavelength transcranial irradiation with approximated cortical surface power densities of 10–25 mW/cm^2 [22]. In rabbits, investigators were able to

P.A. Lapchak, PhD, FAHA (✉)
Department of Neurology and Neurosurgery, Cedars-Sinai Medical Center (CSMC), 127 S. San Vicente Blvd. Suite 8305, Los Angeles, CA 90048, USA
e-mail: Paul.Lapchak@cshs.org

P.D. Boitano, BSc
Department of Neurology, Cedars-Sinai Medical Center (CSMC), 127 S. San Vicente Blvd., Los Angeles, CA 90048, USA

R.L. Applegate et al. (eds.), *Brain Edema XVI: Translate Basic Science into Clinical Practice*, Acta Neurochirurgica Supplement, Vol. 121,
DOI 10.1007/978-3-319-18497-5_2,

demonstrate a 6-h therapeutic widow when efficacy on the primary endpoint, motor function, was measured. When NILT-induced clinical improvement was measured, the effect was permanent (durable) and was measurable up to 21 days after a single treatment [21, 22]. When the therapeutic window of NILT in the RSCEM was compared with the therapeutic window of alteplase (a tissue plasminogen activator, or tPA), the only Food and Drug Administration (FDA)-approved treatment for AIS, NILT was superior in therapeutic window but not in extent of efficacy (i.e., actual increase in behavioral improvement) [19]. In contrast to the rabbit studies described above, NILT studies with a power density 0.9 J/cm^2, done in rats, show no beneficial effect when treatment was initiated 4 h after a stroke, but there was improvement when applied 24 h after the stroke [30]; similar results using an MCAO filament model have been reported [2].

Materials and Methods

All animal skulls were obtained under Institutional Animal Care and Use Committee (IACUC) approved protocols, which were conducted in accordance with the United States Public Health Service's Policy on Humane Care and Use of Laboratory Animals. Mouse skulls were obtained from 12-week-old male C57BL/6 wild-type mice (strain #000664) obtained from Jackson Laboratory (Bar Harbor, ME, USA). Rat skulls were obtained from 12- to 16-week-old male Sprague-Dawley rats obtained from Harlan, Inc. (Hayward, CA, USA). *Oryctolagus cuniculus* rabbit skulls were obtained from 10- to 14-week-old male New Zealand white rabbits obtained from LFPS, Inc. (Norco, CA, USA). Human skulls were obtained from the University of California, San Diego, Department of Anatomy skull bank.

Skull Thickness Measurements

For animal skull thickness, we used a Mitutoyo Ratchet Digimatic Micrometer. Human skull thickness and density were measured using the methods developed and described in detail by Voie et al. [36]. Briefly, the skull was placed in the bore of a Discovery CT750 HD (GE Medical Systems, Waukesha, WI, USA) computed tomography (CT) scanner and scanned to create a set of DICOM images (OsiriX, OsiriX Foundation, Geneva, Switzerland), which were read into MATLAB (MathWorks, Inc., Natick, MA, USA) to create a three-dimensional (3D) matrix of CT values, along with the voxel coordinates. Parametric skull maps are presented to show how each skull has a unique spatial distribution of thickness and density.

NILT Penetration Measurements

For laser penetration studies, we used a K-Laser (Franklin, TN, USA) model K-1200 dual-wavelength (800/970 nm) Class IV laser. The laser light was coupled to a 3 m, 600 µm fiber (FT600UMT, NA 0.39, Thorlabs, Inc., Newton, NJ, USA) that was connected to a Thorlabs collimator (F220SMA-780, 780 nm, $f=11.07$ mm, NA = 0.26). The distance from the lens was adjusted to obtain an 11.7 mm diameter beam with an area of 107.5 mm^2 (1.075 cm^2) to achieve power densities of 200–700 mW/cm^2 for all species except mouse. For mouse skulls, an area of 2.5 mm was utilized. The laser energy was detected using an Integrating Sphere Photodiode Power Sensor (S142C, Thorlabs, Inc., Newton, NJ, USA).

Photographic Images

Photos were taken using a Canon EOS Rebel T3 black (Melville, NY, USA). The color-enhanced NILT diffusion pattern through the rabbit skulls was captured using a JAI (AD130 GE) camera that is capable of simultaneously capturing both near-infrared and visible images. The lens used for capturing the image was a 16 mm lens from Edmund Optics (Techspec VIS-NIR Fixed Focal Length, Barrington, NJ, USA).

Statistical and Correlation Analysis

Descriptive statistics such as means and standard deviations (SD) are reported throughout. Correlation (Pearson) and statistical analysis were done using Statistical Analysis Software (SAS, SAS Institute, Inc., Cary, NC, USA).

Results: Translation from Animals to Humans

NILT Penetration Profiles

NILT penetration of the rabbit skull and brain is achieved to some extent to a depth of approximately 30 mm, almost the complete thickness of the brain [22]. Studies have postulated

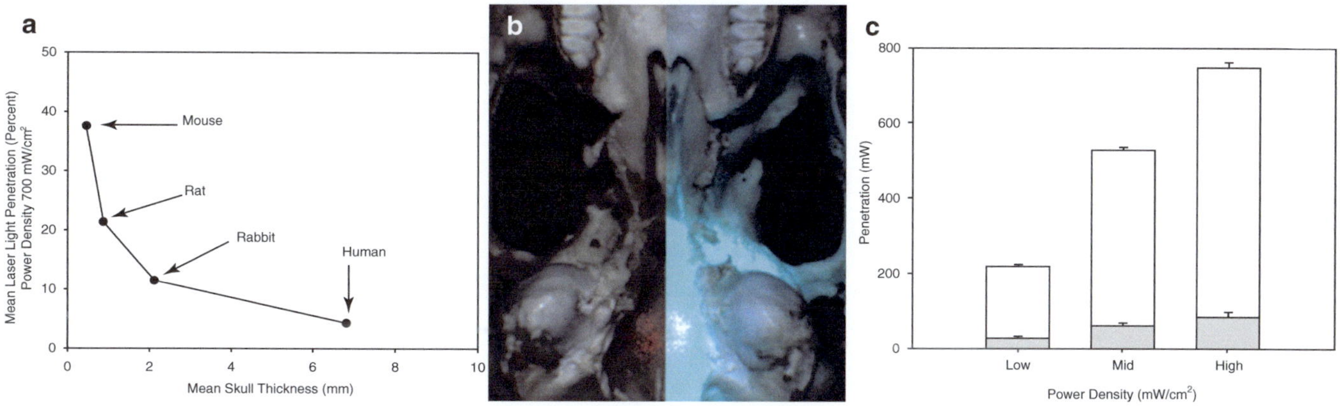

Fig. 1 Laser penetration profiles: (**a**) NILT penetration as a function of skull thickness in four species using a power density of 700 mW/cm². NILT penetration decreased through the skulls of all four species utilized in this study as skull thickness increases. Presented as penetration, calculated based on the area of illumination and the amount of power utilized, (**b**) NILT penetration and scatter through the rabbit skull. *Left,* the red laser spotting beam penetrating the skull. *Right,* blue scatter through the skull. (**c**) NILT penetration as a function of power density: rabbit skull analysis

that the laser beam may encompass most of the brain if placed on the skin surface near the bregma at the midline suture [22]. However, there has been little definitive information published in the literature regarding laser light penetration through the skull and the pattern of scatter once the light beam has penetrated the skull. In Fig. 1a, we show that skulls can greatly attenuate laser light penetration using a skull surface power density of 0.7 W/cm². In Fig. 1a, it is important to note that we present the actual skull thickness (in mm) for all three animal species used in this study. We observed attenuation of laser light penetration as the skull thickness increased from 0.441 mm (mouse) to 0.829 mm (rat) to 2.115 mm (rabbit). As shown in the figure, there is an inverse relationship between laser penetration and skull thickness, which is not linear. Figure 1b shows there is a correlation between laser light penetration (mW) through rabbit skull and Power Density (mW/cm²) on the skull surface. As power density increases, there is incrementally increased laser light penetration. In all cases, approximately 11 % of laser light energy crossed the rabbit skull.

The photograph of the rabbit skull (Fig. 1, panel b, right) shows extensive scatter of laser light once the light has passed through the skull. Numerically, as shown in the line graph (Fig. 1a, b), there is >88 % attenuation of laser light passing from the surface to the interior measured using a Thorlabs power meter. As shown in (c), when using a power density of 200–700 mW/cm² on the skull surface, it is estimated that the ventral surface of the skull has only achieved a power density of 26–85 mW/cm², or approximately 11 % of the applied power. This level of attenuation must be considered when attempting to advance NITL therapy from animals to humans, especially because NILT has never been optimized in any animal species, nor has it been optimized for use in humans.

Using human calvaria, we completed similar measures of actual NILT penetration profiles to determine to what extent

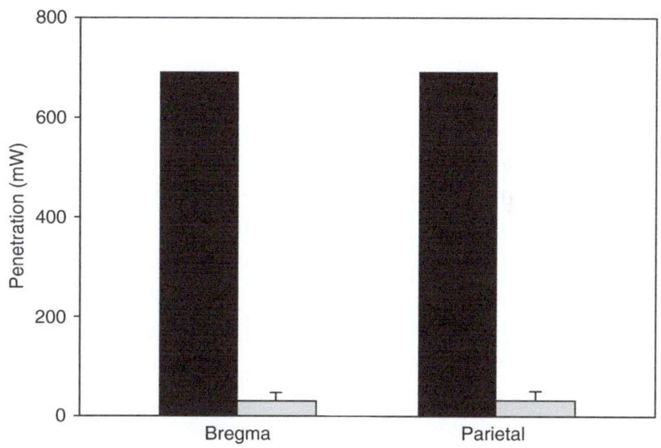

Fig. 2 Human calvaria laser penetration: NILT penetration through the dehydrated human calvaria measured at the bregma and the parietal skull. In both cases, approximately 4.5 % of laser light penetrated the skull bone

penetration was attenuated by the human skull. A sampling of data is presented in Fig. 2. As described above for the rabbit skull, there was extensive attenuation (>95 %) of laser light penetration through human calvaria, which was also measured using a Thorlabs power meter.

Using 18 human calvaria, we were able to accurately measure skull thickness and density by a new CT method described by Voie et al. [36]. We also conducted penetration analysis of every skull using a power density of 700 mW/cm². With both data sets, we determined whether there was a correlation between laser light penetration and either skull thickness or density using Pearson correlation analysis. As shown in Fig. 3a, there was a positive correlation between decreased laser penetration and increased calvaria thickness ($p=0.0127$), but there was no correlation between laser penetration and calvaria density ($p=0.9166$).

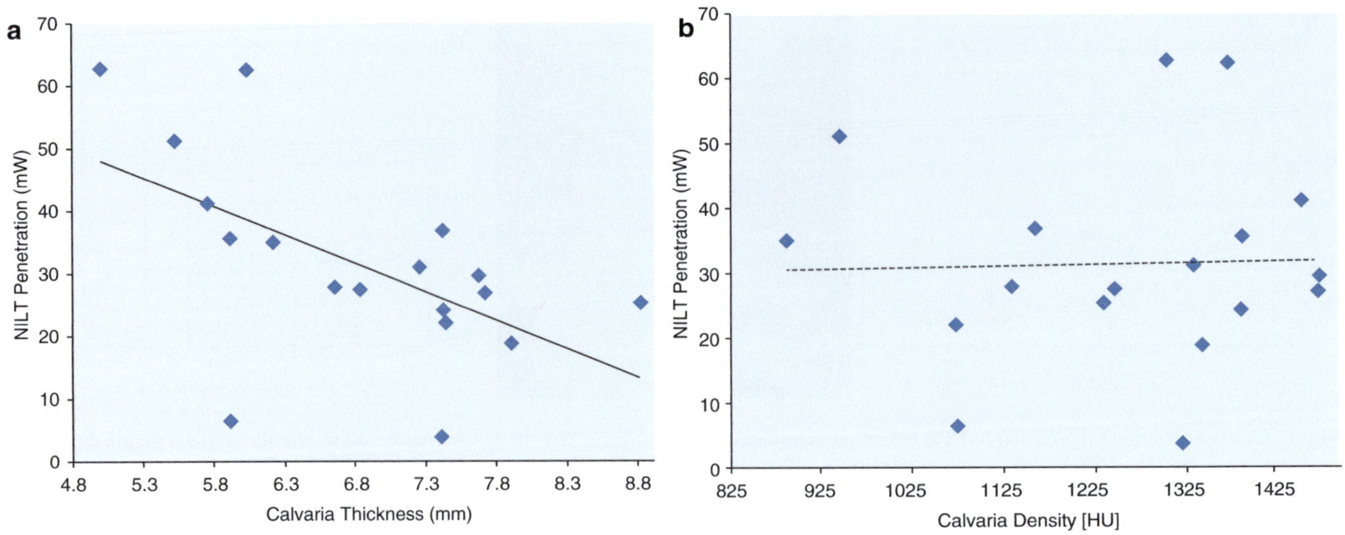

Fig. 3 Correlation analysis of NILT penetration through the dehydrated human calvaria: effect of thickness and density. (**a**) Plots of NILT penetration (mW) vs. thickness (mm) or (**b**) density (HU). Absolute penetration (mW) vs. thickness (mm) or density (HU). Correlation analysis was used to calculate R^2 values for each measurement point. In Panel **a** the R^2 values and Pearson correlations were 0.33433 (–0.57409, $p=0.0127$) for thickness at the bregma. In Panel **b**, the R^2 values and Pearson correlations were 0.00071 (0.02658, $p=0.9166$) for density at the bregma. There was a significant correlation between NILT penetration and skull thickness but not density

There is some literature on possible depth of penetration across the human skull and limited information on the rabbit skull. Using the RSCEM, NILT penetration of the rabbit skull and brain is achieved to a depth of 25–30 mm, almost the complete thickness, and the NILT beam would encompass the majority of the brain if placed on the skin surface posterior to the bregma at the midline [22]. In human studies, the investigators also indicate that NILT would penetrate the brain to approximately 20 mm depth using a power density of 10 mW/cm² (1.2 J/cm² on the cortical surface) [39]. Mathematical estimates indicate an estimated Power density drop from 10 mW/cm² (1.2 J/cm²) to 7.5 μW/cm² (0.9 mJ/cm²) at 18 mm depth from the cortical surface [2]. The extensive power density drop has also been addressed previously [29, 37]. Wan et al. [37] calculated that a power density of 8 J/cm² applied to the "head" will allow for penetration of 2–3 % of laser photons up to 1 cm from the scalp surface; furthermore, only 0.2–0.3 % of photons will reach 2 cm depth. Thus, the overall penetration of continuous wave (CW)-administered near-infrared photons to significant depths is almost negligible.

NeuroThera Effectiveness and Safety Trial (NEST) Efficacy, Failures, and Considerations

NEST-1 was a phase II, double-blind clinical study randomized (2:1) in favor of NILT. The study included 120 patients 40–85 years of age with an average National Institutes of Health Stroke Scale (NIHSS) entry score of 7–22 (mean NIHSS 10), and time to treatment was 16 h 20 min [12]. The primary endpoints were NIHSS and modified Ranking Scale (mRS). As described in detail elsewhere [12], the laser probe was applied to 20 points on the skull for a 2-min duration at each spot, using a power density of 10 mW/cm² delivering a cortical energy density of 1.2 J/cm². The study found that NILT-treated patients showed greater significant improvement from baseline to 90 days ($p=0.021$) than did the sham-treated group and NILT was safe with no differences in mortality rates (placebo 9.8 % vs. NILT 8.9 %) or serious adverse events (SAE: placebo 36.6 % vs. NILT 25.3 %) between the two groups.

NEST-2 was also a phase III, double-blind clinical study with equal randomization (1:1) that enrolled 660 stroke victims 19–95 years of age [39]. The trial was nearly identical to *NEST-1*, but used mRS as the primary endpoint with NIHSS for additional stratification analysis. In NEST-2 the time to treatment was 14 h 38 min. Unlike NEST-1, the trial was not positive ($p=0.094$) for all enrolled patients, with an average NIHSS entry score of 13.1. Interestingly, additional post hoc analysis with severity stratification provided some evidence that stroke patients with NIHSS scores of 7–15 upon enrollment achieved better performance at 90 days ($p=0.044$). Once again, there were no changes in mortality rate or SAEs, but the mortality rate in this trial was almost double that of NEST-1.

The NEST-3 clinical trial [9] was a phase III clinical trial delivering NILT within 24 h of a stroke. The study proposed to include a limited number of patients with an NIHSS baseline score of 7–17, which was based upon "efficacy" in the NEST-2 clinical trial [12, 39]. Moreover, as described in the NIH clinical trial design, only patients with cortical infarcts were enrolled, presumably because of the limited penetration of laser light across the scalp and skull. The trial was ended because of futility at interim analysis [9]. Clearly, with the current information from human skulls, NILT does not effectively cross barriers and must be optimized to promote neuroprotection in humans.

Conclusion

The principal aim of this chapter was to revisit the use of transcranial laser therapy to treat stroke and to discuss important information concerning the extent of NILT penetration through the skull of four species. Our results suggest that the use of small animal species with "thin" skulls, compared to humans, cannot be used to effectively model human diseases because of differential laser penetration and scatter patterns, in Lapchak et al [24]. Based on the scientific information presented here and the efficacy profile of NILT in multiple preclinical translational models, NILT should be further pursued as a possible important neuroprotective or neurorestorative treatment for stroke. It is evident from the literature that neuroprotection must be administered as soon as possible after a stroke [17, 31]. Extensive treatment delays have yet to be found efficacious in any animal model or clinical trial.

It is clear, however, because of significant variances of NILT penetration and skull thickness, that NILT must first be optimized in animals using novel approaches incorporating human skull characteristics. In addition, all future translational studies should incorporate standard STAIR criteria [32, 38], RIGOR guidelines [13, 18, 23], and, most importantly, studies in multiple species [15, 33, 34] for safety [7] and efficacy [15, 33, 34].

Conflict of Interest Statement This study utilized a K-Laser model K-1200 device. K-Laser, Inc. did not have an editorial influence on the study design or scientific content of this article.

Disclosures and Acknowledgments Dr. Lapchak serves as editor-in-chief of the *Journal of Neurology & Neurophysiology* and associate editor of *Translational Stroke Research*. The scientific content of this work was not directly supported by the National Institutes of Health or any other funding source external to Cedars-Sinai Medical Center. He was supported in part by a U01 translational research grant NS060685. Paul D. Boitano has no disclosures.

References

1. Chung H, Dai T, Sharma SK, Huang YY, Carroll JD, Hamblin MR (2012) The nuts and bolts of low-level laser (light) therapy. Ann Biomed Eng 40:516–533
2. Detaboada L, Ilic S, Leichliter-Martha S, Oron U, Oron A, Streeter J (2006) Transcranial application of low-energy laser irradiation improves neurological deficits in rats following acute stroke. Lasers Surg Med 38:70–73
3. De Taboada L, Yu J, El-Amouri S, Gattoni-Celli S, Richieri S, McCarthy T, Streeter J, Kindy MS (2011) Transcranial laser therapy attenuates amyloid-beta peptide neuropathology in amyloid-beta protein precursor transgenic mice. J Alzheimers Dis 23:521–535
4. Desmet KD, Paz DA, Corry JJ, Eells JT, Wong-Riley MT, Henry MM, Buchmann EV, Connelly MP, Dovi JV, Liang HL, Henshel DS, Yeager RL, Millsap DS, Lim J, Gould LJ, Das R, Jett M, Hodgson BD, Margolis D, Whelan HT (2006) Clinical and experimental applications of NIR-LED photobiomodulation. Photomed Laser Surg 24:121–128
5. Drochioiu G (2010) Laser-induced ATP formation: mechanism and consequences. Photomed Laser Surg 28:573–574
6. Eells JT (2003) Therapeutic photobiomodulation for methanol-induced retinal toxicity. Proc Natl Acad Sci U S A 100:3439
7. Fagan SC, Lapchak PA, Liebeskind DS, Ishrat T, Ergul A (2013) Recommendations for preclinical research in hemorrhagic transformation. Transl Stroke Res 4:322–327
8. Farfara D, Tuby H, Trudler D, Doron-Mandel E, Maltz L, Vassar RJ, Frenkel D, Oron U (2015) Low-level laser therapy ameliorates disease progression in a mouse model of Alzheimer's disease. J Mol Neurosci 55(2):430–436
9. Hacke W, Schellinger PD, Albers GW, Bornstein NM, Dahlof BL, Fulton R, Kasner SE, Shuaib A, Richieri SP, Dilly SG, Zivin J, Lees KR; NEST 3 Committees and Investigators (2014) Transcranial laser therapy in acute stroke treatment: results of neurothera effectiveness and safety trial 3, a phase III clinical end point device trial. Stroke 45:3187–3193
10. Huang YY, Chen AC, Carroll JD, Hamblin MR (2009) Biphasic dose response in low level light therapy. Dose Response 7:358–383
11. Karu T (2010) Mitochondrial mechanisms of photobiomodulation in context of new data about multiple roles of ATP. Photomed Laser Surg 28:159–160
12. Lampl Y, Zivin JA, Fisher M, Lew R, Welin L, Dahlof B, Borenstein P, Andersson B, Perez J, Caparo C, Ilic S, Oron U (2007) Infrared laser therapy for ischemic stroke: a new treatment strategy: results of the NeuroThera Effectiveness and Safety Trial-1 (NEST-1). Stroke 38:1843–1849
13. Landis SC, Amara SG, Asadullah K, Austin CP, Blumenstein R, Bradley EW, Crystal RG, Darnell RB, Ferrante RJ, Fillit H, Finkelstein R, Fisher M, Gendelman HE, Golub RM, Goudreau JL, Gross RA, Gubitz AK, Hesterlee SE, Howells DW, Huguenard J, Kelner K, Koroshetz W, Krainc D, Lazic SE, Levine MS, Macleod MR, McCall JM, Moxley RT 3rd, Narasimhan K, Noble LJ, Perrin S, Porter JD, Steward O, Unger E, Utz U, Silberberg SD (2012) A call for transparent reporting to optimize the predictive value of preclinical research. Nature 490:187–191
14. Lapchak PA (2010) Taking a light approach to treating acute ischemic stroke patients: transcranial near-infrared laser therapy translational science. Ann Med 42:576–586
15. Lapchak PA (2010) Translational stroke research using a rabbit embolic stroke model: a correlative analysis hypothesis for novel therapy development. Transl Stroke Res 1:96–107
16. Lapchak PA (2012) Transcranial near-infrared laser therapy applied to promote clinical recovery in acute and chronic neurodegenerative diseases. Expert Rev Med Devices 9:71–83
17. Lapchak PA (2013) Fast neuroprotection (fast-NPRX) for acute ischemic stroke victims: the time for treatment is now. Transl Stroke Res 4:704–709
18. Lapchak PA (2013) Recommendations and practices to optimize stroke therapy: developing effective translational research programs. Stroke 44:841–843

19. Lapchak PA, Araujo DM, Zivin JA (2004) Comparison of Tenecteplase with Alteplase on clinical rating scores following small clot embolic strokes in rabbits. Exp Neurol 185:154–159
20. Lapchak PA, De Taboada L (2010) Transcranial near infrared laser treatment (NILT) increases cortical adenosine-5'-triphosphate (ATP) content following embolic strokes in rabbits. Brain Res 1306:100–105
21. Lapchak PA, Salgado KF, Chao CH, Zivin JA (2007) Transcranial near-infrared light therapy improves motor function following embolic strokes in rabbits: an extended therapeutic window study using continuous and pulse frequency delivery modes. Neuroscience 148:907–914
22. Lapchak PA, Wei J, Zivin JA (2004) Transcranial infrared laser therapy improves clinical rating scores after embolic strokes in rabbits. Stroke 35:1985–1988
23. Lapchak PA, Zhang JH, Noble-Haeusslein LJ (2013) RIGOR guidelines: escalating STAIR and STEPS for effective translational research. Transl Stroke Res 4:279–285
24. Lapchak PA, Boitano PD, Butte PV, Fisher DJ, Hölscher T, Ley EJ, et al. (2015) Transcranial Near-Infrared Laser Transmission (NILT) Profiles (800 nm): Systematic Comparison in Four Common Research Species. PLoS ONE 10(6):e0127580. doi:10.1371/journal.pone.0127580
25. Leung MC, Lo SC, Siu FK, So KF (2002) Treatment of experimentally induced transient cerebral ischemia with low energy laser inhibits nitric oxide synthase activity and up-regulates the expression of transforming growth factor-beta 1. Lasers Surg Med 31:283–288
26. Liang HL, Whelan HT, Eells JT, Wong-Riley MT (2008) Near-infrared light via light-emitting diode treatment is therapeutic against rotenone- and 1-methyl-4-phenylpyridinium ion-induced neurotoxicity. Neuroscience 153:963–974
27. Lyden P, Lu M, Jackson C, Marler J, Kothari R, Brott T, Zivin J, The National Institute of Neurological Disorders and Stroke rt PASSG (1999) Underlying structure of the National Institutes of Health Stroke Scale: results of a factor analysis. Stroke 30: 2347
28. Naeser MA, Hamblin MR (2011) Potential for transcranial laser or LED therapy to treat stroke, traumatic brain injury, and neurodegenerative disease. Photomed Laser Surg 29:443–446
29. Naeser MA, Saltmarche A, Krengel MH, Hamblin MR, Knight JA (2011) Improved cognitive function after transcranial, light-emitting diode treatments in chronic, traumatic brain injury: two case reports. Photomed Laser Surg 29:351–358
30. Oron A, Oron U, Chen J, Eilam A, Zhang C, Sadeh M, Lampl Y, Streeter J, DeTaboada L, Chopp M (2006) Low-level laser therapy applied transcranially to rats after induction of stroke significantly reduces long-term neurological deficits. Stroke 37:2620–2624
31. Saver JL (2006) Time is brain–quantified. Stroke 37:263–266
32. Saver JL, Albers GW, Dunn B, Johnston KC, Fisher M (2009) Stroke Therapy Academic Industry Roundtable (STAIR) recommendations for extended window acute stroke therapy trials. Stroke 40:2594–2600
33. Tajiri N, Dailey T, Metcalf C, Mosley YI, Lau T, Staples M, van Loveren H, Kim SU, Yamashima T, Yasuhara T, Date I, Kaneko Y, Borlongan CV (2013) In vivo animal stroke models: a rationale for rodent and non-human primate models. Transl Stroke Res 4:308–321
34. Turner R, Jickling G, Sharp F (2011) Are underlying assumptions of current animal models of human stroke correct: from STAIRS to high hurdles? Transl Stroke Res 2:138–143
35. Uozumi Y, Nawashiro H, Sato S, Kawauchi S, Shima K, Kikuchi M (2010) Targeted increase in cerebral blood flow by transcranial near-infrared laser irradiation. Lasers Surg Med 42:566–576
36. Voie A, Dirnbacher M, Fisher D, Holscher T (2014). Parametric mapping and quantitative analysis of the human calvarium. Computerized medical imaging and graphics: the official journal of the Computerized Medical Imaging Society. 38(8):675–682. doi: 10.1016/j.compmedimag.2014.06.022. pmid:25069430.
37. Wan S, Parrish JA, Anderson RR, Madden M (1981) Transmittance of nonionizing radiation in human tissues. Photochem Photobiol 34:679–681
38. Wang MM, Xi G, Keep RF (2013) Should the STAIR criteria be modified for preconditioning studies? Transl Stroke Res 4:3–14
39. Zivin JA, Albers GW, Bornstein N, Chippendale T, Dahlof B, Devlin T, Fisher M, Hacke W, Holt W, Ilic S, Kasner S, Lew R, Nash M, Perez J, Rymer M, Schellinger P, Schneider D, Schwab S, Veltkamp R, Walker M, Streeter J (2009) Effectiveness and safety of transcranial laser therapy for acute ischemic stroke. Stroke 40:1359–1364

Human Data Supporting Glyburide in Ischemic Stroke

Kevin N. Sheth, J. Marc Simard, Jordan Elm, Golo Kronenberg, Hagen Kunte, and W. Taylor Kimberly

Introduction

Ischemic stroke afflicts approximately 700,000 people in the United States annually [1]. Malignant infarction, characterized by the syndrome resulting from brain swelling due to rapidly accumulating cerebral edema, occurs in 10 % of ischemic stroke patients [2]. Swelling in these patients often results in case fatality rates as high as 60–80 % [3]. A significant barrier to progress in managing patients with a large stroke is identifying safe and effective pharmacotherapy to prevent brain swelling and the resulting morbidity.

Intravenous (IV) recombinant tissue plasminogen activator (rtPA) administered within 3 h of symptom onset is the only US Food and Drug Administration (FDA)-approved treatment, yet this drug reaches a minority of eligible patients [1]. In the United States, rtPA is not FDA approved for use within 3–4.5 h. Efforts directed at improving outcome through endovascular reperfusion approaches have also been unsuccessful [4]. In patients with large territory infarction, reperfusion may even result in worse outcome, because of swelling or hemorrhagic transformation [5]. Decompressive craniectomy (DC) is the only proven therapy for swelling after ischemia. However, numerous factors limit the usefulness of DC, including limited eligibility for those who have serious comorbidities, and DC itself has a high rate of complications [6, 7].

It is clear that a preventative approach, rather than a reactive one, would be more preferable [8]. Recently, an inducible ion channel, SUR1-TRMP4, was discovered to be transcriptionally upregulated by all cell types in the neurovascular unit following ischemia [9]. Channel blockade reduces edema and hemorrhage, as well as necrotic cell death [10]. Small molecule therapy using glyburide, a well-known drug with an excellent safety profile, is effective in blocking this channel [9]. Multiple preclinical models of ischemic stroke with a similar pattern of findings suggest clinically relevant effects of glyburide [11]. Importantly, the strong, consistent body of preclinical work conforms to all of the major components of the Stroke Treatment Academic Industry Roundtable (STAIR) criteria [11, 12].

The ongoing translation of glyburide administration to human stroke patients has been informed not only by robust basic science data, from cell culture to preclinical models, but also by pertinent human observations, including randomized clinical trials. In this chapter, we summarize the human data available supporting the ongoing translation of glyburide for injection, or RP-1127, in patients with ischemic stroke.

Retrospective Studies of Stroke

The population-level administration of oral glyburide for diabetes for many years facilitates comparative outcome analyses between patients who have been administered sulfonylureas such as glyburide and those who have not. Geographic differences in practice also facilitate yet

K.N. Sheth, MD (✉)
Division of Neurocritical Care and Emergency Neurology, Yale University School of Medicine, 15 York Street, LCI 10th Floor, New Haven, CT 06520, USA
e-mail: kevin.sheth@yale.edu

J.M. Simard, MD, PhD
Department of Neurosurgery, University of Maryland School of Medicine, Baltimore, MD, USA

J. Elm, PhD
Department of Public Health Sciences, Medical School of South Carolina, Charleston, SC, USA

G. Kronenberg, MD • H. Kunte, MD
Department of Neurology, Charité Hospital, Berlin, Germany

W.T. Kimberly, MD, PhD
Department of Neurology, Massachusetts General Hospital, Boston, MA, USA

R.L. Applegate et al. (eds.), *Brain Edema XVI: Translate Basic Science into Clinical Practice*, Acta Neurochirurgica Supplement, Vol. 121,
DOI 10.1007/978-3-319-18497-5_3,

another perspective that relates to the underlying biology of the target channel. In the United States, patients admitted with an ischemic stroke often receive insulin infusions to maintain euglycemia in the hospital, and baseline diabetes medications are withheld. In parts of Europe and Canada, stroke units continue home diabetes medications in the hospital, *after* the stroke. Because SUR1 is not transcriptionally expressed before the onset of ischemia, one would not expect pre-stroke administration of glyburide to be associated with any neurological benefit [13]. In contrast, when sulfonylureas are continued immediately post-stroke onset, channel blockade and neurovascular protection is a possibility.

Two relevant studies were designed to test the association between sulfonylureas and outcome when the medication was given at any time in relation to stroke. The first was by Favilla et al. [14] using the Virtual International Stroke Trials Archive (VISTA), where 1,050 patients with diabetes were analyzed, 298 of whom were taking sulfonylureas. In this study, there was no association between sulfonylurea administration and improved outcome in the overall cohort. Interestingly, in the 28 patients for whom sulfonylureas were continued following stroke, the point estimate favored sulfonylureas. Of note, the stroke subtypes were not known, which is important because patients with lacunar stroke may not receive the same anti-swelling benefit from glyburide. A Danish study using a large administrative database suggested that the 30-day mortality was higher in patients with sulfonylureas [15]. Not only were patients discontinued on sulfonylureas after stroke onset, but the difference in mortality rate did not adjust for stroke severity and was absent at 1 year.

Analyses of post-stroke administration of sulfonylureas, consistent with the de novo expression of the target after the onset of ischemia, produced very different results. A review of diabetic patients hospitalized within 24 h of acute ischemic stroke at Charité Hospital, Berlin, evaluated those patients who were continued on their diabetes medications [16]. The primary outcome, a decrease in the National Institutes of Health Stroke Scale (NIHSS) score of ≥4 points from admission to discharge or a discharge NIHSS score = 0, was reached by 36.4 % of patients in the sulfonylurea group and 7.1 % in the control group ($p = 0.007$). In addition, a separate retrospective study examined the incidence of symptomatic hemorrhagic transformation in diabetic patients with ischemic stroke [17]. Compared with diabetic patients with non-sulfonylurea regimens, those with sulfonylurea exposure had significantly decreased mortality. After matching for baseline imbalances, there was decreased symptomatic hemorrhage (0 % vs. 11 %, $p = 0.016$) in patients taking sulfonylureas. These studies, which carefully adjusted for baseline variables, suggested that glyburide administration after ischemia results in improved outcomes.

Finally, the presence of relevant expression of SUR1 has been explored in brain autopsies of patients with ischemic stroke [18]. In a series of patients with focal infarct, up to 31 days after ischemic stroke, elevated levels of SUR1 were demonstrated in neurons, glial cells, and capillary endothelium.

Phase I and Phase IIa Study of RP-1127 (Glyburide for Injection) in Human Stroke

Oral glyburide has been used for decades in the treatment of diabetes mellitus. Because it was used for patients after consumption of a meal, the drug was developed so that plasma levels would have a rapid peak level, to lower postprandial blood glucose, and then rapidly clear from the plasma (Fig. 1). This is not the desired exposure after acute brain injury, where persistent channel blockade is the goal. Intravenous administration of the drug would allow for sustained, controlled plasma levels aimed at achieving a safe, durable drug effect. The need for achieving rapid steady state levels and maintaining receptor occupancy was demonstrated in preclinical models as well.

Using an IV formulation of glyburide (RP-1127), a phase I trial in health human volunteers (ClinicalTrials.gov identifier: NCT01132703) evaluated the safety, tolerability, and pharmacokinetics of RP-1127. A total of 34 patients were tested at the following doses: 0.4, 3.0, 6.0, and 10.0 mg/day doses. Two patients (one each at 6 and 10 mg/day) discontinued the study because of persistent hypoglycemia. The incidence of blood glucose levels above 80 mg/dL was more frequent in the placebo group than in the 3 mg/day group, while there was no difference in the incidence of blood

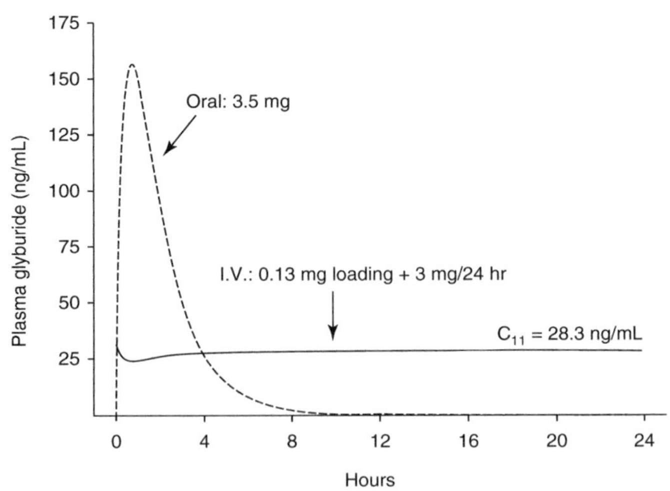

Fig. 1 Time course of plasma glyburide level following oral compared with intravenous bolus followed by 72 h infusion at 3 mg/day dose administration

glucose levels below 70 mg/dL, implying a reduction in blood glucose at the 3 mg/day dose without hypoglycemia. There were no serious adverse events. Steady state plasma glyburide levels were determined to be 27.3 ng/mL. In preclinical experiments, a glyburide dosing regimen that was twice the effective dose average resulted in steady state plasma glyburide levels of 16 ng/mL. These observations suggest that the maximum tolerated dose of 3 mg/day results in human plasma levels that exceed the effective dose in rats.

The Glyburide Advantage in Malignant Edema and Stroke (GAMES) Pilot study [19, 20] (ClinicalTrials.gov identifier: NCT01268683) evaluated the safety and feasibility of administering a 3 mg dose of RP-1127 in patients with severe stroke at high risk for swelling. The primary objective of this prospective, open-label, phase IIa study was to assess the feasibility of enrolling, evaluating, and treating with RP-1127 (bolus followed by 72 h infusion at 3 mg/day dose) patients with severe ischemic stroke, whether or not they were treated with IV rtPA. Patients were enrolled at two centers, using the major inclusion criteria of clinical diagnosis of anterior circulation of ischemic stroke, baseline magnetic resonance imaging (MRI) diffusion weighted imaging (DWI) volume of 82–210 cm^3, age 18–70 years of age, and start of drug infusion ≤10 h from symptom onset. The central inclusion criteria was a DWI lesion volume ≥82 cm^3, chosen because of the high specificity with which it predicts malignant edema [20]. Patients with endovascular treatment for stroke, preexisting evidence of swelling, and recent use of sulfonylureas were excluded. In addition to the baseline MRI, patients underwent follow-up MRI at 72 h after drug infusion and clinical outcome assessment by modified Rankin Scale at 90 days. The mean age of enrolled patients was 51, the median baseline National Institutes of Health Stroke Scale (NIHSS) score was 18, and the mean baseline DWI lesion volume was 102 cm^3. There were no serious adverse events related to the drug, including hypoglycemia. Figure 2 displays representative MRI brain images from a patient treated with RP-1127 (Panel a) and from an untreated historical patient (Panel b) at admission and 72–96 h. The edema and mass effect expected at 72 h are largely absent in the patient treated with RP-1127. Of the 10 patients, 1 patient had a neurological death, even after DC, and only 1 other patient required DC. Furthermore, 8/10 patients did not require any osmotherapy, intubation, or DC. In addition, there were no PH1/PH2 hemorrhages, despite 9/10 patients receiving IV rtPA. Neurological

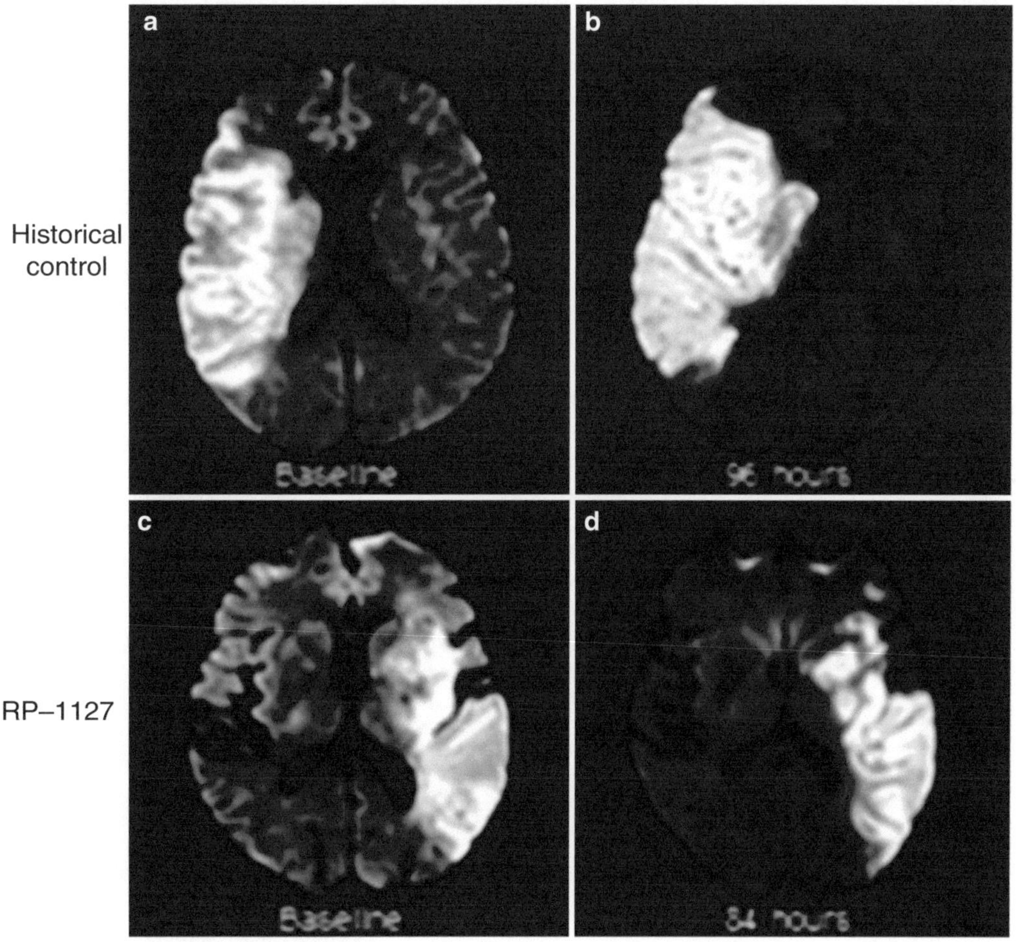

Fig. 2 Magnetic resonance diffusion weighted imaging at baseline (**a**, **c**) and at subacute follow up after stroke (**b**, **d**). The historical control (*top panels*) is from the EPITHET study. The *bottom panels* correspond to a GAMES-Pilot subject treated with RP-1127

outcome at 3 months, overall mortality, need for DC, and hemorrhagic transformation were all improved compared with historical, matched patients [19–21]. GAMES-Pilot was a non-randomized, unblinded study with a small sample size; however, safety at the target dose of 3 mg/day and preliminary signals of efficacy provided the motivation for a randomized, double-blind phase II study.

Effect of RP-1127 on Intermediate Markers of Swelling

Previously, reliable, validated neuroimaging measures of brain swelling after stroke had not been established. Because the treatment effect of glyburide results, in part, from decreased edema formation, the application of a neuroimaging marker of edema is critical to assessing biological effect of the drug.

Our group initially investigated MRI-based ipsilateral hemisphere volumetric determination in stroke patients [22]. Serial MRI studies from stroke patients in the Echoplanar Imaging Thrombolytic Evaluation Trial (EPITHET) [23] with initial DWI lesion volume ≥82 cm^3 were analyzed (baseline and day 3–5). The concordance correlation coefficient between readers was 0.90, and hemisphere volume correlated with early neurological deterioration (area under the curve 0.83; $p=0.04$) Using this method, GAMES-Pilot subjects had an increase of 50 ± 33 cm^3 compared with historical controls of 72 ± 27 cm^3.

While serial change in hemisphere volume is a reasonable surrogate of swelling after ischemia, additional markers of cytotoxic and vasogenic injury can provide insight into the mechanism of action of RP-1127. MRI apparent diffusion coefficient (ADC) sequences vary depending on the restricted diffusion of water between the extracellular and intracellular compartments [24]. T2-based fluid attenuated inversion recovery sequences (FLAIR) may be sensitive to ischemic injury, which depends, in part, on the contribution of swelling from the vasculature [25]. To explore the possible effects of RP-1127 on these MRI signatures, serial MRI from GAMES-Pilot patients were compared with serial MRI from the control arm of the Normobaric Oxygen Therapy in Acute Ischemic Stroke Trial (NBO). Using a case-control design, ADC, FLAIR, and their respective signal intensity ratios (SIR) were obtained by normalizing the value within the stroke region of interest to the contralateral hemisphere.

The baseline characteristics for both groups were the same except more NBO subjects were male and a higher proportion of GAMES Pilot subjects underwent thrombolysis. There were no differences between ADC values or relative intensities in GAMES Pilot versus NBO subjects at baseline or day 1. In contrast, the FLAIR SIR in the NBO cohort was significantly higher as early as 24 h compared with GAMES Pilot subjects. The diminished increase in FLAIR SIR in RP-1127 treated GAMES Pilot subjects appeared to be a durable signal that lasted through the period of drug infusion, and there appeared to be a dose response relationship between the FLAIR ratio and RP-1127 level ($p=0.014$). When patients were dichotomized at a plasma RP-1127 concentration that was associated with mild glucose lowering in the phase I study (25 ng/mL), the FLAIR SIR was lower ($p<0.01$) in the group with high RP-1127 plasma levels (Fig. 3).

An analysis of FLAIR SIR in a cohort of acute stroke subjects suggested that FLAIR SIR was associated with symptomatic hemorrhagic transformation as well as matrix metalloproteinase-9 (MMP-9), an enzyme known to be associated with degradation of the blood-brain barrier, edema, and hemorrhagic transformation [26]. Increased levels of MMP-9 have also been associated with the administration of IV rtPA [27]. When MMP-9 levels were compared between RP-1127 treated patients and control large-stroke patients, glyburide treatment was associated with lower levels of MMP-9 [28]. There were no significant differences in the baseline characteristics, including exposure to rtPA.

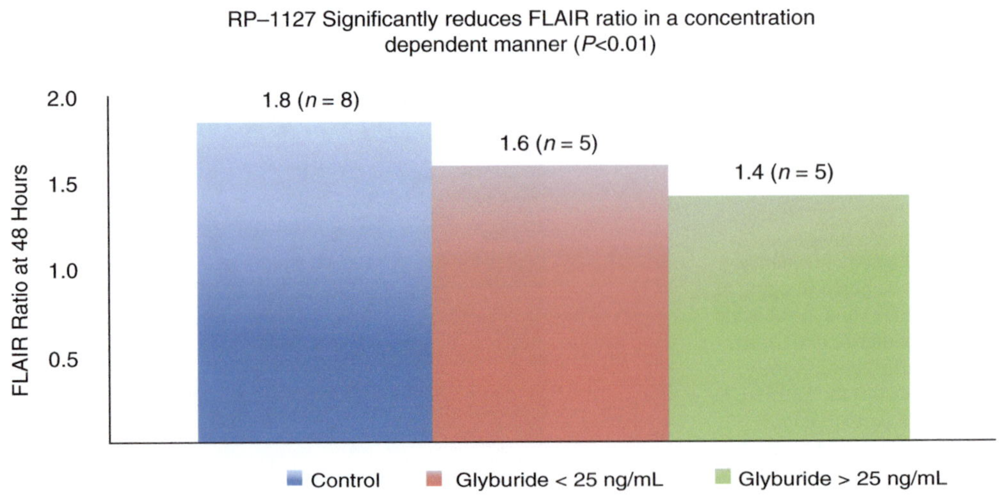

Fig. 3 Dose dependent relationship between RP-1127 and FLAIR Ratio

These results have several important implications for RP-1127 translation. First, there are several candidate MRI signatures that may be modified by RP-1127 administration. In addition, plasma levels of MMP-9 may also decrease in association to RP-1127 exposure. Further, these changes may have a dose-response relationship. The potential biological response of these markers to RP-1127 is even more important considering their prior, established association with brain swelling and hemorrhagic transformation after ischemia, each of which RP-1127 proposes to reduce. The relationship between MRI signatures, MMP-9 levels, and RP-1127 will be further investigated in the ongoing GAMES-RP study; however, there is also an urgent need to further validate these relationships in independent populations of stroke patients, across a broad range of infarct volumes.

Phase II Randomized Trial

The robust preclinical and human data above directly led to the initiation of GAMES-RP (Clinicaltrials.gov identifier: NCT01794182), a randomized, multi-center, prospective, double-blind phase II trial in patients with a severe anterior circulation ischemic stroke who are likely to develop malignant edema. The study population consists of subjects with a clinical diagnosis of acute stroke with a baseline DWI lesion volume of 82–300 cm^3, age 18–80 years, and time of symptom onset to start of drug infusion of ≤10 h. The primary objectives are to demonstrate the safety and efficacy of RP-1127 compared with placebo in patients with a severe anterior circulation ischemic stroke. The primary efficacy objective will be addressed by comparing the proportion of RP-1127 and placebo-treated patients with a day 90 modified Rankin Scale score ≤4 without decompressive craniectomy. The primary safety objective will be measured by comparing the frequency of adverse and severe adverse events in RP-1127 and placebo-treated patients. Subjects are randomized to either RP-1127 or placebo delivered as an IV bolus followed by an IV infusion for 72 h using the same dosing regimen as in GAMES-Pilot. In addition to a baseline MRI, subjects will undergo a 72–96 h follow-up MRI and serial clinical assessments through 1 year, aimed at assessing functional outcome, mood, and quality of life. The primary efficacy endpoint is at 90 days. A multidisciplinary team established clinical standardization guidelines, largely based on the American Heart Association guidelines for the management of patients with severe stroke [3, 29, 30]. This standardization of emergency and intensive care aims to make uniform practices surrounding sedation, use of osmotherapy and sodium management, fluid and insulin administration, and selection of patients for decompressive craniectomy. As of September 23, 2014, 52 subjects across 17 US hospitals have been enrolled, meeting the projected enrollment targets.

Conclusion

The discovery that the SUR-TRPM4 channel may have a crucial role in the development of swelling and hemorrhagic transformation has led to an ongoing effort to translate these findings into an innovative therapy for patients with stroke. Glyburide has been extensively studied in preclinical rodent models of stroke. Several independent lines of inquiry in human stroke now suggest that RP-1127 (intravenous glyburide) is a safe, effective neurovascular protectant. Successful translation of this therapy may result in effective prevention of brain swelling and improvement in the recovery of stroke patients.

References

1. Jauch EC, Saver JL, Adams HP Jr et al (2013) Guidelines for the early management of patients with acute ischemic stroke: a guideline for healthcare professionals from the American Heart Association/American Stroke Association. Stroke 44(3):870–947. doi:10.1161/STR.0b013e318284056a
2. Hacke W, Schwab S, Horn M, Spranger M, De Georgia M, von Kummer R (1996) 'Malignant' middle cerebral artery territory infarction: clinical course and prognostic signs. Arch Neurol 53(4):309–315
3. Wijdicks EF, Sheth KN, Carter BS et al (2014) Recommendations for the management of cerebral and cerebellar infarction with swelling: a statement for healthcare professionals from the American Heart Association/American Stroke Association. Stroke 45(4):1222–1238. doi:10.1161/01.str.0000441965.15164.d6
4. Broderick JP, Palesch YY, Demchuk AM et al (2013) Endovascular therapy after intravenous t-PA versus t-PA alone for stroke. N Engl J Med 368(10):893–903. doi:10.1056/NEJMoa1214300
5. Mlynash M, Lansberg MG, Straka M et al (2011) Refining the definition of the malignant profile: insights from the DEFUSE-EPITHET pooled data set. DEFUSE-EPITHET Investigators. Stroke 42(5):1270–1275. doi:10.1161/STROKEAHA.110.601609. [Epub 2011 Apr 7]
6. Molina CA, Selim MH (2011) Decompressive hemicraniectomy in elderly patients with malignant hemispheric infarction: open questions remain beyond DESTINY. Stroke 42(3):847–848. doi:10.1161/STROKEAHA.110.603613
7. Juttler E, Bosel J, Amiri H et al (2011) DESTINY II: DEcompressive surgery for the treatment of malignant INfarction of the middle cerebral arterYII. Int J Stroke 6(1):79–86. doi:10.1111/j.1747-4949.2010.00544.x
8. Sheth KN (2013) Novel approaches to the primary prevention of edema after ischemia. Stroke 44(6 Suppl 1):S136. doi:10.1161/STROKEAHA.113.001821
9. Simard JM, Chen M, Tarasov KV et al (2006) Newly expressed SUR1-regulated NC(ca-ATP) channel mediates cerebral edema after ischemic stroke. Nat Med 12(4):433–440. doi:10.1038/nm1390
10. Simard JM, Tsymbalyuk N, Tsymbalyuk O, Ivanova S, Yurovsky V, Gerzanich V (2010) Glibenclamide is superior to decompressive craniectomy in a rat model of malignant stroke. Stroke 41(3):531–537. doi:10.1161/STROKEAHA.109.572644
11. Simard JM, Sheth KN, Kimberly WT et al (2013) Glibenclamide in cerebral ischemia and stroke. Neurocrit Care. doi:10.1007/s12028-013-9923-1
12. Fisher M, Feuerstein G, Howells DW et al (2009) Update of the stroke therapy academic industry roundtable preclinical recommendations. Stroke 40(6):2244–2250. doi:10.1161/STROKEAHA.108.541128

13. Simard JM, Kent TA, Kunte H (2011) Letter by Simard et al regarding article, "Sulfonylurea use before stroke does not influence outcome". Stroke. doi:10.1161/STROKEAHA.111.620666
14. Favilla CG, Mullen MT, Ali M, Higgins P, Kasner SE, Virtual International Stroke Trials Archive (VISTA) Collaboration (2011) Sulfonylurea use before stroke does not influence outcome. Stroke 42(3):710–715. doi:10.1161/STROKEAHA.110.599274
15. Horsdal HT, Mehnert F, Rungby J, Johnsen SP (2012) Type of preadmission antidiabetic treatment and outcome among patients with ischemic stroke: a nationwide follow-up study. J Stroke Cerebrovasc Dis 21(8):717–725. doi:10.1016/j.jstrokecerebrovasdis.2011.03.007
16. Kunte H, Schmidt S, Eliasziw M et al (2007) Sulfonylureas improve outcome in patients with type 2 diabetes and acute ischemic stroke. Stroke 38(9):2526–2530. doi:10.1161/STROKEAHA.107.482216
17. Kunte H, Busch M, Trostdorf K et al (2012) Hemorrhagic transformation of ischemic stroke in diabetics on sulfonylureas. Ann Neurol 72:799–806
18. Mehta RI, Ivanova S, Tosun C, Castellani RJ, Gerzanich V, Simard JM (2013) Sulfonylurea receptor 1 expression in human cerebral infarcts. J Neuropathol Exp Neurol 72(9):871–883. doi:10.1097/NEN.0b013e3182a32e40
19. Sheth KN, Taylor Kimberly W, Elm JJ et al (2014) Exploratory analysis of glyburide as a novel therapy for preventing brain swelling. Neurocrit Care 21(1):43–51. doi:10.1007/s12028-014-9970-2
20. Sheth KN, Kimberly WT, Elm JJ et al (2013) Pilot study of intravenous glyburide in patients with a large ischemic stroke. Stroke. doi:10.1161/STROKEAHA.113.003352
21. Thomalla G, Hartmann F, Juettler E et al (2010) Prediction of malignant middle cerebral artery infarction by magnetic resonance imaging within 6 hours of symptom onset: a prospective multicenter observational study. Ann Neurol 68(4):435–445. doi:10.1002/ana.22125
22. Yoo AJ, Sheth KN, Kimberly WT et al (2012) Validating imaging biomarkers of cerebral edema in patients with severe ischemic stroke. J Stroke Cerebrovasc Dis. doi:10.1016/j.jstrokecerebrovasdis.2012.01.002
23. Davis SM, Donnan GA, Parsons MW et al (2008) Effects of alteplase beyond 3 h after stroke in the echoplanar imaging thrombolytic evaluation trial (EPITHET): a placebo-controlled randomised trial. Lancet Neurol 7(4):299–309. doi:10.1016/S1474-4422(08)70044-9
24. Todd NV, Picozzi P, Crockard A, Russell RW (1986) Duration of ischemia influences the development and resolution of ischemic brain edema. Stroke 17(3):466–471
25. Schaefer PW (2000) Diffusion-weighted imaging as a problem-solving tool in the evaluation of patients with acute strokelike syndromes. Top Magn Reson Imaging 11(5):300–309
26. Jha R, Battey TW, Pham L et al (2014) Fluid-attenuated inversion recovery hyperintensity correlates with matrix metalloproteinase-9 level and hemorrhagic transformation in acute ischemic stroke. Stroke 45(4):1040–1045. doi:10.1161/STROKEAHA.113.004627
27. Castellanos M, Leira R, Serena J et al (2003) Plasma metalloproteinase-9 concentration predicts hemorrhagic transformation in acute ischemic stroke. Stroke 34(1):40–46
28. Kimberly WT, Battey TW, Pham L et al (2013) Glyburide is associated with attenuated vasogenic edema in stroke patients. Neurocrit Care. doi:10.1007/s12028-013-9917-z
29. Kimberly WT, Sheth KN (2011) Approach to severe hemispheric stroke. Neurology 76(7 Suppl 2):S50–S56. doi:10.1212/WNL.0b013e31820c35f4
30. Simard JM, Sahuquillo J, Sheth KN, Kahle KT, Walcott BP (2011) Managing malignant cerebral infarction. Curr Treat Options Neurol 13(2):217–229. doi:10.1007/s11940-010-0110-9

Mechanisms Underlying Astrocyte Endfeet Swelling in Stroke

J. Xiang, Y. Tang, C. Li, E.J. Su, D.A. Lawrence, and Richard F. Keep

Introduction

One of the earliest morphological events after an ischemic stroke is swelling of the astrocyte endfeet that surround the cerebral capillaries [1, 2]. Multiple hypotheses have been suggested as to why such swelling occurs [3–7]. These hypotheses have primarily focused on the effects of the parenchymal changes that occur during and after cerebral ischemia (e.g., increased extracellular K^+ and L-glutamate concentrations) and how they may induce astrocyte swelling. In this review, we put forward an alternate or complementary hypothesis that astrocyte endfeet swelling relates to blood-brain barrier (BBB) dysfunction.

Direct Effects of Ischemia on Astrocytes

An example of the astrocyte endfeet swelling that occurs in cerebral ischemia is shown in Fig. 1. One possible cause of such swelling is the direct effects of ischemia, loss of oxygen and glucose supply, on astrocytes. However, experiments mimicking ischemia *in vitro* using oxygen glucose deprivation (OGD) failed to show marked swelling in cultured astrocytes [3], and there is evidence that astrocytes are more resistant to the effects of OGD than neurons [6, 8]. A caveat is that there may be astrocyte heterogeneity, with populations differing in their swelling response to ischemia [9].

Response of Astrocytes to Parenchymal Dysfunction

Under iso-osmotic conditions, cell swelling occurs in response to solute uptake (transporter or channel mediated) or metabolic production of osmoles. Kimelberg [4] reviewed a number of such mechanisms that have been hypothesized to be involved in astrocyte swelling in ischemic stroke. These include the failure of energy metabolism during ischemia causing loss of neuronal K^+ and increased extracellular K^+, with the latter causing astrocyte swelling [6]. Such swelling is, at least in part, due to ion transport via the Na-K-Cl co-transporter, NKCC1 [10]. Astrocytic NKCC1 activity after stroke may also be upregulated by a number of signaling cascades [11].

There is also a release of L-glutamate into the extracellular space during cerebral ischemia [12, 13], and exposure to high L-glutamate concentrations causes astrocyte cell swelling [14]. The astrocyte excitatory amino acid transporters EAAT2 and EAAT1 (GLT-1, GLAST) are involved in clearing L-glutamate from the extracellular space and they cotransport Na^+ and Cl^- into the cell [15].

Given the large electrochemical gradient for Na^+ to enter cells, there has been considerable interest in the possible role of nonselective cation ion channels in brain edema. Thus, there is growing evidence of newly expressed sulfonylurea receptor 1-transient receptor potential melastatin 4 (SUR1-TRPM4) channels having an important role in ischemic brain edema [11]. However, in ischemia, the early expression of this channel is endothelial, with later expression in astro-

J. Xiang • Y. Tang • C. Li
Department of Neurosurgery, University of Michigan, Room 5018, BSRB, Ann Arbor 48109-2200, MI, USA

E.J. Su
Department of Internal Medicine, University of Michigan, Ann Arbor, MI, USA

D.A. Lawrence
Department of Internal Medicine, University of Michigan, Ann Arbor, MI, USA

Department of Molecular and Integrative Physiology, University of Michigan, Ann Arbor, MI, USA

R.F. Keep, PhD (✉)
Department of Neurosurgery, University of Michigan, Room 5018, BSRB, Ann Arbor 48109-2200, MI, USA

Department of Molecular and Integrative Physiology, University of Michigan, Ann Arbor, MI, USA
e-mail: rkeep@umich.edu

R.L. Applegate et al. (eds.), *Brain Edema XVI: Translate Basic Science into Clinical Practice*, Acta Neurochirurgica Supplement, Vol. 121,
DOI 10.1007/978-3-319-18497-5_4,

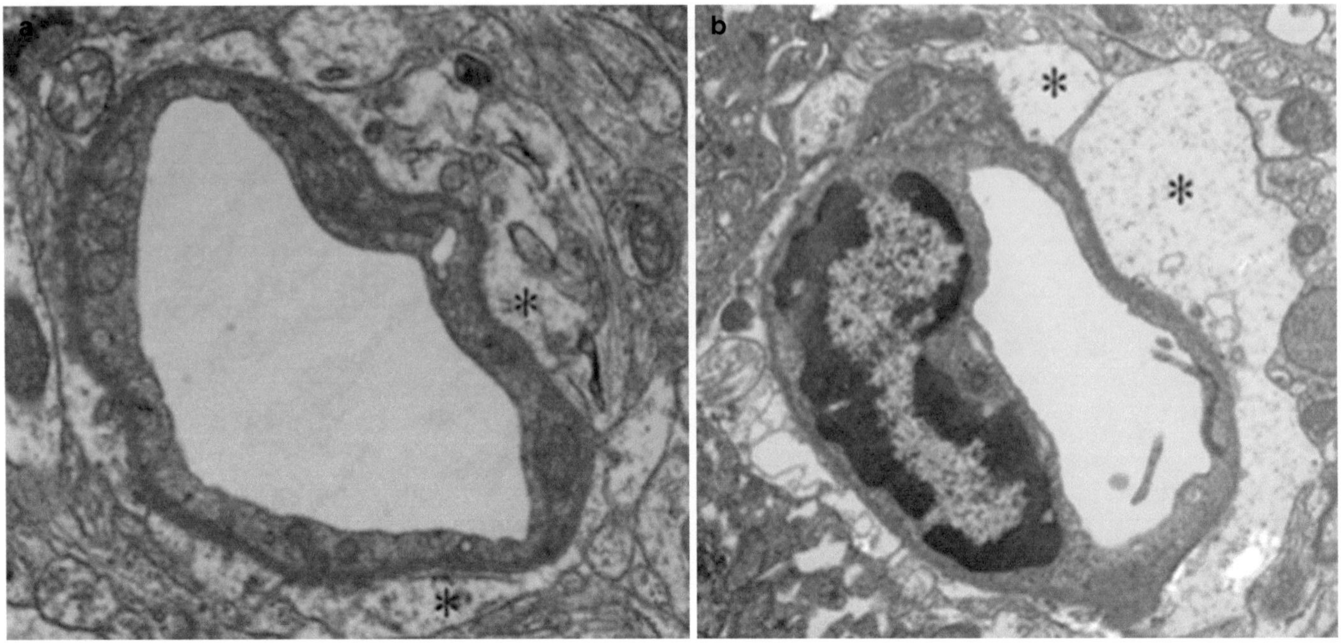

Fig. 1 Electron micrographs from C57BL6/J mouse (**a**) contra- and (**b**) ipsilateral hemispheres 3 h after photothrombotic occlusion of the middle cerebral artery. The micrograph of a capillary from the ipsilateral hemisphere was taken from the ischemic penumbra. The micrograph from the contralateral hemisphere was taken from the corresponding brain region. Note the marked swelling of the astrocyte endfeet (*) that occurred in the ipsilateral hemisphere

cytes [11]. It is therefore unlikely to be involved in early astrocyte endfeet swelling, although other nonselective cation channels might be.

Response to Blood-Brain Barrier Dysfunction

Cerebral ischemia (permanent or transient) causes blood-brain barrier (BBB) disruption, as evinced by increased entry of high molecular weight compounds from blood into brain, compounds normally excluded by the BBB [16, 17]. To examine whether the entry of plasma constituents into brain might induce astrocyte swelling, we examined the effects of serum or plasma on the volume of neonatal astrocytes *in vitro*. Both serum and plasma caused marked cell swelling (Fig. 2).

In vivo, intracarotid injection of hyperosmotic mannitol has been used to disrupt the BBB. Even though this procedure might be expected to transiently shrink cells through osmosis, Al-Sarraf et al. [19] found evidence that this procedure caused swelling of perivascular astrocytes. This data supports the concept that there are some factors that enter the brain upon BBB disruption that can cause astrocyte swelling. However, further *in vivo* validation is needed. In particular, there is the question of when BBB disruption occurs in cerebral ischemia; that is, is it soon enough to participate in early astrocyte swelling? Here, there is conflicting evidence. Markers including a number of large molecular weight tracers and aminoisobutyric acid have shown late BBB disruption (~6 h; e.g., [16, 20]), but some early studies with horseradish peroxidase/electron

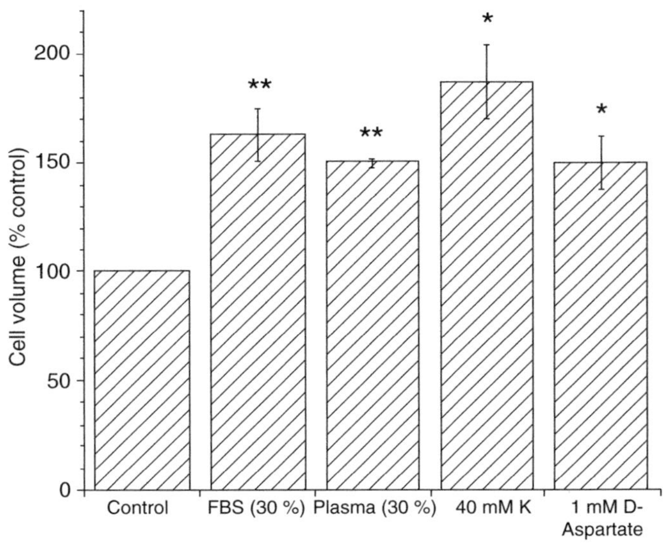

Fig. 2 Effect of different factors on astrocyte cell volume *in vitro*. Neonatal rat astrocytes were cultured in serum-free conditions for 48 h before being exposed to fetal bovine serum (FBS), rat plasma, 1 mM D-aspartate or 40 mM K^+ for 2 h. D-aspartate and high K^+ were included as positive controls known to increase astrocyte cell volume [6, 14]. Astrocyte cell volume was then assessed using 3-0-methyl [^{3}H] D-glucose [18]. Cell volumes are expressed as a percentage of control values (serum free). Values are means± SE, $n = 3$–9 (with each preparation being performed in triplicate). * and ** indicate $p < 0.05$ and $p < 0.01$ vs. control (paired *t*-tests on raw data)

microscopy indicated disruption within minutes [21, 22]. If astrocyte endfeet swelling affects the penetration of tracers away from the vasculature, this could complicate interpretation of different types of tracer data for assessing BBB disruption.

It remain uncertain which factors in plasma (or derived from plasma constituents) may induce cell swelling. It should be noted, however, that plasma L-glutamate and L-aspartate concentrations are much higher than in brain extracellular space/CSF (e.g., [23, 24]), and Westergren et al. [25] found that the concentration of these excitatory amino acids markedly increased (~10–20 fold) in brain extracellular space after BBB disruption with intracarotid infusion of protamine sulfate. Thus, given that excitatory amino acids can induce astrocyte swelling, an influx of those amino acids from plasma after BBB disruption may participate in ischemia-induced astrocyte swelling.

Possible Function of Astrocyte Endfeet Swelling

One possible effect of the swelling of the astrocyte endfeet is occlusion of the extracellular space between the endfeet. This might limit the migration of blood constituents away from a vessel with a disrupted BBB. In particular, the formation of an astrocyte cuff around the vessel may limit the egress of erythrocytes into brain (hemorrhage). In animals, there is evidence that BBB hyperpermeability precedes intracerebral hemorrhage [26], raising the possibility that astrocyte swelling induced by the hyperpermeability may limit potential subsequent hemorrhage.

Limiting hematoma expansion is important clinically, either in preventing the conversion of microbleeds to symptomatic hemorrhage or in reducing the increase in hemorrhage size that occurs in approximately a third of patients during the first day after intracerebral hemorrhage [27, 28]. However, it should also be noted that astrocyte swelling contributes to brain edema, which can cause increased intracranial pressure and brain herniation.

Whether an astrocyte cuff would be complete enough to limit the entry of potentially neurotoxic plasma constituents into brain deserves investigation. A number of studies have reported biphasic opening of the BBB after stroke (e.g., [29]). This is normally attributed to differences in the time courses of various mediators of BBB disruption (e.g., early free radical production and delayed induction of inflammatory mediators). However, it is possible that an astrocyte cuff may participate, at least transiently, in reducing apparent BBB permeability after an initial disruption.

Conclusion

Astrocyte endfeet swelling is an early event in cerebral ischemia. Such swelling may, at least in part, be a response to blood-brain barrier dysfunction and we hypothesize that it may be a mechanism to limit cerebral hemorrhage following an ischemic event.

Acknowledgments This work was supported by the National Institutes of Health grants NS034709, NS079639, and HL55374. The content is solely the responsibility of the authors and does not necessarily represent the official views of the NIH.

Conflicts of Interest None.

References

1. Dodson RF, Chu LW, Welch KM, Achar VS (1977) Acute tissue response to cerebral ischemia in the gerbil. An ultrastructural study. J Neurol Sci 33:161–170
2. Garcia JH, Kalimo H, Kamijyo Y, Trump BF (1977) Cellular events during partial cerebral ischemia. I. Electron microscopy of feline cerebral cortex after middle-cerebral-artery occlusion. Virchows Arch B Cell Pathol 25:191–206
3. Juurlink BH, Chen Y, Hertz L (1992) Use of cell cultures to differentiate among effects of various ischemia factors on astrocytic cell volume. Can J Physiol Pharmacol 70(Suppl):S344–S349
4. Kimelberg HK (2005) Astrocytic swelling in cerebral ischemia as a possible cause of injury and target for therapy. Glia 50:389–397
5. Shigeno T, Mima T, Takakura K (1990) Mechanisms of astroglial swelling in focal cerebral ischemia. Adv Neurol 52:545
6. Walz W, Klimaszewski A, Paterson IA (1993) Glial swelling in ischemia: a hypothesis. Dev Neurosci 15:216–225
7. Walz W, Mukerji S (1990) Simulation of aspects of ischemia in cell culture: changes in lactate compartmentation. Glia 3:522–528
8. Silver IA, Deas J, Erecinska M (1997) Ion homeostasis in brain cells: differences in intracellular ion responses to energy limitation between cultured neurons and glial cells. Neuroscience 78:589–601
9. Benesova J, Hock M, Butenko O, Prajerova I, Anderova M, Chvatal A (2009) Quantification of astrocyte volume changes during ischemia n situ reveals two populations of astrocytes in the cortex of GFAP/EGFP mice. J Neurosci Res 87:96–111
10. Chen H, Sun D (2005) The role of Na-K-Cl co-transporter in cerebral ischemia. Neurol Res 27:280–286
11. Khanna A, Kahle KT, Walcott BP, Gerzanich V, Simard JM (2014) Disruption of ion homeostasis in the neurogliovascular unit underlies the pathogenesis of ischemic cerebral edema. Transl Stroke Res 5:3–16
12. Obrenovitch TP, Richards DA (1995) Extracellular neurotransmitter changes in cerebral ischaemia. Cerebrovasc Brain Metab Rev 7:1–54
13. Obrenovitch TP, Urenjak J, Zilkha E, Jay TM (2000) Excitotoxicity in neurological disorders–the glutamate paradox. Int J Dev Neurosci 18:281–287
14. Bender AS, Schousboe A, Reichelt W, Norenberg MD (1998) Ionic mechanisms in glutamate-induced astrocyte swelling: role of K+ influx. J Neurosci Res 52:307–321
15. Kanai Y, Clemencon B, Simonin A, Leuenberger M, Lochner M, Weisstanner M, Hediger MA (2013) The SLC1 high-affinity gluta-

mate and neutral amino acid transporter family. Mol Aspects Med 34:108–120

16. Knowland D, Arac A, Sekiguchi KJ, Hsu M, Lutz SE, Perrino J, Steinberg GK, Barres BA, Nimmerjahn A, Agalliu D (2014) Stepwise recruitment of transcellular and paracellular pathways underlies blood-brain barrier breakdown in stroke. Neuron 82:603–617
17. Sandoval KE, Witt KA (2008) Blood-brain barrier tight junction permeability and ischemic stroke. Neurobiol Dis 32:200–219
18. Aschner M (2011) Volume measurements in cultured primary astrocytes. Methods Mol Biol 758:391–402
19. Al-Sarraf H, Ghaaedi F, Redzic Z (2007) Time course of hyperosmolar opening of the blood-brain and blood-CSF barriers in spontaneously hypertensive rats. J Vasc Res 44:99–109
20. Betz AL, Keep RF, Beer ME, Ren XD (1994) Blood-brain barrier permeability and brain concentration of sodium, potassium, and chloride during focal ischemia. J Cereb Blood Flow Metab 14:29–37
21. Dietrich WD, Busto R, Watson BD, Scheinberg P, Ginsberg MD (1987) Photochemically induced cerebral infarction. II. Edema and blood-brain barrier disruption. Acta Neuropathol 72:326–334
22. Petito CK (1979) Early and late mechanisms of increased vascular permeability following experimental cerebral infarction. J Neuropathol Exp Neurol 38:222–234
23. Stover JF, Sakowitz OW, Kroppenstedt SN, Thomale UW, Kempski OS, Flugge G, Unterberg AW (2004) Differential effects of prolonged isoflurane anesthesia on plasma, extracellular, and CSF glutamate, neuronal activity, 125I-Mk801 NMDA receptor binding, and brain edema in traumatic brain-injured rats. Acta Neurochir 146:819–830
24. Ye ZC, Sontheimer H (1998) Astrocytes protect neurons from neurotoxic injury by serum glutamate. Glia 22:237–248
25. Westergren I, Nystrom B, Hamberger A, Nordborg C, Johansson BB (1994) Concentrations of amino acids in extracellular fluid after opening of the blood-brain barrier by intracarotid infusion of protamine sulfate. J Neurochem 62:159–165
26. Lee JM, Zhai G, Liu Q, Gonzales ER, Yin K, Yan P, Hsu CY, Vo KD, Lin W (2007) Vascular permeability precedes spontaneous intracerebral hemorrhage in stroke-prone spontaneously hypertensive rats. Stroke 38:3289–3291
27. Keep RF, Hua Y, Xi G (2012) Intracerebral haemorrhage: mechanisms of injury and therapeutic targets. Lancet Neurol 11:720–731
28. Xi G, Keep RF, Hoff JT (2006) Mechanisms of brain injury after intracerebral haemorrhage. Lancet Neurol 5:53–63
29. Haqqani AS, Nesic M, Preston E, Baumann E, Kelly J, Stanimirovic D (2005) Characterization of vascular protein expression patterns in cerebral ischemia/reperfusion using laser capture microdissection and ICAT-nanoLC-MS/MS. FASEB J 19:1809–1821

Hypoxia and Inflammation-Induced Disruptions of the Blood-Brain and Blood-Cerebrospinal Fluid Barriers Assessed Using a Novel T_1-Based MRI Method

Nabeela Nathoo*, Hamza Jalal*, Sirajedin S. Natah, Qiong Zhang, Ying Wu, and Jeff F. Dunn

Introduction

The blood-brain barrier (BBB) protects the brain from potentially harmful elements circulating in the body. Disruption of the BBB is implicated in many neurological conditions, including stroke [1, 2], epilepsy [3, 4], and radiation-induced necrosis [5]. Such BBB disruption can be classified as being either severe or subtle. Severe BBB disruption can be discerned qualitatively as it is localized to specific areas of the brain, and can be assessed by determining the permeability of large molecular weight molecules such as serum proteins [6]. Severe disruption has been demonstrated radiologically with contrast agent extravasation in stroke [7, 8], traumatic brain injury [9, 10], and brain tumors [11].

Subtle disruption is found generalized throughout the brain which requires quantitative methods for assessment. Methods include using smaller molecular weight compounds such as sodium fluorescein (NaF) or Evans blue [12] which are useful in histological studies, but not in whole brain studies. Such subtle BBB disruption may be involved in multiple sclerosis [13] and high-altitude hypoxia exposure [14].

To study BBB disruption that is diffuse and relatively small in magnitude *in vivo*, an MRI method with increased sensitivity to the extravasation of the gadolinium (Gd) contrast agent is needed. Ideally, this method would detect leakage within a single voxel of an image. We propose single voxel analysis and use models of severe and focal disruption contrast with mild and generalized disruption of the BBB to show proof of principle.

Severe disruption is based on the cold injury model which generates a localized region of cortical injury and BBB disruption. Hypoxia leads to nonspecific and diffuse disruptions of the BBB which has been previously demonstrated with enhancement on NaF histology [14]. We also compared this with an established model of lipopolysaccharide (LPS)-associated inflammatory generalized disruption.

Thus, we developed a novel voxel-based analysis facilitating visualization of BBB disruption at the level of a single voxel. This approach would provide the opportunity to quantify diffuse BBB disruption without having to select an arbitrary region of interest (ROI). Using this technique, we propose that mild hypoxia and inflammation resulted in diffuse disruption of the BBB, while more severe insults resulted in prominent leakage in the periventricular area.

Materials and Methods

Animals

Male Wistar rats were used (220–275 g) from Charles River (Montreal, Quebec). Studies were approved by the Animal Care Committee of the University of Calgary.

N. Nathoo* • H. Jalal*
Department of Radiology, University of Calgary,
3330 Hospital Drive, N.W., Calgary, AB T2N 4N1, Canada

Hotchkiss Brain Institute, University of Calgary,
Calgary, AB, Canada

S.S. Natah
Department of Physiology, Umm-Alqura University,
Makkah, Saudi Arabia

Q. Zhang
General Electric, Beijing, China

Y. Wu
Department of Radiology, University of Calgary,
3330 Hospital Drive, N.W., Calgary, AB T2N 4N1, Canada

J.F. Dunn (✉)
Hotchkiss Brain Institute, University of Calgary,
Calgary, AB, Canada

Experimental Imaging Centre, University of Calgary,
Calgary, AB, Canada

Department of Radiology, University of Calgary,
3330 Hospital Drive, N.W., Calgary, AB T2N 4N1, Canada
e-mail: dunnj@ucalgary.ca

R.L. Applegate et al. (eds.), *Brain Edema XVI: Translate Basic Science into Clinical Practice*, Acta Neurochirurgica Supplement, Vol. 121,
DOI 10.1007/978-3-319-18497-5_5,

Cold Injury Model

This method has been described previously [15]. Two rats were anesthetized with 1–2 % isoflurane anesthesia. At approximately 3 mm posterior to the bregma and 2 mm lateral, a 2.5 mm hole was drilled, exposing the dura mater. Using forceps, the dura was removed, exposing the underlying brain. A metal probe (2 mm) cooled in liquid nitrogen for 5 min was applied to the surface for 45 s. For the sham rat, the same probe at room temperature was applied. The scalp was sutured and the animals were given a subcutaneous injection of analgesic (Buprenex; 0.3 mg/kg). Magnetic resonance imaging (MRI) was performed 24 h later.

LPS Treatment

Intraperitoneal (IP) injection was given at 0.1 or 1.0 mg/kg ($n=5$ for each concentration). With this model, increased BBB permeability occurs after 3–6 h [16]. MRI was performed 3 h later.

Hypoxia

For hypobaric (10 %) hypoxia, rats ($n=5$) were placed in a custom-built hypobaric chamber [14] and exposed for 24 h at 375 mmHg and 22 °C, which corresponded to a PO_2 of 78.8 mmHg. For more severe hypoxia (8 %), rats ($n=2$) were placed in a normobaric chamber with an O_2:N_2 (8:92 %) gas mixture, corresponding to PO_2 of 60.8 mmHg. After 24 h, rats were removed from the hypoxic chamber and transported to the imaging center (within 5 min) and administered an O_2:N_2 gas mixture with an equivalent FiO_2 to match the hypobaric chamber PO_2. Animals were anesthetized with 3 % isoflurane for MRI.

MRI Protocol

A 9.4T Bruker Avance console was used with a 35 mm quadrature volume coil. A cannula was placed intravenously for delivery of Gd (Gd; gadodiamide [Omniscan, GE Healthcare, USA]; 0.5 mmol/kg body weight). Hypobaric hypoxia rats were given O_2:N_2 of 10:88.5 %, normobaric hypoxia rats an 8:90.5 % mixture, and control animals were given a 30:68.5 % gas mixture with 1.5 % isoflurane. Body temperature was measured and maintained at 37 °C.

In two animals, Gd was injected in the magnet and a time course study was done to determine how much time needed to pass in order for the signal to reach steady state and to collect the second set of images. After determining this, Gd was injected and T_1-weighted spin echo images were acquired (TR = 500 ms, TE = 6 ms, matrix = 256 × 256, number of averages = 2, FOV = 3 × 3 cm, slice thickness = 1.5 mm).

NaF Histology

After MRI and while sedated, animals were given 1.0 mL of sodium fluorescein (2 % NaF (w/v) in normal saline 0.9 %; Sigma) intravenously. After 10 min, the animal was injected with ketamine (intraperitoneally; 1 mL/kg), and perfusion fixed with saline and 4 % paraformaldehyde. Brains were extracted and stored at 4 °C until sectioning, at which time brains were frozen in the cryostat for 30 min at −20 °C. Cryostat sections were cut at 50 μm and imaged using a fluorescent microscope (Olympus BX61). Analysis was done using StereoInvestigator (MBF Bioscience, Williston, VT, USA).

Voxel-Based Analysis

Average signal intensity from the same voxel in a series of 6 pre-Gd, T_1-weighted standard spin echo images was compared with a series of 10 post-Gd images using a custom MATLAB code. Images were aligned to ensure co-registration of voxels. Absolute values of signal intensity (16-bit) were used for processing to eliminate automatic normalization and scaling effects by the software. The average signal intensity of the pre-Gd and post-Gd series of voxels was compared using the one-tailed *Z*-test. A map of probability values of obtaining the observed mean difference in intensities was created for each voxel.

Bonferroni's correction for multiple comparisons was used. A range of *p*-values were tested. The resultant *p*-value of 5×10^{-4} was used as the significance level for individual comparisons of voxels. Following statistical testing, voxels that were significantly enhanced ($p < 5 \times 10^{-4}$) post-Gd appeared white.

Results

Validation of Voxel-Based Analysis Using Cold-Injury Model

Following induction of the cold-injury model, enhancement was qualitatively observed in the area of injury with Gd (Fig. 1a). This enhancement corresponded to the voxel-map

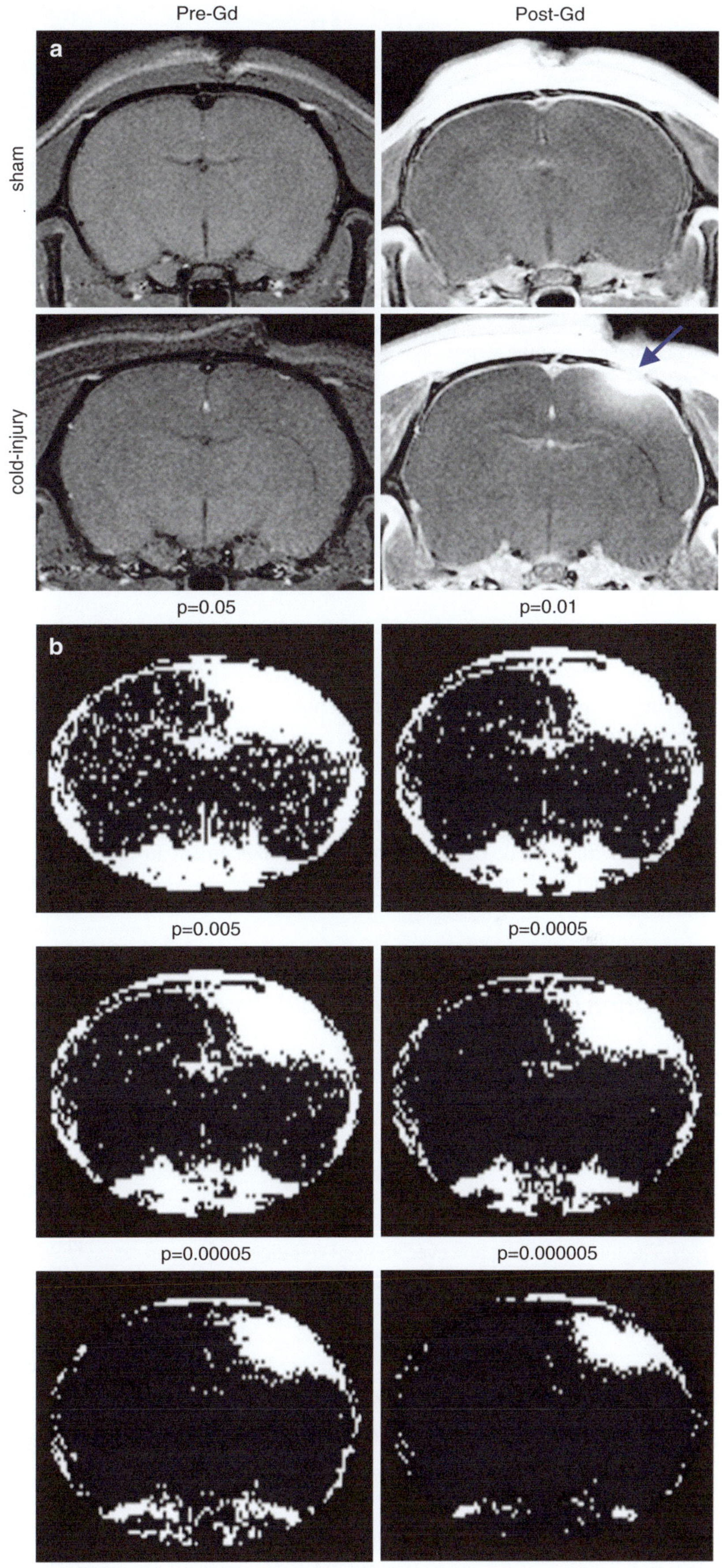

Fig. 1 Selection of significance value for voxel enhancement maps using T_1-weighted spin echo brain MRIs in the cold-injury model. Significantly enhanced voxels after Gd administration appear white. (**a**) Representative pre- and post-Gd T_1-weighted images for a sham rat and a cold injury rat. Area of injury in the cold injury model appears hyperintense post-Gd (*blue arrow*). (**b**) Signal intensities for post-Gd images were compared voxel-by-voxel using the *Z*-test with Bonferroni's correction for multiple comparisons. The effect of testing for statistical significance at different probability values based on the number of voxels included in the multiple comparisons is shown. Groups of 100 voxels were selected for statistical comparisons based on a qualitative analysis of background noise and phantoms resulting in significance inferred for changes in signal intensities of voxels at $p < 0.0005$

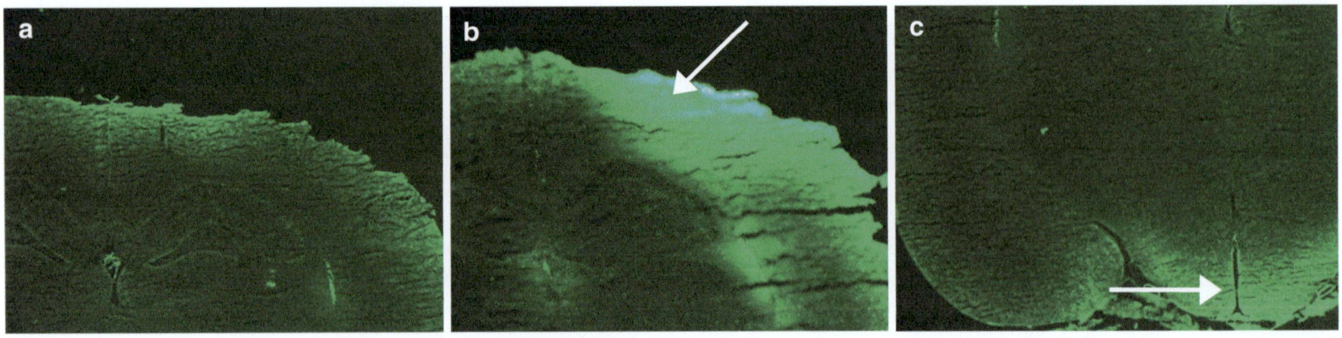

Fig. 2 Representative sodium fluorescein (NaF) histology for sham and cold-injury rats. (**a**) NaF histology for a sham rat with no obvious enhancement. (**b**) NaF histology for a rat that underwent cold injury. Intense focal enhancement is seen at the surgery site and adjacent area (*white arrow*). (**c**) NaF histology of a sham rat showing visible enhancement near the median eminence of the hypothalamus (area of weak BBB) (*white arrow*); this was seen for both conditions

that shows that significantly different voxels are clustered around the site of surgery and the surrounding area (Fig. 1b). A p-value of 5×10^{-4} was selected. Voxels that were significantly enhanced post-Gd appeared white.

NaF Histology for Cold-Injury Model

In sham animals, NaF enhancement was not observed at the surgery site (Fig. 2a). In cold injury animals, NaF enhancement was observed in the region surrounding the site of surgery (Fig. 2b); no enhancement was observed on the contralateral side. The median eminence, a circumventricular organ with a weak BBB, showed NaF enhancement in both sham and cold-injury animals (Fig. 2c).

Voxel-Based Analysis Shows Diffuse BBB Disruption in Low-Dose LPS and Mild Hypoxia

In control (Fig. 3a), low-dose LPS (Fig. 3b), and hypobaric hypoxia animals (Fig. 3d), no obvious areas of enhancement were observed. Furthermore, ROIs were drawn in the cortex, corpus callosum, and thalamus, and numbers of significant voxels were compared with controls. There was no significant difference ($p > 0.05$, one-way ANOVA with Dunnett's test post hoc). The third ventricle, however, showed significant enhancement; the fraction of significant voxels in the hypoxia group was 0.11 ± 0.01, while controls was 0.08 ± 0.01 (mean ± SEM).

Voxel-Based Analysis Shows Enhancement of the Periventricular Area in High-Dose LPS and Severe Hypoxia

In high-dose LPS animals, two responses were observed (Fig. 3c). The first was seen in two animals and consisted of significant periventricular disruption ($p < 0.0005$, Z-test) accompanied by enhancement throughout the parenchyma. The second was seen in the other three animals, where there was no obvious disruption of the BBB. Thus, it appears that once a threshold has been reached, the BBB becomes disrupted throughout the brain with a focus on leakage in the periventricular area.

Rats exposed to 8 % normobaric hypoxia also showed significant enhancement in the ventricles and periventricular area ($p < 0.0005$, Z-test) (Fig. 3e). Furthermore, there were increased numbers of individual voxels showing Gd enhancement throughout the parenchyma in severe hypoxia.

Discussion

It is fairly straightforward to detect major localized BBB disruption such as that in tumors or stroke with Gd-enhanced MRI [17]. Such disruptions cause enough T_1 signal change that regions can be seen without image processing. More quantitative methods, such as modeling the time course of enhancement or quantifying T_1, lead to voxel-based data that, theoretically, can be used to detect changes in a single voxel. However, these methods require modeling assumptions, and it may be difficult to identify changes within one voxel with a high degree of statistical confidence.

The method proposed here does not include a modeling assumption. The main statistical limitation is that the high number of comparisons made in a single test can lead to a type 1 error (differences are detected when none exist). To minimize this problem, we examined BBB disruption in a cold-injury model where we knew there would be significant focal disruption. When using a probability threshold often used in biological studies (i.e., $p < 0.05$), most of the brain showed significant change. This may, in part, be due to the fact that the blood T_1 was being shortened throughout the brain. The final p-value was selected to result in a statistical map that closely mapped the disruption observed using

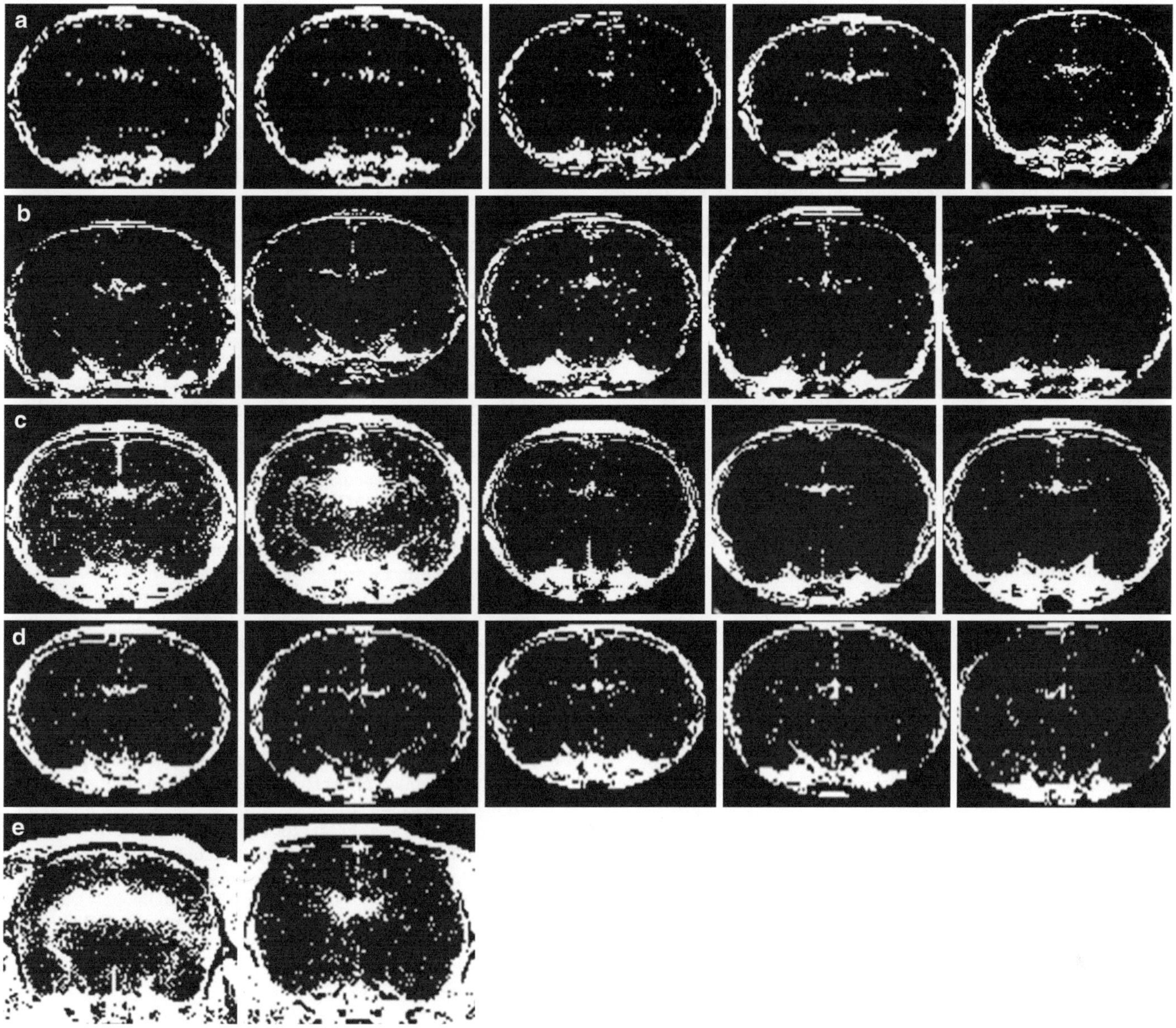

Fig. 3 Voxel-based analysis identified major enhancement in the periventricular area in the brains of rats exposed to high-dose lipopolysaccharide (LPS) and normobaric hypoxic conditions. Voxels with statistically increased signal after Gd administration are hyperintense. (**a**) Control rats that were exposed to 21 % O_2. (**b**) Rats exposed to low-dose LPS (0.1 mg/kg). (**c**) Rats exposed to high-dose LPS (1 mg/kg). In two rats (*leftmost* images in the row), periventricular enhancement is obvious. (**d**) Rats exposed to hypobaric hypoxia (1/2 atm, equivalent to approximately 10 % O_2 at sea level). (**e**) Rats exposed to normobaric hypoxia with 8 % O_2. Periventricular enhancement was substantial in both rats. Statistical significance was set as $p<0.0005$ using a *Z*-test

fluorescent microscopy. In the future, should this method be adapted for human use, such a threshold will require further validation and identification of an appropriate statistical threshold.

It should be noted that we did not observe significant parenchymal enhancement in hypobaric hypoxia nor in low-dose LPS within the tissue. However, we detected changes in the ventricle indicating that there is increased transfer of contrast agent to the ventricle with this mild perturbation.

Moreover, we detected major disruption in the blood-CSF barrier in normobaric hypoxia and high-dose LPS. This is indicated by the fact that most changes were periventricular. Compared with the BBB, the blood-CSF barrier is relatively leakier as it lacks the same tight junction configuration [18].

Limitations of this study include the use of a conservative threshold value for significance ($p<0.0005$), leading to a high degree of false-negative voxels. However, this allowed for a significant reduction of type 1 errors, thereby strengthening our findings of the affected regions. Also, isoflurane during imaging may have exacerbated damage in hypoxic conditions, where the interaction between hypoxia and isoflurane was lethal in a number of animals. This possible confounder was minimized by using the same anesthetic in control animals, though future studies may consider exploring different agents. Finally, this proof-of-principle concept requires validation in larger studies.

There are a number of advantages to using the voxel-based analysis method. It is a post-MRI acquisition method that provides high spatial resolution and it does not require specific ROIs, as it can detect enhancement anywhere in a given MR image. The steps to generate a voxel map can be compiled with computer software, so it could easily be applied clinically. Also, Gd is regularly administered to patients undergoing MRIs, so this method could be applied for such scans to highlight areas of BBB disruption.

In this study, we have shown that voxel-based analysis can be used to detect subtle disruptions to the BBB and blood-CSF barrier. We showed that there are changes in both inflammation and hypoxia models that are consistent with disruption of the blood-CSF barrier. Thus, further investigation of periventricular disruption in conditions where hypoxia and inflammation play a role is warranted.

Acknowledgments This work was supported by Alberta-Innovates Health Solutions and the National Science and Engineering Research Council Canada.

Conflict of Interest None.

References

1. Chen B et al (2009) Severe blood-brain barrier disruption and surrounding tissue injury. Stroke 40(12):e666–e674
2. Hom J et al (2011) Blood-brain barrier permeability assessed by perfusion CT predicts symptomatic hemorrhagic transformation and malignant edema in acute ischemic stroke. AJNR Am J Neuroradiol 32(1):41–48
3. Oby E, Janigro D (2006) The blood-brain barrier and epilepsy. Epilepsia 47(11):1761–1774
4. Seiffert E et al (2004) Lasting blood-brain barrier disruption induces epileptic focus in the rat somatosensory cortex. J Neurosci 24(36):7829–7836
5. Kumar AJ et al (2000) Malignant gliomas: MR imaging spectrum of radiation therapy- and chemotherapy-induced necrosis of the brain after treatment. Radiology 217(2):377–384
6. Broadwell RD, Sofroniew MV (1993) Serum proteins bypass the blood-brain fluid barriers for extracellular entry to the central nervous system. Exp Neurol 120(2):245–263
7. Fujioka M et al (1999) Novel brain ischemic change on MRI. Delayed ischemic hyperintensity on T1-weighted images and selective neuronal death in the caudoputamen of rats after brief focal ischemia. Stroke 30(5):1043–1046
8. Moseley ME et al (1990) Early detection of regional cerebral ischemia in cats: comparison of diffusion- and T2-weighted MRI and spectroscopy. Magn Reson Med 14(2):330–346
9. Habgood MD et al (2007) Changes in blood-brain barrier permeability to large and small molecules following traumatic brain injury in mice. Eur J Neurosci 25(1):231–238
10. Schneider G et al (2002) Pathophysiological changes after traumatic brain injury: comparison of two experimental animal models by means of MRI. MAGMA 14(3):233–241
11. Provenzale JM, Mukundan S, Dewhirst M (2005) The role of blood-brain barrier permeability in brain tumor imaging and therapeutics. AJR Am J Roentgenol 185(3):763–767
12. Kaya M, Ahishali B (2011) Assessment of permeability in barrier type of endothelium in brain using tracers: Evans blue, sodium fluorescein, and horseradish peroxidase. Methods Mol Biol 763:369–382
13. Soon D et al (2007) Quantification of subtle blood-brain barrier disruption in non-enhancing lesions in multiple sclerosis: a study of disease and lesion subtypes. Mult Scler 13(7):884–894
14. Natah SS et al (2009) Effects of acute hypoxia and hyperthermia on the permeability of the blood-brain barrier in adult rats. J Appl Physiol 107(4):1348–1356
15. Nag S, Picard P, Stewart DJ (2001) Expression of nitric oxide synthases and nitrotyrosine during blood-brain barrier breakdown and repair after cold injury. Lab Invest 81(1):41–49
16. Singh AK, Jiang Y (2004) How does peripheral lipopolysaccharide induce gene expression in the brain of rats? Toxicology 201(1–3):197–207
17. Mikulis DJ, Roberts TP (2007) Neuro MR: protocols. J Magn Reson Imaging 26(4):838–847
18. Redzic Z (2011) Molecular biology of the blood-brain and the blood-cerebrospinal fluid barriers: similarities and differences. Fluids Barriers CNS 8(1):3

Vascular Integrity in the Pathogenesis of Brain Arteriovenous Malformation

Rui Zhang, Wan Zhu, and Hua Su

Introduction

Patients harboring brain arteriovenous malformation (bAVM) are at life-threatening risk of vessel rupture and intracranial hemorrhage (ICH) [1, 2], and the malformed vessels are fragile and prone to rupture, causing bleeding into the brain. ICH is the first clinical symptom in about 50 % of bAVM patients. In a past study, we showed that 30 % of unruptured and non-hemorrhagic bAVMs demonstrated microscopic evidence of hemosiderin deposition in the vascular wall [3]. The presence of silent intralesional microhemorrhage may be a biomarker for the risk of ICH. However, the underlying mechanisms for bAVM rupture and microhemorrhage are not fully understood.

Current treatment options for bAVM are invasive. Approximately 20 % of patients are not offered interventional therapy because of excessive treatment-related risks [4, 5]. Furthermore, treatment of unruptured bAVMs—half of all cases—has become increasingly controversial because the natural history for these patients may be less morbid than invasive therapy [6–10]. So far, there is no specific medical therapy to treat bAVMs.

Previous studies have focused on the association of bAVM angioarchitecture and the risk of hemorrhage. These studies have found that a small number of draining veins, excessive deep-draining veins, vein stenosis, deep locations in the brain, and diffused bAVM morphology are risk factors for bAVM rupture [11–16]. Analysis of mean pressure of feeding arteries, in conjunction with other morphological or clinical risk factors, indicates that high arterial input pressure and venous outflow restriction (exclusively deep venous drainage) are the most powerful risk predictors for hemorrhagic bAVM presentation [17]. Previously, because of the lack of an animal model, the biology behind the abnormal vascular remodeling could not be tested.

We have established several bAVM mouse models through conditional knockout of endoglin (*Eng*) or Activin-like kinase 1 (*Alk1*; *Acvlr1*) genes, causative genes for an autosomal-dominated genetic disorder, Hereditary hemorrhagic telangiectasia (HHT) [18–21]. HHT is characterized by solid organ AVMs (i.e., in the lung, liver, and brain) and mucocutaneous telangiectasias [22]. As much as 5 % of bAVMs may be due to HHT [23]. As a familial form, bAVM in HHT possesses a similar phenotype to sporadic bAVM so that knowledge of these inherited gene pathways can shed light on sporadic disease pathogenesis [24]. Our mouse models resemble some phenotypes of human bAVM that are related to rupture risk, for example, iron deposition from red blood cell (RBC) extravasation [3] and macrophage infiltration [25–27].

In this review, we provide evidence that vascular structure is abnormal in bAVM, which might be formatted through the following pathways (Fig. 1): (1) ALK1, ENG, or matrix Gla protein (MGP) deletion leads to reduced expression of the Notch ligand, delta-like ligand-4 (DLL4), in microvascular endothelial cells; (2) decreased DLL4 results in a reduction of platelet-derived growth factor-B (PDGFB) signaling. As a result, mural cell recruitment is impaired [19, 28].

Impaired Vessel Wall Structure Correlates with Vascular Leakage and Microhemorrhage

Structural imperfection and immaturity of the vascular wall in bAVM suggest that vessels are histoembryogenically maldeveloped. Prominent caliber dilation, hypertrophy of muscular layer, hyalinization, and an abnormal increase of elastic fibers might be the result of vascular remodeling in response to changed cerebral hemodynamics caused by an arteriovenous shunt [29].

R. Zhang, PhD • W. Zhu, PhD • H. Su, MD (✉)
Department of Anesthesia and Perioperative Care, Center for Cerebrovascular Research, University of California, San Francisco, 1001 Potrero Avenue, Box 1363, San Francisco, CA 94110, USA
e-mail: hua.su@ucsf.edu

R.L. Applegate et al. (eds.), *Brain Edema XVI: Translate Basic Science into Clinical Practice*, Acta Neurochirurgica Supplement, Vol. 121,
DOI 10.1007/978-3-319-18497-5_6,

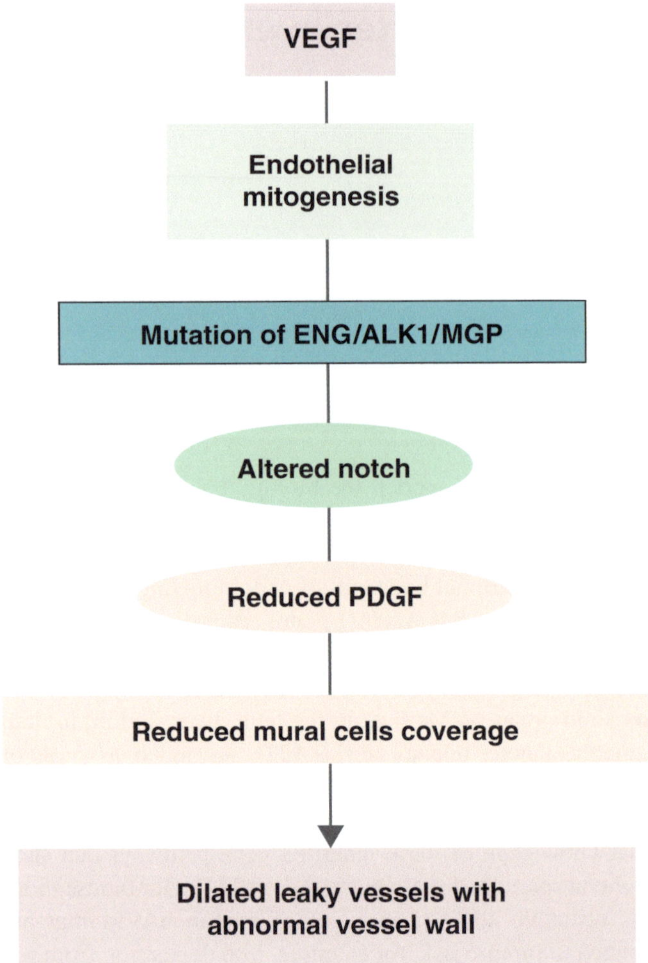

Fig. 1 Speculated pathways involved in AVM pathogenesis. Angiogenic factors, such as VEGF, induce endothelial mitogenesis. When mutation of AVM causative genes occurs, the angiogenic response leads to the formation of leaky vessels with abnormal vessel wall structure through altered Notch signaling and reduced Pdgf-b signaling

Abnormal expression pattern of collagen (Col) I and Col III has been found in bAVMs [30]. Compared with control brain samples, bAVMs have a higher level of Col I and a lower level of Col III. The collagen fibers in bAVM vessels are disorganized and interrupted in the internal elastic lamina. Col I is a stiff fibrillar protein that provides resistance to tension, whereas Col III forms an elastic network [31] that prevents rupture of the vessel wall. Col I/Col III ratio is markedly increased in bAVM, which can increase the stiffness of the bAVM vessels. Interestingly, ruptured AVMs have higher type-I and -III collagen content than unruptured AVMs [32].

In a study analyzing surgical specimens of four adult cases of cerebral pial AVM [33], severe mural fibrosis was found in arteriovenous shunts larger than 700 μm located in the subarachnoid space. The authors found that vessels adjacent to shunting segments were arterialized veins and have segmental loss of the internal elastic membrane (IEM) and/or smooth muscle cells (SMCs). The smaller shunts in the cerebral parenchyma were dilated small arteries, which showed abrupt loss of IEM and gradual loss of SMCs and transformed into dilated and tortuous veins [33]. These findings suggest that AVM rupture is caused not only by dilated veins but also by a segmental loss of IEM and SMCs.

SMCs in AVMs are in various stages of differentiation [34]. The expression of smoothelin is less prevalent in large AVM vessels than in the normal brain, which may reflect the loss of contractile property associated with hemodynamic stress [34]. Hoya et al. [35] analyzed the expression of SMC marker proteins, including smooth muscle alpha-actin and four myosin heavy chain isoforms (SM1, SM2, SMemb, and NMHC-A) in bAVM specimens. Although the arterial components of AVM showed the same staining pattern as mature normal arteries, two different types of abnormal veins were noticed in the AVM specimens: large veins with a thick and fibrous wall (so-called "arterialized" veins) and intraparenchymal thin-walled sinusoidal veins. The former express alpha-actin, SM1, SM2, and SMemb, and the latter, alpha-actin, SM1, and SM2. These markers are normally expressed in cerebral arteries. The results were compatible with arterialization of the cerebral veins caused by arteriovenous shunting [35, 36].

Abnormal vessel wall structure has also been noticed in the bAVM vessels in our mouse models [18, 37]. Compared with normal brain angiogenic foci, the lesion in bAVM mouse models have more vessels with diameters larger than 15 μm that lack α-SMA positive cells and have fewer pericytes. Reduced SMC and pericyte coverage is associated with increased vascular permeability and microhemorrhage.

All of the data cited thus far suggest that vessels in bAVMs have impaired wall structure, which may be the cause of AVM microhemorrhage and rupture. Currently, it is not clear which molecular signaling pathway is involved in the formation of these abnormal vascular structures. Through analysis of the surgically sectioned human bAVM specimens and bAVM in the HHT mouse models, we found Notch and Pdgf-b signaling pathways are involved in abnormal vascular formation and remodeling.

Altered Notch Signaling Causes Abnormal Angiogenesis in bAVM

There is empirical evidence that proteins involved in Notch signaling—including receptors, ligands, and downstream signals—are expressed in excised surgical specimens [38, 39]. Animal experiments support a potential link between Notch signaling and human diseases. In mice, both gain and loss of Notch function cause arteriovenous shunts to form during prenatal development [40]. Endothelial overexpression of a constitutive active Notch-4 intracellular domain (Notch 4*) results in bAVMs in young mice [41, 42], and normalizing Notch 4* expression results in lesion regression [43]. In addition, the expression of Notch ligands, Jagged 1 and 2, are increased in Mgp deficient mice [44]. All these data indicate that Notch signaling is involved in bAVM pathogenesis.

In mammals, there are 4 Notch receptors (Notch-1, -2, -3 and -4) and 5 ligands (Jagged1 and 2, Dll1, 3, and 4). Notch interacts with VEGF signaling during tip-cell and stalk-cell specification [45]. Dll4 is predominantly expressed in tip cells, and Jagged-1 in stalk cells. Dll4-Notch1 signaling suppresses tip cell formation leading to nonproductive sprouting, whereas Jagged-1 antagonizes the Dll4 ligand, thereby promoting sprouting angiogenesis [46]. We and others have found through analysis of human bAVM specimens and animal model development that a pro-angiogenic signal is needed for bAVM development [18, 47–51]. Without Dll4 signaling, a pro-angiogenic state is favored, for example, proliferation of tip at the expense of stalk cells [46, 52]. Blocking Dll4 in tumor models leads to an excessively branched, chaotic vascular network and impaired mural cell recruitment [53, 54].

In addition to its interaction with angiogenesis, Notch signaling is also essential in regulating arterial fate specification [55]. Notch and its downstream signaling are important in directing arterial-venous segregation and stabilizing brain endothelial-pericyte interaction during vasculogenesis in the embryos [55–57]. Absence of Notch results in expression of venous markers in the arteries [58]. We found that endothelial cells in some vessels in the bAVM lesion in a mouse model express both arterial and venous markers [18], suggesting that *Alk1* deletion impairs the endothelial cell specification during angiogenesis. This altered specification may be the cause of irregular SMC coverage of AVM vessels.

The interaction of Alk1 or Eng with Notch signaling is just beginning to be examined [52, 59]. Notch signaling is important in vascular homeostasis and response to injury (angiogenesis) [59–62].

Gain and loss of Notch function may affect venous and arterial cells differently [63]. *ALK1* knockdown in human umbilical artery endothelial cells (HUAEC) causes a reduction in EPHRIN B2, a marker for artery endothelial cells [63]. Deficiency of Mgp, a bone morphogenetic protein (Bmp) inhibitor, causes alternation of Notch ligand-expression, dysregulation of endothelial differentiation, and development of bAVM [44]. Increased Bmp activity due to the lack of Mgp induces the expression of Alk1 in the cerebrovascular endothelium, which enhances the expression of Notch ligands (Jagged 1 and 2) and alters the expression of arterial and venous endothelial markers (Ephrin B2 and Eph B4). Expression of Alk1 does not change when Jagged expression is reduced [44], suggesting that Jagged 1 and 2 act downstream of Alk1.

Together, the data above suggest that Notch signaling is located downstream of bAVM causative genes, such as Alk1 or Mgp. Notch and its downstream signaling participate in bAVM pathogenesis in several ways: (1) enhancement of angiogenesis; (2) impairment of vessel wall structure; and (3) alteration of arterial and venous specification in endothelial cells.

Reduced PDGF-B Signaling Results in Abnormal Mural Cell Coverage in Brain AVM

PDGFs are important mitogens for various types of mesenchymal cells, such as fibroblasts, SMC, and pericytes [64]. They exert critical function during organogenesis in mammalian embryonic and early postnatal development. Increase or loss of function of PDGF is also noticed in diseases such as cancer, tissue fibrosis, and cardiovascular diseases in adults [65]. The PDGF family includes PDGF-A, -B, -C and -D, which are assembled as disulfide-linked homo- or heterodimers. PDGFs have two types of receptors: PDGFR-α and -β [64, 66]. Among PDGFs, PDGF-B has intrinsic pro-angiogenic effects. Microvascular integrity can be compromised when PDGF-B expression is too high [67] or too low [68, 69]. PDGF-B signaling through PDGFR-β regulates pericyte recruitment and differentiation to nascent capillaries. The differentiation of mesenchymal cells into the pericyte/SMC- lineage is dependent on PDGFR-β expression in mice [70].

Knockout *Pdgf-b* or *Pdgfr-β* in mice results in loss of pericytes from the microvessels [68]. The absence of pericytes also leads to endothelial hyperplasia (associated with abnormal endothelial junctions), and excessive endothelial luminal membrane folds [69]. *Pdgfr-β* or *Pdgf-b* null mice have cerebral hemorrhage with an absence of microvascular pericytes in the brain vessels and endothelial hyperplasia [69]. Reduction of vascular pericytes correlates with impairment of vascular integrity [71, 72]. Higher PDGF-B expression has been detected in some, but not all, resected sporadic human bAVM specimens compared with control tissue [73, 74]. Other cells in the brain can also express PDGF-B, which could obscure the analysis of PDGF-B expression [75].

We have demonstrated that expression of Pdgfr-β is reduced in the bAVM lesions of *Alk1*-deficient mice [19], suggesting a possible link between Alk1 and Pdfgr-β/Pdgf-b signaling pathways. However, it is not clear whether the reduced expression of Pdfgr-β is caused by the reduced number of pericytes in the tissue. Many AVM vessels in Alk1-deficient mice do not have the SMC-layer and have less pericyte coverage.

PDGF-B/PDGFR-β has also been implicated in skin and retina AVMs, as well as Eng-associated signaling pathway.

Oral administration of thalidomide reduces the frequency and the duration of nosebleeds and blood transfusion requirements in a small group of HHT patients [28]. Thalidomide treatment does not inhibit endothelial cell proliferation and migration, but increases mural cell coverage of the vasculature through increasing Pdgf-b expression in endothelial cells [28].

The data above indicate that: (1) AVM-causative genes, such as Alk1 and Eng, play an important role in maintaining cerebrovascular integrity; (2) mutations of these genes result in abnormal angiogenic response, which leads to abnormal vessel formation; (3) PDGF-B signaling is one of the downstream signaling pathways involved in brain AVM pathogenesis; (4) upregulation of PDGF-B signaling may reduce the severity of bAVM phenotype, and thus could be developed into a therapeutic strategy to treat bAVM.

Other Signalings

Angiopoietin/TIE2 signaling also plays a role in the recruitment of peri-endothelial support structures. Alternations of angiopoietin/TIE2 expression in human bAVM specimens have been noticed [76], which could be a cause of defective vessel wall in bAVM. For example, angiopoietin-2 (ANG-2), which allows loosening of cell-to-cell contacts, is overexpressed in the perivascular region in AVM vascular channels [76].

A key downstream consequence of VEGF and ANG-2 signaling contributing to the angiogenic phenotype is matrix metalloproteinase (MMP) expression. MMP-9 expression, in particular, appears to be higher in bAVM than in control tissue [27, 77]. Similarly, TIMP-1 and TIMP-3, which are naturally occurring MMP inhibitors, are also increased in bAVM but to a lesser degree.

Exactly how the dysplastic response propagates and leads to bAVM formation is not known. Recruitment of progenitor cell populations may be one source influencing AVM growth and development, an area that needs further exploration. For example, endothelial progenitor cells are present in the nidus of the brain and spinal cord AVMs, and may mediate pathological vascular remodeling and impact the clinical course of AVMs.

More generally, circulating bone marrow-derived cells have a major role in both microcirculatory angiogenesis [78, 79] and conductance vessel remodeling [80, 81]. If bAVM pathogenesis involves these two processes, it is reasonable to infer that bone marrow-derived cells may have an underappreciated role in lesion formation and growth. An unresolved issue with stem cell interaction is the extent to which progenitor cells actually integrate into existing tissue compartments, or whether they provide a nursing function by supplying critical components of the repair response, such as cytokines, growth factors, and enzymes, to the tissue.

In summary, we have reviewed the possible roles of Notch and Pdgf-b signaling in bAVM pathogenesis. In both brain and non-brain endothelial cells, Alk1 is upstream of Notch signaling [59], and Notch signaling is upstream of Pdgf-b, which appears to be an important regulator of cerebrovascular Pdgf-b expression [67]. The relationship between Eng function and Pdgf-β [28] and Notch signaling is not as well understood [52]. However, animal studies show that either correcting Notch signaling [43] or increasing Pdgf-b [28] expression resumes abnormal vascular structure in bAVM. Thus, by modulating these two pathways, new therapies could be developed.

Acknowledgments We thank members of the UCSF BAVM Study Project (http://avm.ucsf.edu) for their support, and Voltaire Gungab for assistance with manuscript preparation. This study was supported by grants to Hua Su from the National Institutes of Health (R01 NS027713, R01 HL122774, and 1R21NS083788) and from the Michael Ryan Zodda Foundation and UCSF Research Evaluation and Allocation Committee (REAC).

References

1. Fleetwood IG, Steinberg GK (2002) Arteriovenous malformations. Lancet 359(9309):863–873
2. Arteriovenous Malformation Study Group (1999) Arteriovenous malformations of the brain in adults. N Engl J Med 340(23):1812–1818
3. Guo Y, Saunders T, Su H, Kim H, Akkoc D, Saloner DA, Hetts SW, Hess C, Lawton MT, Bollen AW, Pourmohamad T, McCulloch CE, Tihan T, Young WL (2012) Silent intralesional microhemorrhage as a risk factor for brain arteriovenous malformation rupture. Stroke 43(5):1240–1246
4. Spetzler RF, Martin NA (1986) A proposed grading system for arteriovenous malformations. J Neurosurg 65(4):476–483
5. Han PP, Ponce FA, Spetzler RF (2003) Intention-to-treat analysis of Spetzler-Martin grades IV and V arteriovenous malformations: natural history and treatment paradigm. J Neurosurg 98(1):3–7
6. Stapf C, Mohr JP, Choi JH, Hartmann A, Mast H (2006) Invasive treatment of unruptured brain arteriovenous malformations is experimental therapy. Curr Opin Neurol 19(1):63–68
7. Cockroft KM, Jayaraman MV, Amin-Hanjani S, Derdeyn CP, McDougall CG, Wilson JA (2012) A perfect storm: how a randomized trial of unruptured brain arteriovenous malformations' (ARUBA's) trial design challenges notions of external validity. Stroke 43(7):1979–1981
8. Mohr JP, Moskowitz AJ, Stapf C, Hartmann A, Lord K, Marshall SM, Mast H, Moquete E, Moy CS, Parides M, Pile-Spellman J, Al-Shahi Salman R, Weinberg A, Young WL, Estevez A, Kureshi I, Brisman JL (2010) The ARUBA trial: current status, future hopes. Stroke 41(8):e537–e540
9. Mohr JP, Moskowitz AJ, Parides M, Stapf C, Young WL (2012) Hull down on the horizon: a randomized trial of unruptured brain arteriovenous malformations (ARUBA) trial. Stroke 43(7):1744–1745
10. Mohr JP, Parides MK, Stapf C, Moquete E, Moy CS, Overbey JR, Salman RA, Vicaut E, Young WL, Houdart E, Cordonnier C, Stefani MA, Hartmann A, von Kummer R, Biondi A, Berkefeld J,

Klijn CJ, Harkness K, Libman R, Barreau X, Moskowitz AJ (2014) Medical management with or without interventional therapy for unruptured brain arteriovenous malformations (ARUBA): a multicentre, non-blinded, randomised trial. Lancet 383(9917):614–621
11. Mansmann U, Meisel J, Brock M, Rodesch G, Alvarez H, Lasjaunias P (2000) Factors associated with intracranial hemorrhage in cases of cerebral arteriovenous malformation. Neurosurgery 46(2):272–279
12. Stefani MA, Porter PJ, terBrugge KG, Montanera W, Willinsky RA, Wallace MC (2002) Angioarchitectural factors present in brain arteriovenous malformations associated with hemorrhagic presentation. Stroke 33(4):920–924
13. Stefani MA, Porter PJ, terBrugge KG, Montanera W, Willinsky RA, Wallace MC (2002) Large and deep brain arteriovenous malformations are associated with risk of future hemorrhage. Stroke 33(5):1220–1224
14. Pollock BE, Flickinger JC, Lunsford LD, Bissonette DJ, Kondziolka D (1996) Factors that predict the bleeding risk of cerebral arteriovenous malformations. Stroke 27(1):1–6
15. Hademenos GJ, Massoud TF (1996) Risk of intracranial arteriovenous malformation rupture due to venous drainage impairment. A theoretical analysis. Stroke 27(6):1072–1083
16. Stapf C, Mast H, Sciacca RR, Choi JH, Khaw AV, Connolly ES, Pile-Spellman J, Mohr JP (2006) Predictors of hemorrhage in patients with untreated brain arteriovenous malformation. Neurology 66(9):1350–1355
17. Duong DH, Young WL, Vang MC, Sciacca RR, Mast H, Koennecke HC, Hartmann A, Joshi S, Mohr JP, Pile-Spellman J (1998) Feeding artery pressure and venous drainage pattern are primary determinants of hemorrhage from cerebral arteriovenous malformations. Stroke 29(6):1167–1176
18. Walker EJ, Su H, Shen F, Choi EJ, Oh SP, Chen G, Lawton MT, Kim H, Chen Y, Chen W, Young WL (2011) Arteriovenous malformation in the adult mouse brain resembling the human disease. Ann Neurol 69(6):954–962
19. Chen W, Guo Y, Walker EJ, Shen F, Jun K, Oh SP, Degos V, Lawton MT, Tihan T, Davalos D, Akassoglou K, Nelson J, Pile-Spellman J, Su H, Young WL (2013) Reduced mural cell coverage and impaired vessel integrity after angiogenic stimulation in the *Alk1*-deficient brain. Arterioscler Thromb Vasc Biol 33(2):305–310
20. Chen W, Sun Z, Han Z, Jun K, Camus M, Wankhede M, Mao L, Arnold T, Young WL, Su H (2014) De novo cerebrovascular malformation in the adult mouse after endothelial Alk1 deletion and angiogenic stimulation. Stroke 45(3):900–902
21. Choi EJ, Chen W, Jun K, Arthur HM, Young WL, Su H (2014) Novel brain arteriovenous malformation mouse models for type 1 hereditary hemorrhagic telangiectasia. PLoS One 9(2), e88511
22. Braverman IM, Keh A, Jacobson BS (1990) Ultrastructure and three-dimensional organization of the telangiectases of hereditary hemorrhagic telangiectasia. J Invest Dermatol 95(4):422–427
23. Bharatha A, Faughnan ME, Kim H, Pourmohamad T, Krings T, Bayrak-Toydemir P, Pawlikowska L, McCulloch CE, Lawton MT, Dowd CF, Young WL, Terbrugge KG (2012) Brain arteriovenous malformation multiplicity predicts the diagnosis of hereditary hemorrhagic telangiectasia: quantitative assessment. Stroke 43(1):72–78
24. Shovlin CL (2010) Hereditary haemorrhagic telangiectasia: pathophysiology, diagnosis and treatment. Blood Rev 24(6):203–219
25. Chen Y, Zhu W, Bollen AW, Lawton MT, Barbaro NM, Dowd CF, Hashimoto T, Yang GY, Young WL (2008) Evidence of inflammatory cell involvement in brain arteriovenous malformations. Neurosurgery 62(6):1340–1349
26. Chen Y, Pawlikowska L, Yao JS, Shen F, Zhai W, Achrol AS, Lawton MT, Kwok PY, Yang GY, Young WL (2006) Interleukin-6 involvement in brain arteriovenous malformations. Ann Neurol 59(1):72–80
27. Chen Y, Fan Y, Poon KY, Achrol AS, Lawton MT, Zhu Y, McCulloch CE, Hashimoto T, Lee C, Barbaro NM, Bollen AW, Yang GY, Young WL (2006) MMP-9 expression is associated with leukocytic but not endothelial markers in brain arteriovenous malformations. Front Biosci 11:3121–3128
28. Lebrin F, Srun S, Raymond K, Martin S, van den Brink S, Freitas C, Breant C, Mathivet T, Larrivee B, Thomas JL, Arthur HM, Westermann CJ, Disch F, Mager JJ, Snijder RJ, Eichmann A, Mummery CL (2010) Thalidomide stimulates vessel maturation and reduces epistaxis in individuals with hereditary hemorrhagic telangiectasia. Nat Med 16(4):420–428
29. Isoda K, Fukuda H, Takamura N, Hamamoto Y (1981) Arteriovenous malformation of the brain – histological study and micrometric measurement of abnormal vessels. Acta Pathol Jpn 31(5):883–893
30. Guo Y, Qumu SW, Nacar OA, Yang JY, Du J, Belen D, Pan L, Zhao YL (2013) Human brain arteriovenous malformations are associated with interruptions in elastic fibers and changes in collagen content. Turk Neurosurg 23(1):10–15
31. Lee RM (1995) Morphology of cerebral arteries. Pharmacol Ther 66(1):149–173
32. Niu H, Cao Y, Wang X, Xue X, Yu L, Yang M, Wang R (2012) Relationships between hemorrhage, angioarchitectural factors and collagen of arteriovenous malformations. Neurosci Bull 28(5):595–605
33. Meng JS, Okeda R (2001) Histopathological structure of the pial arteriovenous malformation in adults: observation by reconstruction of serial sections of four surgical specimens. Acta Neuropathol 102(1):63–68
34. Uranishi R, Baev NI, Kim JH, Awad IA (2001) Vascular smooth muscle cell differentiation in human cerebral vascular malformations. Neurosurgery 49(3):671–679
35. Hoya K, Asai A, Sasaki T, Nagata K, Kimura K, Kirino T (2003) Expression of myosin heavy chain isoforms by smooth muscle cells in cerebral arteriovenous malformations. Acta Neuropathol 105(5):455–461
36. Hoya K, Asai A, Sasaki T, Kimura K, Kirino T (2001) Expression of smooth muscle proteins in cavernous and arteriovenous malformations. Acta Neuropathol 102(3):257–263
37. Chen W, Guo Y, Walker EJ, Shen F, Jun K, Oh SP, Degos V, Lawton MT, Tihan T, Davalos D, Akassoglou K, Nelson J, Pile-Spellman J, Su H, Young WL (2013). Reduced mural cell coverage and impaired vessel integrity after angiogenic stimulation in the *Alk1*-deficient brain. Arterioscler Thromb Vasc Biol 33(2):305–310
38. ZhuGe Q, Zhong M, Zheng W, Yang GY, Mao X, Xie L, Chen G, Chen Y, Lawton MT, Young WL, Greenberg DA, Jin K (2009) Notch1 signaling is activated in brain arteriovenous malformation in humans. Brain 132(Pt 12):3231–3241
39. Murphy PA, Lu G, Shiah S, Bollen AW, Wang RA (2009) Endothelial Notch signaling is upregulated in human brain arteriovenous malformations and a mouse model of the disease. Lab Invest 89(9):971–982
40. Gridley T (2010) Notch signaling in the vasculature. Curr Top Dev Biol 92:277–309
41. Murphy PA, Lam MT, Wu X, Kim TN, Vartanian SM, Bollen AW, Carlson TR, Wang RA (2008) Endothelial Notch4 signaling induces hallmarks of brain arteriovenous malformations in mice. Proc Natl Acad Sci U S A 105(31):10901–10906
42. Murphy PA, Kim TN, Huang L, Nielsen CM, Lawton MT, Adams RH, Schaffer CB, Wang RA (2014) Constitutively active Notch4 receptor elicits brain arteriovenous malformations through enlargement of capillary-like vessels. Proc Natl Acad Sci U S A 111(50):18007–18012
43. Murphy PA, Kim TN, Lu G, Bollen AW, Schaffer CB, Wang RA (2012) Notch4 normalization reduced blood vessel size in arteriovenous malformations. Sci Transl Med 4(117):117ra118

44. Yao Y, Yao J, Radparvar M, Blazquez-Medela AM, Guihard PJ, Jumabay M, Bostrom KI (2013) Reducing Jagged 1 and 2 levels prevents cerebral arteriovenous malformations in matrix Gla protein deficiency. Proc Natl Acad Sci U S A 110(47):19071–19076
45. Phng LK, Potente M, Leslie JD, Babbage J, Nyqvist D, Lobov I, Ondr JK, Rao S, Lang RA, Thurston G, Gerhardt H (2009) Nrarp coordinates endothelial Notch and Wnt signaling to control vessel density in angiogenesis. Dev Cell 16(1):70–82
46. Benedito R, Roca C, Sorensen I, Adams S, Gossler A, Fruttiger M, Adams RH (2009) The notch ligands Dll4 and Jagged1 have opposing effects on angiogenesis. Cell 137(6):1124–1135
47. Kim H, Su H, Weinsheimer S, Pawlikowska L, Young WL (2011) Brain arteriovenous malformation pathogenesis: a response-to-injury paradigm. Acta Neurochir Suppl 111:83–92
48. Xu B, Wu YQ, Huey M, Arthur HM, Marchuk DA, Hashimoto T, Young WL, Yang GY (2004) Vascular endothelial growth factor induces abnormal microvasculature in the endoglin heterozygous mouse brain. J Cereb Blood Flow Metab 24(2):237–244
49. Hao Q, Su H, Marchuk DA, Rola R, Wang Y, Liu W, Young WL, Yang GY (2008) Increased tissue perfusion promotes capillary dysplasia in the ALK1-deficient mouse brain following VEGF stimulation. Am J Physiol Heart Circ Physiol 295(6):H2250–H2256
50. Hao Q, Zhu Y, Su H, Shen F, Yang GY, Kim H, Young WL (2010) VEGF induces more severe cerebrovascular dysplasia in Endoglin$^{+/-}$ than in Alk1$^{+/-}$ mice. Transl Stroke Res 1(3):197–201
51. Walker EJ, Su H, Shen F, Degos V, Amend G, Jun K, Young WL (2012) Bevacizumab attenuates VEGF-induced angiogenesis and vascular malformations in the adult mouse brain. Stroke 43(7):1925–1930
52. Benedito R, Trindade A, Hirashima M, Henrique D, da Costa LL, Rossant J, Gill PS, Duarte A (2008) Loss of Notch signalling induced by Dll4 causes arterial calibre reduction by increasing endothelial cell response to angiogenic stimuli. BMC Dev Biol 8:117
53. Djokovic D, Trindade A, Gigante J, Badenes M, Silva L, Liu R, Li X, Gong M, Krasnoperov V, Gill PS, Duarte A (2010) Combination of Dll4/Notch and Ephrin-B2/EphB4 targeted therapy is highly effective in disrupting tumor angiogenesis. BMC Cancer 10(1):641
54. Trindade A, Djokovic D, Gigante J, Badenes M, Pedrosa AR, Fernandes AC, Lopes-da-Costa L, Krasnoperov V, Liu R, Gill PS, Duarte A (2012) Low-dosage inhibition of Dll4 signaling promotes wound healing by inducing functional neo-angiogenesis. PLoS One 7(1), e29863
55. Gridley T (2007) Notch signaling in vascular development and physiology. Development 134(15):2709–2718
56. Herbert SP, Huisken J, Kim TN, Feldman ME, Houseman BT, Wang RA, Shokat KM, Stainier DY (2009) Arterial-venous segregation by selective cell sprouting: an alternative mode of blood vessel formation. Science 326(5950):294–298
57. Li F, Lan Y, Wang Y, Wang J, Yang G, Meng F, Han H, Meng A, Wang Y, Yang X (2011) Endothelial Smad4 maintains cerebrovascular integrity by activating N-cadherin through cooperation with Notch. Dev Cell 20(3):291–302
58. Hofmann JJ, Iruela-Arispe ML (2007) Notch signaling in blood vessels: who is talking to whom about what? Circ Res 100(11):1556–1568
59. Larrivee B, Prahst C, Gordon E, Del Toro R, Mathivet T, Duarte A, Simons M, Eichmann A (2012) ALK1 signaling inhibits angiogenesis by cooperating with the Notch pathway. Dev Cell 22(3):489–500
60. Outtz HH, Tattersall IW, Kofler NM, Steinbach N, Kitajewski J (2011) Notch1 controls macrophage recruitment and Notch signaling is activated at sites of endothelial cell anastomosis during retinal angiogenesis in mice. Blood 118(12):3436–3439
61. Outtz HH, Wu JK, Wang X, Kitajewski J (2010) Notch1 deficiency results in decreased inflammation during wound healing and regulates vascular endothelial growth factor receptor-1 and inflammatory cytokine expression in macrophages. J Immunol 185(7):4363–4373
62. Moya IM, Umans L, Maas E, Pereira PN, Beets K, Francis A, Sents W, Robertson EJ, Mummery CL, Huylebroeck D, Zwijsen A (2012) Stalk cell phenotype depends on integration of notch and smad1/5 signaling cascades. Dev Cell 22(3):501–514
63. Kim JH, Peacock MR, George SC, Hughes CC (2012) BMP9 induces EphrinB2 expression in endothelial cells through an Alk1-BMPRII/ActRII-ID1/ID3-dependent pathway: implications for hereditary hemorrhagic telangiectasia type II. Angiogenesis 15(3):497–509
64. Heldin CH, Westermark B (1999) Mechanism of action and in vivo role of platelet-derived growth factor. Physiol Rev 79(4):1283–1316
65. Betsholtz C, Keller A (2014) PDGF, pericytes and the pathogenesis of idiopathic basal ganglia calcification (IBGC). Brain Pathol 24(4):387–395
66. Shim AH, Liu H, Focia PJ, Chen X, Lin PC, He X (2010) Structures of a platelet-derived growth factor/propeptide complex and a platelet-derived growth factor/receptor complex. Proc Natl Acad Sci U S A 107(25):11307–11312
67. Yao H, Duan M, Hu G, Buch S (2011) Platelet-derived growth factor B chain is a novel target gene of cocaine-mediated Notch1 signaling: implications for HIV-associated neurological disorders. J Neurosci Meth 31(35):12449–12454
68. Lindahl P, Johansson BR, Leveen P, Betsholtz C (1997) Pericyte loss and microaneurysm formation in PDGF-B-deficient mice. Science 277(5323):242–245
69. Hellstrom M, Gerhardt H, Kalen M, Li X, Eriksson U, Wolburg H, Betsholtz C (2001) Lack of pericytes leads to endothelial hyperplasia and abnormal vascular morphogenesis. J Cell Biol 153(3):543–553
70. Crosby JR, Seifert RA, Soriano P, Bowen-Pope DF (1998) Chimaeric analysis reveals role of Pdgf receptors in all muscle lineages. Nat Genet 18(4):385–388
71. Bell RD, Winkler EA, Sagare AP, Singh I, LaRue B, Deane R, Zlokovic BV (2010) Pericytes control key neurovascular functions and neuronal phenotype in the adult brain and during brain aging. Neuron 68(3):409–427
72. Armulik A, Genove G, Mae M, Nisancioglu MH, Wallgard E, Niaudet C, He L, Norlin J, Lindblom P, Strittmatter K, Johansson BR, Betsholtz C (2010) Pericytes regulate the blood–brain barrier. Nature 468(7323):557–561
73. Hashimoto T, Wu Y, Lawton MT, Yang GY, Barbaro NM, Young WL (2005) Co-expression of angiogenic factors in brain arteriovenous malformations. Neurosurgery 56(5):1058–1065
74. Yildirim O, Bicer A, Ozkan A, Kurtkaya O, Cirakoglu B, Kilic T (2010) Expression of platelet-derived growth factor ligand and receptor in cerebral arteriovenous and cavernous malformations. J Clin Neurosci 17(12):1557–1562
75. Sasahara M, Sato H, Iihara K, Wang J, Chue CH, Takayama S, Hayase Y, Hazama F (1995) Expression of platelet-derived growth factor B-chain in the mature rat brain and pituitary gland. Brain Res Mol Brain Res 32(1):63–74
76. Hashimoto T, Lam T, Boudreau NJ, Bollen AW, Lawton MT, Young WL (2001) Abnormal balance in the angiopoietin-tie2 system in human brain arteriovenous malformations. Circ Res 89(2):111–113
77. Hashimoto T, Wen G, Lawton MT, Boudreau NJ, Bollen AW, Yang GY, Barbaro NM, Higashida RT, Dowd CF, Halbach VV, Young WL (2003) Abnormal expression of matrix metalloproteinases and tissue inhibitors of metalloproteinases in brain arteriovenous malformations. Stroke 34(4):925–931
78. Hao Q, Liu J, Pappu R, Su H, Rola R, Gabriel RA, Lee CZ, Young WL, Yang GY (2008) Contribution of bone marrow-derived cells associated with brain angiogenesis is primarily through leucocytes

and macrophages. Arterioscler Thromb Vasc Biol 28(12):2151–2157

79. Hao Q, Chen Y, Zhu Y, Fan Y, Palmer D, Su H, Young WL, Yang GY (2007) Neutrophil depletion decreases VEGF-induced focal angiogenesis in the mature mouse brain. J Cereb Blood Flow Metab 27(11):1853–1860
80. Ota R, Kurihara C, Tsou TL, Young WL, Yeghiazarians Y, Chang M, Mobashery S, Sakamoto A, Hashimoto T (2009) Roles of matrix metalloproteinases in flow-induced outward vascular remodeling. J Cereb Blood Flow Metab 29(9):1547–1558
81. Nuki Y, Matsumoto MM, Tsang E, Young WL, van Rooijen N, Kurihara C, Hashimoto T (2009) Roles of macrophages in flow-induced outward vascular remodeling. J Cereb Blood Flow Metab 29(3):495–503

Preconditioning Section

Role of Circulating Immune Cells in Stroke and Preconditioning-Induced Protection

Raffaella Gesuete, Susan L. Stevens, and Mary P. Stenzel-Poore

The Good and the Bad of Immune Cell Activation in Stroke

Brain injury caused by ischemic stroke is characterized by complex spatial and temporal events evolving over several days in which inflammation plays a key role. The inflammatory response is a complex regulatory process that begins early and lasts for days and even weeks after ischemia, involving many different cell types, inflammatory mediators, and extracellular receptors. The sudden loss of oxygen and glucose causes cells in the ischemic area to be rapidly killed by lipolysis and proteolysis resulting from total bioenergetic failure. As cells die, they release intracellular components that activate neighboring cells to produce pro-inflammatory mediators such as cytokines and chemokines, and promote transmigration of inflammatory cells from the periphery to the ischemic brain area, resulting in exacerbation of damage [1]. The critical role of inflammatory cells in stroke-induced brain injury has been demonstrated by the attenuation of ischemic damage in mice that are unable to mount an inflammatory response [2, 3]. However, certain aspects of the inflammatory response are critical to remove dead cells and promote regeneration after ischemic injury [4]. Thus, the inflammatory cascade can be beneficial or damaging, depending on the stage of tissue injury, the magnitude of the response, and whether the inflammatory response also activates neuroprotective pathways [4].

Recent studies indicate that brain injury activates populations of inflammatory-related cells that can limit ischemic damage. For example, subpopulations of regulatory lymphocytes are induced after stroke that *suppress* inflammation, thus promoting protection against injury [5, 6]. In addition, peripheral inflammatory cells have been implicated in the induction of protection associated with preconditioning [7]. Preconditioning is a phenomenon whereby exposure to a small but potentially harmful stimulus is able to induce protection against a subsequent ischemic event. These studies point to a role for inflammatory cells prior to an ischemic event in mediating the evolution of injury.

This review discusses the role of circulating immune cell activation in the pathology of stroke injury and neuroprotection, and reports data from our laboratory supporting the role of circulating cells in mediating preconditioning.

Peripheral Immune Cells Contribute to Ischemic Injury Following Stroke

Following ischemia, neutrophils, macrophages, and lymphocytes have been shown to infiltrate the brain [8]. Neutrophils are the most abundant cell population present at the site of injury, with a peak influx between 1 and 3 days after ischemia [8, 9]. They have been widely considered key contributors to inflammatory brain injury because they are a main source of free oxygen radicals that can directly cause neuronal death. In addition neutrophils cause endothelial cell dysfunction and blood-brain barrier disruption through release of matrix metalloproteinase 9 [10]. Multiple studies using both neutrophil-depleted animals and antagonists or blocking antibodies support neutrophils as key players in inflammatory-induced ischemic injury [11–16]. However, other studies report no effect on infarct size when neutrophils are depleted or blocked [2, 17]. Some of these differences may be attributed to the particular experimental model system employed, with those models involving reperfusion more likely to demonstrate a role for neutrophils in the exacerbation of injury. Clinical trials reflect these differences

R. Gesuete • S.L. Stevens
Department of Molecular Microbiology and Immunology, Oregon Health and Science University, Portland, OR, USA

M.P. Stenzel-Poore (✉)
Department of Molecular Microbiology and Immunology, L220, Oregon Health and Science University,
3181 Sam Jackson Park Road, Portland, OR 97239, USA
e-mail: poorem@ohsu.edu

DOI 10.1007/978-3-319-18497-5_7,

with slight improvement seen with an antagonist for CD11b, an integrin highly expressed on neutrophils, used in combination with tissue plasminogen activator, an inducer of reperfusion [18]. However, other clinical trials have shown no effect on stroke outcome when neutrophil infiltration is blocked [19, 20]. These results suggest that neutrophils may not be the only contributors to ischemic injury, but instead a complex interaction of multiple cell populations may mediate inflammatory damage.

Resident microglia and infiltrating macrophages also represent a significant immune population identified in ischemic tissue following stroke. These cells appear as early as 12 h after ischemia and peak between 3 and 7 days [8, 9]. Macrophages and microglia produce reactive oxygen species (ROS), nitric oxide, and other cytokines that can have direct toxic effects on brain tissue following stroke. In addition, macrophages and microglia amplify the inflammatory response through recruitment of other immune cells such as lymphocytes. Involvement of macrophages and microglia in the development of infarct damage after stroke was demonstrated by Tang et al. [21]. In this study, attenuation of proliferation and infiltration of microglia and macrophages was obtained by knocking down the chemokine receptor 1 (CX3CR1), which is highly expressed on resident brain microglia and peripheral macrophages. Knockout animals demonstrated a significant decrease in the ischemic lesion, number of apoptotic cells, and post-ischemic brain inflammatory responses (including ROS and pro-inflammatory cytokine production), indicating that suppression of macrophage and microglia activation reduces ischemia-induced inflammation and neurotoxicity.

The importance of lymphocytes (B and T cells) to the inflammatory response following ischemia has become increasingly evident. Although lymphocyte infiltration in the brain after ischemia peaks around day 3 [8, 9], several studies have found both B and T lymphocytes in the brain as early as 4–6 h after ischemia, suggesting a role in the development of inflammation in the ischemic area [2, 9]. Severe combined immunodeficient (SCID) mice lacking both T and B cells showed significant reduction of ischemic volume and suppression of post-ischemic induction of inflammatory mediators in the brain, demonstrating the important role of T and B cells in development of the ischemic damage [3].

Protective Role of Peripheral Immune Cells Responding to Stroke

In addition to the damaging effects of peripheral immune cells, studies have shown that inflammatory cells also play a role in protecting the brain from ischemic injury. Downes et al. [22] showed that hematopoietic cells have a critical role in mitigating the extent of injury following stroke. In particular, they showed that hematopoietic cells exhibit a neuroprotective function after stroke that is mediated by myeloid differentiation factor-88 (MyD88), the adaptor protein for Toll-like receptors (TLRs), and IL-1 signaling cascades. They demonstrated that mice lacking MyD88 signaling on hematopoietic cells had exacerbated ischemic volume, indicating that particular peripheral cell populations can promote protection against brain injury.

Microglia and macrophages have also been implicated in neuroprotection after stroke. These cells phagocytize debris and dead cells, and microglia can produce neurotrophic factors that can promote neuronal growth and survival, both mechanisms that are important in resolution of inflammation and tissue regeneration after injury. Selective ablation of proliferating microglia has been shown to exacerbate ischemic injury [23], indicating an important role of microglia in modulating protection against ischemia. In addition, exogenous microglial cells administered peripherally 24 h before or after global ischemia have been shown to reach the ischemic area and protect against neuronal injury by releasing neurotrophic factors [24].

B cells may represent another hematopoietic population with potential to confer protection against ischemic injury. Two conflicting reports using B cell-deficient mice have defined a neutral or protective role for B cells in ischemic injury. Yilmaz et al. [2] reported no difference in infarct size in mice deficient in B cells, whereas Ren et al. [25] found exacerbation of injury in B cell-deficient mice, supporting a protective role for B cells. Ren et al. were also able to reduce the infarct size in their model by adoptively transferring B cells into the deficient mice, further supporting a protective role for B cells in ischemic injury. Further work in this model has defined IL10 secreting B cells (B regulatory cells; Bregs) as the subset of B cells mediating protection [6, 26].

Regulatory lymphocytes represent a small percentage of infiltrating B and T lymphocytes—referred to as Bregs and Tregs, respectively. They are characterized by their ability to control immune responses, regulate the function of effector T cells, and regulate the activity of antigen-presenting cells. The anti-inflammatory cytokine, IL10, is the primary effector of regulatory lymphocytes. A growing amount of evidence points to the importance of these regulatory cells in modulating the inflammatory response after stroke, leading to suppressed inflammation and added protection against ischemic injury. Similar to the protective role of Bregs, Liesz et al. [5] found that depletion of Tregs significantly increased brain infarct volume and worsened functional outcome, indicating a protective effect of Tregs. Protection was mediated through Treg induction of IL10 and the subsequent suppression of inflammatory cytokines and modulation of the invasion and activation of lymphocytes and microglia in the ischemic brain [5].

It is not clear whether regulatory cells need to infiltrate the brain to induce the protective phenotype. Tregs, for example, have been detected in the brain 3 days after stroke, while their effect on modulating cytokine levels in the brain is already evident 6 h after ischemia [5]. Therefore, it is more likely that Tregs are able to monitor and regulate the inflammatory response from the periphery. Understanding the mechanisms by which peripheral cells communicate with the central nervous system in the context of injury as well as how they may mediate protection may be critical to the development of new therapeutic strategies against stroke.

Involvement of Peripheral Immune Cells in Preconditioning Induced Neuroprotection

Peripheral immune cells have been implicated as contributors to the induction of neuroprotection associated with preconditioning. Preconditioning involves mild treatment with an otherwise harmful stimulus to reprogram the cellular response to injury, thereby leading to a reduction of damage. A particularly effective means of inducing systemic preconditioning against cerebral ischemia occurs through activation of the innate immune response with ligands for TLR. We have shown that prior systemic administration using one of several TLR agonists (e.g., lipopolysaccharide, CpG oligonucleotides) induces robust neuroprotection against subsequent cerebral ischemia in a mouse stroke model [27–30]. We have also shown significant protection with the TLR9 agonist, CpG, in a nonhuman primate model of cerebral ischemia [31]. TLR9 is expressed on multiple cells both in the periphery (i.e., leukocytes) and in the brain (i.e., neurons, astrocytes, microglia, endothelium). We have published that effective preconditioning and neuroprotection with CpG stimulation requires TLR9 expression on at least two distinct cell populations, one of hematopoietic origin and one of nonhematopoietic origin [32]. We generated bone marrow chimeric mice by irradiating WT mice and repopulating their leukocytes with cells from TLR9-deficient mice. Thus, these animals lacked TLR9 expression on leukocytes, while still expressing TLR9 on parenchymal cells such as endothelial cells, astrocytes, microglia, and neurons. We found that mice lacking TLR9 expression on leukocytes were not protected by CpG preconditioning, demonstrating that TLR9-mediated leukocyte responses are required to confer CpG-induced neuroprotection. In addition, irradiated TLR9KO mice repopulated with leukocytes from WT mice also were not protected by CpG preconditioning, demonstrating that TLR9 expression on leukocytes was not sufficient for CpG-induced neuroprotection. These data indicate a strict requirement for TLR9-mediated responses on both leukocytes and parenchymal cells for protection induced by systemic CpG preconditioning and suggest a need for cross-talk between these compartments to achieve neuroprotection [32].

Systemic administration of CpG allows direct contact with brain microvascular endothelial cells belonging to the blood-brain barrier (BBB). The BBB is the interface between the blood and the brain and strictly regulates the passage of molecules and cells between the periphery and the CNS compartment [33]. Stroke dramatically impairs BBB integrity, leading to increased permeability and expression of endothelial adhesion molecules, resulting in increased leukocyte adhesion and transmigration [1]. We have found, using an *in vitro* BBB model consisting of a co-culture of primary brain microvascular endothelial cells (BMECs) and mixed glial cells (Fig. 1a), that CpG preconditioning can signal and protect the endothelium from ischemic injury. Cell cultures were preconditioned with CpG 24 h before modeled ischemia consisting of 5 h of oxygen-glucose deprivation (OGD). CpG significantly attenuated both the drop in trans-endothelial-electrical resistance (TEER) (Fig. 1b) and the increase of BBB permeability to Na-fluorescein induced by OGD (Fig.1c). These results indicate that CpG preconditioning stabilizes the BBB, possibly by affecting endothelial interactions with circulating immune cells that could alter the inflammatory response to ischemia. In support of this, we have found, using *in vivo* 2-photon microscopy, that CpG preconditioning induces leukocyte rolling and adhesion to brain microvascular endothelium before an ischemic event that may contribute to neuroprotection (Fig. 2).

It remains to be elucidated which leukocyte populations are required for CpG induction of neuroprotection. Bregs offer potential as they are known to be immunosuppressive, and CpG has been reported to drive the differentiation of B cells into Bregs [34]. In line with a protective role for Bregs prior to stroke, Bodhankar et al. [26] showed that adoptive transfer of Bregs 24 h before cerebral ischemia reduces infarct size. Mice receiving IL-10-secreting B cells showed an increase of regulatory cell populations in the periphery and reduced infiltration of T cells and proinflammatory cytokines levels in the ischemic hemisphere. These results show that the increased presence of Bregs before stroke can modulate the inflammatory response, potentially contributing to protection against subsequent ischemia. In further support, Monson et al. [7] found that repetitive hypoxic preconditioning (RHP) induces an immunosuppressive phenotype in resident B cells before stroke and results in decreased infiltration of leukocytes in the brain following stroke. It appeared that RHP reprograms B cells to downregulate genes involved in T cell differentiation and B-T cell interactions [7].

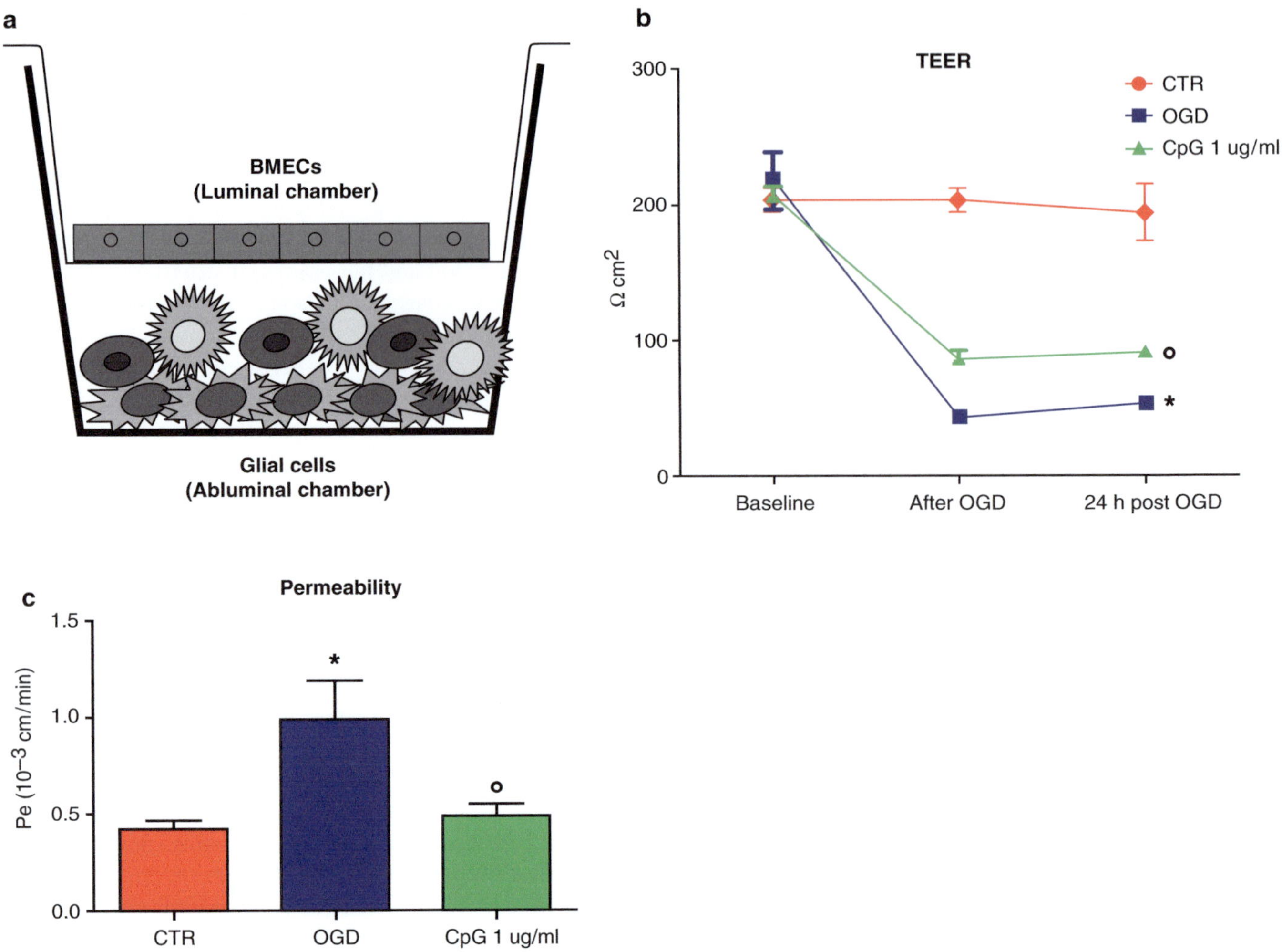

Fig. 1 CpG protects the BBB in an *in vitro* model of ischemic injury. (**a**) Schematic diagram of *in vitro* BBB model consisting of brain microvascular endothelial cells (BMECs) co-cultured with glial cells. Pretreatment with CpG attenuates OGD-induced decrease of trans-endothelial-electrical resistance (TEER) (**b**) and increase of permeability for Na Fluorescein (**c**) in an *in vitro* BBB model of ischemic injury. Values are group means ± SEM; *$p<0.001$ versus control (CTR) and °$p<0.01$ versus OGD

Conclusions

These studies clearly demonstrate the complex nature of the inflammatory response associated with stroke. The interplay between damaging and protective effects is a delicate balancing act that determines the extent of injury. Understanding this interplay and developing ways to modulate the immune cell effectors could greatly advance therapeutic treatment of ischemic brain injury, including stroke. Recent data suggest that endogenous mechanisms engaged by preconditioning include modulation of immune cells, highlighting the effectiveness of targeting these responses in mitigating cerebral ischemic injury.

Conflict of Interest Statement The authors declare no conflict of interest.

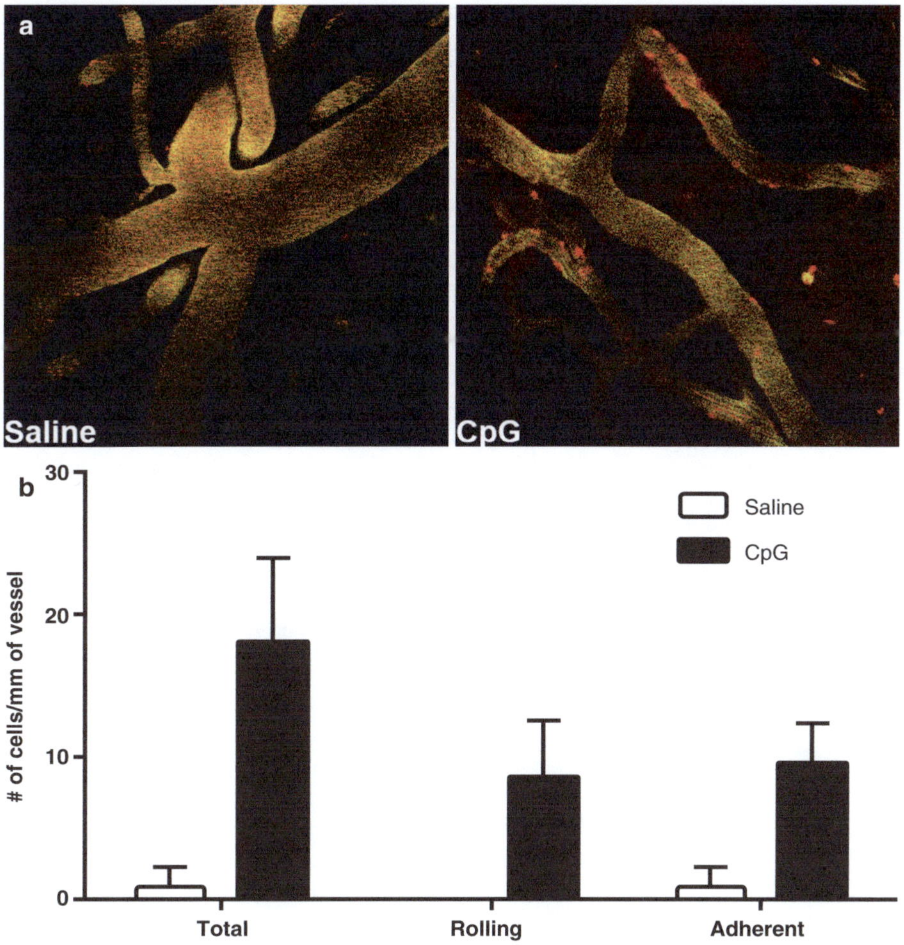

Fig. 2 CpG-induces leukocyte-endothelial interactions. (**a**) Representative images of cortical vessels in mice acquired by *in vivo* two-photon microscopy 24 h after treatment with saline or CpG (0.8 mg/kg). Leukocytes stained in red. (**b**) Quantification of leukocytes per mm of vessel from five separate video clips +/– SEM of an individual mouse for each treatment

References

1. Huang J, Upadhyay UM, Tamargo RJ (2006) Inflammation in stroke and focal cerebral ischemia. Surg Neurol 66(3):232–245
2. Yilmaz G et al (2006) Role of T lymphocytes and interferon-gamma in ischemic stroke. Circulation 113(17):2105–2112
3. Hurn PD et al (2007) T- and B-cell-deficient mice with experimental stroke have reduced lesion size and inflammation. J Cereb Blood Flow Metab 27(11):1798–1805
4. Iadecola C, Anrather J (2011) The immunology of stroke: from mechanisms to translation. Nat Med 17(7):796–808
5. Liesz A et al (2009) Regulatory T cells are key cerebroprotective immunomodulators in acute experimental stroke. Nat Med 15(2):192–199
6. Bodhankar S et al (2013) IL-10-producing B-cells limit CNS inflammation and infarct volume in experimental stroke. Metab Brain Dis 28(3):375–386
7. Monson NL et al (2014) Repetitive hypoxic preconditioning induces an immunosuppressed B cell phenotype during endogenous protection from stroke. J Neuroinflammation 11:22
8. Gelderblom M et al (2009) Temporal and spatial dynamics of cerebral immune cell accumulation in stroke. Stroke 40(5):1849–1857
9. Gronberg NV et al (2013) Leukocyte infiltration in experimental stroke. J Neuroinflammation 10:115
10. Rosell A et al (2008) MMP-9-positive neutrophil infiltration is associated to blood–brain barrier breakdown and basal lamina type IV collagen degradation during hemorrhagic transformation after human ischemic stroke. Stroke 39(4):1121–1126
11. Matsuo Y et al (1994) Correlation between myeloperoxidase-quantified neutrophil accumulation and ischemic brain injury in the rat. Effects of neutrophil depletion. Stroke 25(7):1469–1475
12. Matsuo Y et al (1994) Role of cell adhesion molecules in brain injury after transient middle cerebral artery occlusion in the rat. Brain Res 656(2):344–352
13. Hudome S et al (1997) The role of neutrophils in the production of hypoxic-ischemic brain injury in the neonatal rat. Pediatr Res 41(5):607–616
14. Mori E et al (1992) Inhibition of polymorphonuclear leukocyte adherence suppresses no-reflow after focal cerebral ischemia in baboons. Stroke 23(5):712–718
15. Zhang Y et al (1996) Propentofylline inhibits polymorphonuclear leukocyte recruitment in vivo by a mechanism involving adenosine A2A receptors. Eur J Pharmacol 313(3):237–242
16. McCarter JF et al (2001) FK 506 protects brain tissue in animal models of stroke. Transplant Proc 33(3):2390–2392
17. Harris AK et al (2005) Effect of neutrophil depletion on gelatinase expression, edema formation and hemorrhagic transformation after focal ischemic stroke. BMC Neurosci 6:49
18. Krams M et al (2003) Acute Stroke Therapy by Inhibition of Neutrophils (ASTIN): an adaptive dose–response study of UK-279,276 in acute ischemic stroke. Stroke 34(11):2543–2548
19. Becker KJ (2002) Anti-leukocyte antibodies: LeukArrest (Hu23F2G) and Enlimomab (R6.5) in acute stroke. Curr Med Res Opin 18(Suppl 2):s18–s22

20. Enlimomab Acute Stroke Trial Investigators (2001) Use of anti-ICAM-1 therapy in ischemic stroke: results of the Enlimomab Acute Stroke Trial. Neurology 57(8):1428–1434
21. Tang Z et al (2014) CX3CR1 deficiency suppresses activation and neurotoxicity of microglia/macrophage in experimental ischemic stroke. J Neuroinflammation 11:26
22. Downes CE et al (2013) MyD88 is a critical regulator of hematopoietic cell-mediated neuroprotection seen after stroke. PLoS One 8(3), e57948
23. Lalancette-Hebert M et al (2007) Selective ablation of proliferating microglial cells exacerbates ischemic injury in the brain. J Neurosci 27(10):2596–2605
24. Imai F et al (2007) Neuroprotective effect of exogenous microglia in global brain ischemia. J Cereb Blood Flow Metab 27(3):488–500
25. Ren X et al (2011) Regulatory B cells limit CNS inflammation and neurologic deficits in murine experimental stroke. J Neurosci 31(23):8556–8563
26. Bodhankar S et al (2014) Treatment of experimental stroke with IL-10-producing B-cells reduces infarct size and peripheral and CNS inflammation in wild-type B-cell-sufficient mice. Metab Brain Dis 29(1):59–73
27. Rosenzweig HL et al (2004) Endotoxin preconditioning prevents cellular inflammatory response during ischemic neuroprotection in mice. Stroke 35(11):2576–2581
28. Rosenzweig HL et al (2007) Endotoxin preconditioning protects against the cytotoxic effects of TNFalpha after stroke: a novel role for TNFalpha in LPS-ischemic tolerance. J Cereb Blood Flow Metab 27(10):1663–1674
29. Stevens SL et al (2008) Toll-like receptor 9: a new target of ischemic preconditioning in the brain. J Cereb Blood Flow Metab 28(5):1040–1047
30. Marsh B et al (2009) Systemic lipopolysaccharide protects the brain from ischemic injury by reprogramming the response of the brain to stroke: a critical role for IRF3. J Neurosci 29(31):9839–9849
31. Bahjat FR et al (2011) Proof of concept: pharmacological preconditioning with a Toll-like receptor agonist protects against cerebrovascular injury in a primate model of stroke. J Cereb Blood Flow Metab 31(5):1229–1242
32. Packard AE et al (2012) TLR9 bone marrow chimeric mice define a role for cerebral TNF in neuroprotection induced by CpG preconditioning. J Cereb Blood Flow Metab 32(12):2193–2200
33. Abbott NJ et al (2010) Structure and function of the blood-brain barrier. Neurobiol Dis 37(1):13–25
34. Miyazaki D et al (2009) Regulatory function of CpG-activated B cells in late-phase experimental allergic conjunctivitis. Invest Ophthalmol Vis Sci 50(4):1626–1635

Humoral Mediators of Remote Ischemic Conditioning: Important Role of eNOS/NO/Nitrite

David C. Hess, Mohammad Nasrul Hoda, and Mohammad B. Khan

The history of ischemic preconditioning dates back to pivotal studies in Kurt Reimer's laboratory, with the demonstration that brief repetitive cycles (four) of 5-min periods of occlusion and 5-min periods of reperfusion of the left anterior descending artery (LAD) reduced infarction after a subsequent 45-min period of occlusion of the LAD [1]. Six years later, Pryzklenk and colleagues [2] showed "regional" preconditioning when they discovered that brief repetitive occlusion of the circumflex artery protected the territory of the LAD during a 60-min occlusion, implying a role for a humoral blood-borne substance. Other investigators found that the cardioprotective conditioning stimulus could be applied at a distance to the kidneys or bowel [3] and eventually the limb [4]. Finally, the conditioning stimulus could be applied during the occlusion "perconditioning," rather than before (pre-) and still protect the heart [5].

There have been two broad theories of how the peripheral signal from the limb is transmitted to a distant organ—neural and humoral—with the suggestion that both are required in some models. Findings that blockade of the autonomic ganglia with hexamethonium blocked the conditioning effect in the heart and brain suggested involvement of the autonomic nervous system [3, 6]. However, experiments demonstrating that transfer of blood from conditioned animals to isolated hearts (Langendorff preparation) mediates cardioprotection [7] and the finding that transplanted, denervated hearts can still be conditioned strongly suggests the key role of humoral factors [8].

D.C. Hess, MD (✉) • M.B. Khan, PhD
Department of Neurology, Medical College of Georgia, Georgia Regent's University, Augusta, GA 30912, USA
e-mail: dhess@gru.edu

M.N. Hoda, PhD
Department of Medical Laboratory, Imaging and Radiological Sciences College of Allied Health Sciences, Georgia Regent's University, Augusta, GA 30912, USA

Putative Circulating Mediators

A number of circulating mediators and biomarkers of the conditioning response have been reported in cardiac injury models, including stromal-derived factor −1 (SDF-1), IL-10, microRNA 144 (miR144), and nitrite (Table 1). SDF-1 (CXCL12) is increased in the plasma after remote ischemic conditioning (RIC) in a rat cardiac model and is cardioprotective. Blockade of SDF-1 with its antagonist AMD3100 abrogates the protective effect [9]. IL-10 is increased in the plasma in mice after RIC and is also cardioprotective. Genetic deletion of IL10 and blockade with an IL-10 antibody abrogates the protective effect of RIC [10]. Redington and colleagues [11] found miR144 increased in the plasma of rats and humans after RIC and a specific antisense oligonucleotide to miR144 blocked the protective effect of RIC. Moreover, miR 144 was protective itself, thereby providing evidence that miRNA144 may be a circulating effector of RIC. Strong evidence exists for plasma nitrite as a mediator [12].

Cerebral Blood Flow (CBF) after RIC

In the cardiac studies of RIC, coronary blood flow is seldom directly measured. Many cardiac studies of RIC use the Langendorff heart perfusion model, an *in vitro* technique where the heart is removed and reverse perfused through the aorta, negating any ability to study regulation of coronary blood flow. However, in other model systems, there is evidence that RIC improves coronary blood flow. In a pig model of LAD occlusion, coronary resistance was decreased and coronary blood flow was increased by remote ischemic preconditioning [13]. Moreover, in healthy subjects and humans with congestive heart failure (CHF), RIC increased coronary microvascular perfusion as measured by transthoracic Doppler echocardiography [14].

R.L. Applegate et al. (eds.), *Brain Edema XVI: Translate Basic Science into Clinical Practice*, Acta Neurochirurgica Supplement, Vol. 121,
DOI 10.1007/978-3-319-18497-5_8,

In some of the earliest studies of preconditioning in the brain, improvements in microvascular perfusion and CBF were shown to contribute to the protective effect. Administration of lipopolysaccharide (LPS) protects against permanent MCA occlusion 72 h later with a reduction in infarct size. Microvascular flow was increased at 4 and 24 h after MCA occlusion in the LPS-treated mice compared with control mice, indicating that preservation of blood flow partially accounted for the protective effect [15].

In a permanent occlusion model, Zhao and Nowak [16] showed that ischemic preconditioning 24 h prior to permanent ischemia increased CBF and reduced infarct size in accord with preservation of local CBF. Brief episodes of ischemia (15 min) protected against a subsequent 45-min duration of ischemia in mice and increased CBF as measured by laser Doppler and MRI arterial spin labeling (ASL), demonstrating the critical importance of CBF as a mediator of protection [17].

In an autologous thromboembolic clot model in the mouse, we found that RIC increased CBF as measured by laser Doppler flowmetry and laser contrast speckle imaging (LCSI) in mice treated with tissue plasminogen activator (tPA) and in mice not treated with IV tPA [18–20]. This effect was seen in young males, ovariectomized females, and aged male mice (12 months old). We have also found that remote ischemic postconditioning daily for 2 weeks increases CBF in a mouse bilateral carotid artery stenosis (BCAS) model (Fig. 1) [21]. This increase in CBF persists at least 1 week beyond the cessation of remote limb postconditioning.

Table 1 Putative circulating mediators of RIC

SDF-1 [9]
IL-10 [10]
Nitrite/NO bioactivity [12]
microRNA 144 [11]

Nitric Oxide

Early work in preconditioning implicated NO in the mechanism of action. In a study of hypoxic preconditioning in a neonatal rodent hypoxia ischemia (HI) model, previous hypoxia (8 % oxygen) for 3 h completely protected against a subsequent HI-induced injury 24 h later. This was dependent on NO as the effect was abolished with L nitroarginine, a nonselective inhibitor of NOS but not with the selective nNOS (7-nitroindazole) or iNOS inhibitor (aminoguanidine), suggesting that preconditioning was dependent on eNOS (NOS3) [22]. In a permanent middle cerebral artery (MCA) occlusion model, brief occlusion of the MCA for 5 min repeated 3 times reduced infarct size in wild-type mice but not in eNOS or nNOS knockout mice indicating a role for NO and implicating both eNOS and nNOS [23]. NO generation via eNOS or nNOS is also required for the preconditioning effect of LPS [24].

In RIC, the NO system also appears to play a role in the mechanism of protection. In a mouse liver ischemia-reperfusion model, NO plays an essential role in mediating protection from RIC. Mice treated with RIC are protected from liver ischemic damage and have elevated microvascular blood flow. This protection is abolished with PTIO, a NO scavenger [25]. The mice treated with RIC have elevated NOx levels in the blood. Moreover, eNOS knockouts are not protected by RIC in this model [26].

NO and nitrite are also a key signaling pathway mediating RIC-induced cardioprotection. Rassaf et al. [12] reported that RIC protected hearts during 30-min LAD occlusion and increased nitrite levels in the plasma and hearts in mice. Nitrite levels also increased in the plasma of healthy human volunteers during RIC of the arm. The nitrite increase was dependent on reactive hyperremia during the reperfusion phase and related to shear stress-induced upregulation of eNOS. Cardioprotection with RIC in mice was lost in eNOS knockouts. Transfer experiments in the Langendorff heart

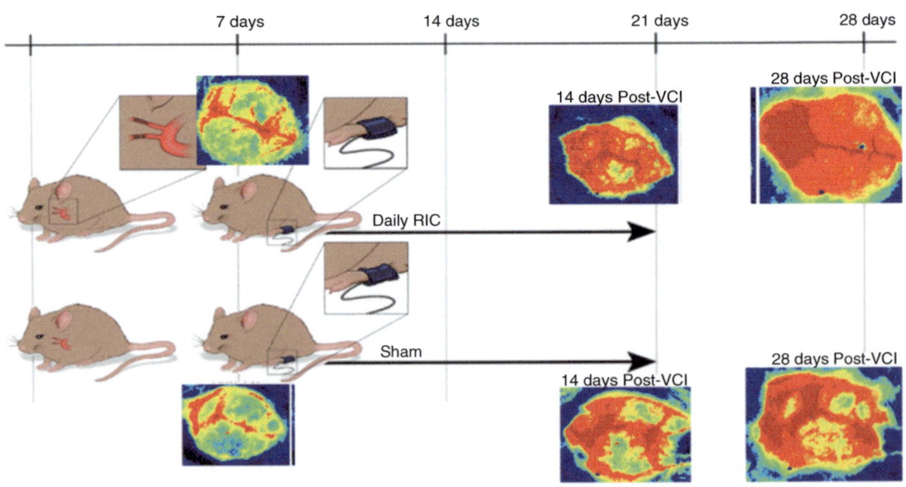

Fig. 1 Mice had microcoils applied to both internal carotid arteries. After 1 week, CBF was measured by laser contrast speckle imaging (LCSI) and showed a severe drop in CBF. Mice were randomized to RIC (*top*) or sham RIC daily (*bottom*) for 2 weeks. CBF was measured 21 and 28 days after placement of the coils. CBF was improved in the RIC mice at 21 and 28 days (7 days after stopping of RIC) (see Khan et al. [21] for details)

model showed that plasma from conditioned humans was protective. Administration of exogenous nitrite was protective in mice. Myoglobin was essential to the protection, as myoglobin knockouts were not protected and myoglobin appeared to mediate nitrite reductase activity in the heart. These data meet the criteria to establish plasma nitrite as a mediator of RIC according the Working Group of the Cellular Biology of the Heart of the European Society of Cardiology [27].

In the mouse BCAS model where there are increases in CBF with chronic daily RIC, we measured plasma nitrite by ozone-chemiluminesence (GE Sievers NOA 280) in mice subjected to sham coiling, to mice with coiling and sham RIC, and in mice with BCAS with RIC ($N=6$ per group) at 28 days post coiling. Mice subjected to BCAS had reduced plasma nitrite but RIC administered daily for 2 weeks dramatically and significantly increased plasma nitrite (Fig. 2). This increase was associated with increased CBF by LSCI in these mice and improved cognitive outcome.

Nitrite serves a "storage" pool of NO derived from endogenous eNOS that circulates in the blood associated with RBC/ hemoglobin and is reduced to NO in areas of hypoxemia, mediating hypoxic vasodilatation [28, 29]. As nitrite is a known vasodilator and increases CBF, upregulation of nitrite by RIC may explain the increase of CBF. Nitrite also is involved in the nitrosylation of key mitochondria proteins including complex I [12]. Therefore, increases of plasma nitrite likely increase CBF and protect mitochondria from oxidative stress.

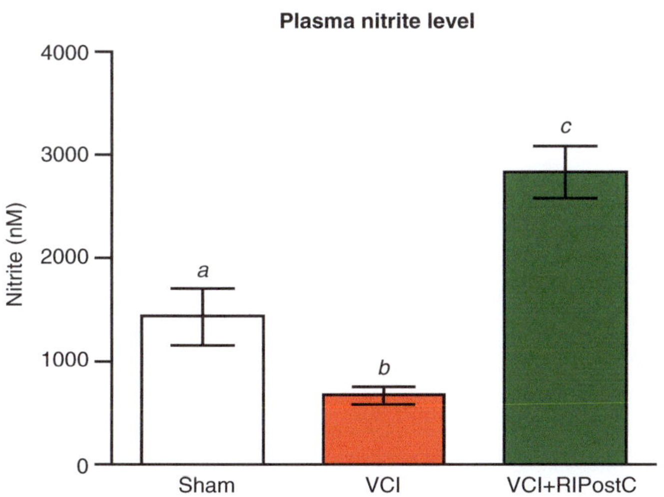

Fig. 2 Mice were randomized to BCAS surgery (as in Fig. 1) or to sham surgery. The BCAS mice (model for vascular cognitive impairment (VCI)) were randomized to RIC or sham RIC (N-6 per group). Plasma nitrite (measured at 28 days) was reduced in the mice with BCAS (**b**) compared with those with sham surgery (**a**), and there was a significant increase in mice randomized to RIC (**c**) compared with sham RIC (**b**) ($p<.05$)

Conclusions

Biomarkers of the conditioning response are needed in clinical trials of RIC to help select dose and duration of therapy. We propose that CBF as measured by MRI ASL and plasma nitrite could serve as imaging and blood biomarkers in clinical trials of RIC in acute ischemic stroke, subarachnoid hemorrhage, intracranial atherosclerosis, and vascular cognitive impairment.

Acknowledgments The authors would like to acknowledge Colby Polonsky, medical illustrator, Georgia Regent's University for Fig. 1. This work is supported by NIH-NINDS R21 NS081143.

Conflict of Interest The authors have no conflicts of interest to report.

References

1. Murry CE, Jennings RB, Reimer KA (1986) Preconditioning with ischemia: a delay of lethal cell injury in ischemic myocardium. Circulation 74(5):1124–1136
2. Przyklenk K, Bauer B, Ovize M, Kloner RA, Whittaker P (1993) Regional ischemic 'preconditioning' protects remote virgin myocardium from subsequent sustained coronary occlusion. Circulation 87(3):893–899
3. Gho BC, Schoemaker RG, van den Doel MA, Duncker DJ, Verdouw PD (1996) Myocardial protection by brief ischemia in noncardiac tissue. Circulation 94(9):2193–2200
4. Birnbaum Y, Hale SL, Kloner RA (1997) Ischemic preconditioning at a distance: reduction of myocardial infarct size by partial reduction of blood supply combined with rapid stimulation of the gastrocnemius muscle in the rabbit. Circulation 96(5):1641–1646
5. Schmidt MR, Smerup M, Konstantinov IE, Shimizu M, Li J, Cheung M et al (2007) Intermittent peripheral tissue ischemia during coronary ischemia reduces myocardial infarction through a KATP-dependent mechanism: first demonstration of remote ischemic perconditioning. Am J Physiol Heart Circ Physiol 292(4):H1883–H1890
6. Malhotra S, Naggar I, Stewart M, Rosenbaum DM (2011) Neurogenic pathway mediated remote preconditioning protects the brain from transient focal ischemic injury. Brain Res 1386:184–190
7. Shimizu M, Tropak M, Diaz RJ, Suto F, Surendra H, Kuzmin E et al (2009) Transient limb ischaemia remotely preconditions through a humoral mechanism acting directly on the myocardium: evidence suggesting cross-species protection. Clin Sci (Lond) 117(5):191–200
8. Konstantinov IE, Li J, Cheung MM, Shimizu M, Stokoe J, Kharbanda RK et al (2005) Remote ischemic preconditioning of the recipient reduces myocardial ischemia-reperfusion injury of the denervated donor heart via a Katp channel-dependent mechanism. Transplantation 79(12):1691–1695
9. Davidson SM, Selvaraj P, He D, Boi-Doku C, Yellon RL, Vicencio JM et al (2013) Remote ischaemic preconditioning involves signalling through the SDF-1alpha/CXCR4 signalling axis. Basic Res Cardiol 108(5):377
10. Cai ZP, Parajuli N, Zheng X, Becker L (2012) Remote ischemic preconditioning confers late protection against myocardial ischemia-reperfusion injury in mice by upregulating interleukin-10. Basic Res Cardiol 107(4):277

11. Li J, Rohailla S, Gelber N, Rutka J, Sabah N, Gladstone RA et al (2014) MicroRNA-144 is a circulating effector of remote ischemic preconditioning. Basic Res Cardiol 109(5):423
12. Rassaf T, Totzeck M, Hendgen-Cotta UB, Shiva S, Heusch G, Kelm M (2014) Circulating nitrite contributes to cardioprotection by remote ischemic preconditioning. Circ Res 114(10):1601–1610
13. Shimizu M, Konstantinov IE, Kharbanda RK, Cheung MH, Redington AN (2007) Effects of intermittent lower limb ischaemia on coronary blood flow and coronary resistance in pigs. Acta Physiol (Oxf) 190(2):103–109
14. Kono Y, Fukuda S, Hanatani A, Nakanishi K, Otsuka K, Taguchi H et al (2014) Remote ischemic conditioning improves coronary microcirculation in healthy subjects and patients with heart failure. Drug Des Devel Ther 8:1175–1181
15. Dawson DA, Furuya K, Gotoh J, Nakao Y, Hallenbeck JM (1999) Cerebrovascular hemodynamics and ischemic tolerance: lipopolysaccharide-induced resistance to focal cerebral ischemia is not due to changes in severity of the initial ischemic insult, but is associated with preservation of microvascular perfusion. J Cereb Blood Flow Metab 19(6):616–623
16. Zhao L, Nowak TS Jr (2006) CBF changes associated with focal ischemic preconditioning in the spontaneously hypertensive rat. J Cereb Blood Flow Metab 26(9):1128–1140
17. Hoyte LC, Papadakis M, Barber PA, Buchan AM (2006) Improved regional cerebral blood flow is important for the protection seen in a mouse model of late phase ischemic preconditioning. Brain Res 1121(1):231–237
18. Hoda MN, Bhatia K, Hafez SS, Johnson MH, Siddiqui S, Ergul A et al (2014) Remote ischemic perconditioning is effective after embolic stroke in ovariectomized female mice. Transl Stroke Res 5:484–490
19. Hoda MN, Fagan SC, Khan MB, Vaibhav K, Chaudhary A, Wang P et al (2014) A 2 x 2 factorial design for the combination therapy of minocycline and remote ischemic perconditioning: efficacy in a preclinical trial in murine thromboembolic stroke model. Exp Transl Stroke Med 6:10
20. Hoda MN, Siddiqui S, Herberg S, Periyasamy-Thandavan S, Bhatia K, Hafez SS et al (2012) Remote ischemic perconditioning is effective alone and in combination with intravenous tissue-type plasminogen activator in murine model of embolic stroke. Stroke 43(10):2794–2799
21. Khan MB, Hoda MN, Vaibhav K, Giri S, Wang P, Waller JL et al (2015) Remote ischemic postconditioning: harnessing endogenous protection in a murine model of vascular cognitive impairment. Transl Stroke Res 6(1):69–77
22. Gidday JM, Shah AR, Maceren RG, Wang Q, Pelligrino DA, Holtzman DM et al (1999) Nitric oxide mediates cerebral ischemic tolerance in a neonatal rat model of hypoxic preconditioning. J Cereb Blood Flow Metab 19(3):331–340
23. Atochin DN, Clark J, Demchenko IT, Moskowitz MA, Huang PL (2003) Rapid cerebral ischemic preconditioning in mice deficient in endothelial and neuronal nitric oxide synthases. Stroke 34(5):1299–1303
24. Orio M, Kunz A, Kawano T, Anrather J, Zhou P, Iadecola C (2007) Lipopolysaccharide induces early tolerance to excitotoxicity via nitric oxide and cGMP. Stroke 38(10):2812–2817
25. Abu-Amara M, Yang SY, Quaglia A, Rowley P, de Mel A, Tapuria N et al (2011) Nitric oxide is an essential mediator of the protective effects of remote ischaemic preconditioning in a mouse model of liver ischaemia/reperfusion injury. Clin Sci (Lond) 121(6):257–266
26. Abu-Amara M, Yang SY, Quaglia A, Rowley P, Fuller B, Seifalian A et al (2011) Role of endothelial nitric oxide synthase in remote ischemic preconditioning of the mouse liver. Liver Transpl 17(5):610–619
27. Ovize M, Baxter GF, Di Lisa F, Ferdinandy P, Garcia-Dorado D, Hausenloy DJ et al (2010) Postconditioning and protection from reperfusion injury: where do we stand? Position paper from the Working Group of Cellular Biology of the Heart of the European Society of Cardiology. Cardiovasc Res 87(3):406–423
28. Kim-Shapiro DB, Gladwin MT (2014) Mechanisms of nitrite bioactivation. Nitric Oxide 38:58–68
29. Liu C, Wajih N, Liu X, Basu S, Janes J, Marvel M et al (2015) Mechanisms of human erythrocytic bioactivation of nitrite. J Biol Chem 290(2):1281–1294

Exsanguination Postconditioning of ICH (EPIC-H) Using the Lancet for Brain Bleed in Rodents, Preliminary Study

Tim Lekic and John H. Zhang

Introduction

Cerebral iron overload contributes to free-radical damage and secondary brain injury following intracerebral hemorrhage (ICH) [1–12]. Among experts of clinical medicine [13, 14], it is well known that phlebotomy most effectively removes iron from the human body, with greater efficacy on human physiology than any currently known pharmacological chelator [13–15], including deferoxamine [16]. For centuries, this ancient method, called "bloodletting," was the treatment for stroke, among many other maladies. Fortunately, for most medical applications the practice was abandoned, but this was done without any actual scientific investigation [14, 15, 17]. Today, translational ICH research is a potential beneficiary of phlebotomy therapy, as this is the standard of care for other proven iron overload conditions [13, 14]. This is the first controlled scientific evaluation of the phlebotomy approach after ICH. In this study, femoral catheterization followed intraparenchymal collagenase infusion, and different exsanguination volumes were compared with untreated controls.

T. Lekic
Division of Physiology and Pharmacology, Loma Linda University School of Medicine, 11041 Campus Street, Risley Hall Rm 219, Loma Linda, CA 92354, USA

J.H. Zhang, MD, PhD (✉)
Division of Physiology and Pharmacology, Loma Linda University School of Medicine, 11041 Campus Street, Risley Hall Rm 219, Loma Linda, CA 92354, USA

Department of Neurosurgery, School of Medicine, Loma Linda, CA, USA
e-mail: johnzhang3910@yahoo.com

Methods

In brief, femoral catheterization occurred 30 min after collagenase infusion. Three different exsanguination volumes (1, 2, and 3 ml) were compared with ICH (0 ml) and sham controls (as below), representing about 5–15 % of the total blood volume. Routine studies included hemorrhage size, brain water content, and neuroscore measured 24 h later.

Animals and General Procedures

Adult male Sprague-Dawley rats (~300 g; Harlan, Indianapolis, IN, USA) were used in the study. All procedures were in compliance with the *Guide for the Care and Use of Laboratory Animals* and approved by the Animal Care and Use Committee at Loma Linda University. An aseptic technique was used for all surgeries. Rats were anesthetized with isoflurane (4 % induction, 2 % maintenance, 70 % N_2O, and 30 % O_2). Animals were allowed free access to food and water after recovery from anesthesia.

Intracerebral Hemorrhage

Anesthetized animals were placed prone in a stereotaxic frame (Kopf Instruments, Tujunga, CA, USA), as described previously [11, 18]. A midline incision was made over the scalp, under which the following stereotactic coordinates localized the right basal ganglia: 0.2 mm anterior, 5.6 mm ventral, and 2.9 mm lateral to the bregma. A posterior cranial burr hole (1 mm) was drilled over the right cerebral hemisphere, and a 27 gauge needle was inserted at a rate of 1 mm/min, followed by a microinfusion pump (Harvard Apparatus, Holliston, MA, USA) infusion of bacterial collagenase (VII-S; Sigma, St Louis, MO, USA; 0.2 U in 1 μl

R.L. Applegate et al. (eds.), *Brain Edema XVI: Translate Basic Science into Clinical Practice*, Acta Neurochirurgica Supplement, Vol. 121, DOI 10.1007/978-3-319-18497-5_9, © Springer International Publishing Switzerland 2016

saline) through a Hamilton syringe at a rate of 0.2 μl/min. The needle remained in place for an additional 10 min after injection to prevent "back-leakage." To maintain a core temperature within 37.0 ± 0.5 °C, an electronic thermostat-controlled warming blanket was used throughout the operation. After needle removal, the burr hole was sealed with bone wax, the incision sutured closed, and the animal was allowed to recover. Sham surgeries consisted of needle insertion alone.

Phlebotomy

Using standard antiseptic techniques while under general anesthesia (i.e., perioperatively) [19], the right femoral artery was catheterized [20, 21] for therapeutic exsanguination (volumes included 0, 1, 2, or 3 ml) of whole femoral arterial blood. These hematological products were then appropriately discarded following retrieval.

Hematoma Size

The hemorrhagic injury size was quantified using computer-assisted outlining of brain slices, as described previously [22]. Briefly, the brains were removed and cut into slices using a 1-mm rat brain matrix. Under standardized conditions, images of the brain slices were taken with a digital camera, which were then converted into a binary image for area delineation analysis using Image J software (National Institutes of Health, Bethesda, MD, USA), with further details and validation published elsewhere [23, 24].

Neuroscore

Neurological evaluations [25] were performed in all groups at 24 h by highly experienced and blinded examiners. The scoring system consists of six tests with possible scores of 0–3 for each test (0 = worst, 3 = best), including: (a) spontaneous activity, (b) symmetry of movement, (c) forepaw outstretching, (d) climbing, (e) body proprioception, and (f) response to vibrissae touch. Scores were given to each rat at the completion of the evaluation, for a total summation of all six individual tests.

Percent Edema

Animals were re-anesthetized and brain samples were collected. Brain edema was measured by methods described previously [19–21, 26]. Briefly, the rats were decapitated and brains removed immediately, then divided into five parts: ipsilateral and contralateral basal ganglia, ipsilateral and contralateral cortex, and cerebellum. Tissue samples were weighed on an analytical balance (model AE 100; Mettler Instrument Co., Columbus, OH, USA) to the nearest 0.01 mg to obtain wet weight (WW). The brain tissue was then dried at 100 °C for 24 h to find the dry weight (DW) measurement. Finally, the brain water (%) was calculated using the formula $(WW-DW)/WW \times 100$, as described previously [19–21, 26].

Results

Preliminary analysis of serial brain sections (Fig. 1) demonstrated that therapeutic phlebotomy (occurring shortly after ICH in adult rats) subjectively reduced the appearance of hemorrhagic brain injury 24 h after collagenase infusion. There was a significant reduction in hematoma size (Fig. 2) in comparing 2 ml exsanguination treatment to the control (0 ml ICH non-exsanguination) group. However, at 1 day after ICH, there was no difference in neurological ability between groups (Fig. 2). Percentage of brain edema (Fig. 3), however, was significantly reduced in a dose-response fashion after exsanguination therapy, compared with ICH control.

Conclusion

Translational stroke studies, including animal modeling, are needed to safely integrate basic preclinical scientific principles ahead of clinical application [27–31]. Exsanguination therapy following ICH in rodents, using the traditional phlebotomy approach, may ameliorate the early brain injury (hemorrhage and edema), despite equivocal changes in the short-term neurological functional ability. This study forms the basis to justify further investigation into the preclinical application of this safe and broadly available clinical therapy as a potential therapeutic modality for this devastated patient population. Future studies will need to further delineate the involvement of specific neuroprotective molecules, sympathetic responses, hemodynamic molecules, or neuro-endocrine factors involved in this apparent postconditioning of rat ICH.

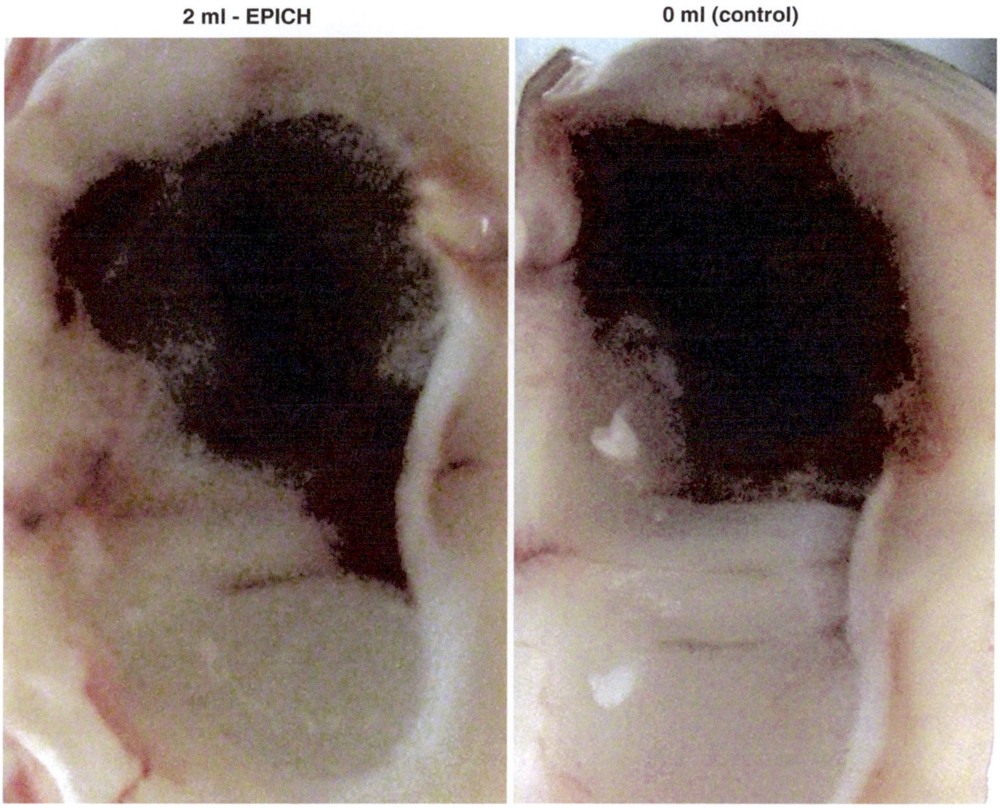

Fig. 1 Pictographs showing representative relative hemorrhage between groups

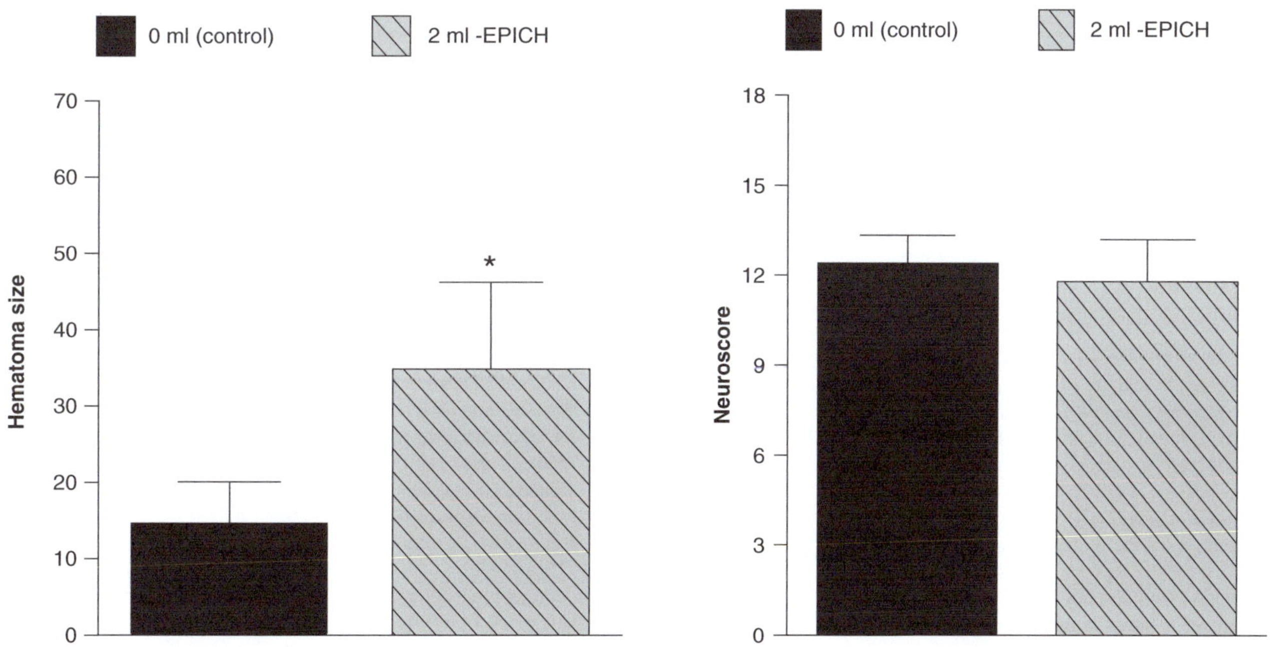

Fig. 2 (*Left panel*) Hematoma expansion; (*Right panel*) neurological deficits (sensorimotor skill) measured 24 h following collagenase infusion; *SEM*, standard error of the mean (*asterisk*) <0.05 compared with vehicle

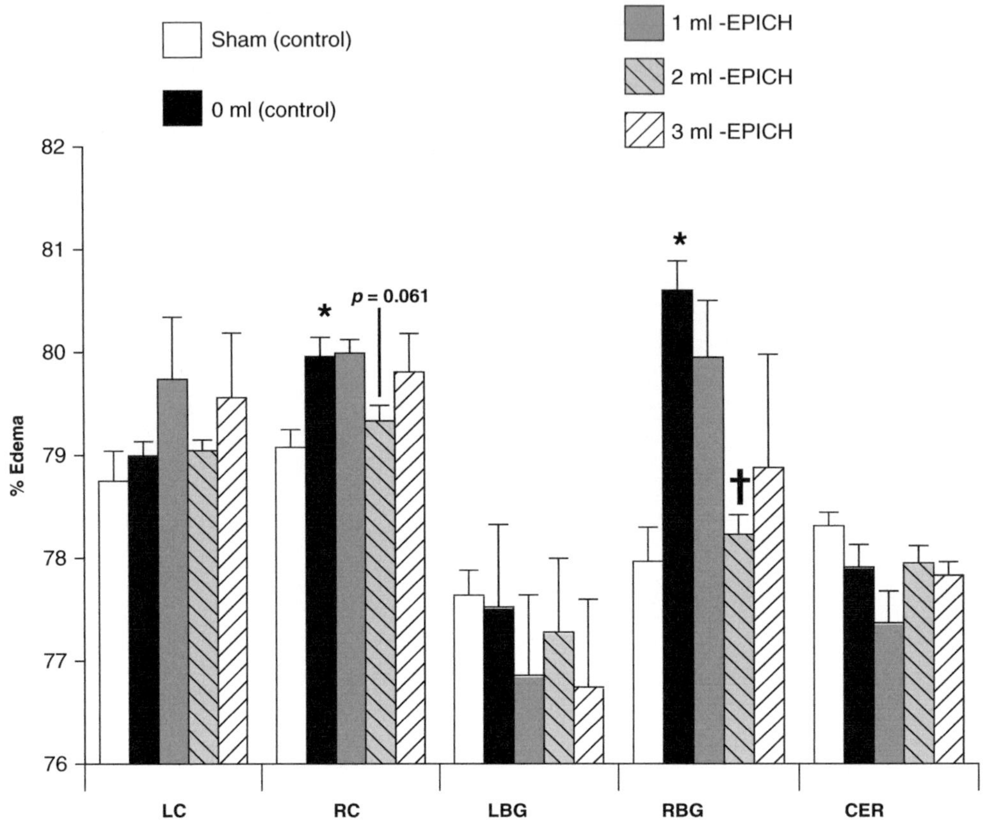

Fig. 3 Percent edema 24 h following collagenase infusion, (*asterisk*) <0.05 compared to sham; (*cross*) <0.05 to 0 ml control; *SEM* standard error of the mean

Acknowledgment This study was partially supported by National Institutes of Health grant RO1 NS078755 (Dr Zhang). We wish to thank William Rolland for his handling of a few samples.

Disclosures None

References

1. Nakamura T, Keep RF, Hua Y, Nagao S, Hoff JT, Xi G (2006) Iron-induced oxidative brain injury after experimental intracerebral hemorrhage. Acta Neurochir Suppl 96:194–198
2. Gao C, Du H, Hua Y, Keep RF, Strahle J, Xi G (2014) Role of red blood cell lysis and iron in hydrocephalus after intraventricular hemorrhage. J Cereb Blood Flow Metab 34:1070–1075
3. Zhao J, Chen Z, Xi G, Keep RF, Hua Y (2014) Deferoxamine attenuates acute hydrocephalus after traumatic brain injury in rats. Transl Stroke Res 5:586–594
4. Chen Z, Gao C, Hua Y, Keep RF, Muraszko K, Xi G (2011) Role of iron in brain injury after intraventricular hemorrhage. Stroke 42:465–470
5. Hua Y, Keep RF, Hoff JT, Xi G (2007) Brain injury after intracerebral hemorrhage: the role of thrombin and iron. Stroke 38:759–762
6. Hua Y, Nakamura T, Keep RF, Wu J, Schallert T, Hoff JT, Xi G (2006) Long-term effects of experimental intracerebral hemorrhage: the role of iron. J Neurosurg 104:305–312
7. Wu J, Hua Y, Keep RF, Nakamura T, Hoff JT, Xi G (2003) Iron and iron-handling proteins in the brain after intracerebral hemorrhage. Stroke 34:2964–2969
8. Huang FP, Xi G, Keep RF, Hua Y, Nemoianu A, Hoff JT (2002) Brain edema after experimental intracerebral hemorrhage: role of hemoglobin degradation products. J Neurosurg 96:287–293
9. Okauchi M, Hua Y, Keep RF, Morgenstern LB, Xi G (2009) Effects of deferoxamine on intracerebral hemorrhage-induced brain injury in aged rats. Stroke 40:1858–1863
10. Xiong XY, Wang J, Qian ZM, Yang QW (2014) Iron and intracerebral hemorrhage: from mechanism to translation. Transl Stroke Res 5:429–441
11. Klahr AC, Dickson CT, Colbourne F (2015) Seizure activity occurs in the collagenase but not the blood infusion model of Striatal hemorrhagic stroke in rats. Transl Stroke Res 6:29–38
12. Cheng Y, Xi G, Jin H, Keep RF, Feng J, Hua Y (2014) Thrombin-induced cerebral hemorrhage: role of protease-activated receptor-1. Transl Stroke Res 5:472–475
13. Adams PC, Barton JC (2010) How I treat hemochromatosis. Blood 116:317–325
14. Parapia LA (2008) History of bloodletting by phlebotomy. Br J Haematol 143:490–495
15. Weinberg F (1994) Bloodletting. Can Fam Physician 40:131–134
16. Warkentin LM, Auriat AM, Wowk S, Colbourne F (2010) Failure of deferoxamine, an iron chelator, to improve outcome after collagenase-induced intracerebral hemorrhage in rats. Brain Res 1309:95–103
17. Morabia A (2006) Pierre-Charles-Alexandre Louis and the evaluation of bloodletting. J R Soc Med 99:158–160

18. Schlunk F, Schulz E, Lauer A, Yigitkanli K, Pfeilschifter W, Steinmetz H, Lo EH, Foerch C (2014) Warfarin pretreatment reduces cell death and MMP-9 activity in experimental intracerebral hemorrhage. Transl Stroke Res. doi:10.1007/s12975-014-0377-3
19. Lekic T, Hartman R, Rojas H, Manaenko A, Chen W, Ayer R, Tang J, Zhang JH (2010) Protective effect of melatonin upon neuropathology, striatal function, and memory ability after intracerebral hemorrhage in rats. J Neurotrauma 27:627–637
20. Lekic T, Rolland W, Manaenko A, Krafft PR, Kamper JE, Suzuki H, Hartman RE, Tang J, Zhang JH (2013) Evaluation of the hematoma consequences, neurobehavioral profiles, and histopathology in a rat model of pontine hemorrhage. J Neurosurg 118:465–477
21. Lekic T, Rolland W, Hartman R, Kamper J, Suzuki H, Tang J, Zhang JH (2011) Characterization of the brain injury, neurobehavioral profiles, and histopathology in a rat model of cerebellar hemorrhage. Exp Neurol 227:96–103
22. Lekic T, Manaenko A, Rolland W, Krafft PR, Peters R, Hartman RE, Altay O, Tang J, Zhang JH (2012) Rodent neonatal germinal matrix hemorrhage mimics the human brain injury, neurological consequences, and post-hemorrhagic hydrocephalus. Exp Neurol 236:69–78
23. Chang CF, Chen SF, Lee TS, Lee HF, Shyue SK (2011) Caveolin-1 deletion reduces early brain injury after experimental intracerebral hemorrhage. Am J Pathol 178:1749–1761
24. Foerch C, Arai K, Jin G, Park KP, Pallast S, van Leyen K, Lo EH (2008) Experimental model of warfarin-associated intracerebral hemorrhage. Stroke 39:3397–3404
25. Garcia JH, Wagner S, Liu KF, Hu XJ (1995) Neurological deficit and extent of neuronal necrosis attributable to middle cerebral artery occlusion in rats. Statistical validation. Stroke 26:627–634
26. Tang J, Liu J, Zhou C, Ostanin D, Grisham MB, Neil Granger D, Zhang JH (2005) Role of NADPH oxidase in the brain injury of intracerebral hemorrhage. J Neurochem 94:1342–1350
27. Tso MK, Macdonald RL (2014) Subarachnoid hemorrhage: a review of experimental studies on the microcirculation and the neurovascular unit. Transl Stroke Res 5:174–189
28. Marbacher S, Nevzati E, Croci D, Erhardt S, Muroi C, Jakob SM, Fandino J (2014) The rabbit shunt model of subarachnoid haemorrhage. Transl Stroke Res 5:669–680
29. Pluta RM, Bacher J, Skopets B, Hoffmann V (2014) A non-human primate model of aneurismal subarachnoid hemorrhage (SAH). Transl Stroke Res 5:681–691
30. Zhang YP, Cai J, Shields LB, Liu N, Xu XM, Shields CB (2014) Traumatic brain injury using mouse models. Transl Stroke Res 5:454–471
31. Wada K, Makino H, Shimada K, Shikata F, Kuwabara A, Hashimoto T (2014) Translational research using a mouse model of intracranial aneurysm. Transl Stroke Res 5:248–251

Sevoflurane Preconditioning Confers Neuroprotection *via* Anti-apoptosis Effects

Hailian Wang, Hong Shi, Qiong Yu, Jun Chen, Feng Zhang, and Yanqin Gao

Introduction

The phenomenon whereby preconditioning with volatile anesthetics mimics ischemic preconditioning was first reported in heart in 1997 [1]. Since then, the neuroprotective effect of volatile anesthetic preconditioning (APC) against cerebral ischemia has been demonstrated in both *in vivo* and *in vitro* settings [2–13]. APC appears to confer biphasic protection, one in an early window (which occurs within minutes and subsides within hours) and another in a delayed window (which is manifested after 24 h and is maintained for days). Edmands et al. [13] reported that delayed preconditioning with isoflurane lasted 72–96 h *in vitro*. The protective mechanisms of APC are not fully understand thus far, although previous studies show that the mechanisms underlying APC involve attenuating neuronal apoptosis [14–16] and oxidative stress [17], opening of adenosine triphosphate-sensitive potassium channels [10], activation of adenosine A1 receptor and protein kinase C [4], or activating the Akt pathway [4, 6, 18].

Suppressing apoptotic pathways could be the primary mechanism for APC, as apoptosis contributes to ischemic brain injury [14, 15, 19–22]. Among signaling cascades leading to the activation of apoptotic execution following ischemia, the mitochondrial death pathway appears to play a central role [20–22]. After ischemic injury, a number of damaging stimuli may activate the mitochondrial death pathway, such as oxidative stress and the pro-apoptotic molecules, including Bid, Bax, and Bad, leading to the release of cytochrome *c* and other pro-apoptotic factors. Among those factors, cytochrome *c* plays a key role in the activation of caspases, whereas AIF causes cell death via caspase-independent mechanisms. Mitogen-activated protein kinases (MAPK) are an evolutionary conserved family of signal transduction proteins, which regulate differentiation, proliferation, and survival/apoptosis. The principal MAPK pathways include ERK, JNK, and p38, which are activated by many putative stimuli such as stress, cytokines, and growth factors [23]. In addition, DNA damage can trigger apoptosis by inducing the expression of the transcription factor p53 [23], and p53 expression can alter transcription of several genes that result in the initiation of apoptosis, including Bax and Puma [24, 25].

In the present study, to test our hypothesis that caspase3, AIF, Bcl-2 family, JNK, and p53 pathway contribute to the neuroprotective effect of sevoflurane-induced preconditioning, we performed *in vivo* experiments to determine the effects of APC with sevoflurane on changes in apoptotic factors in the brain after ischemic insult.

Materials and Methods

Experimental Groups and APC with Sevoflurane

All animal experiments were performed in accordance with institutional guidelines and all efforts were made to minimize the number of animals. Rats were randomized into

H. Wang • Q. Yu
Department of Anesthesiology, Huashan Hospital, Shanghai, China

State Key Laboratory of Medical Neurobiology, Institutes of Brain Science, Fudan University, 138 Yixueyuan Road, Shanghai 200032, China

H. Shi
Department of Anesthesiology of Shanghai Pulmonary Hospital, Tongji University, Shanghai 200433, China

J. Chen • F. Zhang (✉) • Y. Gao (✉)
State Key Laboratory of Medical Neurobiology, Institutes of Brain Science, Fudan University, 138 Yixueyuan Road, Shanghai 200032, China

Department of Neurology, University of Pittsburgh School of Medicine, Pittsburgh, PA 15261, USA
e-mail: ZhanFx2@upmc.edu; yqgao@shmu.edu.cn

R.L. Applegate et al. (eds.), *Brain Edema XVI: Translate Basic Science into Clinical Practice*, Acta Neurochirurgica Supplement, Vol. 121,
DOI 10.1007/978-3-319-18497-5_10, © Springer International Publishing Switzerland 2016

three experimental groups: sham-operated (branches of external cervical artery dissected without ischemia and APC exposure); vehicle (exposed to ambient air before ischemia); and sevoflurane (Baxter) APC groups (exposed to sevoflurane before ischemia). There were four rats in each group per time point.

In the preconditioning group, the rats received 1 minimum alveolar concentration (MAC) sevoflurane (97.6 % air/2.4 % sevoflurane) in an anesthetic chamber for 30 min after 15 min equilibrium on 4 consecutive days. End-tidal concentration of sevoflurane was monitored with a Datex-Ohmeda AS/3 monitoring device. Twenty-four hours after a four-cycle preconditoning with sevoflurane, rats were anesthetized, intubated, catheterized, and exposed to transient focal cerebral ischemia.

Animal Model of Transient Focal Cerebral Ischemia

Transient focal cerebral ischemia was induced by middle cerebral artery occlusion (MCAO) as previously described [26]. In brief, adult male Sprague-Dawley rats (SD, 250–300 g; Shanghai SLAC Laboratory Animal Co. Ltd.) were anesthetized with 1.5 % isoflurane (Forene, Abbott) in air and mechanically ventilated with an endotracheal tube. Rectal temperature was maintained at 37.0 °C during and shortly after surgery with a temperature-regulated heat lamp. The left femoral artery and vein were cannulated and used for blood pressure monitoring, blood sampling, and fluid administration. Arterial blood gas was analyzed 15 min after induction of ischemia and 15 min after reperfusion. A 3–0 monofilament with a blunt end was inserted into left internal carotid artery to the origin of middle cerebral artery for 60 min, and then reperfusion was established by withdrawing the suture. To confirm the induction of ischemia and successful reperfusion, changes in regional cerebral blood flow (rCBF) before, during, and after MCAO were evaluated in rats by laser Doppler flowmetry.

PANT Staining

The DNA polymerase I-mediated biotin-dATP nick-translation (PANT) assay was performed on coronal sections from the brains subjected to 1 h of MCAO and 24 h of reperfusion. The procedures for PANT have been described previously [27]. In brief, sections were air-dried, fixed in ethanol/acetic acid (2:1 vol/vol) for 5 min, and washed three times in PBS. The sections were permeabilized with 1 % Triton X-100 for 20 min, and were then incubated in a moist-air chamber at 37 °C for 90 min with the PANT reaction mixture containing 5 mmol/L $MgCl_2$; 10 mmol/L 2-mer-captoethanol; 20 mg/mL bovine serum albumin; dGTP, dCTP, and dTTP at 30 mmol/L each; 29 mmol/L biotinylated dATP; 1 mmol/L dATP; and 40U/mL *Escherichia coli* DNA polymerase I (Sigma) in phosphate-buffered saline (PBS) (pH 7.4). The biotin-dATP incorporated in DNA was detected using Texas Red Avidin D (cell sorting grade; Vector Laboratories, Burlingame, CA, USA). Polymerase I-mediated biotin-dATP nick-translation-positive cells were quantified using a computerized scanning program (MCID, St. Catharines, Ontario, Canada).

Immunofluorescence Staining

At the indicated time points after ischemia ($n=3$ per condition), rabbit anti-cleaved caspase3 monoclonal antibody (Cell Signaling Technology, Danvers, MA, USA), rabbit anti-cytochrome *c* antibody, rabbit anti-Puma, and rabbit anti-p-JNK antibody (Santa Cruz Biotechnology, Santa Cruz, CA, USA) were used as the primary antibodies. The procedures for immunohistochemistry were the same as described previously [27, 28]. Sections were then stained for 30 min with Hoechst 33258 at 37 °C for counterstaining.

Western Blots

Rat cortical tissues were collected at the indicated time points after ischemia ($n=4$ per condition), and Western blot analyses were performed as previously described [27, 28]. The primary antibodies used in this study were rabbit anti-caspase3 monoclonal antibody, rabbit anti-Bcl-2 polycolonal antibody (Cell Signaling Technology, Danvers, MA, USA), rabbit anti-cytochrome *c* antibody, rabbit anti-Bcl-xL, rabbit anti-Bax, goat anti-Bid, rabbit anti-p53, rabbit anti-p-c-jun, and rabbit anti-p-JNK antibody (Santa Cruz Biotechnology, Santa Cruz, CA, USA). The blots were semi-quantified with gel densitometry with the BIO-RAD system.

Statistical Analysis

Data were presented mean ± SD. Differences in Western blotting and immunofluorescence staining were determined with one-way analysis of variance (ANOVA) followed by post hoc tests. A p-value < 0.05 was considered statistically significant.

Results

Sevoflurane Preconditioning Suppresses Apoptotic Cell Death after MCAO

To determine the protective effect of sevoflurane preconditioning on MCAO-induced apoptosis, PANT staining was applied to detect DNA damage induced by ischemic insult. As shown in Fig. 1a&c, fewer PANT-positive cells were detected in the sevoflurane-preconditioned group compared with the control. Further studies (Fig. 1b–f) showed that the APC group demonstrated reduced cleavage of caspase-3 and release of cytochrome *c* compared with the control group, indicating that sevoflurane preconditioning protects the brain by suppressing apoptotic cell death after ischemia.

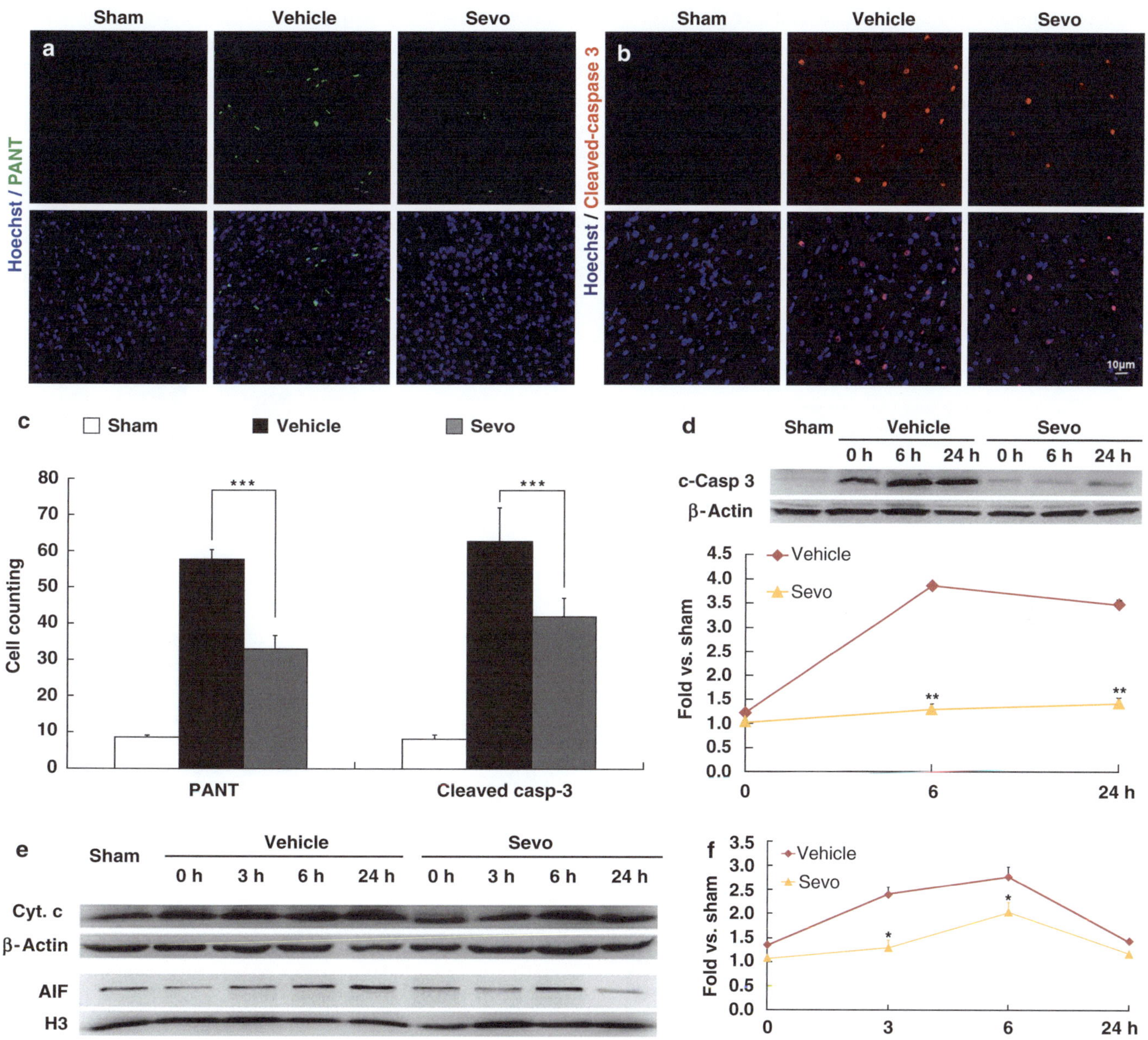

Fig. 1 Sevoflurane preconditioning suppresses the apoptotic death pathway. (**a**) PANT staining and (**b**) immunofluorescence photomicrographs of cleaved caspase-3 (*red*) with Hoechst counterstaining (*blue*) of the infarct at 24 h after MCAO. Scale bar = 10 μm. (**c**) Counting of PANT positive and caspase-3 positive cell numbers, showing reduced apoptotic cell death after APC. $***p<0.001$ compared with control group. (**d**) Representative Western blot and semi-quantitation of cleaved ccaspase-3 in the brain at various time points after MCAO. $**p<0.01$ compared with control group. (**e**) Representative Western blot and (**f**) semi-quantitation of cytochrome *c* in the brain at various time points after MCAO. $*p<0.05$ compared with control group

Sevoflurane Preconditioning Increases the Ratio of Anti-apoptotic Proteins over Pro-apoptotic Proteins of the Bcl-2 Family

As shown above, sevoflurane preconditioning suppresses mitochondrial apoptotic pathways. We next detected whether sevoflurane preconditioning influences the ratio of anti-apoptotic proteins over pro-apoptotic proteins of the Bcl-2 family, the upper stream of the mitochondrial apoptotic pathway. As shown in Fig. 2, both anti-apoptotic proteins and pro-apoptotic proteins of the Bcl-2 family increased after ischemic insult; however, the levels of Bcl-2 and Bcl-xL increases were greater than the levels of Bax and Bid increases, indicating that sevoflurane preconditioning suppresses apoptotic death by regulating Bcl-2 family members.

Inhibition of JNK and p53 Was Involved in the Neuroprotection of Sevoflurane

Activation of JNK and p53 is a contributing factor in the pathophysiology of cerebral ischemia [23]. Therefore, we further investigated whether sevoflurane preconditioning inhibits these two pathways. We collected the cortical tissues and extracted the cytosolic and nuclear proteins and then subjected the proteins to Western blots. As shown in Fig. 3a, sevoflurane preconditioning significantly decreased the

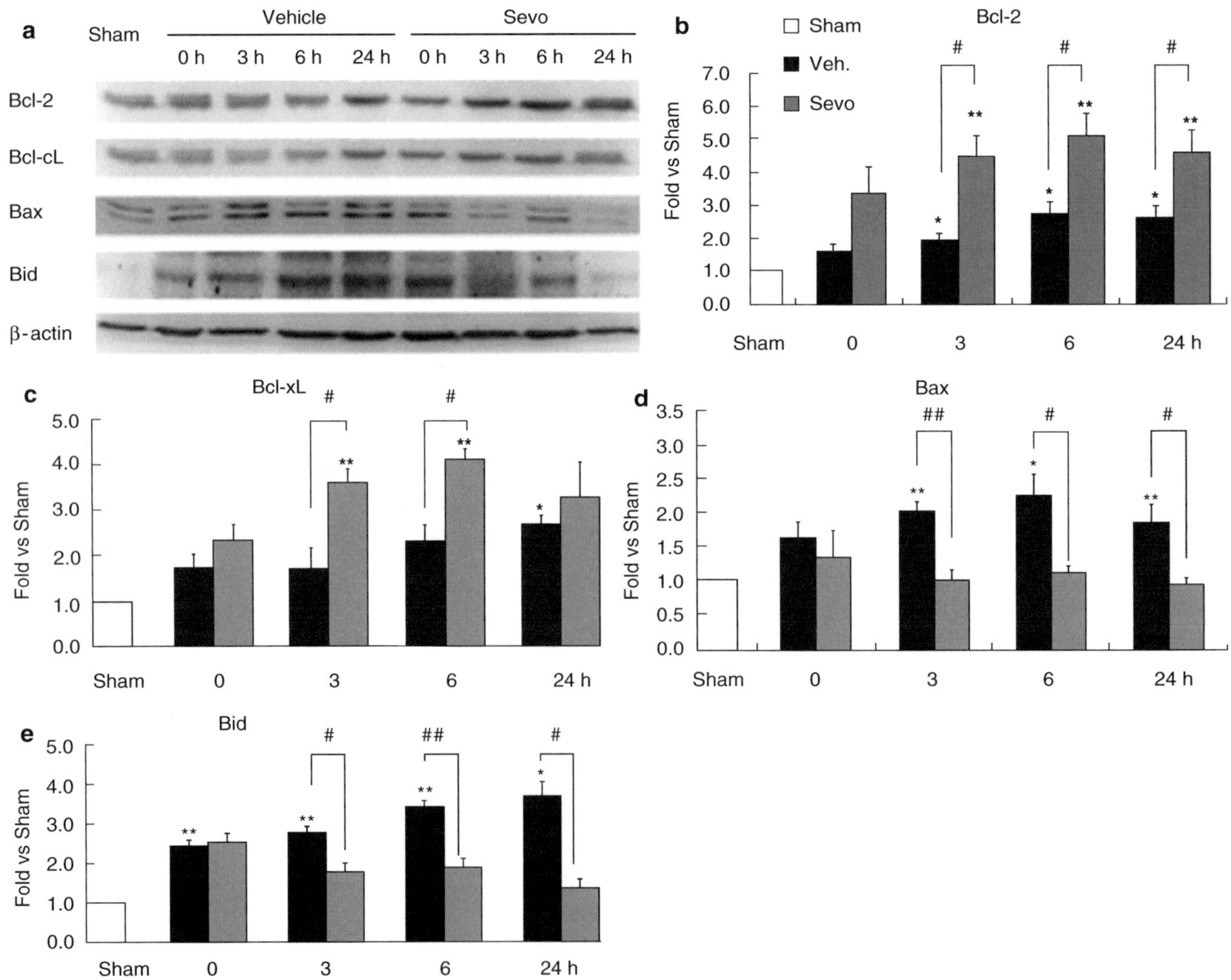

Fig. 2 Sevoflurane preconditioning enhances anti-apoptotic machinery. (**a**) Representative Western blots of Bcl-2 family members and semi-quantitative analysis of (**b**) Bcl-2, (**c**) Bcl-xL, (**d**) Bax, and (**e**) Bid levels in the cortex after MCAO, showing that sevoflurane preconditioning increased the ratio of anti-apoptotic proteins over pro-apoptotic proteins. $n=4$; $^{**}p<0.01$, $^{*}p<0.05$ compared with sham group and $^{\#\#}p<0.01$, $^{\#}p<0.05$ compared with vehicle group

levels of p-JNK compared with the control; consequently, the levels of p-c-jun, a downstream molecule of JNK, were also reduced (Fig. 3b). Similarly, sevoflurane preconditioning also significantly decreased the levels of p53 nuclear translocation and Puma, one of its target gene products. Collectively, these findings suggested that the neuroprotection of sevoflurane preconditioning involves the inhibition of JNK and p53 pathways.

Discussion

We have previously reported that repeated pretreatment with 1 MAC sevoflurane 24 h before MCAO exerts a neuroprotective effect [29]. In the current study, we further demonstrated that the repetitive preconditioning of sevoflurane markedly reduced apoptotic cell death, caspase-3 cleavage, and cytochrome *c* release. Sevoflurane preconditioning also robustly suppressed pro-apoptotic proteins and increased anti-apoptotic proteins of the Bcl-2 super family. Furthermore, APC with sevoflurane attenuated JNK and p53 pathways.

In agreement with previous reports [14, 15, 19], our finding also showed that apoptotic suppression plays an important role in APC. Although the exact regulative mechanisms remain unclear, influence on mitochondrial apoptotic pathways appears to be important [14, 15, 19, 21, 30]. For example, sevoflurane preconditioning inhibited mitochondrial permeability transition pore opening after cerebral ischemia [30], and desflurane preserved mitochondrial function after cerebral ischemia reperfusion injury [16]. In support, our

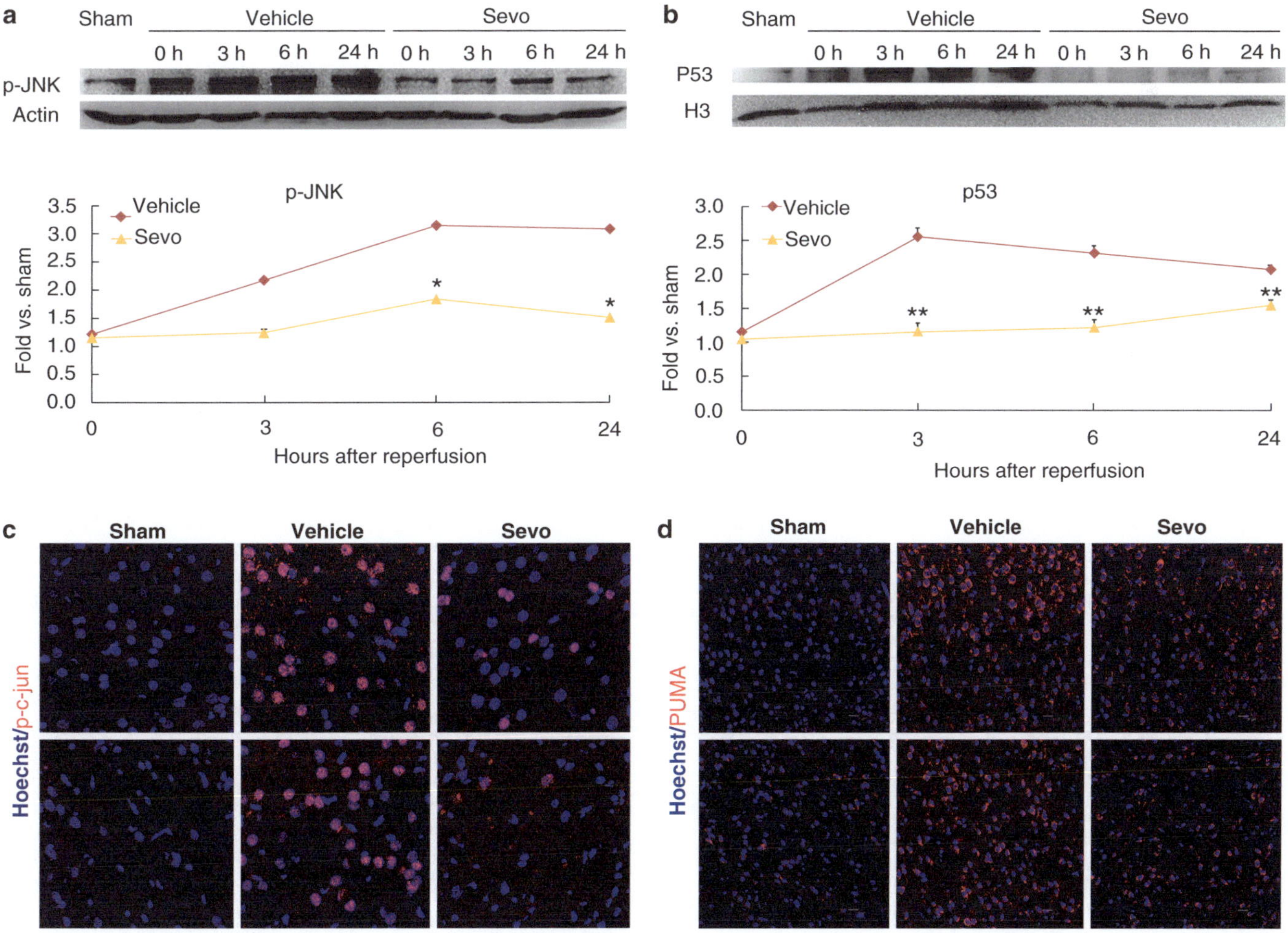

Fig. 3 Sevoflurane preconditioning attenuates the JNK and p53 pathways. (**a**) Representative Western blots and semi-quantitative analysis of p-JNK in cortex at various time points after MCAO. $n=4$, $*p<0.05$ compared with vehicle group. (**b**) Immunofluorescence photomicrographs of p-c-jun at 24 h after MCAO, scale bar = 20 μm. (**c**) Representative Western blots and semi-quantitative analysis of p53 in the nuclei at various time points after MCAO. $**p<0.01$ compared with vehicle group. (**d**) Immunofluorescence photomicrographs of Puma at 24 h after MCAO, scale bar = 20 μm

data clearly demonstrated that sevoflurane preconditioning reduced cytochrome *c* release, a marker for the mitochondrial apoptotic pathway, further indicating that sevoflurane preconditioning largely inhibits mitochondrial apoptotic pathway.

One of the checkpoints of the mitochondrial apoptotic pathway is regulated by the balance between anti-apoptotic proteins and pro-apoptotic proteins of the Bcl-2 family [20, 22, 31]. Previous reports suggested that APC might regulate Bcl-2 family proteins. Sevoflurane exposure during 30 min MCAO in rats reduced the Bax level as early as 4 h after ischemic insult [15]. In a rat forebrain ischemia model, sevoflurane increased the levels of Bcl-2 and Mdm-2 and reduced the Bax level in the first 3 days after ischemia [32]. Sevoflurane preconditioning was also reported to increase Bcl-2 in rat brain following focal ischemia [19]. In this study, we systemically analyzed both anti-apoptotic and pro-apoptotic protein levels of Bcl-2 family and found that the overall effect of sevoflurane preconditioning was to increase the ratio of anti-apoptotic proteins over pro-apoptotic proteins of Bcl-2 family, therefore inhibiting apoptotic cell death after cerebral ischemia.

It is unclear how sevoflurane preconditioning influences the expression of Bcl-2 family proteins. Among the transcription factors that regulate the Bcl-2 family, c-jun and p53 are noticeable [23, 24, 33]. JNK pathway activates Bad and Bax [34–36]; JNK can also induce the expression of p53 [37]. The activation of p53 promotes apoptosis. In mice deficient in p53, Bcl-2 increases but Bax decreases in several tissues, suggesting a possible mechanism by which p53 regulates apoptosis [33]. In addition, p53 induces Puma, which interacts with Bcl-xL and promotes mitochondrial translocation and multimerization of Bax [25]. We observed that sevoflurane preconditioning inhibited JNK and p53 pathways, which could be contributing factors in sevoflurane preconditioning attenuation of apoptotic cell death after stroke.

In summary, we demonstrated that sevoflurane preconditioning protected the brain against brain ischemia and suppressed apoptotic cell death following MCAO in rats by regulating Bcl-2 family members. Sevoflurane preconditioning could be a useful method to induce ischemic tolerance.

Acknowledgments This work was supported by NSFC 81301123 (to HW), 81171149, 81371306 (to YG), and 81228008 (to JC); the Shanghai Committee of Science and Technology Support Program 14431907002 (to YG); the Doctoral Fund of the Chinese Ministry of Education 20120071110042 (JC); National Institutes of Health/National Institute of Neurological Disorders and Stroke grants NS36736, NS43802, and NS45048 (to JC); and the Natural Science Foundation of Shanghai 14ZR1434600 (to HS).

References

1. Kersten JR, Schmeling TJ, Pagel PS, Gross GJ, Warltier DC (1997) Isoflurane mimics ischemic preconditioning via activation of K(ATP) channels: reduction of myocardial infarct size with an acute memory phase. Anesthesiology 87:361–370
2. Stetler RA, Leak RK, Gan Y, Li P, Zhang F, Hu X et al (2014) Preconditioning provides neuroprotection in models of CNS disease: paradigms and clinical significance. Prog Neurobiol 114:58–83
3. Chen F, Qi Z, Luo Y, Hinchliffe T, Ding G, Xia Y et al (2014) Non-pharmaceutical therapies for stroke: mechanisms and clinical implications. Prog Neurobiol 115:246–269
4. Deng J, Lei C, Chen Y, Fang Z, Yang Q, Zhang H et al (2014) Neuroprotective gases – fantasy or reality for clinical use? Prog Neurobiol 115:210–245
5. Anrather J, Hallenbeck J (2013) Biological networks in ischemic tolerance — rethinking the approach to clinical conditioning. Transl Stroke Res 4:114–129
6. Gao X, Zhang H, Steinberg G, Zhao H (2010) The Akt pathway is involved in rapid ischemic tolerance in focal ischemia in rats. Transl Stroke Res 1:202–209
7. Koch S (2013) Moving towards preconditioning for neurological disorders: are we ready for clinical trials? Transl Stroke Res 4:15–18
8. Meller R, Simon R (2013) Tolerance to ischemia—an increasingly complex biology. Transl Stroke Res 4:40–50
9. Seifert H, Pennypacker K (2014) Molecular and cellular immune responses to ischemic brain injury. Transl Stroke Res 5:543–553
10. Kehl F, Payne RS, Roewer N, Schurr A (2004) Sevoflurane-induced preconditioning of rat brain in vitro and the role of KATP channels. Brain Res 1021:76–81
11. Payne RS, Akca O, Roewer N, Schurr A, Kehl F (2005) Sevoflurane-induced preconditioning protects against cerebral ischemic neuronal damage in rats. Brain Res 1034:147–152
12. Zuo Z, Wang Y, Huang Y (2006) Isoflurane preconditioning protects human neuroblastoma SH-SY5Y cells against in vitro simulated ischemia-reperfusion through the activation of extracellular signal-regulated kinases pathway. Eur J Pharmacol 542:84–91
13. Bickler PE, Zhan X, Fahlman CS (2005) Isoflurane preconditions hippocampal neurons against oxygen-glucose deprivation: role of intracellular Ca2+ and mitogen-activated protein kinase signaling. Anesthesiology 103:532–539
14. Codaccioni JL, Velly LJ, Moubarik C, Bruder NJ, Pisano PS, Guillet BA (2009) Sevoflurane preconditioning against focal cerebral ischemia: inhibition of apoptosis in the face of transient improvement of neurological outcome. Anesthesiology 110:1271–1278
15. Engelhard K, Werner C, Eberspacher E, Pape M, Blobner M, Hutzler P et al (2004) Sevoflurane and propofol influence the expression of apoptosis-regulating proteins after cerebral ischaemia and reperfusion in rats. Eur J Anaesthesiol 21:530–537
16. Wise-Faberowski L, Raizada MK, Sumners C (2003) Desflurane and sevoflurane attenuate oxygen and glucose deprivation-induced neuronal cell death. J Neurosurg Anesthesiol 15:193–199
17. Yang Q, Dong H, Deng J, Wang Q, Ye R, Li X et al (2011) Sevoflurane preconditioning induces neuroprotection through reactive oxygen species-mediated up-regulation of antioxidant enzymes in rats. Anesth Analg 112:931–937
18. Chen Y, Nie H, Tian L, Tong L, Deng J, Zhang Y et al (2015) Sevoflurane preconditioning-induced neuroprotection is associated with Akt activation via carboxy-terminal modulator protein inhibition. Br J Anaesth 114:327–335

19. Bedirli N, Bagriacik EU, Emmez H, Yilmaz G, Unal Y, Ozkose Z (2012) Sevoflurane and isoflurane preconditioning provides neuroprotection by inhibition of apoptosis-related mRNA expression in a rat model of focal cerebral ischemia. J Neurosurg Anesthesiol 24:336–344
20. Graham SH, Chen J (2001) Programmed cell death in cerebral ischemia. J Cereb Blood Flow Metab 21:99–109
21. Yu Q, Wang H, Chen J, Gao Y, Liang W (2010) Neuroprotections and mechanisms of inhalational anesthetics against brain ischemia. Front Biosci (Elite Ed) 2:1275–1298
22. Zhang F, Yin W, Chen J (2004) Apoptosis in cerebral ischemia: executional and regulatory signaling mechanisms. Neurol Res 26:835–845
23. Liou AK, Clark RS, Henshall DC, Yin XM, Chen J (2003) To die or not to die for neurons in ischemia, traumatic brain injury and epilepsy: a review on the stress-activated signaling pathways and apoptotic pathways. Prog Neurobiol 69:103–142
24. Miyashita T, Harigai M, Hanada M, Reed JC (1994) Identification of a p53-dependent negative response element in the bcl-2 gene. Cancer Res 54:3131–3135
25. Yu J, Wang Z, Kinzler KW, Vogelstein B, Zhang L (2003) PUMA mediates the apoptotic response to p53 in colorectal cancer cells. Proc Natl Acad Sci 100:1931–1936
26. Zhang F, Wang S, Luo Y, Ji X, Nemoto EM, Chen J (2009) When hypothermia meets hypotension and hyperglycemia: the diverse effects of adenosine 5'-monophosphate on cerebral ischemia in rats. J Cereb Blood Flow Metab 29:1022–1034
27. Zhang F, Signore AP, Zhou Z, Wang S, Cao G, Chen J (2006) Erythropoietin protects CA1 neurons against global cerebral ischemia in rat: potential signaling mechanisms. J Neurosci Res 83:1241–1251
28. Yu Q, Chu M, Wang H, Lu S, Gao H, Li P et al (2011) Sevoflurane preconditioning protects blood–brain-barrier against brain ischemia. Front Biosci (Elite Ed) 3:978–88
29. Wang H, Lu S, Yu Q, Liang W, Gao H, Li P et al (2011) Sevoflurane preconditioning confers neuroprotection via anti-inflammatory effects. Front Biosci (Elite Ed) 3:604–15
30. Ye R, Yang Q, Kong X, Li N, Zhang Y, Han J et al (2012) Sevoflurane preconditioning improves mitochondrial function and long-term neurologic sequelae after transient cerebral ischemia: role of mitochondrial permeability transition. Crit Care Med 40:2685–2693
31. Zhang SD, Zhai J, Zhang H, Wan H, Li DZ (2006) Protective effect of isoflurane and sevoflurane on ischemic neurons and expression of Bcl-2 and ICE genes in rat brain. Biomed Environ Sci 19:143–146
32. Pape M, Engelhard K, Eberspacher E, Hollweck R, Kellermann K, Zintner S et al (2006) The long-term effect of sevoflurane on neuronal cell damage and expression of apoptotic factors after cerebral ischemia and reperfusion in rats. Anesth Analg 103:173–9, table of contents
33. Miyashita T, Krajewski S, Krajewska M, Wang HG, Lin HK, Liebermann DA et al (1994) Tumor suppressor p53 is a regulator of bcl-2 and bax gene expression in vitro and in vivo. Oncogene 9:1799–1805
34. Kamada H, Nito C, Endo H, Chan PH (2007) Bad as a converging signaling molecule between survival PI3-K/Akt and death JNK in neurons after transient focal cerebral ischemia in rats. J Cereb Blood Flow Metab 27:521–533
35. Cerezo-Guisado MI, Alvarez-Barrientos A, Argent R, Garcia-Marin LJ, Bragado MJ, Lorenzo MJ (2007) c-Jun N-terminal protein kinase signalling pathway mediates lovastatin-induced rat brain neuroblast apoptosis. Biochim Biophys Acta 1771:164–176
36. Eilers A, Whitfield J, Vekrellis K, Neame SJ, Shah B, Ham J (1999) c-Jun and Bax: regulators of programmed cell death in developing neurons. Biochem Soc Trans 27:790–797
37. Hong MY, Gao JL, Cui JZ, Wang KJ, Tian YX, Li R et al (2012) Effect of c-Jun NH(2)-terminal kinase-mediated p53 expression on neuron autophagy following traumatic brain injury in rats. Chin Med J (Engl) 125:2019–2024

Remote Ischemic Postconditioning (RIPC) After GMH in Rodents

Tim Lekic, Damon Klebe, Jerry Flores, Regina Peters, William B. Rolland, Jiping Tang, and John H. Zhang

Introduction

Germinal matrix hemorrhage (GMH) is the most common neurological disease of premature infants, partly because this germinal region is most vulnerable to spontaneous bleeding within the first 3 days of preterm life [1]. Intracerebroventricular expansion partly contributes to long-term brain injury through mechanical compression of surrounding tissues [2–4]. Devastating outcomes include hydrocephalus, mental retardation, and cerebral palsy [1, 5, 6]. Current treatment modalities are largely ineffective, and GMH has been thus far not preventable [7].

Remote ischemic postconditioning (RIPC) is a method by which brief limb ischemic stimuli protect the injured brain that has been shown to be neuroprotective in multiple stroke animal models [8–12]. Therefore, we hypothesized that modulation of brain injury through RIPC could be an eventual strategy to help improve outcomes after GMH.

Methods

All studies, protocols, and procedures were approved by the Institutional Animal Care and Use Committee at Loma Linda University. Postnatal day 7 (P7) neonatal rats were subjected to stereotactic ganglionic eminence collagenase infusion. Neonatal rats (P7) were subjected to either stereotactic ganglionic eminence collagenase infusion or sham surgery. Groups were as follows: sham ($n = 10$), GMH non-RIPC ($n = 10$), GMH + 1 week RIPC ($n = 10$), and GMH + 2 week RIPC ($n = 10$). Neurobehavior analysis at the fourth week consisted of Morris water maze (MWM) and rotarod (RR). This was followed by euthanasia for histopathology on day 28 as routinely performed [13].

Animal Surgeries

P7 Sprague-Dawley rat pups (14–19 g) were randomly allocated to either GMH or sham operation. A stereotactically guided, 0.3 U bacterial collagenase infusion model was used to model preterm right-sided ganglionic eminence bleeds [14–16]. Timed pregnant rats were purchased from Harlan Laboratories (Indianapolis, IN, USA) and pups of equally both genders were subjected to collagenase infusion [15]. Briefly, general anesthesia was obtained by using isoflurane (3 % in 30/70 % oxygen/medical air). Anesthetized pups were positioned prone, with heads secured onto the neonatal stereotactic frame (Kopf Instruments, Tujunga, CA, USA). The scalp was then sterilized (using betadine solution), and a small midline incision was made to expose the bregma. A 1-mm cranial burr hole was made using a standard dental drill (bregma coordinates: 1.8 mm anterior, 1.5 mm lateral, 2.8 mm deep) through which a 26-gauge needle was lowered, and at this position, clostridial collagenase VII-S (0.3 U; Sigma, St. Louis, MO, USA) was infused at 0.25 μl/min into the right basal ganglion. The needle was left in place for 10 min after infusion to prevent backflow. Thereafter, the needle was slowly withdrawn at rate of 1 mm/min, the burr hole was sealed with bone wax, and the scalp was sutured closed. All animals were allowed to recover under observation on a 37 °C warm heating blanket before being returned to their dams. Shams received all of the above without collagenase infusion, as routinely performed [13].

T. Lekic • D. Klebe • J. Flores • R. Peters • W.B. Rolland • J. Tang
Division of Physiology and Pharmacology, School of Medicine, Loma Linda, CA, USA

J.H. Zhang, MD, PhD (✉)
Department of Neurosurgery, School of Medicine, Loma Linda, CA, USA

Division of Physiology and Pharmacology, Loma Linda University School of Medicine, 11041 Campus Street, Risley Hall Rm 219, Loma Linda, CA 92354, USA
e-mail: johnzhang3910@yahoo.com

R.L. Applegate et al. (eds.), *Brain Edema XVI: Translate Basic Science into Clinical Practice*, Acta Neurochirurgica Supplement, Vol. 121,
DOI 10.1007/978-3-319-18497-5_11, © Springer International Publishing Switzerland 2016

Neurobehavior

For motor function, the rotarod measured striatal ability through a standard apparatus (Columbus Instruments) consisting of horizontal rotating cylinder (7 cm-diameter × 9.5 cm-wide) with accelerating ability to 2 rpm/5 s requiring continuous walking and balance to avoid falling off. Latency to fall was recorded by a photo beam circuit [17, 18]. MWM measured spatial learning and memory on three daily blocks, as per our prior studies [17, 18]. The apparatus consisted of a metal pool (110 cm diameter) filled with water to within 15 cm of the upper edge, containing a small platform (11 cm diameter) for the animal to climb onto. The animal swim path length was digitally analyzed by Noldus EthoVision tracking software. Cued trials (maximum of 60 s/trial) measured general associative learning, sensorimotor abilities, and motivation to escape the water with the escape platform obviously visible from above the water's surface. The platform's location was changed with every trial. Spatial trials (maximum of 60 s/trial) measured spatial learning given the platform was submerged, hidden, but discoverable. Probe trials measured spatial memory by recording time spent in the target quadrant once the platform was removed.

Animal Perfusion, Tissue Extraction, and Histology

Rodents were fatally anesthetized with isoflurane (≥5 %) followed by cardiovascular perfusion with ice-cold PBS and 10 % paraformaldehyde. Brains were removed and separated from surrounding tissues and post-fixed in 10 % paraformaldehyde and then 30 % sucrose (weight/volume) for total of 3 days. Histopathological pictographs used 10-μm thick coronal sections, caudally cut every 600 μm on a cryostat (Leica Microsystems LM3050S), then mounted and stained on poly-L-lysine-coated slides. Morphometric analysis of slides [13] involved computer-assisted (ImageJ 4.0, Media Cybernetics, Silver Spring, MD, USA) hand delineation of the ventricle system, hemisphere, caudate, thalamus, hippocampus, and corpus callosum. Borderlines of these structures are based on stereologic pathology studies using optical dissector anatomical principles [19–24]. Volumes were then calculated using an established formula: [(Average) (Area of coronal section) × Interval × Number of sections)] [25].

Statistical Analysis

Significance was based on $p < 0.05$. Neurobehavior was statistically analyzed by Kruskal-Wallis one-way analysis of variance (ANOVA) on ranks, followed by the Student-Newman-Keuls method, then repeated-measures ANOVA for long-term study. Other data were analyzed using one-way ANOVA, followed by Tukey post hoc test when appropriate. Analyses were performed using SigmaPlot version 10.0 for Windows.

Results

Both 1- and 2-week RIPC showed a tendency of improvement in rotarod motor testing (not shown) compared with untreated animals (i.e., GMH without RIPC), however, RIPC treatment significantly ($p < 0.05$) improved cognition ability (MWM; Fig. 1) and mostly attenuated neuropathological ventricular enlargement (hydrocephalus; Figs. 2 and 3) in juvenile animals following GMH.

Conclusion

Translational stroke studies, in particular animal modeling, are greatly needed to safely integrate basic preclinical scientific principles ahead of clinical application [26–30]. This study, in summary, showed that treatment with RIPC is a safe and noninvasive approach and this animal model demonstrated improved sensorimotor and neuropathological outcomes following GMH in rats. Further studies are needed to evaluate the actual mechanisms of RIPC neuroprotection.

Acknowledgment This study was partially supported by the National Institutes of Health grant RO1 NS078755 (Dr Zhang).

Disclosures None

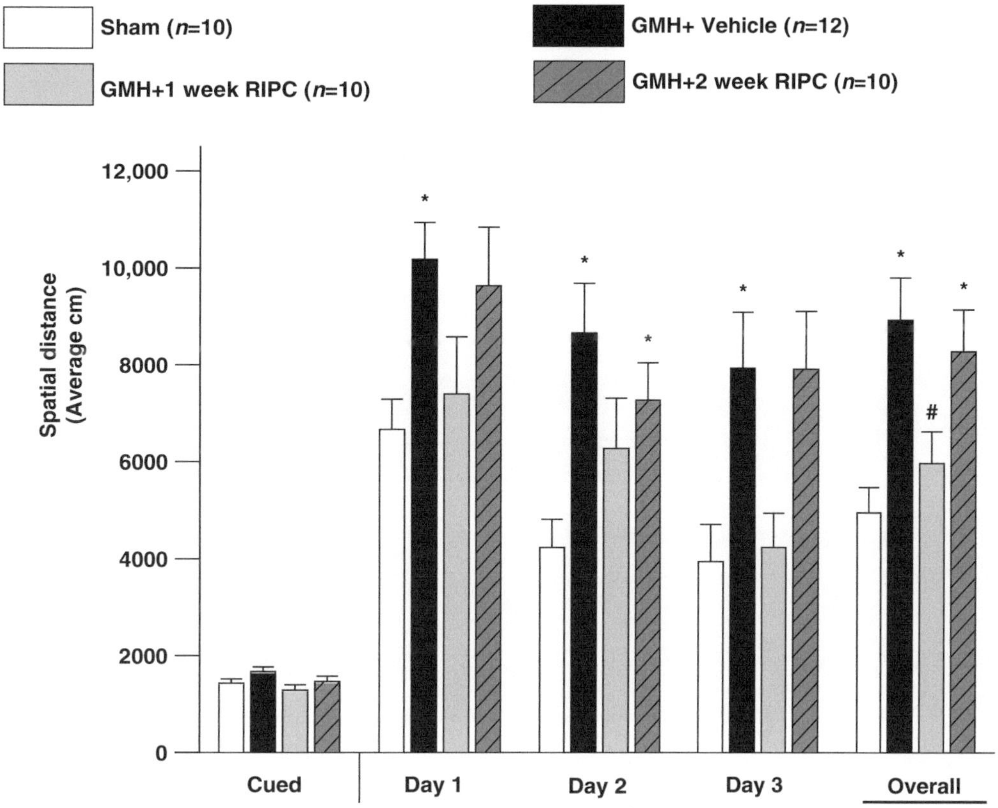

Fig. 1 Water-maze analysis at one month after GMH. Animals were tested using progressive levels, from cued to spatial trials. (*) <0.05 compared with sham; (#) <0.05 compared with vehicle. Data expressed as standard error of mean; $n=10$–12/group

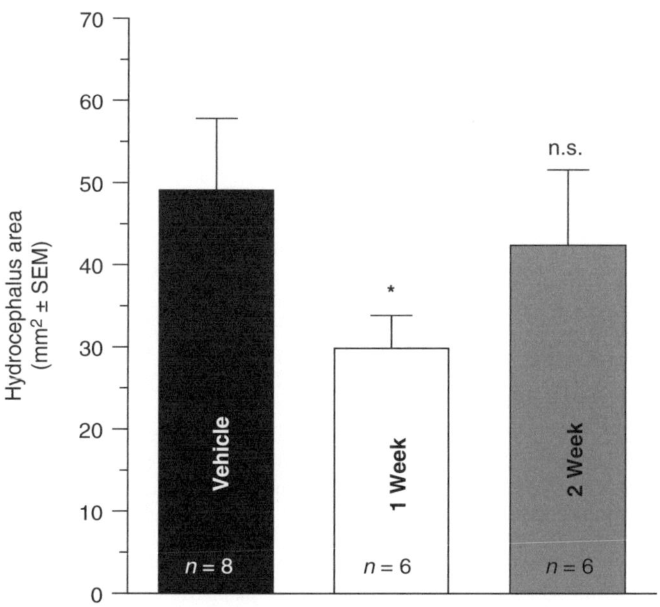

Fig. 2 Ventricular area (extent of hydrocephalus) at 1 month after GMH. (*)<0.05 compared with vehicle. Data expressed as standard error of mean; $n=6$–8/group

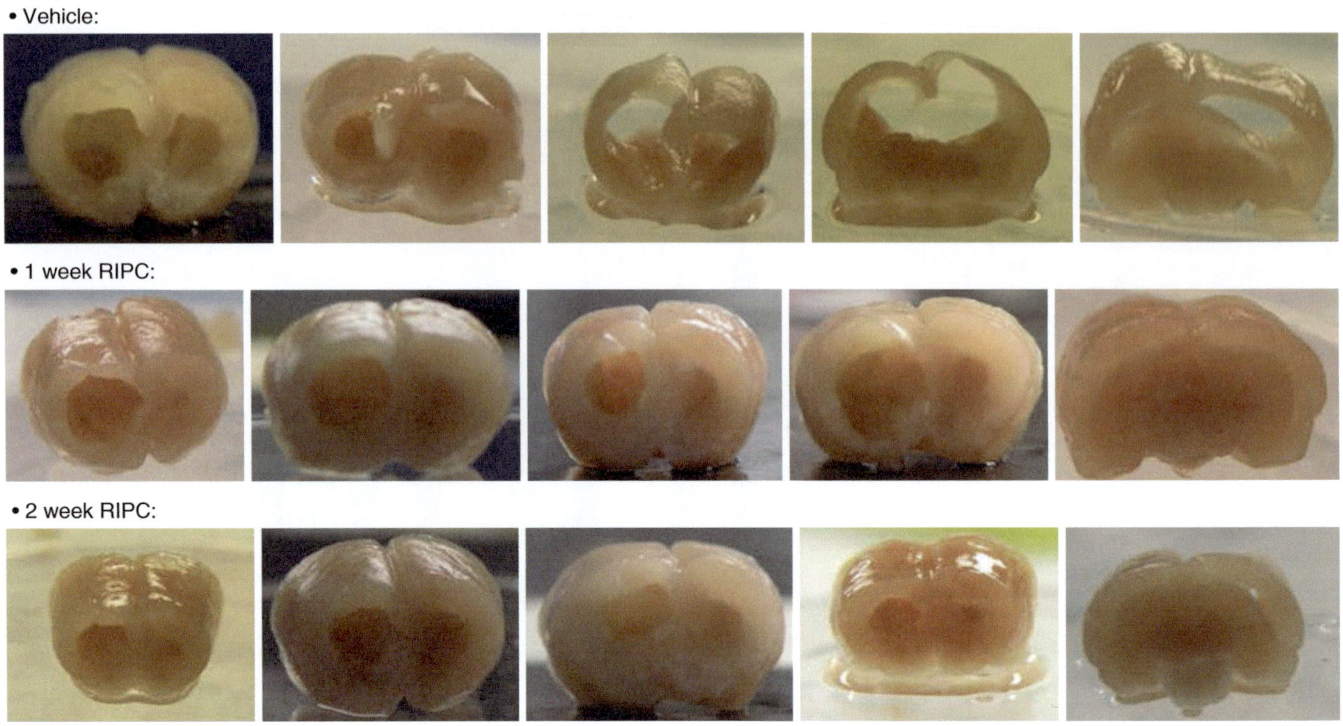

Fig. 3 Pictographs showing relative cortical thickness and ventricular and overall brain size between groups

References

1. Ballabh P (2010) Intraventricular hemorrhage in premature infants: mechanism of disease. Pediatr Res 67:1–8
2. Aquilina K, Chakkarapani E, Love S, Thoresen M (2011) Neonatal rat model of intraventricular haemorrhage and post-haemorrhagic ventricular dilatation with long-term survival into adulthood. Neuropathol Appl Neurobiol 37:156–165
3. Chen Q, Zhang J, Guo J, Tang J, Tao Y, Li L, Feng H, Chen Z (2014) Chronic hydrocephalus and perihematomal tissue injury developed in a rat model of intracerebral hemorrhage with ventricular extension. Transl Stroke Res. doi:10.1007/s12975-014-0367-5
4. Zhao J, Chen Z, Xi G, Keep RF, Hua Y (2014) Deferoxamine attenuates acute hydrocephalus after traumatic brain injury in rats. Transl Stroke Res 5:586–594
5. Heron M, Sutton PD, Xu J, Ventura SJ, Strobino DM, Guyer B (2010) Annual summary of vital statistics: 2007. Pediatrics 125:4–15
6. Uria-Avellanal C, Robertson NJ (2014) Na(+)/H(+) exchangers and intracellular pH in perinatal brain injury. Transl Stroke Res 5:79–98. doi:10.1007/s12975-013-0322-x
7. Whitelaw A (2001) Intraventricular haemorrhage and posthaemorrhagic hydrocephalus: pathogenesis, prevention and future interventions. Semin Neonatol 6:135–146
8. Keep RF, Wang MM, Xiang J, Hua Y, Xi G (2014) Full steam ahead with remote ischemic conditioning for stroke. Transl Stroke Res 5:535–537
9. Liu X, Zhao S, Liu F, Kang J, Xiao A, Li F, Zhang C, Yan F, Zhao H, Luo M, Luo Y, Ji X (2014) Remote ischemic postconditioning alleviates cerebral ischemic injury by attenuating endoplasmic reticulum stress-mediated apoptosis. Transl Stroke Res 5:692–700
10. Khan MB, Hoda MN, Vaibhav K, Giri S, Wang P, Waller JL, Ergul A, Dhandapani KM, Fagan SC, Hess DC (2015) Remote ischemic postconditioning: harnessing endogenous protection in a murine model of vascular cognitive impairment. Transl Stroke Res 6:69–77
11. Hoda MN, Bhatia K, Hafez SS, Johnson MH, Siddiqui S, Ergul A, Zaidi SK, Fagan SC, Hess DC (2014) Remote ischemic perconditioning is effective after embolic stroke in ovariectomized female mice. Transl Stroke Res 5:484–490
12. Zhou Y, Fathali N, Lekic T, Ostrowski RP, Chen C, Martin RD, Tang J, Zhang JH (2011) Remote limb ischemic postconditioning protects against neonatal hypoxic-ischemic brain injury in rat pups by the opioid receptor/Akt pathway. Stroke 42:439–444
13. Lekic T, Rolland W, Hartman R, Kamper J, Suzuki H, Tang J, Zhang JH (2011) Characterization of the brain injury, neurobehavioral profiles, and histopathology in a rat model of cerebellar hemorrhage. Exp Neurol 227:96–103
14. Manaenko A, Lekic T, Barnhart M, Hartman R, Zhang JH (2014) Inhibition of transforming growth factor-beta attenuates brain injury and neurological deficits in a rat model of germinal matrix hemorrhage. Stroke 45:828–834
15. Lekic T, Manaenko A, Rolland W, Krafft PR, Peters R, Hartman RE, Altay O, Tang J, Zhang JH (2012) Rodent neonatal germinal matrix hemorrhage mimics the human brain injury, neurological consequences, and post-hemorrhagic hydrocephalus. Exp Neurol 236:69–78
16. Leitzke AS, Rolland WB, Krafft PR, Lekic T, Klebe D, Flores JJ, Van Allen NR, Applegate RL 2nd, Zhang JH (2013) Isoflurane post-treatment ameliorates GMH-induced brain injury in neonatal rats. Stroke 44:3587–3590
17. Lekic T, Hartman R, Rojas H, Manaenko A, Chen W, Ayer R, Tang J, Zhang JH (2010) Protective effect of melatonin upon neuropathology, striatal function, and memory ability after intracerebral hemorrhage in rats. J Neurotrauma 27:627–637
18. Hartman R, Lekic T, Rojas H, Tang J, Zhang JH (2009) Assessing functional outcomes following intracerebral hemorrhage in rats. Brain Res 1280:148–157

19. Oorschot DE (1996) Total number of neurons in the neostriatal, pallidal, subthalamic, and substantia nigral nuclei of the rat basal ganglia: a stereological study using the cavalieri and optical disector methods. J Comp Neurol 366:580–599
20. Bermejo PE, Jimenez CE, Torres CV, Avendano C (2003) Quantitative stereological evaluation of the gracile and cuneate nuclei and their projection neurons in the rat. J Comp Neurol 463:419–433
21. Ekinci N, Acer N, Akkaya A, Sankur S, Kabadayi T, Sahin B (2008) Volumetric evaluation of the relations among the cerebrum, cerebellum and brain stem in young subjects: a combination of stereology and magnetic resonance imaging. Surg Radiol Anat 30:489–494
22. Reisert I, Wildemann G, Grab D, Pilgrim C (1984) The glial reaction in the course of axon regeneration: a stereological study of the rat hypoglossal nucleus. J Comp Neurol 229:121–128
23. Avendano C, Machin R, Bermejo PE, Lagares A (2005) Neuron numbers in the sensory trigeminal nuclei of the rat: A GABA- and glycine-immunocytochemical and stereological analysis. J Comp Neurol 493:538–553
24. Tang Y, Lopez I, Baloh RW (2001) Age-related change of the neuronal number in the human medial vestibular nucleus: a stereological investigation. J Vestib Res 11:357–363
25. MacLellan CL, Silasi G, Poon CC, Edmundson CL, Buist R, Peeling J, Colbourne F (2008) Intracerebral hemorrhage models in rat: comparing collagenase to blood infusion. J Cereb Blood Flow Metab 28:516–525
26. Tso MK, Macdonald RL (2014) Subarachnoid hemorrhage: a review of experimental studies on the microcirculation and the neurovascular unit. Transl Stroke Res 5:174–189
27. Marbacher S, Nevzati E, Croci D, Erhardt S, Muroi C, Jakob SM, Fandino J (2014) The rabbit shunt model of subarachnoid haemorrhage. Transl Stroke Res 5:669–680
28. Pluta RM, Bacher J, Skopets B, Hoffmann V (2014) A non-human primate model of aneurismal subarachnoid hemorrhage (SAH). Transl Stroke Res 5:681–691
29. Zhang YP, Cai J, Shields LB, Liu N, Xu XM, Shields CB (2014) Traumatic brain injury using mouse models. Transl Stroke Res 5:454–471
30. Wada K, Makino H, Shimada K, Shikata F, Kuwabara A, Hashimoto T (2014) Translational research using a mouse model of intracranial aneurysm. Transl Stroke Res 5:248–251

Animal Model Section

Patterns of Behavioral Deficits in Rodents Following Brain Injury Across Species, Gender, and Experimental Model

Richard E. Hartman and Earl C. Thorndyke III

Introduction

Although rats and mice are the most commonly used lab animals for models of brain injury, few studies have focused on comparative behavioral analyses between the species, and fewer still have assessed gender by species interactions. Rodents, like humans, can perform complex behaviors across a variety of situational demands. However, due in part to their remarkable resiliency, demonstration of consistent and significant behavioral deficits following brain injury can often prove challenging. Variations in testing protocols within and across laboratories, as well as innate differences between rats and mice and their interaction with gender, have muddied the waters even further.

A long history of research has suggested that rats may provide a better model of human behavior than mice, despite their increased cost for experimentation. For decades, rats were the preferred species for studying the effects of brain injury. There are a number of reasons for this preference, including a larger brain (making surgeries somewhat easier) and seemingly more complex behavioral abilities. A review by Wishaw and colleagues [31] concluded that mice present with a simpler, more reflexive repertoire and fewer complex social behaviors. Neuroanatomical differences between rats and mice may account for some of these differences [7, 28]. However, the benefits of mice include lower initial and housing costs, ease of transportation, and the increasing availability of transgenic and knockout mice. For these reasons, many behavioral laboratories, including our own, now test mice more often than rats. Fortunately, behavioral protocols specific to mice are being refined [6]. Furthermore, males are represented in the both the rat and mouse literature to a much larger extent than females. Although avoidance of behavioral variance due to estrous cycles is often cited as a reason to *not* use females, the lack of female representation in the literature presents a broad gap in knowledge, especially in light of the consistent behavioral and neuroanatomical differences observed between human males and females [29].

Our group has tested rodent models of traumatic brain injury to the cortex [1, 3, 8, 9, 14, 16, 23, 24], as well as subcortical injuries such as intracerebral hemorrhage [11–13, 17–19, 21, 26] and hypoxic ischemia encephalopathy [2, 4, 5, 10, 22, 25]. Although these individual studies have provided many insights into the deficits following these injuries and their mechanisms, we have become increasingly interested in comparing the similarities and differences among the behavioral and neuropathological phenotypes induced by different types of brain injury. Because the ultimate goal of these studies is to elucidate the sequelae and mechanisms of brain injury in humans, it is important to determine whether our models' endpoints accurately reflect those observed in humans.

Materials and Methods

For these analyses, water maze and rotarod data from several experiments performed in Loma Linda University's Behavioral Neuroscience Laboratory were combined into a common database consisting of 700 animals (~70 % mice vs. ~30 % rats; ~75 % male vs. ~25 % female). Although the majority of these animals were noninjured or "sham" controls, a subset (~15 %) sustained either traumatic brain injury ("cortical") or intracerebral hemorrhage/ischemia ("subcortical"). Various strains were used for each species, although Sprague-Dawley was the most commonly used rat, and c57Bl/6 was the most commonly used mouse.

The water maze is a test of spatial learning and memory in rodents, requiring the animal to find a slightly submerged platform within a large pool of opaque water. Cumulative distance to the platform (measured 5×/s) was used as the water maze outcome to control for potential differences in swim speed.

R.E. Hartman (✉) • E.C. Thorndyke III
Behavioral Neuroscience Laboratory, Department of Psychology, School of Behavioral Health, Loma Linda University, 11130 Anderson St., Loma Linda, CA 92354, USA
e-mail: behavioralneuroscience@gmail.com

R.L. Applegate et al. (eds.), *Brain Edema XVI: Translate Basic Science into Clinical Practice*, Acta Neurochirurgica Supplement, Vol. 121,
DOI 10.1007/978-3-319-18497-5_12,

The rotarod test consists of a rotating cylinder placed approximately 30 cm above a tray. The animal is required to walk forward to stay on this cylinder as it rotates to avoid falling. Latency to fall off the rotating cylinder was used as the rotarod outcome. Because the data were gathered over a period of several years and in multiple laboratory environments with diverse research goals, exact implementations of behavioral tests have varied, as have the specific equipment used. Although these differences have increased the variance within the data, the large number of subjects in the database to some extent counteracts these effects. Within- and between-subject ANOVAs were used to analyze the data. For homogeneity of variance and sphericity violations, the appropriate corrections were applied, and significant effects were analyzed with the Scheffé post hoc test.

Results

Overall water maze data suggest that control animals demonstrated an obvious and significant spatial learning curve, in which performance improved with each trial (Fig. 1a). Animals with subcortical injuries and cortical injuries were both significantly impaired. Although both injury groups performed similarly by the end of testing, animals with subcortical injuries started off significantly more impaired. By the end of testing, both types of injury were associated with severe deficits compared with controls. In a comparison of performance by species, both rats and mice started off with similar performance and demonstrated significant learning curves, but the mice reached asymptote earlier than the rats, which continued to improve (Fig. 1b). Across species, males showed slightly, but significantly, improved spatial learning performance compared with females (Fig. 1c). However, when broken down by species and gender (Fig. 1d), it becomes obvious that the effect was driven more by rats, in which males performed significantly better than females. In mice, however, the water maze performance of males and females did not significantly differ.

Overall rotarod performance suggests that cortical injuries produced profound deficits compared with subcortical injuries, which do not differ significantly from controls (Fig. 2a). Similar to the superior cognitive performance of rats in the water maze, rats also demonstrated superior

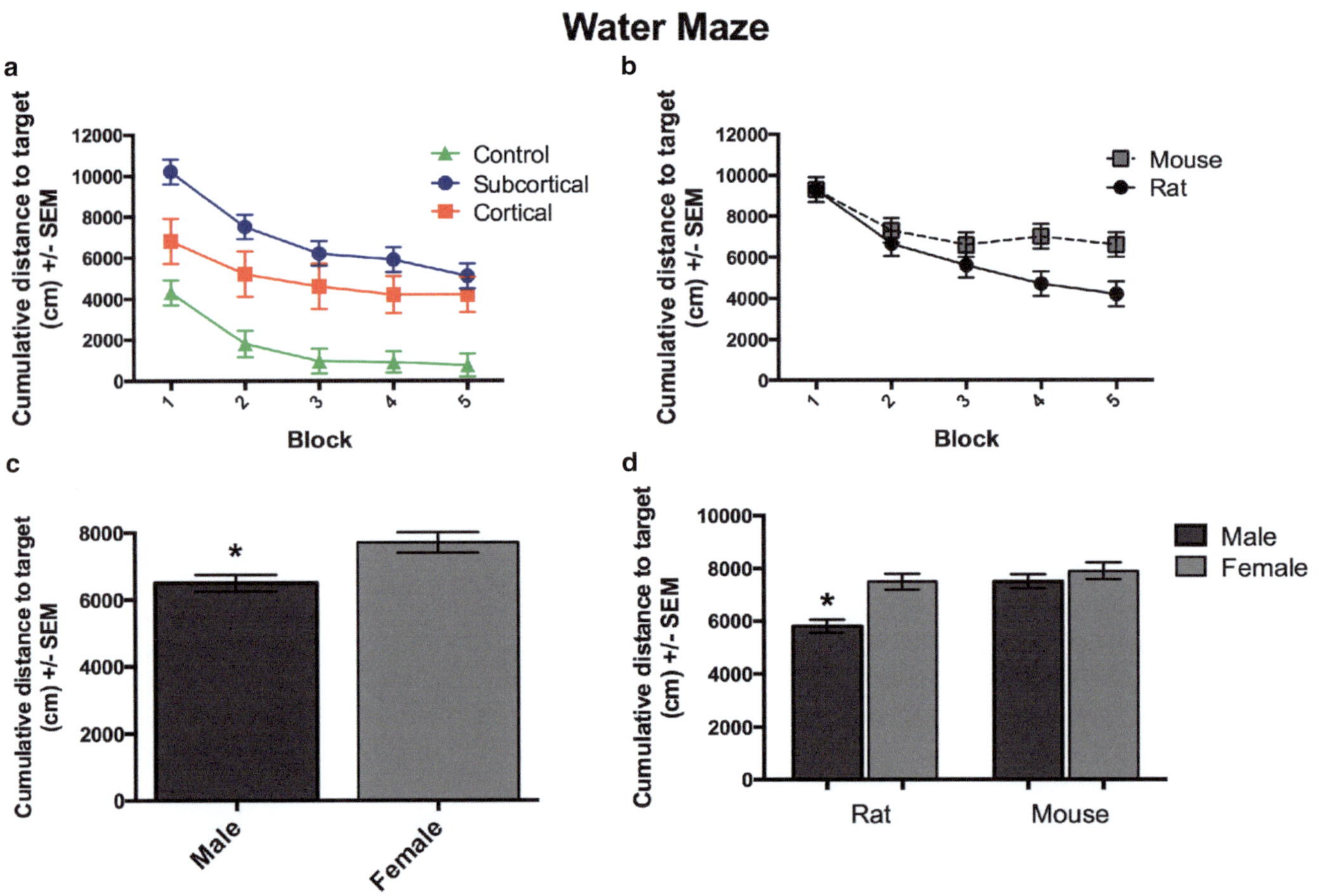

Fig. 1 Spatial learning performance as assessed by the water maze. (**a**) Control animals performed better across the spatial learning trials than cortical animals ($p<.05$), which performed better than subcortical animals ($p<.05$). (**b**) Rats performed better than mice ($p<.05$). (**c**) Males performed better than females ($p<.05$). (**d**) Male rats performed better ($p<.05$) than female rats, male mice, and female mice, which did not differ

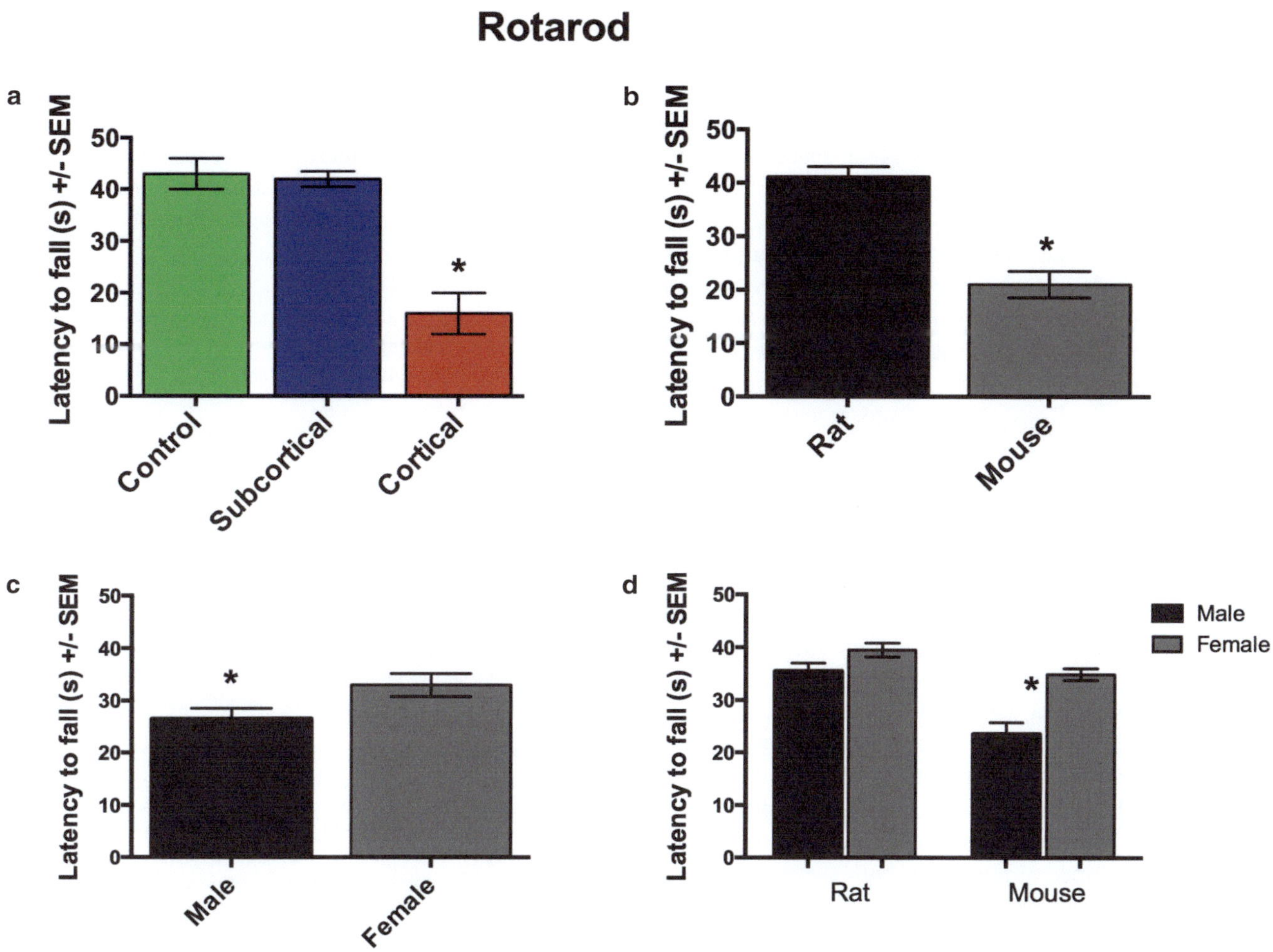

Fig. 2 Sensorimotor balance and coordination performance as assessed by the rotarod. (**a**) Cortical animals performed worse ($p < .05$) than control or subcortical animals, which did not differ. (**b**) Mice performed worse than rats ($p < .05$). (**c**) Males performed worse than females ($p < .05$). (**d**) Male mice performed worse ($p < .05$) than female mice, male rats, and female rats, which did not differ

sensorimotor coordination and balance on the rotarod by staying on the rotating cylinder significantly longer than mice (Fig. 2b). Across species, females showed slightly, but significantly, improved performance compared with males (Fig. 2c). However, when broken down by species and gender (Fig. 2d), it becomes obvious that the effect was driven more by mice, in which males performed significantly worse than females. In rats, however, males performed only slightly worse than females.

Discussion

These findings extend the existing body of literature by making comparisons among species, gender, and injury model across cognitive and sensorimotor behavioral domains. We have also shown that cortical injuries, such as those induced by a traumatic brain injury, were associated with profound sensorimotor and cognitive deficits. In contrast, subcortical injuries, such as those induced by intracerebral hemorrhage, hypoxic-ischemia, or both, were associated with even more profound cognitive deficits in the absence of significant sensorimotor deficits. The observed patterns of performance indicate the similarities of the broad pattern of neurocognitive deficits associated with these rodent brain injury models and those observed following human brain injury.

Likewise, we observed subtle gender differences that proved to be species-dependent. As often reported in humans, males performed subtly, but significantly, better than females on a task of spatial learning. However, this phenomenon was only observed in rats, and mice of both genders performed more like female rats in the water maze. The opposite pattern was observed on a test of sensorimotor coordination and balance. In general, males performed subtly, but significantly, worse than females on the rotarod. However, this phenomenon was most evident in mice, and rats of both genders performed similarly to female mice. Although many studies from our laboratory have not found statistically significant differences in gender, these results suggest that consistent, but subtle, differences exist. Indeed, a meta-analysis of rodent sex differences by Jonasson [15] concluded that there was evidence for gender differences in spatial learning, despite the fact that the majority of reviewed studies reported no significant differences.

Finally, we observed that, in general, rats performed better across both cognitive and sensorimotor behavioral domains. However, as noted for spatial learning in the water maze, this was only true for male rats. For sensorimotor coordination and balance on the rotarod, only male mice performed worse than rats. These results at least partly corroborate those reported in the literature. When Wishaw and Tomie [32] used the water maze to assess spatial learning in rats and mice, rats performed significantly better. Moreover, the rats demonstrated improved problem-solving strategies over time relative to mice, indicating that they were learning to learn, whereas mice showed no such problem-solving strategy improvement. Even though strain differences have been observed in both rats [20] and mice [27] due to varying swim speeds and visual acuity, rats' ability to conduct an organized search with high accuracy suggests that they are better problem solvers in the water. Even though it has been suggested that the Barnes maze, a dry land alternative to the water maze, may be more appropriate for mice, mice in our hands have performed similarly on both the Barnes maze and the water maze. Additionally, similar to our rotarod results, rats have demonstrated a greater ability to learn complex and coordinated asymmetrical motor behavior than mice in a test of reaching behavior and environmental manipulation [30].

Significant differences in task performance and trends in performance could indicate that particular species and gender combinations could provide better models for humans, or reveal the most important controls to consider, depending on the behavior of interest. Notably, gender differences were present, but were not the same for rats and mice. Mice demonstrated more pronounced gender differences in motor ability than rats, whereas rats demonstrated more pronounced gender differences in spatial learning. These findings have implications for study design. The extensive time and budget resources required for administration of a comprehensive battery requires that researchers use the most efficient design. Strategically designed batteries could identify initial behavioral outcomes and indicate the need for future behavioral testing while consuming the fewest resources. Depending on the nature of the injury and the deficits produced, the economic benefits of using mice over rats may be offset by the larger number of animals required to attain sufficient statistical power.

In summary, this study showed that the cognitive and sensorimotor abilities of rodents differ according to species, gender, and type of injury. This study also characterized distinct behavioral profiles for animals with cortical and subcortical brain injury models that resemble injury profiles in humans. Additional covariates, such as edema and lesion size, may further clarify these phenotypes. Overall, we provide evidence that abbreviated test batteries may be specifically designed to test deficits depending on the species, gender, and model.

Acknowledgments We would like to thank our collaborators at Loma Linda University, including the laboratories of Drs. John Zhang, Andre Obenaus, Jiping Tang, Stephen Ashwal, and Jerome Badaut.

Conflict of Interest The authors declare that they have no conflict of interest.

References

1. Ajao DO, Pop V, Kamper JE et al (2012) Traumatic brain injury in young rats leads to progressive behavioral deficits coincident with altered tissue properties in adulthood. J Neurotrauma 29(11):2060–2074
2. Ashwal S, Ghosh N, Turenius CI, Dulcich M, Denham CM, Tone B, Hartman R, Snyder EY, Obenaus A (2014) Reparative effects of neural stem cells in neonatal rats with hypoxic ischemic injury are not influenced by host gender. Pediatr Res 75(5):603–611
3. Bertolizio G, Bissonnette B, Mason L, Ashwal S, Hartman R, Marcantonio S, Obenaus A (2011) Effects of hemodilution after traumatic brain injury in juvenile rats. Paediatr Anaesth. doi:10.1111/j.1460-9592.2011.03695.x
4. Chen W, Hartman RE, Ayer R, Marcantonio S, Kamper J, Tang J, Zhang JH (2009) Matrix metalloproteinases inhibition provides neuroprotection against hypoxia-ischemia in the developing brain. J Neurochem 111(3):726–736
5. Chen W, Ma Q, Suzuki H, Hartman RE, Tang J, Zhang JH (2011) Osteopontin reduced hypoxia-ischemia neonatal brain injury by suppression of apoptosis in a rat pup model. Stroke 42(3):764–769
6. Crawley J (2008) What's wrong with my mouse – chapter 13. B chapter 1–20. Wiley-Liss, New York
7. Defelipe J (2011) The evolution of the brain, the human nature of cortical circuits, and intellectual creativity. Front Neuroanat 5:29
8. Donovan V, Bianchi A, Hartman R, Bhanu B, Carson MJ, Obenaus A (2012) Computational analysis reveals increased blood deposition following repeated mild traumatic brain injury. NeuroImage Clin 1(1):18–28
9. Fukuda AM, Adami A, Pop V, Bellone JA, Coats JS, Hartman RE, Ashwal S, Obenaus A, Badaut J (2013) Posttraumatic reduction of edema with aquaporin-4 RNA interference improves acute and chronic functional recovery. J Cereb Blood Flow Metab 33(0923559):1621–1632
10. Hartman RE, Lee JM, Zipfel GJ, Wozniak DF (2005) Characterizing learning deficits and hippocampal neuron loss following transient global cerebral ischemia in rats. Brain Res 1043(1–2):48–56
11. Hartman RE, Lekic T, Rojas H, Tang J, Zhang JH (2009) Assessing functional outcomes following intracerebral hemorrhage in rats. Brain Res 1280:148–157
12. Hartman RE, Rojas HA, Lekic T, Ayer R, Lee S, Jadhav V, Titova E, Tang J, Zhang JH (2008) Long-term effects of melatonin after intracerebral hemorrhage in rats. Acta Neurochir (Wien) 105:99–100

13. Hartman RE, Rojas H, Tang J, Zhang JH (2008) Long-term behavioral characterization of a rat model of intracerebral hemorrhage. Acta Neurochir (Wien) 105:125–126
14. Huang L, Coats JS, Mohd-Yusof A et al (2013) Tissue vulnerability is increased following repetitive mild traumatic brain injury in the rat. Brain Res 1499:109–120
15. Jonasson Z (2005) Meta-analysis of sex differences in rodent models of learning and memory: a review of behavioral and biological data. Neurosci Biobehav Rev 28:811–825
16. Kamper JE, Pop V, Fukuda AM, Ajao DO, Hartman RE, Badaut J (2013) Juvenile traumatic brain injury evolves into a chronic brain disorder: behavioral and histological changes over 6months. Exp Neurol 250:8–19
17. Lekic T, Hartman RE, Rojas H, Manaenko A, Chen W, Ayer R, Tang J, Zhang JH (2010) Protective effect of melatonin upon neuropathology, striatal function, and memory ability after intracerebral hemorrhage in rats. J Neurotrauma 27(3):627–637
18. Lekic T, Manaenko A, Rolland W, Krafft PR, Peters R, Hartman RE, Altay O, Tang J, Zhang JH (2012) Rodent neonatal germinal matrix hemorrhage mimics the human brain injury, neurological consequences, and post-hemorrhagic hydrocephalus. Exp Neurol 236(1):69–78
19. Lekic T, Manaenko A, Rolland W, Virbel K, Hartman RE, Tang J, Zhang J (2011) Neuroprotection by melatonin after germinal matrix hemorrhage in neonatal rats. Acta Neurochir (Wien) 111:201–206
20. Lindner MD, Schallert T (1988) Aging and atropine effects on spatial navigation in the Morris water task. Behav Neurosci 102:621–634
21. Manaenko A, Lekic T, Barnhart M, Hartman R, Zhang JH (2014) Inhibition of transforming growth factor-β attenuates brain injury and neurological deficits in a rat model of germinal matrix hemorrhage. Stroke 45:828–834
22. Obenaus A, Dilmac N, Tone B, Tian HR, Hartman R, Digicaylioglu M, Snyder EY, Ashwal S (2011) Long-term magnetic resonance imaging of stem cells in neonatal ischemic injury. Ann Neurol 69:282–291
23. Pop V, Sorensen DW, Kamper JE, Ajao DO, Murphy MP, Head E, Hartman RE, Badaut J (2013) Early brain injury alters the blood–brain barrier phenotype in parallel with β-amyloid and cognitive changes in adulthood. J Cereb Blood Flow Metab 33(2):205–214
24. Pop V, Sorensen DW, Kamper JE, Ajao DO, Paul Murphy M, Head E, Hartman RE, Badaut J, Murphy PM (2013) Early brain injury alters the blood – brain barrier phenotype in parallel with β-amyloid and cognitive changes in adulthood. J Cereb Blood Flow Metab 33(2):205–214
25. Recker R, Adami A, Tone B, Tian HR, Lalas S, Hartman RE, Obenaus A, Ashwal S (2009) Rodent neonatal bilateral carotid artery occlusion with hypoxia mimics human hypoxic-ischemic injury. J Cereb Blood Flow Metab 29:1305–1316
26. Rolland WB, Lekic T, Krafft PR, Hasegawa Y, Altay O, Hartman R, Ostrowski R, Manaenko A, Tang J, Zhang JH (2013) Fingolimod reduces cerebral lymphocyte infiltration in experimental models of rodent intracerebral hemorrhage. Exp Neurol 241:45–55
27. Royle SJ, Collins FC, Rupniak HT, Barnes JC, Anderson R (1999) Behavioural analysis and susceptibility to CNS injury of four inbred strains of mice. Brain Res 816:337–349
28. Snyder JS, Choe JS, Clifford MA, Jeurling SI, Hurley P, Brown A, Kamhi JF, Cameron HA (2009) Adult-born hippocampal neurons are more numerous, faster maturing, and more involved in behavior in rats than in mice. J Neurosci 29:14484–14495
29. Voyer D, Voyer S, Bryden MP (1995) Magnitude of sex differences in spatial abilities: a meta-analysis and consideration of critical variables. Psychol Bull 117:250–270
30. Whishaw IQ (1996) An endpoint, descriptive, and kinematic comparison of skilled reaching in mice (*Mus musculus*) with rats (*Rattus norvegicus*). Behav Brain Res 78:101–111
31. Whishaw IQ, Metz GAS, Kolb B, Pellis SM (2001) Accelerated nervous system development contributes to behavioral efficiency in the laboratory mouse: a behavioral review and theoretical proposal. Dev Psychobiol 39:151–170
32. Whishaw IQ, Tomie JA (1997) Of mice and mazes: similarities between mice and rats on dry land but not water mazes. Physiol Behav 60:1191–1197

Large Animal Stroke Models vs. Rodent Stroke Models, Pros and Cons, and Combination?

Bin Cai and Ning Wang

Review

Stroke is a leading cause of serious long-term disability worldwide and the second leading cause of death in many countries [12, 36]. Effective drugs for acute cerebral infarction are lacking, and only thrombolytic treatments have been proven effective by evidence-based medicine [8, 18]. However, the narrow time window of thrombolysis greatly limits its clinical application. Mechanical embolectomy is another method that has been approved by the US Food and Drug Administration (FDA), but its application is restricted because of the time window and technical conditions of hospitals [1]. Hence, finding effective neuroprotective agents remains a hot topic in neuroscience research. Rodent stroke models have been widely used in stroke research because of their advantages, such as cost, logistical ease, and ethical standards [26]. To date, more than 1,000 neuroprotective agents have been proven effective in animal studies, but all have failed in subsequent clinical trials [17, 24, 29]. One important reason for these failures is the huge gap between the studies using stroke animal models and those in patients with stroke (Table 1). Stroke models using small animals have tremendous differences from humans with respect to physiological and pathophysiological characteristics and so are very different from stroke in clinical practice [8, 21]. Narrowing the gap between stroke models and human stroke and promoting clinical translation of neuroprotective agents has become an urgent issue. The advantages and disadvantages of both large animal stroke models and rodent stroke models are reviewed below.

B. Cai, MD, PhD • N. Wang, MD, PhD (✉)
Department of Neurology and Institute of Neurology, First Affiliated Hospital, Fujian Medical University, 20 Chazhong Road, Fuzhou 350005, China
e-mail: caibin929@163.com; ningwang@mail.fjmu.edu.cn

The use of large animal stroke models is expected to narrow the gap between clinical trials and studies using small animal models and promote the clinical translation of achievements of basic stroke research because large animals, especially nonhuman primates, possess a variety of advantages when used for stroke models, detailed below and in Table 2.

Large animals are analogous to humans in genetic background, behavioral characteristics, concurrent complications, risk factors for cerebrovascular diseases, and anatomical structure of brain tissues and blood vessels [8]. In particular, their physiological features, such as vascular reactivity, inflammatory response, stroke recovery, and blood components [19, 31] are close to those of humans. Therefore, large animals better resemble human pathophysiological and clinical manifestations of stroke [28]. Similar to humans, most large animals have a gyrencephalic brain, and subcortical white matter accounts for a higher proportion of the brain than in small animals [8]. Because the white matter and gray matter exhibit different sensitivities to cerebral ischemic injury, models prepared with large animals more closely

Table 1 Gap between animal studies and clinical trials of stroke

	Stroke animal research	Stroke clinical trials
Condition control	Easy	Difficult
Subject	Animal	Human
Cerebral ischemia	Heterogeneity	Homogeneity
Reperfusion	Consistent	Inconsistent
Physiological parameter	Stable	Inconsistent
Administration time of drug	Narrow	Longer and different
Dosage of drug	Consistent	Inconsistent
Observation time point	Curative effect	Long term effect
Sample size	Small	Large

R.L. Applegate et al. (eds.), *Brain Edema XVI: Translate Basic Science into Clinical Practice*, Acta Neurochirurgica Supplement, Vol. 121,
DOI 10.1007/978-3-319-18497-5_13,

Table 2 Advantages of large animals and disadvantages of rodents in stroke model

	Advantages of large animal	Disadvantages of rodent
Physiological characteristics (genetic background, behavioral characteristics, concurrent complications, risk factors)	Analogous to humans	Great difference from humans
Brain	Gyrencephalic	Lissencephalic
Cerebral volume	Large	Small
Proportion of white matter	High	Low
Cerebral vascular diameter	Large	Small
Model resembles human stroke	Better	Poorly
Instruments in surgery, anesthesia, and monitoring designed for humans can be used	Yes	No
Neurological examinations, neurological behaviors are analogous to humans	Yes	No
Pathophysiological and clinical manifestations of stroke are analogous to humans	Yes	No
Drug safety is analogous to humans	Yes	No
Structural and functional imaging	Clear	Blurry

resemble stroke in humans. Although the failure to translate preclinical pharmacological insight into therapy is multifactorial, Dewar [10] proposes that failure to ameliorate ischemic damage to white matter has been a major factor.

Large animals have a larger cerebral volume and greater vascular diameter and are therefore suitable for complicated surgeries. Models for different needs can be prepared based on different surgical approaches, obstructed blood vessels, obstruction methods, and whether reperfusion is involved [33]. Large animals have larger cerebral vascular diameter; as a result, a reproducible model of brainstem stroke can be induced in rabbits using selective endovascular occlusion of the basilar artery [2]. With the assistance of superselective angiography, a catheter can be inserted into the middle cerebral artery (MCA) to induce an MCA embolism via injection of a thrombus, followed by thrombolysis with rTPA injected through the catheter, and the entire process of MCA embolism and recanalization can be clearly visualized [22]. Moreover, larger animals have a large venous diameter and are suitable for research on diseases such as venous sinus thrombosis.

Instruments that are designed for human use can be used to monitor physiological parameters, such as blood pressure, heart rate, and respiration. With the sufficient blood volume of large animals, repeated routine blood tests, clinical chemistry tests, and blood gas analysis are possible, which ensures consistent physiological parameters in the preparation of animal models.

Integrated analyses of neurological examinations, neurological behaviors, neurochemistry, and neuropathology are available in the same individual large animal [7, 16, 23].

Large animals are accessible for in vivo structural and functional brain imaging, including brain CT [3, 27], brain magnetic resonance imaging (MRI) [4, 7, 13], MR spectroscopy [9], brain positron emission tomography (PET) [5, 32], in vivo fluorescence, and ultrasound. It is feasible to qualitatively measure cerebral blood volume (CBV) and cerebral blood flow (CBF) by using robot-arm-mounted flat panel computed tomography (CT) in a large-animal model [3]. Correlation of cerebral metabolites with functional outcome suggest that MR spectroscopy may play a role in outcome prediction following cerebral infarction in higher primates [9]. Steady-state (15)O continuous inhalation was used for assessment of local cerebral blood flow, cerebral metabolic rate of oxygen, and oxygen extraction fraction using high-resolution PET [32]. These in vivo molecular imaging analytical techniques are important tools for research on stroke and the assessment of drug treatments and play a crucial role in the study of the mechanisms of pathogenesis and drug research and development.

Finally, using large animals is more conducive to monitoring drug safety because of their physiological characteristics, which closely resemble those of humans.

The Stroke Treatment Academic Industry Roundtable (STAIR) has recommended using cats or primates to verify the efficacy of drugs that have been proven effective in rodents before clinical trials [14, 30]. In addition, according to the regulations of the US FDA and the China State Food and Drug Administration (SFDA), all new drugs above Class 2 are allowed to enter clinical trials only after primate studies that meet the requirements. In a report published in *Lancet Neurology* in 2012, one of the most promising neuroprotective agents, TAT-NR2B9c, was studied in cynomolgus monkeys, which are closely related to humans, following the STAIR standards. In the study, the animal model was prepared under MRI guidance with dynamic monitoring of

Table 3 Advantages of rodents and disadvantages of large animals in stroke model

	Advantages of rodent	Disadvantages of large animal
Strains	Diverse	Few
Physiological information	Abundant	Lacking
Costs	Lower	High
Care	Easy	Difficult
Ethical issues	Simpler	Complicated
Transgenic and gene knockout	Accessible	Difficult
MCAO model by suture	Easy	Difficult
Surgery, anesthesia, and monitoring	Easy	Complicated
Operative injuries	Severe	Mild
Cerebral infarction volume	Stable	Unstable
Neurological function impairment	Stable	Unstable

changes in animal behavior, imaging, genomics, and pathology, as well as a comprehensive analysis of the results [7]. Such animal studies have narrowed the gap with clinical conditions and will thus facilitate the discovery of clinically translatable neuroprotective agents. In fact, the Phase II clinical trials of TAT-NR2B9c were also reported in the *Lancet Neurology* in 2012 and showed that TAT-NR2B9c reduced the number of small infarction foci and alleviated ischemic cerebral injury following endovascular treatment of aneurysms [20]. This clinical trial provided the first evidence for the feasibility and measurability of neuroprotection in ischemic patients.

Before the first use of the suture occlusion method to prepare middle cerebral artery occlusions (MCAO) in small animals in the mid-1980s, large animal stroke models were actually employed more frequently. Why has the use of large animal stroke models decreased? Mainly because rodent models possess some advantages (Table 3) that many large animal stroke models do not have, such as diverse strains, lower maintenance costs, ease of care, abundant physiological information, fewer ethical issues, and accessibility to transgenic and gene knockout technology [26]. Moreover, a variety of model preparation methods are available for rodents, and the MCAO model is easy to prepare using the suture occlusion method and shows stable features. In contrast, large animal stroke models possess some disadvantages, detailed below and in Table 3.

First, it is more difficult to prepare stroke models with large animals. Because of the highly tortuous blood vessels that are responsible for the blood supply to the brain in large animals, sutures cannot be inserted into the middle cerebral artery. Therefore, unlike small animals, the suture occlusion method is difficult to use in large animals. In the embolic model using blood clots, the location and extent of the embolism, as well as the possibility of spontaneous recanalization, is difficult to control, leading to unstable models. Thus, invasive procedures, such as opening the dura, are frequently required in large animals to generate and monitor cerebral ischemia. These procedures result in more severe injuries and postoperative exhaustion in animals and thus in difficulties in monitoring neurological functions [15]. Although opening the dura can be avoided when the middle cerebral artery is accessed through the orbital-cranial approach, it requires removal of the eye, making it impossible to assess visual spatial neglect after a stroke [35].

Large animal stroke models usually have variations in cerebral infarction volume and neurological function impairment grading, which are mainly related to large fluctuations of physiological parameters, variability of the brain collateral circulation, and the use of anesthesia, which may affect the outcome of cerebral ischemia, leading to higher mortality [25].

Large animals must undergo major surgeries for model preparation, which requires large amounts of specialized equipment and personnel for the surgery, anesthesia, and monitoring, and onerous intraoperative and postoperative monitoring.

Large animals undergo slow reproduction and have less information regarding their physiological parameters and pathological manifestations, leading to a lack of experimental data available for analysis and comparison. Transgenic models are still relatively rare in large animals.

The public is more concerned about the welfare of large animals, especially nonhuman primates, and the related ethical issues are thus more complicated, which seriously affects the undertaking of experiments involving large animals.

Finally, high costs are an important factor that hinders the use of large animals, especially nonhuman primates.

Which species of animals will be selected in future stroke studies? Rodents should be selected as stroke models for initial testing because rodent stroke models are easy to prepare and have a high success rate, highly stable infarct volume, and a close resemblance to humans with respect to cerebrovascular anatomy and physiology [6, 11]. In addition, the availability of various strains, low cost, and accessibility of gene knockout and transgenic technology also make rodents a desirable model for research on the pathophysiology and recovery mechanisms of stroke.

After protective effects have been shown in small animals such as rodents, the efficacy should then be confirmed in large animals, especially nonprimate large animals such as rabbits, cats, dogs, pigs, cattle, and sheep [34]. The characteristics of the animals should be considered in the selection of animal models. For example, rabbits have less tortuous cerebral blood vessels and can be used for the preparation of MCA embolic and thrombolytic models through intervention. However, similar to rats, rabbits do not have a gyrencephalic brain structure. In contrast, even though they have gyrencephalic brain structure, cats are not suitable for preparing models through interventions due to their tortuous blood vessels.

Nonhuman primates can be considered for further validation after efficacy has been demonstrated in nonprimate large animals. As we design nonhuman primate stroke models, several factors, including the choice of species, the method of inducing the stroke, and the choice of outcome measures, should be considered [8]. Different primate species possess different characteristics. For example, marmosets have the advantage of low body weight. The animals should be selected according to the needs of the study.

Continuous exploration is needed to improve model preparation methods and establish stable large animal stroke models that more closely resemble human stroke. For example, the use of a less invasive method for preparing models and dosing enables more accurate control of the ischemic location, extent of ischemia, and the subsequent reperfusion, eventually leading to better translation into clinical interventions. Finally, attention should be paid to establishing large transgenic animals for stroke research.

The use of large animals, especially nonhuman primates, in China has a variety of advantages. China has rich primate resources, with many primate animal study centers that have the capacity for large-scale primate care and breeding. Genetic engineering of economic animal models, such as mature technology developed for transgenic pigs and cattle, has made rapid progress in China. At present, animal rights activists in China are not as active, and thus, there is less resistance to studies using large animals. Therefore, these advantages will facilitate studies with large animal stroke models in China.

Acknowledgments This work was supported by grant No. 81171114 of Natural Science Foundation of China (BC), grant No. 2014-ZQN-ZD-18 of Fujian Provincial Medical Project for Middle-aged and Young Talents (BC), and the National key clinical specialty discipline construction program and the Fujian key clinical specialty discipline construction program.

Conflicts of Interest The authors declare that they have no conflict of interest.

References

1. Adams HP Jr, del Zoppo G, Alberts MJ, Bhatt DL, Brass L, Furlan A, Grubb RL, Higashida RT, Jauch EC, Kidwell C, Lyden PD, Morgenstern LB, Qureshi AI, Rosenwasser RH, Scott PA, Wijdicks EF, American Heart Association; American Stroke Association Stroke Council; Clinical Cardiology Council; Cardiovascular Radiology and Intervention Council; Atherosclerotic Peripheral Vascular Disease and Quality of Care Outcomes in Research Interdisciplinary Working Groups (2007) Guidelines for the early management of adults with ischemic stroke: a guideline from the American Heart Association/American Stroke Association Stroke Council, Clinical Cardiology Council, Cardiovascular Radiology and Intervention Council, and the Atherosclerotic Peripheral Vascular Disease and Quality of Care Outcomes in Research Interdisciplinary Working Groups: the American Academy of Neurology affirms the value of this guideline as an educational tool for neurologists. Stroke 38:1655–1711
2. Amiridze N, Gullapalli R, Hoffman G, Darwish R (2009) Experimental model of brainstem stroke in rabbits via endovascular occlusion of the basilar artery. J Stroke Cerebrovasc Dis 18:281–287
3. Beuing O, Boese A, Kyriakou Y, Deuerling-Zengh Y, Jollenbeck B, Scherlach C, Lenz A, Serowy S, Gugel S, Rose G, Skalej M (2014) A novel technique for the measurement of CBF and CBV with robot-arm-mounted flat panel CT in a large-animal model. AJNR Am J Neuroradiol 35:1740–1745
4. Bihel E, Pro-Sistiaga P, Letourneur A, Toutain J, Saulnier R, Insausti R, Bernaudin M, Roussel S, Touzani O (2010) Permanent or transient chronic ischemic stroke in the non-human primate: behavioral, neuroimaging, histological, and immunohistochemical investigations. J Cereb Blood Flow Metab 30:273–285
5. Boltze J, Forschler A, Nitzsche B, Waldmin D, Hoffmann A, Boltze CM, Dreyer AY, Goldammer A, Reischauer A, Hartig W, Geiger KD, Barthel H, Emmrich F, Gille U (2008) Permanent middle cerebral artery occlusion in sheep: a novel large animal model of focal cerebral ischemia. J Cereb Blood Flow Metab 28:1951–1964
6. Cai B, Lin Y, Xue XH, Fang L, Wang N, Wu ZY (2011) TAT-mediated delivery of neuroglobin protects against focal cerebral ischemia in mice. Exp Neurol 227:224–231
7. Cook DJ, Teves L, Tymianski M (2012) Treatment of stroke with a PSD-95 inhibitor in the gyrencephalic primate brain. Nature 483:213–217
8. Cook DJ, Tymianski M (2011) Translating promising preclinical neuroprotective therapies to human stroke trials. Expert Rev Cardiovasc Ther 9:433–449
9. Coon AL, Arias-Mendoza F, Colby GP, Cruz-Lobo J, Mocco J, Mack WJ, Komotar RJ, Brown TR, Connolly ES Jr (2006) Correlation of cerebral metabolites with functional outcome in experimental primate stroke using in vivo 1H-magnetic resonance spectroscopy. AJNR Am J Neuroradiol 27:1053–1058
10. Dewar D, Yam P, McCulloch J (1999) Drug development for stroke: importance of protecting cerebral white matter. Eur J Pharmacol 375:41–50
11. Dietz GP (2011) Protection by neuroglobin and cell-penetrating peptide-mediated delivery in vivo: a decade of research. Comment on Cai, et al: TAT-mediated delivery of neuroglobin protects against focal cerebral ischemia in mice. Exp Neurol. 227(1): 224–31. Exp Neurol 231:1–10
12. Donnan GA, Fisher M, Macleod M, Davis SM (2008) Stroke. Lancet 371:1612–1623
13. Duong TQ (2013) Magnetic resonance imaging of perfusion-diffusion mismatch in rodent and non-human primate stroke models. Neurol Res 35:465–469
14. Fisher M, Feuerstein G, Howells DW, Hurn PD, Kent TA, Savitz SI, Lo EH, Group S (2009) Update of the stroke therapy academic industry roundtable preclinical recommendations. Stroke 40:2244–2250
15. Fukuda S, del Zoppo GJ (2003) Models of focal cerebral ischemia in the nonhuman primate. ILAR J 44:96–104
16. Furuichi Y, Maeda M, Matsuoka N, Mutoh S, Yanagihara T (2007) Therapeutic time window of tacrolimus (FK506) in a nonhuman

primate stroke model: comparison with tissue plasminogen activator. Exp Neurol 204:138–146
17. Gladstone DJ, Black SE, Hakim AM, Stroke Foundation Heart of Ontario Centre of Excellence in Stroke R (2002) Toward wisdom from failure: lessons from neuroprotective stroke trials and new therapeutic directions. Stroke 33:2123–2136
18. Hacke W, Kaste M, Bluhmki E, Brozman M, Davalos A, Guidetti D, Larrue V, Lees KR, Medeghri Z, Machnig T, Schneider D, von Kummer R, Wahlgren N, Toni D, Investigators E (2008) Thrombolysis with alteplase 3 to 4.5 hours after acute ischemic stroke. N Engl J Med 359:1317–1329
19. Hanson SR, Harker LA (1987) Baboon models of acute arterial thrombosis. Thromb Haemost 58:801–805
20. Hill MD, Martin RH, Mikulis D, Wong JH, Silver FL, Terbrugge KG, Milot G, Clark WM, Macdonald RL, Kelly ME, Boulton M, Fleetwood I, McDougall C, Gunnarsson T, Chow M, Lum C, Dodd R, Poublanc J, Krings T, Demchuk AM, Goyal M, Anderson R, Bishop J, Garman D, Tymianski M, ENACT trial investigators (2012) Safety and efficacy of NA-1 in patients with iatrogenic stroke after endovascular aneurysm repair (ENACT): a phase 2, randomised, double-blind, placebo-controlled trial. Lancet Neurol 11:942–950
21. Howells DW, Porritt MJ, Rewell SS, O'Collins V, Sena ES, van der Worp HB, Traystman RJ, Macleod MR (2010) Different strokes for different folks: the rich diversity of animal models of focal cerebral ischemia. J Cereb Blood Flow Metab 30: 1412–1431
22. Jahan R, Stewart D, Vinters HV, Yong W, Vinuela F, Vandeberg P, Marder VJ (2008) Middle cerebral artery occlusion in the rabbit using selective angiography: application for assessment of thrombolysis. Stroke 39:1613–1615
23. Kito G, Nishimura A, Susumu T, Nagata R, Kuge Y, Yokota C, Minematsu K (2001) Experimental thromboembolic stroke in cynomolgus monkey. J Neurosci Methods 105:45–53
24. Lo EH, Dalkara T, Moskowitz MA (2003) Mechanisms, challenges and opportunities in stroke. Nat Rev Neurosci 4:399–415
25. Mehra M, Henninger N, Hirsch JA, Chueh J, Wakhloo AK, Gounis MJ (2012) Preclinical acute ischemic stroke modeling. J Neurointervent Surg 4:307–313
26. Mhairi Macrae I (1992) New models of focal cerebral ischaemia. Br J Clin Pharmacol 34:302–308
27. Moustafa RR, Baron JC (2008) Pathophysiology of ischaemic stroke: insights from imaging, and implications for therapy and drug discovery. Br J Pharmacol 153(Suppl 1):S44–S54
28. Nudo RJ, Larson D, Plautz EJ, Friel KM, Barbay S, Frost SB (2003) A squirrel monkey model of poststroke motor recovery. ILAR J 44:161–174
29. O'Collins VE, Macleod MR, Donnan GA, Horky LL, van der Worp BH, Howells DW (2006) 1,026 experimental treatments in acute stroke. Ann Neurol 59:467–477
30. Stroke Therapy Academic Industry Roundtable (STAIR) (1999) Recommendations for standards regarding preclinical neuroprotective and restorative drug development. Stroke 30:2752–2758
31. Traystman RJ (2003) Animal models of focal and global cerebral ischemia. ILAR J 44:85–95
32. Umemura K, Tsukada H, Kakiuchi T, Yamada N, Matsuura H (2005) PET study of the neuroprotective effect of TRA-418, an antiplatelet agent, in a monkey model of stroke. J Nucl Med 46:1931–1936
33. Watanabe O, Bremer AM, West CR (1977) Experimental regional cerebral ischemia in the middle cerebral artery territory in primates. Part 1: Angio-anatomy and description of an experimental model with selective embolization of the internal carotid artery bifurcation. Stroke 8:61–70
34. Wells AJ, Vink R, Blumbergs PC, Brophy BP, Helps SC, Knox SJ, Turner RJ (2012) A surgical model of permanent and transient middle cerebral artery stroke in the sheep. PLoS One 7, e42157
35. West GA, Golshani KJ, Doyle KP, Lessov NS, Hobbs TR, Kohama SG, Pike MM, Kroenke CD, Grafe MR, Spector MD, Tobar ET, Simon RP, Stenzel-Poore MP (2009) A new model of cortical stroke in the rhesus macaque. J Cereb Blood Flow Metab 29:1175–1186
36. Writing Group Members, Lloyd-Jones D, Adams RJ, Brown TM, Carnethon M, Dai S, De Simone G, Ferguson TB, Ford E, Furie K, Gillespie C, Go A, Greenlund K, Haase N, Hailpern S, Ho PM, Howard V, Kissela B, Kittner S, Lackland D, Lisabeth L, Marelli A, McDermott MM, Meigs J, Mozaffarian D, Mussolino M, Nichol G, Roger VL, Rosamond W, Sacco R, Sorlie P, Roger VL, Thom T, Wasserthiel-Smoller S, Wong ND, Wylie-Rosett J; American Heart Association Statistics Committee and Stroke Statistics Subcommittee (2010) Heart disease and stroke statistics--2010 update: a report from the American Heart Association. Circulation 121:e46–e215

Endovascular Perforation Murine Model of Subarachnoid Hemorrhage

Guo Jia Du, Gang Lu, Zhi Yuan Zheng, Wai Sang Poon, and Kwok Chu George Wong

Background

Subarachnoid hemorrhage (SAH) is a devastating condition caused by bleeding into the space surrounding the brain. It is a common cerebrovascular disease and one of the subtypes of hemorrhagic stroke. SAH accounts for about 5 % of all strokes, which is reported to be the second leading cause of death in the world. Patients with SAH are left with high rates of disability and mortality with regard to of brain injury [12, 20]. The causes of SAH mainly include ruptured aneurysms and nonaneurysmal perimesencephalic hemorrhage, with ruptured aneurysms accounting for 85 % of patients. The risks of rebleeding and de novo aneurysms contribute to the difficulty in curing the disease. Therefore, a standardized SAH model is needed so that exploration of the treatment of SAH can proceed [2, 13].

To better investigate pathophysiological mechanisms and treatment strategies after SAH, a variety of laboratory techniques have been developed to induce a SAH animal model. Reports in the literature suggest that three surgical procedures are commonly used for inducing SAH animal models: autologous blood or hemolysate injection or infusion, blood clot placement, or endovascular perforation. Injection of autologous fresh blood into the cistern or subarachnoid space is easy to perform and reproducible as the blood volume can be directly determined. In addition, it allows saline injection as a sham control. Unfortunately, there are some aspects of the SAH pathophysiology that cannot be mimicked by this procedure, such as mechanical trauma.

The blood clot placement method mimics some late events, to a certain extent, including delayed vasospasm and ischemia by surgically placed *ex vivo* clot, which is from autologously withdrawn blood on the adventitial surface of arteries. This permits investigation of late pathophysiological mechanisms and pharmacological intervention. The method was determined to have low animal mortality, however, it fails to reproduce early injuries of SAH and mechanical trauma, which is a limitation in these experiments.

Endovascular perforation is demonstrated by puncture of the intracranial artery on the skull base by an endovascular filament. It mimics the pathophysiology in humans most closely. Disadvantages are the inherent technical difficulties in establishing a simple, reliable, and reproducible model in a small rodent and high mortality caused by poor control of bleeding [11, 19].

Establishment of a SAH model in the mouse would be of particularly valuable because the mouse is a common mammalian species available for study; it has a well-characterized genome, making genetic manipulation and generation of genetically modified strains possible; and the species is relatively inexpensive to purchase and house. Thus, increasing efforts have been directed toward establishing a stable and reproducible SAH mouse model with limited surgical procedures and low mortality. Herein, we present an endovascular filament SAH model in C57/BL6 mice, which simulates human cerebral aneurysmal rupture near the bifurcation of the anterior cerebral artery (ACA) and the middle cerebral artery (MCA).

G.J. Du, MD[$]
Department of Neurosurgery,
the First Teaching Hospital of Xinjiang Medical University,
Urumqi 830054, Xinjiang Uygur Autonomous Region, China

Division of Neurosurgery, Department of Surgery,
The Chinese University of Hong Kong, Hong Kong, China

G. Lu, MD[$] • Z.Y. Zheng, MSc • W.S. Poon, FRCS
K.C.G. Wong, MD (✉)
Division of Neurosurgery, Department of Surgery,
The Chinese University of Hong Kong, Hong Kong, China
e-mail: georgewong@surgery.cuhk.edu.hk

[$]Author contributed equally with all other contributors.

R.L. Applegate et al. (eds.), *Brain Edema XVI: Translate Basic Science into Clinical Practice*, Acta Neurochirurgica Supplement, Vol. 121,
DOI 10.1007/978-3-319-18497-5_14,

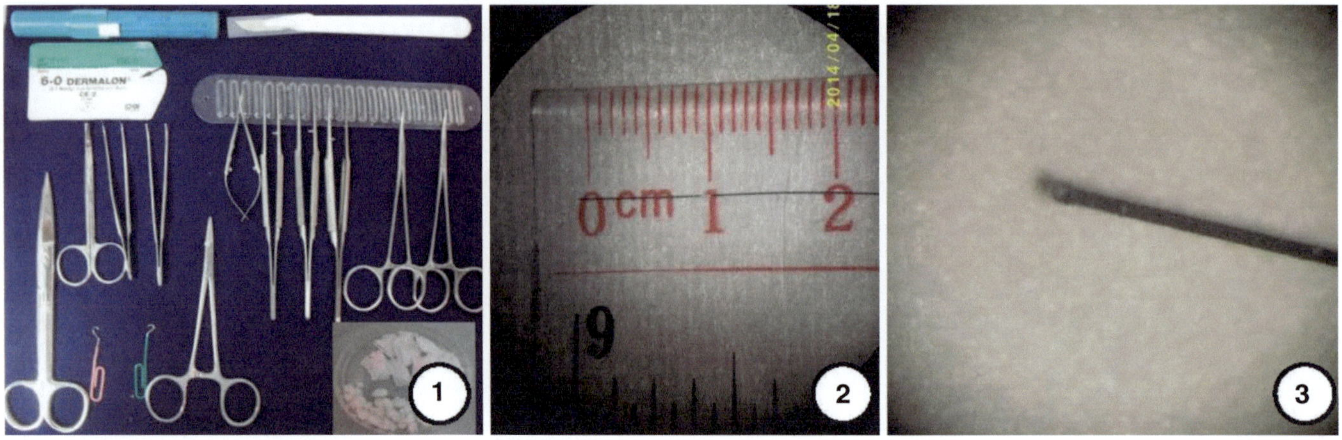

Fig. 1 Microsurgical instruments (①) and the filament (② and ③) used in inducing SAH

Materials and Methods

Animals

Pathogen-free, adult male mice C57BL/6, average weight 23–26 g, were obtained from the Experimental Animal Center of the Lo Kwee Seong Integrated Biomedical Science Building of the Chinese University of Hong Kong. All animals were housed in cages under a temperature-controlled environment at 21 °C with access to food and water. Animals were accepted pretrained by researchers 4 days before any experiment. The protocols for the experimental study received the approval of the Ethics Committee of the Chinese University of Hong Kong.

Experiment Approach

An endovascular perforation procedure was applied to establish the SAH model (n = 15) on the same day and observed for up to 14 days. Ten mice underwent sham surgery. Mice in the model of SAH underwent post-mortem examination to demonstrate evidence of SAH.

SAH Model Establishment

Preoperative Preparation of Instruments (Fig. 1)

A set of micro-neurosurgical apparatus included a microscope, microsurgical scissors, elbow microsurgical forceps, straight microsurgical forceps, bipolar coagulation, and micro-clips. Other equipment included a razor for shaving animal fur, normal forceps, ophthalmological scissors, needle-holder, scalpel, and sutures. Filaments (ShaDong Biological Tech. Co., Ltd., Beijing) marked with a certain scale were smoothed to blunt the top in advance under the microscope. Small cotton balls and gauzes were prepared to stop bleeding during the operation.

Anesthesia

C57BL/6 mice were anesthetized with intraperitoneal administration of 0.2 mL/100 g of a mixed solution consisting of 5 mg/mL ketamine and 2.5 mg/mL xylazine. Under anesthesia, the mice stayed still and unresponsive to any external stimuli, including cutaneous pinching and tail pinching with a sharp forceps, which the mouse would withdraw when pinched. For the righting reflex, mice did not right themselves from dorsal to sternal recumbency and muscles were relaxed when picked up by the tail. Mice had constant breath and heart beat. The absence of the palpebral reflex is considered a respectable depth. Because body temperature is reported to suddenly decrease after induction and remains diminished during anesthesia, hypothermia is considered a potentially fatal injury in small rodents. Therefore, maintenance of body temperature was included in anesthesia management. Mice were placed on a heating pad that was preheated to 37 °C and maintained until termination of surgery [1, 8].

Operation Procedures (Fig. 2)

Mice were fixed in a supine position and shaved of neck fur. A rectal temperature probe was inserted to monitor and maintain the body constantly at 37 °C with a heating pad during surgery. The neck region was disinfected with 70 % ethanol. Under a microscope (Zeiss), a midline neck incision was made and the skin was cut with a pair of scissors from sternum to chin (1 cm). The surrounding tissue was dissected bluntly and the salivary glands pushed aside. The left common carotid artery (CCA) was exposed and gently mobilized . Great care was taken not to harm the vagal nerve, which runs in the same surrounding tissue sheath as the CCA. Using the same technique, the left external carotid artery (ECA) was exposed and mobilized. The first ECA branch, which is the occipital artery, was mobilized and coagulated. The ECA was ligated as far cranially as possible and pulled to the other side of long ligation to the right side and fixed with adhesive plaster. Two 5–0 silk sutures were prearranged (1.5 cm segments)

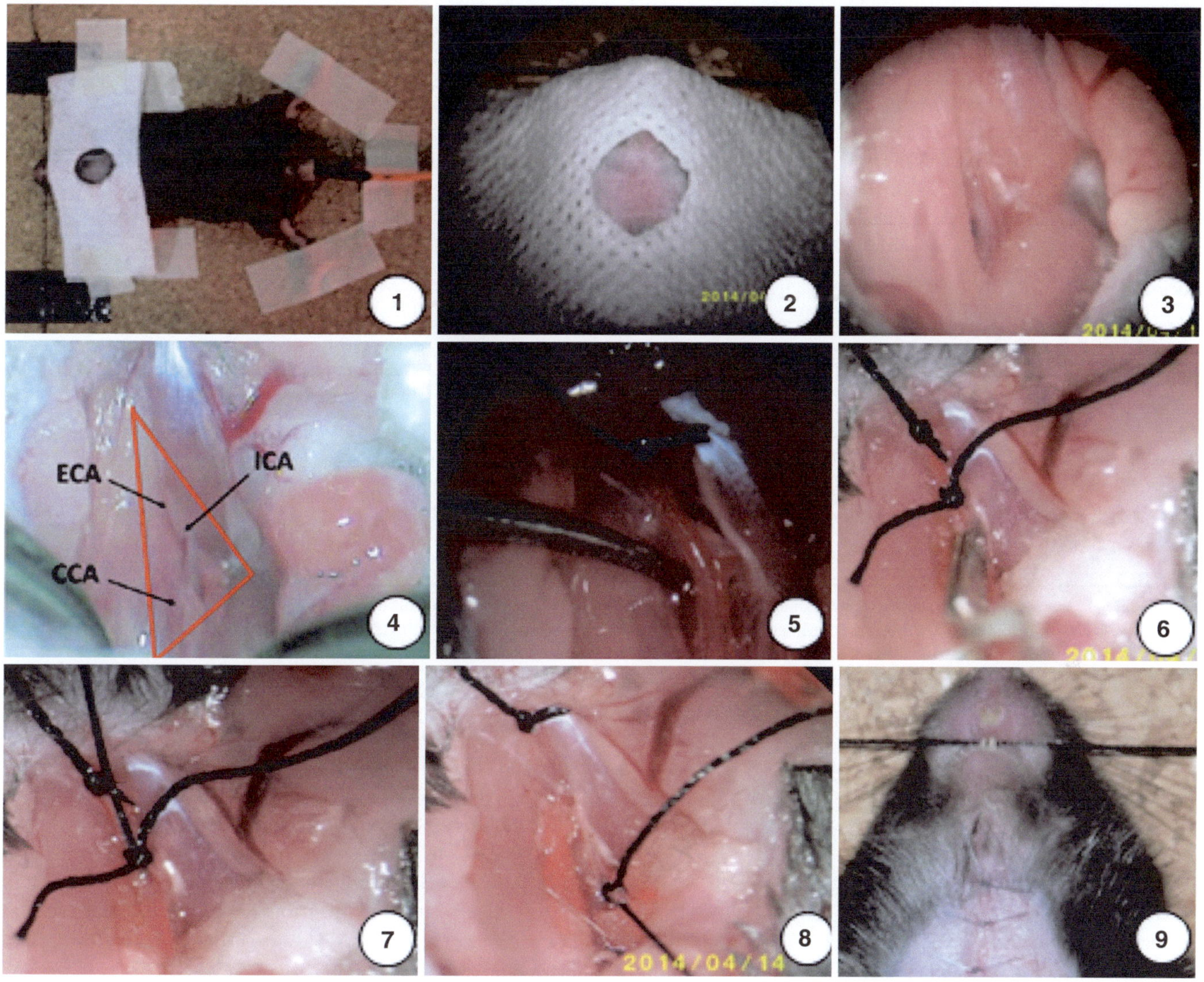

Fig. 2 Surgical steps for inducing SAH model in the mouse (as described in the text)

for the filament around the ECA. The distal of the left internal carotid artery (ICA) was gently exposed. The origin of the ECA was temporarily occluded with one micro-clip. A hole was cut as near as possible to the previous ligation for the filament insertion with a vessel micro-scissors. A 20-mm-long blunted 5–0 monofilament nylon suture was inserted into the ECA. Two prearranged sutures were knotted with the appropriate intensity and then the ECA was cut at thr hole point. The micro-clip from the ECA was removed and the filament was advanced with a forceps into the ICA to its bifurcations, where resistance was encountered. The filament was immediately withdrawn after advancing another 2 mm further to perforate the vessel. The total length inserted into the artery was defined to be 10 mm. The ECA was ligated by knotting the prearranged ligations tightly. The skin wound was closed immediately with suture after the removal of the filament. Mice were continuously observed under 23 °C until recovery and were then returned to their cages. Subcutaneous injections of 0.5 ml saline were given twice per day to all mice to standardize hydration. All of SAH mice were analgesized with buprenorphine (0.03 mg/kg body weight intraperitoneally) once per day for at least three days after surgery [3, 14, 17].

Mouse Motor and Sensory Scale (MMSS)

The Mouse Motor and Sensory Scale (MMSS) was used to evaluate the neurologic deficits of SAH mice before operation and at day 3, 7, and 14 after SAH induction [15]. The scale was combined from the prior scales in previously described examinations [4, 7, 9], which were comprised of motor (0–12) (spontaneous activity, symmetry of limb movements, climbing, balance) and sensory (5–15) (proprioception, vibrissae, visual, olfactory, and tactile responses) (Table 1). Neurologic function is graded on a scale of 5–27, with 5 indicating maximum functional deficits and 27 normal neurologic functions; the lower the score, the more severe the brain injury.

Table 1 A Mouse Motor and Sensory Scale (Parra et al. [15], 5–27)

Function		0	1	2	3
Motor	*Activity* (5 min open field)	No movement	Moves, no walls approached	1–2 walls approached	3–4 walls approached
	Limb symmetry (suspended by tail)	Left forelimb, no movement	Minimal movement	Abnormal forelimb walk	Symmetrical extension
	Climbing (on inverted metal mesh)	Fails to hold	Hold < 4 s	Holds, no displacement	Displaces across mesh
	Balance	Falls < 2 s	Falls > 2 s	Holds, no displacement	Displaces across rod
Sensory	*Proprioception* (cotton tip to both sides of neck)		No reaction	Asymmetrical head turning	Symmetric head turning
	Vibrissae (cotton tip to vibrissae)		No reaction	Asymmetrical head turning	Symmetric head turning
	Visual (tip toward each eye)		No reaction	Unilateral blink	Bilateral blink
	Olfactory (lemon juice on tip)		No sniffing	Brief sniff	Sniff >2 s
	Tactile (needle stick to palm)		No reaction	Delayed withdrawal	Immediate withdrawal

Parra scale [15] was combined from two prior scales: Garcia [7] and Crawley [4] comprised of motor (0–12)—spontaneous activity, symmetry of limb movements, climbing, balance—and coordination and sensory (5–15)—proprioception, vibrissae, visual, olfactory, and tactile responses

Results

Mortality

Two mice died in the first 24 h, two mice died with 2 days of SAH induction, and one mouse died within 5 days of SAH induction. In total, five mice died after SAH induction, with most dying in the first 48 h after the surgery, yielding a surgery-associated mortality of 33.3 % in our study.

General Observations and MMSS

Intraoperatively, the mice demonstrated deep breathing and evanescent hyperspasmia when there was a "give" during the puncture of artery. The mice exhibited signs of inspiratory dyspnea with depressed or paradoxical chest and abdomen movement with tachycardia, resulting in high mortality when the vagus nerve was irritated during the operative procedure. Postoperatively, all experimental animals were drowsy in the first 48 h after SAH, with no feeding and drinking behavior. Six mice moaned for about 1 week. Five mice exhibited ischemic symptoms, of which three mice showed ipsilateral drooping eyelids, similar to Horner's syndrome, due to a deficiency of sympathetic activity. Those with severe ischemia symptoms, including hemiplegia and rotation when picked up by the tail, were prone to die. The ischemia symptoms emerged variably from either the left or right side. The body weight of the SAH mice decreased significantly at day 3 after SAH procedure. The average body weight decreased more than 3 g. At day 7, body weight returned to the level of original states in the SAH group.

In the MMSS score analysis, mice showed a significant neurologic dysfunction from day 3 to day 14, with lowest scores on day 3 ($p < 0.05$). However, the sham control group showed an almost normal score of MMSS.

Post-mortem Determination

Immediately after death by sacrifice, isolated brains were examined under magnification. The distribution of hemorrhage was along the Circle of Willis around the cerebral space. The sham-operated mice were sacrificed as controls. There was no visible blood surrounding the cerebral space (Fig. 3).

Discussion

It is important to establish an ideal SAH animal model simulating clinical aneurysm rupture in humans. The SAH murine model depicted in this experiment exhibited the typical signs of SAH with comparable mortality to previous literature

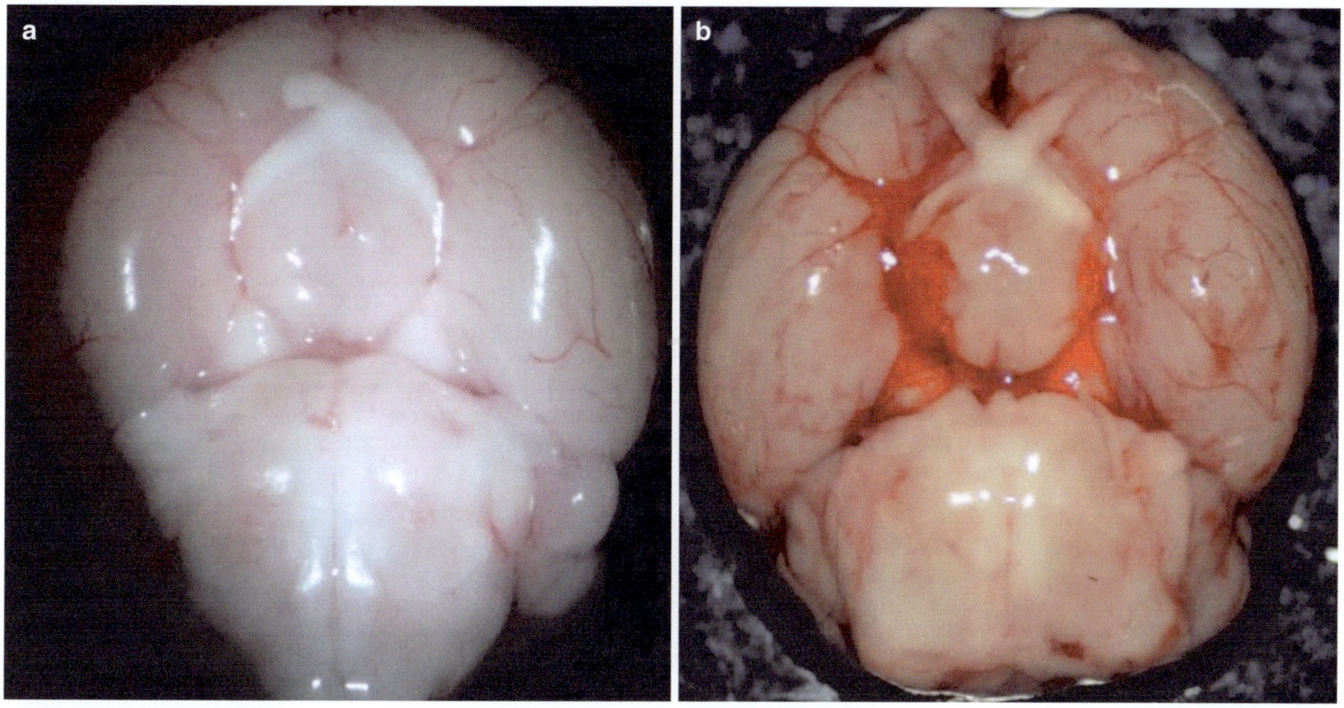

Fig. 3 General appearance of the subarachnoid hemorrhage under microscope. The isolated brains were shown on the ventral surface in sham (**a**) and SAH (**b**) mice

[6, 21]. The evanescent hyperspasmia presented during the operation was probably caused by the sudden increased intracerebral pressure (ICP), which is induced by bleeding into the subarachnoid space. The temporary increased ICP increased signs and symptoms in the animal model similar to the Cushing reflex. This can be considered as a sign by which to judge the condition of vessel perforation. The ischemia symptoms could be the result of hemorrhage-induced delayed cerebral vasospasm [5, 10, 15, 16].

An ideal SAH experimental model exhibits the following important characteristics [18]: (1) consistent and reproducible clot deposition in the space surrounding the brain; (2) uniform and controlled degree of hemorrhage; (3) mechanism of hemorrhage closely mimicking aneurismal rupture and blood distribution connecting with aneurysmal SAH; and (4) performance and reasonable cost. The SAH murine model reported herein satisfied several criteria above. The most frequently mentioned drawback of the filament perforation model in the literature is that bleeding volume cannot be directly controlled.

This problem can be resolved, to some extent, by ensuring the following: (1) suitable marked filament with heparin immersion is used; (2) a minimally invasive procedure; (3) operators capable of skilled microsurgical technique during SAH induction; and (4) good postoperative care. High mortality is a characteristic of SAH in humans. Endovascular puncture in the murine model has a relatively high mortality compared with the blood injection model, which indicates that this model closely mimics aneurismal rupture in humans. The limited attention afforded to mice in this context derives from the inherent technical difficulties in establishing a simple, reliable, and reproducible model in a small rodent. Despite the apparent technical impediments, establishment of a mouse model of SAH would be of considerable value.

Acknowledgment This work was supported by a direct grant from the Chinese University of Hong Kong (Reference no. 2013.1.105).

Conflict of Interest Statement All authors read and approved the final manuscript. The authors declare that they have no conflicts of interests.

References

1. Arras M, Autenried P, Rettich A, Spaeni D, Rulicke T (2001) Optimization of intraperitoneal injection anesthesia in mice: drugs, dosages, adverse effects, and anesthesia depth. Comp Med 51:443–456
2. Bassel Zebian GC (2012) Spontaneous intracranial haemorrhage. Surgery (Oxford) 30:136–141
3. Buhler D, Schuller K, Plesnila N (2014) Protocol for the induction of subarachnoid hemorrhage in mice by perforation of the circle of Willis with an endovascular filament. Transl Stroke Res 5(6): 653–659
4. Crawley JN (1999) Behavioral phenotyping of transgenic and knockout mice: experimental design and evaluation of general health, sensory functions, motor abilities, and specific behavioral tests. Brain Res 835:18–26

5. Dietrich HH, Dacey RG Jr (2000) Molecular keys to the problems of cerebral vasospasm. Neurosurgery 46:517–530
6. Feiler S, Friedrich B, Scholler K, Thal SC, Plesnila N (2010) Standardized induction of subarachnoid hemorrhage in mice by intracranial pressure monitoring. J Neurosci Methods 190:164–170
7. Garcia JH, Wagner S, Liu KF, Hu XJ (1995) Neurological deficit and extent of neuronal necrosis attributable to middle cerebral artery occlusion in rats. Statistical validation. Stroke 26:627–634; discussion 635
8. Gargiulo S, Greco A, Gramanzini M, Esposito S, Affuso A, Brunetti A, Vesce G (2012) Mice anesthesia, analgesia, and care, Part I: anesthetic considerations in preclinical research. ILAR J 53:E55–E69
9. Hamers FP, Lankhorst AJ, van Laar TJ, Veldhuis WB, Gispen WH (2001) Automated quantitative gait analysis during overground locomotion in the rat: its application to spinal cord contusion and transection injuries. J Neurotrauma 18:187–201
10. Hanafy KA (2013) The role of microglia and the TLR4 pathway in neuronal apoptosis and vasospasm after subarachnoid hemorrhage. J Neuroinflammation 10:83
11. Kamii H, Kato I, Kinouchi H, Chan PH, Epstein CJ, Akabane A, Okamoto H, Yoshimoto T (1999) Amelioration of vasospasm after subarachnoid hemorrhage in transgenic mice overexpressing CuZn-superoxide dismutase. Stroke 30:867–871; discussion 872
12. Kooijman E, Nijboer CH, van Velthoven CT, Kavelaars A, Kesecioglu J, Heijnen CJ (2014) The rodent endovascular puncture model of subarachnoid hemorrhage: mechanisms of brain damage and therapeutic strategies. J Neuroinflammation 11:2
13. Marder CP (2014) Subarachnoid hemorrhage: beyond aneurysms. AJR Am J Roentgenol 202:25–37
14. Park IS, Meno JR, Witt CE, Suttle TK, Chowdhary A, Nguyen TS, Ngai AC, Britz GW (2008) Subarachnoid hemorrhage model in the rat: modification of the endovascular filament model. J Neurosci Methods 172:195–200
15. Parra A, McGirt MJ, Sheng H, Laskowitz DT, Pearlstein RD, Warner DS (2002) Mouse model of subarachnoid hemorrhage associated cerebral vasospasm: methodological analysis. Neurol Res 24:510–516
16. Rowland MJ, Hadjipavlou G, Kelly M, Westbrook J, Pattinson KT (2012) Delayed cerebral ischaemia after subarachnoid haemorrhage: looking beyond vasospasm. Br J Anaesth 109:315–329
17. Schüller K, Bühler D, Plesnila N (2013) A murine model of subarachnoid hemorrhage. J Vis Ex (81):e50845
18. Schwartz AY, Masago A, Sehba FA, Bederson JB (2000) Experimental models of subarachnoid hemorrhage in the rat: a refinement of the endovascular filament model. J Neurosci Methods 96:161–167
19. Sehba FA, Pluta RM (2013) Aneurysmal subarachnoid hemorrhage models: do they need a fix? Stroke Res Treat 2013:615154
20. Sehba FA, Pluta RM, Zhang JH (2011) Metamorphosis of subarachnoid hemorrhage research: from delayed vasospasm to early brain injury. Mol Neurobiol 43:27–40
21. Sozen T, Tsuchiyama R, Hasegawa Y, Suzuki H, Jadhav V, Nishizawa S, Zhang JH (2009) Role of interleukin-1beta in early brain injury after subarachnoid hemorrhage in mice. Stroke 40:2519–2525

Assessment of the Correlations Between Brain Weight and Brain Edema in Experimental Subarachnoid Hemorrhage

Yu Hasegawa, Hidenori Suzuki, Takashi Nakagawa, Ken Uekawa, Nobutaka Koibuchi, Takayuki Kawano, and Shokei Kim-Mitsuyama

Introduction

Subarachnoid hemorrhage (SAH) is a life-threatening disease. The main pathogenesis of death and disability in the acute phase of SAH is early brain injury, with a major component being brain edema [1]. Because brain edema after SAH can be an independent risk factor for mortality and poor outcome [2], it is important to evaluate brain edema as a prognostic assessment in experimental SAH.

Brain edema is classically distinguished by two factors, cytotoxic and vasogenic edema. Those two factors usually overlap after stroke, and brain edema is defined as an abnormal accumulation of fluid associated with volumetric enlargement of the brain [3]. Therefore, brain water content (BWC), which reflects increasing water content, is widely used to evaluate brain edema in experimental stroke studies [4, 5]. Conversely, the weight of the brain (wet brain) should reflect increasing water content and not be influenced by differences in various protocols, such as incubation time and degree. However, it is unclear whether the weight of the brain is useful for the evaluation of brain edema in experimental SAH.

To address the usefulness of the weight of the brain for the severity of brain edema in experimental SAH studies, we determined the correlations between the weight of wet cerebrum (WWC) and BWC, and compared those values in sham-operated and SAH groups. Moreover, we examined the implication of body weight (BW) and the weight of the dry cerebrum (WDC), which is measured as a substitute for the original brain weight of the animals for the values of WWC and BWC.

Materials and Methods

Experimental Animals

All experiments were approved by the institutional animal care and use committee of Kumamoto University. Twenty-five male Sprague-Dawley rats (Japan SLC, Shizuoka, Japan) weighing 348–464 g were assigned to the sham- or SAH-operation groups. The animals were operated on under 2 % isoflurane through a facemask or mechanical ventilation with a tracheostomy and underwent SAH modeling by endovascular perforation methods using a hollow polytetrafluoroethylene tube (SUBL-120; Braintree Scientific, Braintree, MA, USA) and a tungsten rod (diameter, .004 in.; A-M systems, Sequim, WA, USA), as previously described [4, 6]. The sham operation followed the same procedure without the arterial puncture.

Neurological Findings

Neurological scoring (NS) of all of the animals was determined at 1 h before euthanasia using a modified 22-pointed scoring system mixed with composite sensorimotor scoring and a beam walking test [4]. A higher score indicates greater function.

Y. Hasegawa, MD, PhD (✉) • T. Nakagawa, MD
K. Uekawa, MD, PhD • N. Koibuchi, PhD
S. Kim-Mitsuyama, MD, PhD
Department of Pharmacology and Molecular Therapeutics, Graduate School of Medical Sciences, Kumamoto University, 1-1-1, Honjo, Chuo-ku, Kumamoto-shi, Kumamoto -ken 8608556, Japan
e-mail: fpmhasse@yahoo.co.jp

H. Suzuki, MD, PhD
Department of Neurosurgery, Mie University Graduate School of Medicine, Kumamoto, Japan

T. Kawano, MD, PhD
Department of Neurosurgery, Kumamoto University School of Medicine, Kumamoto, Japan

R.L. Applegate et al. (eds.), *Brain Edema XVI: Translate Basic Science into Clinical Practice*, Acta Neurochirurgica Supplement, Vol. 121, DOI 10.1007/978-3-319-18497-5_15, © Springer International Publishing Switzerland 2016

Brain Water Content

The rats were killed at 24 h after SAH induction with deep anesthesia. The brains were removed and their cerebra were collected. After quickly measuring the WWC, the samples were kept in an oven at 105 °C for 72 h and were then weighed to determine WDC. The following formula was used for calculating the BWC: [(WWC − WDC)/WWC] × 100 % [4].

Statistical Analysis

All values are expressed as the mean ± SD. The comparisons of WWC, BWC, and NS in sham-operated and SAH rats were assessed with an unpaired *t*-test or a Mann-Whitney *U* test in the presence or absence of normal distribution and equal variance. In addition, the correlations among the NS, WWC, BWC, BW, and WDC were evaluated using the Pearson or Spearman rank correlation coefficient in the presence or absence of a normal distribution and were calculated using Graphpad Prism version 6 for Windows (Graphpad Software). A $p < 0.05$ was considered significant.

Results

Comparisons of Neurological Scoring, Weight of Wet Cerebrum, and Brain Water Content

Because one rat appeared to be an outlier in the BWC data, the rats were assigned to the sham-operated ($n = 8$) and SAH ($n = 16$) groups. Although significant deteriorations of NS and BWC were seen in the SAH group (16.3 ± 4.4, 79.1 ± 0.3 %) compared with the sham group (21.7 ± 0.6, 78.6 ± 0.2 %; $p < 0.01$, $p < 0.01$, respectively), there was no significant difference in WWC between the sham-operated (1.49 ± 0.05g) and SAH (1.51 ± 0.06g) rats ($p = 0.61$).

Correlations Among Neurological Scoring, Weight of Wet Cerebrum, and Brain Water Content

To address whether the weight of the wet brain was suitable for the evaluation of brain edema, we evaluated the correlations among the NS, WWC, and BWC of all animals (Fig. 1 and Table 1). Although there were clear correlations between WWC and BWC, and NS and BWC, the NS had no relationship to WWC. Conversely, subanalyses of the correlations showed clear relationships among them in the SAH rats.

The Implication of Body Weight and Original Brain Weight for the Values of Weight of Wet Cerebrum and Brain Water Content

Next, the brains of all rats were examined for the influence of BW and WDC, both of which could affect the values of WWC and BWC (Fig. 2 and Table 1). WWC had a strong correlation to WDC and a moderate correlation to BW in all rats. Conversely, BWC had no relationship to BW or WDC.

Discussion

Brain weight has been examined as a substratum for evaluating brain atrophy in a chronic phase in an experimental stroke model [7]. Conversely, the usefulness of increasing brain weight and the relation to brain edema has been undetermined, although it is possible that the weight of the wet brain is a good candidate measurement for edema in experimental SAH.

The major findings of this study were that WWC was not useful to evaluate brain edema, although WWC was correlated with BWC. The reasons are the influence of BW and original brain weight. Although we intended to separate a cerebrum in a similar fashion each time, small differences in original brain volume induced large variances in the value of WWC. Thus, the usefulness of brain weight for evaluating brain edema is limited. However, as there was a clear correlation between WWC and NS in SAH brains, we thought that brain weight might be useful for detecting brain edema if the range of BW and the method of removing the brain are strictly established.

Conversely, BWC was correlated with NS in all animals and was not affected by BW and original brain weight. A major pathogenesis of brain edema after SAH is increasing intracranial pressure, and the severity of brain edema is not influenced by differences in BW. Although it has been reported that the values of BWC can be changeable and misleading in a small change [8, 9], BWC is a suitable method for detecting brain edema if it is processed by the same protocol throughout the study.

In conclusion, WWC cannot be a major method of evaluation, unlike BWC, for the severity of brain edema in SAH studies. Because the strength of the measurement of brain weight is its simple evaluation, which should not be affected by different protocols, further study is needed to clarify the significant roles of brain weight in SAH studies.

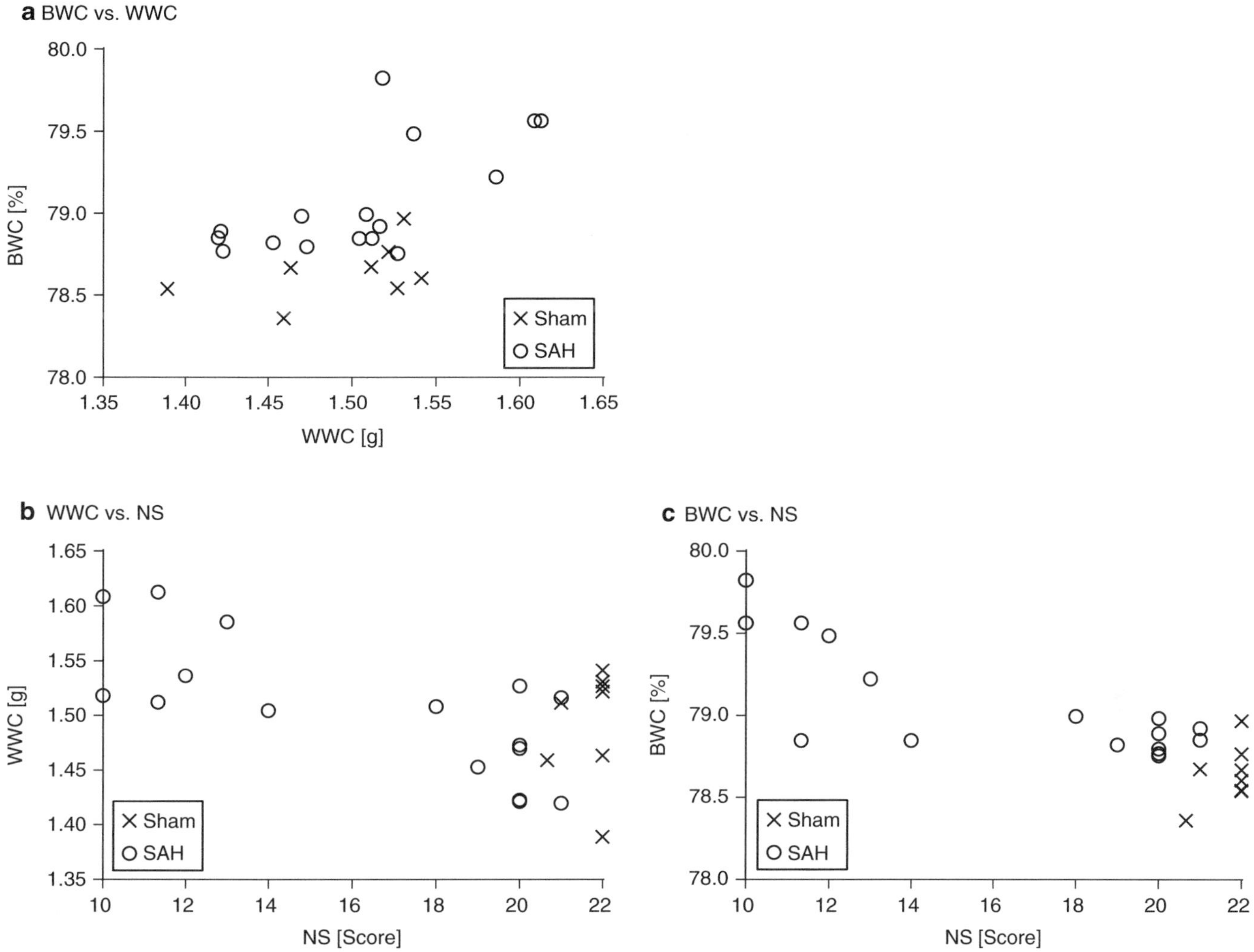

Fig. 1 Graphs showing the correlations of the weight of wet cerebrum (WWC), brain water content (BWC), and neurological scoring (NS)

Table 1 Correlations among neurological scoring (NS), weight of wet cerebrum (WWC), brain water content (BWC), body weight (BW), and weight of dry cerebrum (WDC)

	WWC vs. BWC	WWC vs. NS	BWC vs. NS	WWC vs. BW	WWC vs. WDC	BWC vs. BW	BWC vs. WDC
All rats ($n=24$)	$r=0.41, p=0.05$	$r=-0.28, p=0.18$	$r=-0.73, p<0.01$	$r=0.44, p=0.03$	$r=0.89, p<0.01$	$r=-0.02, p=0.91$	$r=-0.05, p=0.80$
Sham-operated rats ($n=8$)	$r=0.47, p=0.24$	$r=0.41, p=0.28$	$r=0.33, p=0.39$	$r=0.47, p=0.24$	$r=0.97, p<0.01$	$r=0.08, p=0.85$	$r=0.25, p=0.55$
SAH rats ($n=16$)	$r=0.58, p=0.02$	$r=-0.67, p<0.01$	$r=-0.62, p=0.02$	$r=0.47, p=0.06$	$r=0.92, p<0.01$	$r=0.24, p=0.35$	$r=0.25, p=0.33$

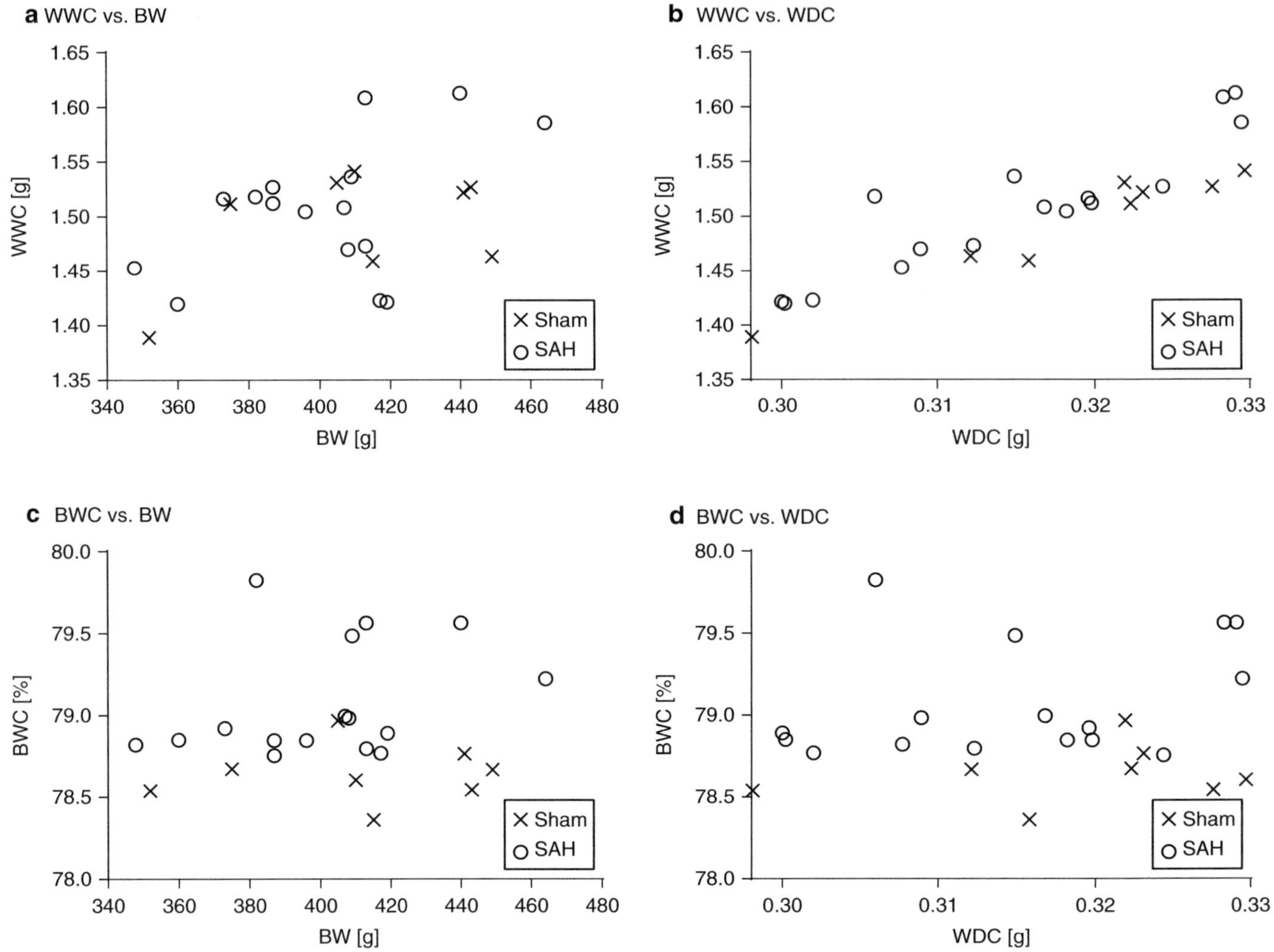

Fig. 2 Graphs showing the correlations of the weight of wet cerebrum (WWC), brain water content (BWC), body weight (BW), and weight of dry cerebrum (WDC)

Conflict of Interests This study was supported by JSPS KAKENHI Grant Number 24592135.

References

1. Ostrowski RP, Colohan AR, Zhang JH (2006) Molecular mechanisms of early brain injury after subarachnoid hemorrhage. Neurol Res 28:399–414
2. Claassen J, Carhuapoma JR, Kreiter KT, Du EY, Connolly ES, Mayer SA (2002) Global cerebral edema after subarachnoid hemorrhage: frequency, predictors, and impact on outcome. Stroke 33:1225–1232
3. Xiao F (2002) Bench to bedside: brain edema and cerebral resuscitation: the present and future. Acad Emerg Med 9:933–946
4. Hasegawa Y, Suzuki H, Altay O, Zhang JH (2011) Preservation of tropomyosin-related kinase B (TrkB) signaling by sodium orthovanadate attenuates early brain injury after subarachnoid hemorrhage in rats. Stroke 42:477–483
5. Rolland WB, Lekic T, Krafft PR, Hasegawa Y, Altay O, Hartman R, Ostrowski R, Manaenko A, Tang J, Zhang JH (2013) Fingolimod reduces cerebral lymphocyte infiltration in experimental models of rodent intracerebral hemorrhage. Exp Neurol 241: 45–55
6. Uekawa K, Hasegawa Y, Ma M, Nakagawa T, Katayama T, Sueta D, Toyama K, Kataoka K, Koibuchi N, Kawano T, Kuratsu J, Kim-Mitsuyama S (2014) Rosuvastatin ameliorates early brain injury after subarachnoid hemorrhage via suppression of superoxide formation and nuclear factor-kappa B activation in rats. J Stroke Cerebrovasc Dis 23:1429–1439
7. Fathali N, Ostrowski RP, Hasegawa Y, Lekic T, Tang J, Zhang JH (2013) Splenic immune cells in experimental neonatal hypoxia-ischemia. Transl Stroke Res 4:208–219
8. Duris K, Manaenko A, Suzuki H, Rolland W, Tang J, Zhang JH (2011) Sampling of CSF via the cisterna magna and blood collection via the heart affects brain water content in a rat SAH model. Transl Stroke Res 2:232–237
9. Keep RF, Hua Y, Xi G (2012) Brain water content. A misunderstood measurement? Transl Stroke Res 3:263–265

Analysis of Small Ischemic Lesions in the Examinees of a Brain Dock and Neurological Examination of Animals Subjected to Cortical or Basal Ganglia Photothrombotic Infarction

Toshihiko Kuroiwa, Hitoshi Tabata, Guohua Xi, Ya Hua, Timothy Schallert, and Richard F. Keep

Introduction

Small cerebral ischemic lesions are frequently found in the elderly by magnetic resonance imaging (MRI). Such lesions are distributed widely in the brain, from the deep brain structures to cortical and subcortical areas. Photothrombosis has been used to induce ischemia in the cortex but not in deep brain structures [1, 8]. To reproduce the small ischemic lesions frequently found in clinical cases, we have developed an animal model of photothrombotic ischemia induced by a thin optic fiber installed stereotaxically to a region of interest [5]. We have examined differences in neurological deficits between cortical and caudate nucleus infarction in this model [6]. We found the duration of neurological deficits was longer in animals with larger infarctions. Neurological deficits showed location-dependent differences.

T. Kuroiwa, MD (✉)
Laboratory of Clinical Medicine,
Namegata District General Hospital,
98-8 Inouefujii, Namegata, Ibaraki 311-3516, Japan
e-mail: tkuroiwa-nsu@umin.ac.jp

H. Tabata
Department of Neurosurgery, Namegata District General Hospital, Ibaraki, Japan

G. Xi • Y. Hua • R.F. Keep
Department of Neurosurgery, University of Michigan, Ann Arbor, MI, USA

T. Schallert
Department of Psychology and Neurobiology, Institute for Neuroscience, University of Texas at Austin, Austin, TX, USA

Materials and Methods

Clinical Study

We analyzed cases of small brain ischemic lesions found in the examinees of a brain dock (a neurological health screening center). MRI (3.0 T MRI scanner) was performed in 733 examinees. The distribution of incidental brain infarction and cerebral white matter lesion [3] was analyzed.

Animal Study

Male Sprague-Dawley rats or male Mongolian gerbils were used. Anesthesia was induced by inhalation of 4 % isoflurane in a mixture of nitrous oxide/oxygen mixture (70 %/30 %) and maintained by 2 % isoflurane. Rectal temperature was maintained at 37.5 °C with the use of a feedback-controlled heating pad. The left femoral vein and artery were cannulated for drug injection and for monitoring blood gases and blood pressure. Rose Bengal dye (20 mg/kg) was intravenously injected. The left caudate nucleus or left parietal cortex was exposed to cold white light for 5–10 min by using an optic fiber of 0.5 or 0.75 mm diameter. Neurological deficits were examined by forelimb placing and corner turn tests [4], as well as adhesive tape removal [2] and open field tests [7] in gerbils. In the forelimb placing test, the occurrence of forelimb placing on the edge of the countertop in response to the vibrissae stimulation was counted. In the corner turn test, the number of left and right turns when exiting a corner was counted. In the adhesive removal test, adhesive tape was applied to each forepaw of animals and the time required to remove the tape was measured. In the open field test, the animals were placed in an open field 90 × 90 cm in size and their spontaneous locomotion was traced with a video-tracking system for 5 min. The length of time spent in the

R.L. Applegate et al. (eds.), *Brain Edema XVI: Translate Basic Science into Clinical Practice*, Acta Neurochirurgica Supplement, Vol. 121,
DOI 10.1007/978-3-319-18497-5_16,

center and the periphery of the open field, both equal to 50 % of total area, was calculated. For histopathology, rodents were reanesthetized with 4 % isoflurane and transcardially perfused with 4 % paraformaldehyde at various times from 4 h to 6 weeks following photothrombosis. The fixed brains were removed and kept in 4 % paraformaldehyde. A coronal slab of brain tissue containing the center of the lesion was cut, embedded in paraffin, sectioned, and prepared for hematoxylin and eosin staining.

Results

Clinical Study

Small cerebral infarctions were found in 17 % of examinees (124 of 733 cases). White matter lesions, defined as hyperintense lesions on both proton and T2-weighted images but not hypointense on T1-weighted images [3], were found in 24 % of cases. The ischemic lesions were located in the cortex or subcortical white matter in 31 % of cases and in the basal ganglia in 44 %. Infratentorial infarction was found in 1.6 % (Fig. 1)

Animal Study

Histological examination revealed that a round infarct with thrombosed parenchymal vessels surrounded by a layer of selective neuronal death formed around the tip of the optic fiber both in caudate and cortical infarct animals (Fig. 2) The lesion volume 1 day after photothrombosis was 7.04 ± 1.18 mm^3 (mean ± SD) in rats with 10 min light exposure with an optic fiber 0.75 mm in diameter. The volume was 4.2 ± 1.24 mm^3 and 1.2 ± 0.25 mm^3 using a 0.5 mm diameter optic fiber with 10 and 5 min exposure, respectively. Ischemic lesions turned into cystic cavities (lacune) over 6 weeks.

Lesioned animals showed reduced right forelimb placing compared with the left forelimb (Fig. 3 left) Thus, successful placing of the right forelimb 1 day after a caudate photothrombotic lesion was 45 ± 21 % compared with 95 ± 8.5 % in sham-operated animals. In the corner turn test, 1 day after lesioning (10 min exposure with 0.5 mm optic fiber) right turns were 6.7 ± 8.3 % compared with 53.3 ± 10.5 % in sham-operated animals (Fig. 3 middle). Deficits were observed for 6 weeks in animals with large lesion volumes (7.0 ± 1.2 mm^3), but only for 3 days with small lesion volumes (1.2 ± 0.3 mm^3). In the adhesive tape removal test, lesioned animals took longer to remove adhesive tape from the right forepaw compared with the left. Recording of locomotion in gerbil after photothrombosis revealed a different pattern and distribution between caudate and cortical lesions. Animals before photothrombosis moved evenly in both the center and the periphery of the open field. Tracking showed circling after caudate photothrombosis. After cortical photothrombosis, animals developed linear locomotion, mainly in the periphery of the open field.

Discussion

The Rotterdam Scan Study revealed that the severity of chronic ischemic lesions detected by MRI is closely associated with cognitive impairment in elderly subjects [3]. The relationship between cognitive dysfunction and lesion severity differed between subcortical and periventricular lesions.

In rodents, early after caudate photothrombosis, histological examination showed a spherical infarct around the tip of the optic fiber surrounded by a peripheral area of selective neuronal death and ischemic edema. The ischemia was caused by thrombotic occlusion of small parenchymal vessels found in the center and periphery of the lesion [5]. Local cerebral blood flow was decreased to approximately 15 % of control levels. The infarcted area turned into a small cyst "lacune" 6 weeks after photothrombosis. These histological changes were also found in cortical photothrombosis. Thus, by placing an optic fiber stereotaxically, it was possible to induce a small photothrombotic ischemic lesion in a region of interest, and this technique can be used to model the small cerebral ischemic lesions frequently found by MRI in the elderly.

In the present study, the severity of neurological deficits correlated with lesion size. Results also revealed that the pattern of neurological deficit in rodent differed between basal ganglia and cortical infarction. Thus, photothrombotic infarction is a useful model for future studies on location- and size-dependent neurological changes in cerebral infarction.

Conflict of Interest Statement The authors declare that there are no conflicts of interest associated with the present study.

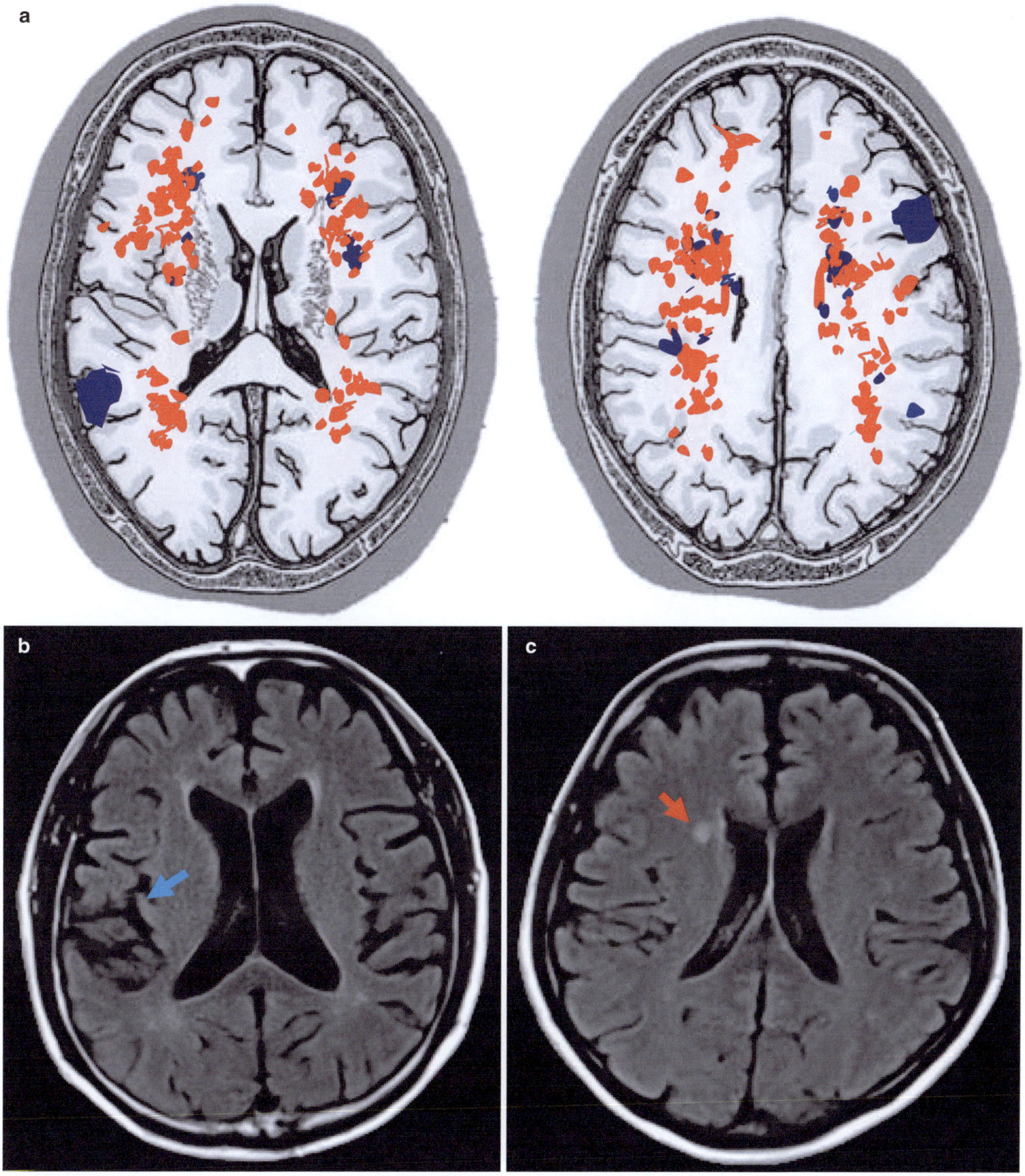

Fig. 1 (**a**) Distribution of small ischemic lesions in brain detected by MRI in examinees of a brain dock. White matter lesion (*red*) and infarction (*blue*). (**b**) A cortical infarction (*blue arrow*) incidentally found in an examinee of a brain dock. (**c**) A cerebral white matter lesion (*red arrow*) located in the centrum semiovale

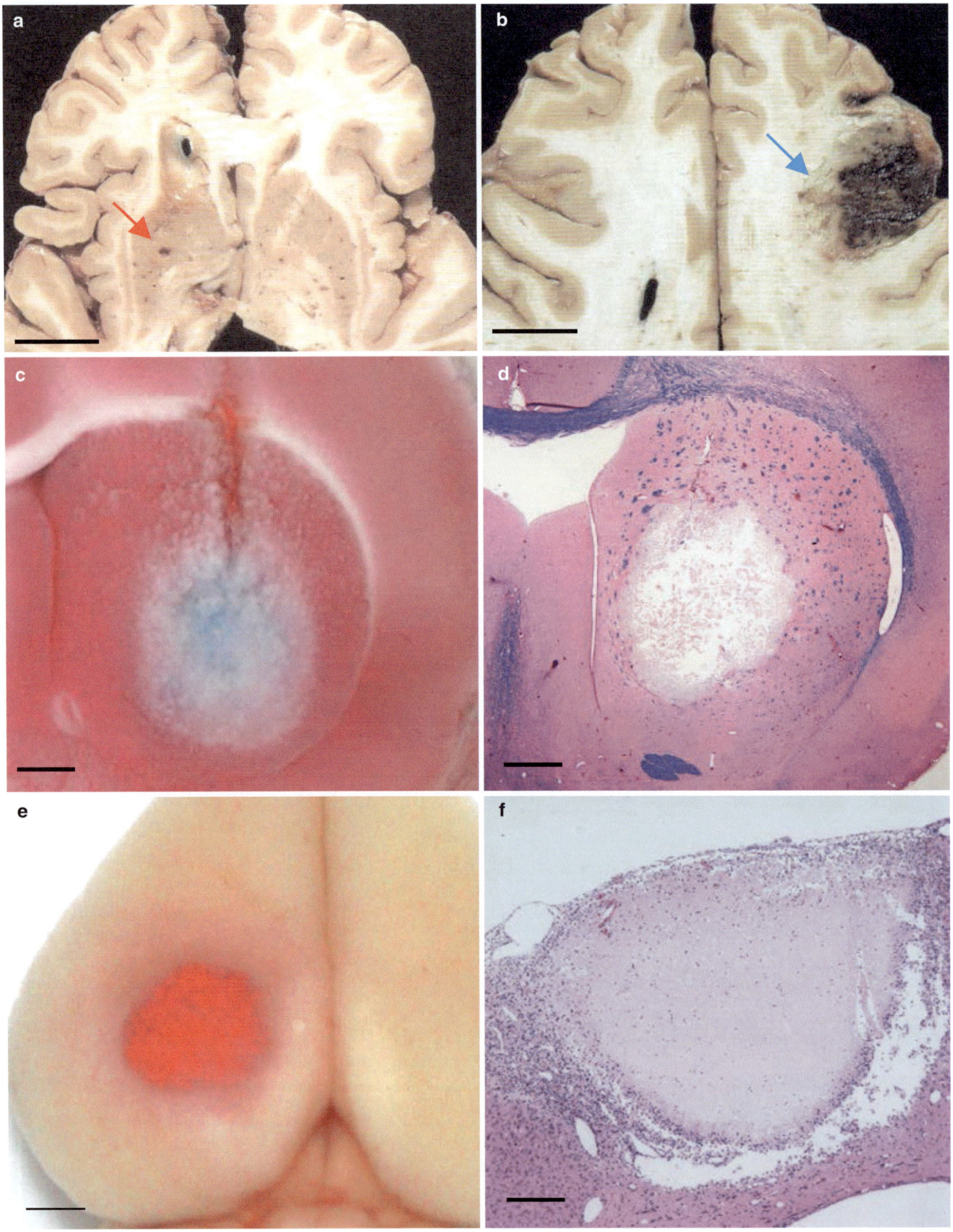

Fig. 2 (**a**) A lacunar infarct in the striatum in a clinical case (*red arrow*). (**b**) A hemorrhagic infarct in the frontal cortex in a clinical case (*blue arrow*). (**c**) A round infarction was induced by photothrombosis in the caudate nucleus in gerbil. The brain was stained with TTC (triphenyl tetrazolium chloride) solution. (**d**) Hematoxylin eosin staining of the caudate photothrombotic infarction. (**e**) A cortical ischemic lesion induced by photothrombosis in gerbil. (**f**) Hematoxylin eosin staining of the cortical photothrombotic infarction. Bar=2 cm in figs (**a**, **b**), Bar=5 mm in figs (**c**–**f**)

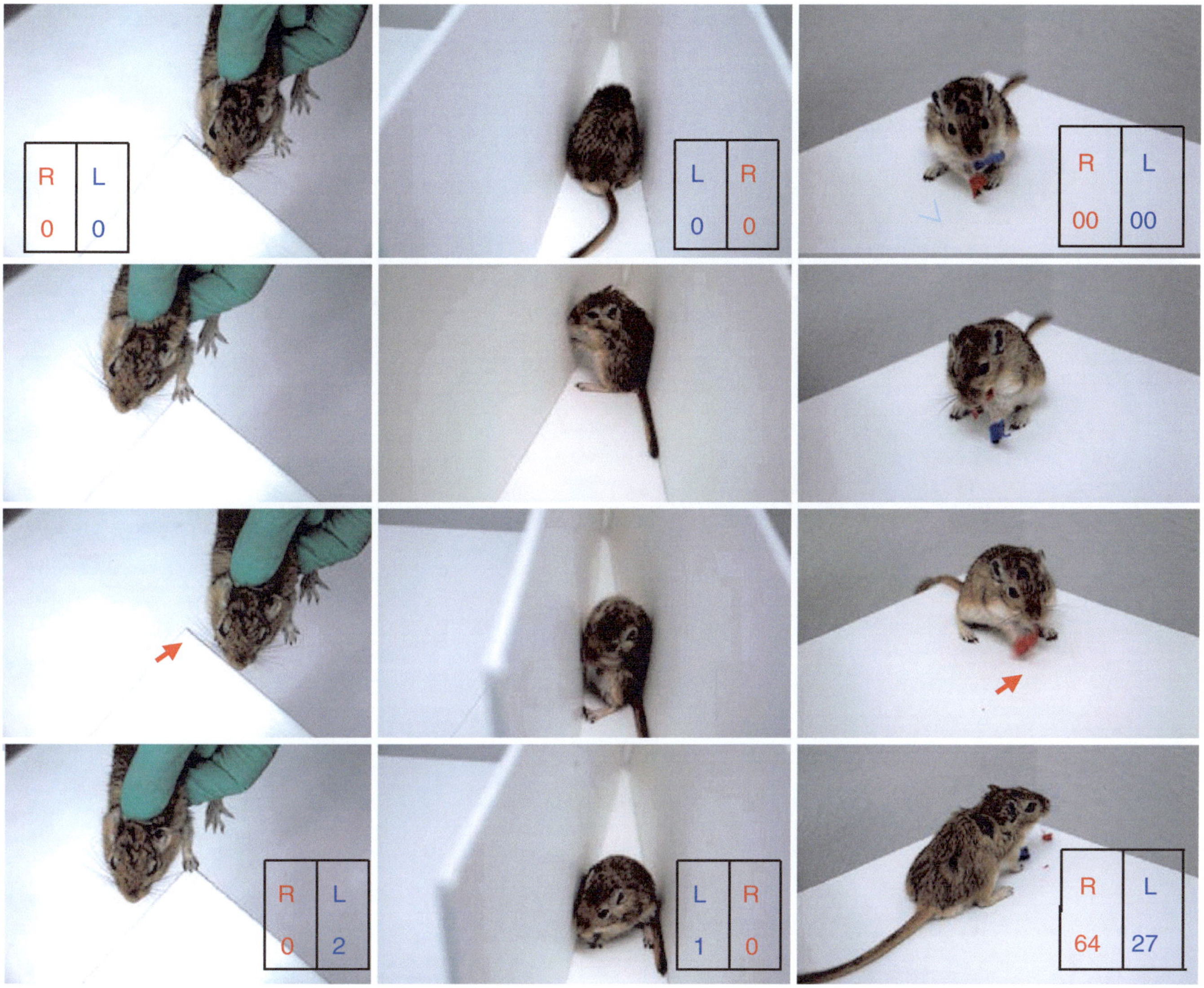

Fig. 3 In a gerbil with left caudate photothrombotic infarction, occurrence of successful placing of right forelimb (*red arrow*) was smaller than left (*left column*), the number of left turns at a corner was larger than right turns (*middle column*), and the time to remove adhesive tape from the right forepaw (*red arrow*) was longer than for the left (*right column*)

References

1. Boquillon M, Boquillon JP, Bralet J (1992) Photochemically induced, graded cerebral infarction in the mouse by laser irradiation evolution of brain edema. J Pharmacol Toxicol Methods 27:1–6
2. Bouet V, Boulouard M, Toutain J, Divoux D, Bernaudin M, Schumann-Bard P, Freret T (2009) The adhesive removal test: a sensitive method to assess sensorimotor deficits in mice. Nat Protoc 4(10):1560–1564
3. de Groot JC, de Leeuw FE, Oudkerk M, van Gijn J, Hofman A, Jolles J, Breteler MM (2000) Cerebral white matter lesions and cognitive function: the Rotterdam Scan Study. Ann Neurol 47(2): 145–151
4. Hua Y, Schallert T, Keep RF, Hoff JT, Xi G (2002) Behavioral tests after intracerebral hemorrhage in rat. Stroke 33:2478–2484
5. Kuroiwa T, Xi G, Hua Y, Nagaraja TN, Fenstermacher JD, Keep RF (2009) Development of a rat model of photothrombotic ischemia and infarction within the caudoputamen. Stroke 40:248–253
6. Kuroiwa T, Keep RF (2011) Photothrombotic infarction of caudate nucleus and parietal cortex. In: Lane EL, Dunnett SB (eds) Animal models of movement disorders, vol II. Humana Press, New York, pp 183–192
7. Gould TD, Dao DT, Kovacsics CE (2009) The open field test. Neuromethods 42:1–20
8. Watson BD, Dietrich WD, Busto R, Wachtel MS, Ginsberg MD (1985) Induction of reproducible brain infarction by photochemically initiated thrombosis. Ann Neurol 17:497–504

Brain Volume Determination in Subarachnoid Hemorrhage Using Rats

Tim Lekic, Maurice Hardy, Mutsumi Fujii, Devin W. McBride, and John H. Zhang

Introduction

Brain edema is routinely measured using the wet-dry method [1]. This measure is used in multiple studies [2–9]. Because volume is the sum total of all cerebral tissues [10–12], including water, by extension, volumetric changes following brain injury may not be adequately quantified using measurements of edema [13–24]. Therefore, in this short preliminary study we tested the hypothesis that dried brains reconstituted with water could be carefully and successfully reconstituted to determine the actual volume.

Methods

Subarachnoid hemorrhage (SAH) was induced by endovascular perforation in adult male Sprague-Dawley rats ($n=30$). Animals were euthanized at 24 and 72 h after evaluation of neurobehavior and brain water content was determined. Dried brains were thereafter reconstituted with equal parts of water (lost from brain edema) and centrifuged to remove air bubbles. The total volume was quantified using hydrostatic (underwater) physics principles that 1 mL water (mass) = 1 cm^3 (volume). The amount of additional water needed to reach a preset level marked on 2 mL test tubes was added to that lost from brain edema, and from the brain itself, to determine the final volume.

T. Lekic • M. Hardy • M. Fujii • D.W. McBride
Division of Physiology and Pharmacology,
School of Medicine, Loma Linda, CA, USA

J.H. Zhang, MD, PhD (✉)
Department of Neurosurgery, School of Medicine,
Loma Linda, CA, USA

Department of Physiology and Pharmacology,
Loma Linda University School of Medicine,
11041 Campus Street, Risley Hall Rm 219,
Loma Linda, CA 92354, USA
e-mail: johnzhang3910@yahoo.com

Experimental Animals

All protocols used in the study were approved by the Institutional Animal Care and Use Committee at Loma Linda University. Adult male Sprague-Dawley rats (Harlan, Indianapolis, IN, USA) weighing between 280 and 350 g were randomly assigned.

Subarachnoid Hemorrhage Modeling

The endovascular perforation SAH rat model was produced as previously described [25]. Briefly, anesthesia was induced with 3 % isoflurane, and then maintained with 2–3 % isoflurane. Animals were trans-orally intubated and their respiration maintained with respirator (Harvard Apparatus, Holliston, MA, USA). The left common carotid artery was then exposed and the external carotid artery (ECA) divided into a 3-mm stump. A 4–0 monofilament nylon suture was advanced into the internal carotid artery (ICA) from the ECA stump until resistance was felt. The suture was then advanced another 3 mm to perforate the bifurcation of the anterior-middle cerebral arteries. The suture was then immediately withdrawn to reperfuse ICA territories. Sham operations involved animals in which the suture was advanced until resistance was felt and then withdrawn without perforation of the artery. Animals were returned to their cages after recovery from anesthesia with access to food and water.

Garcia Test

We used this test with modifications [25, 26] to evaluate the neurobehavioral deficits after SAH. Briefly, neurological evaluations were performed in all groups by highly experienced and blinded examiners [26]. The scoring system consisted of six tests with possible scores of 0–3 for each test (0 = worst; 3 = best), including: (a) spontaneous activity, (b) symmetry of

R.L. Applegate et al. (eds.), *Brain Edema XVI: Translate Basic Science into Clinical Practice*, Acta Neurochirurgica Supplement, Vol. 121,
DOI 10.1007/978-3-319-18497-5_17, © Springer International Publishing Switzerland 2016

movement, (c) forepaw outstretching, (d) climbing, (e) body proprioception, and (f) response to vibrissae touch. Scores were given to each rat at the completion of the evaluation, for a total summation of all six individual tests.

SAH Grading

SAH grading was determined by assessing high-resolution photographs of the brains at time of sacrifice, as described [27]. Animals received a total score ranging from 0 to 18

Brain Edema

Animals were re-anesthetized and brain samples were collected. Brain edema was measured by methods described previously [28–31]. Briefly, the rats were decapitated and brains removed immediately, then divided into five parts: ipsilateral and contralateral basal ganglia, ipsilateral and contralateral cortex, and cerebellum. Tissue samples were weighed on an analytical balance (model AE 100; Mettler Instrument Co., Columbus, OH, USA) to the nearest 0.01 mg to obtain wet weight (WW). The brain tissue was then dried at 100 °C for 24 h to find the dry weight (DW) measurement. Finally, the brain water (%) was calculated using the formula (WW − DW)/WW × 100, as previously described [28–31].

Reconstituted Brain Volume Determination (Technical Procedure)

1. Weigh samples in previously weighed 1.5 mL centrifuge tubes
2. Quickly transfer wet brain tissue to a graduated cylinder filled to a known level
3. Using a syringe with gradations, draw water from the graduated cylinder to the known level
4. Quickly place the wet brain tissue in a premeasured centrifuge tube and put it in the oven (approximately 100 °C)
5. Make note of the amount of water in the syringe
6. Place dried brain tissue in 1.5 mL centrifuge tubes
7. Place dried brain tissue in oven for ~12 h+
8. Remove from the oven and weigh dried brain tissue
9. Add 1 mL to each of the centrifuge tubes
10. Centrifuge the samples for 20 min at 4 °C and 14,000 rpm
11. Using a 1-mL syringe with a needle, fill the syringe up to 1 mL
12. Carefully add water to the tube until the bottom of the meniscus reaches the 1.5 mL mark on the centrifuge tube
13. Record the amount of water left in the syringe
14. Calculate the total volume of water needed for reconstitution

Results

SAH significantly increased both brain water and volume while worsening neurological function in affected rats. Volumetric measurements demonstrated significant brain swelling after SAH. This value was unchanged despite additional use of the same tissues for the wet-dry brain edema approach (Figs. 1, 2, and 3).

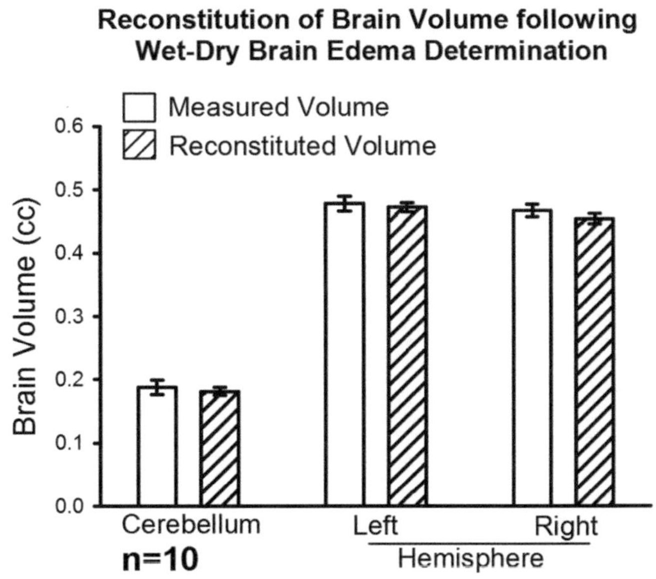

Fig. 1 Comparison of brain volume determination between those directly measured versus reconstitution after the brain edema procedure; *SEM* standard error of the mean; $n = 10$/group

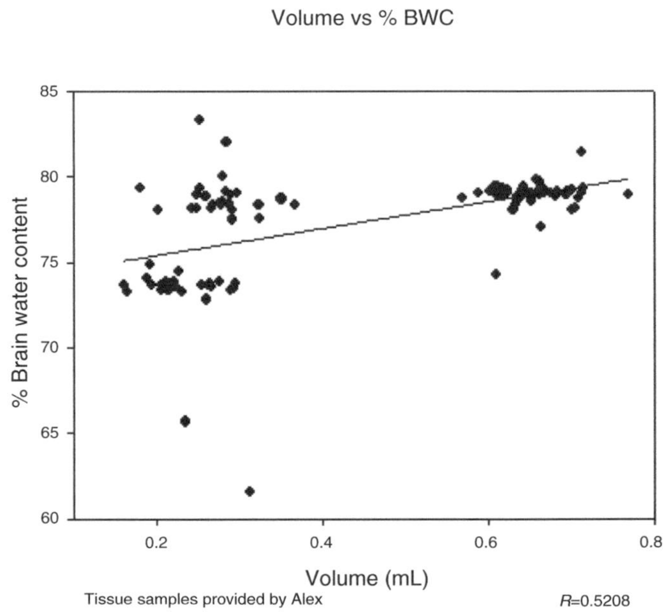

Fig. 2 Demonstration of correlation between percentage brain water content and volume. Note fold changes in volume for each percentage edema. *Left cluster* infratentorial, *right cluster* supratentorial (i.e., cerebral hemispheres)

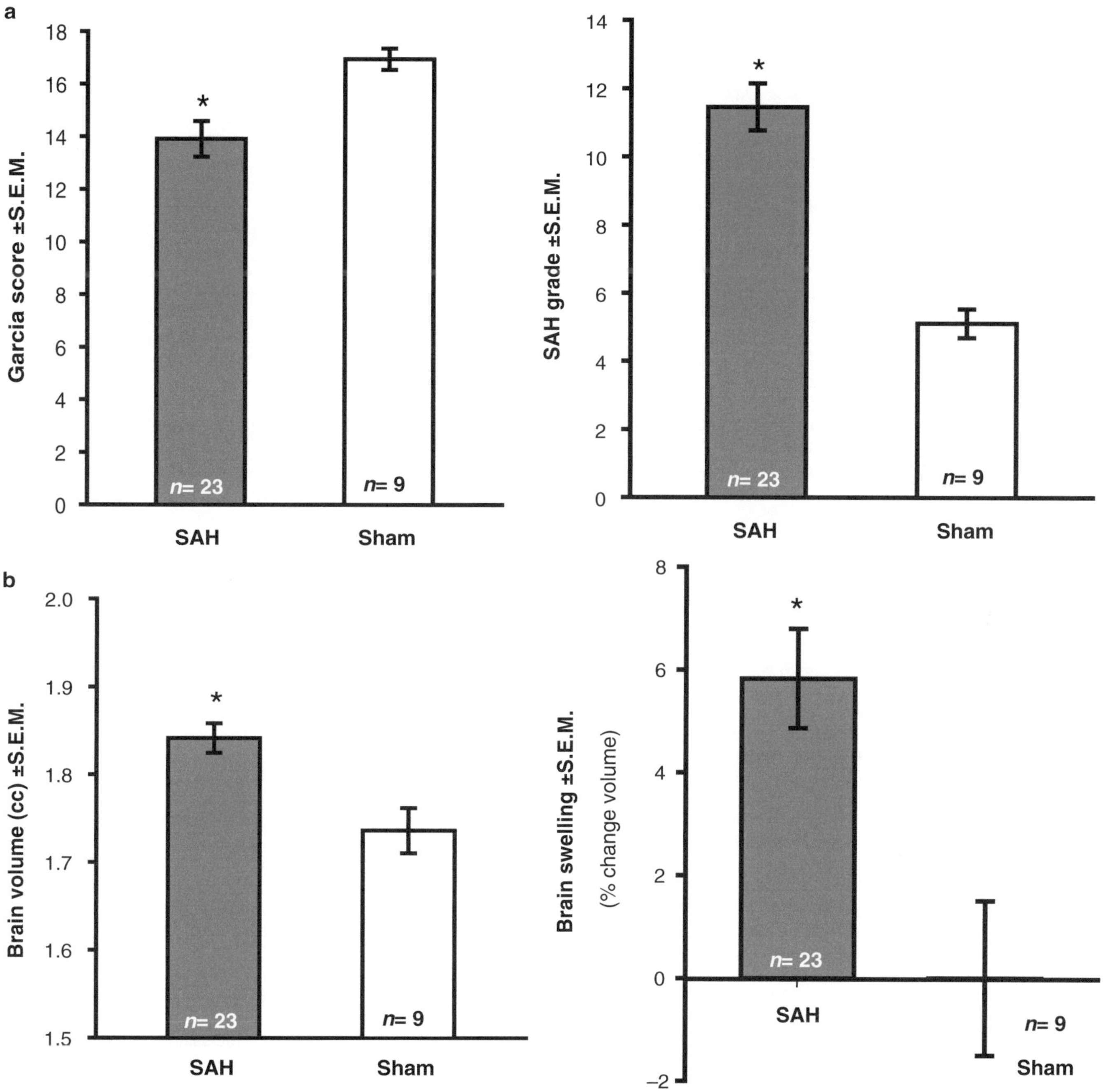

Fig. 3 (**a**) Neurological deficit (Garcia score; *left panel*), SAH grade (*right panel*) measured following SAH; (**b**) calculated brain volume (*left panel*), and mathematical conversion into percentage swelling (*right panel*) measured following SAH; (*asterisk*) <0.05 versus sham; *SEM* standard error of mean; $n = 9–23$/group

Conclusion

Translational stroke studies, including animal modeling, are greatly needed to safely integrate basic preclinical scientific principles ahead of clinical application [32–36]. Thus, this modification of the "wet-dry" brain edema method permits brain volume determination using valuable post hoc dried brain tissue. Perhaps the greatest strength of this approach is the acquisition of additional valuable data without greatly added expense to neuroscience laboratories. Nonetheless, the application of these volumetric measurements needs validation in other studies, across models and species. In the meantime, this breakthrough technique remains a hammer without a nail but we hope not for much longer.

Acknowledgment This study was partially supported by the National Institutes of Health grant RO1 NS078755 (Dr Zhang).

Disclosures None

References

1. Keep RF, Hua Y, Xi G (2012) Brain water content. A misunderstood measurement? Transl Stroke Res 3:263–265
2. Hasegawa Y, Nakagawa T, Uekawa K, Ma M, Lin B, Kusaka H, Katayama T, Sueta D, Toyama K, Koibuchi N, Kim-Mitsuyama S (2014) Therapy with the combination of amlodipine and irbesartan has persistent preventative effects on stroke onset associated with BDNF preservation on cerebral vessels in hypertensive rats. Transl Stroke Res. doi:10.1007/s12975-014-0383-5
3. Schlunk F, Schulz E, Lauer A, Yigitkanli K, Pfeilschifter W, Steinmetz H, Lo EH, Foerch C (2014) Warfarin pretreatment reduces cell death and MMP-9 activity in experimental intracerebral hemorrhage. Transl Stroke Res. doi:10.1007/s12975-014- 0377–3
4. Chen Q, Zhang J, Guo J, Tang J, Tao Y, Li L, Feng H, Chen Z (2014) Chronic hydrocephalus and perihematomal tissue injury developed in a rat model of intracerebral hemorrhage with ventricular extension. Transl Stroke Res. doi:10.1007/s12975-014-0367-5
5. Merali Z, Leung J, Mikulis D, Silver F, Kassner A (2015) Longitudinal assessment of Imatinib's effect on the blood–brain barrier after ischemia/reperfusion injury with permeability MRI. Transl Stroke Res 6:39–49
6. Li Q, Khatibi N, Zhang JH (2014) Vascular neural network: the importance of vein drainage in stroke. Transl Stroke Res 5:163–166
7. Jayakumar AR, Valdes V, Tong XY, Shamaladevi N, Gonzalez W, Norenberg MD (2014) Sulfonylurea receptor 1 contributes to the astrocyte swelling and brain edema in acute liver failure. Transl Stroke Res 5:28–37
8. Hoda MN, Bhatia K, Hafez SS, Johnson MH, Siddiqui S, Ergul A, Zaidi SK, Fagan SC, Hess DC (2014) Remote ischemic perconditioning is effective after embolic stroke in ovariectomized female mice. Transl Stroke Res 5:484–490
9. Khanna A, Kahle KT, Walcott BP, Gerzanich V, Simard JM (2014) Disruption of ion homeostasis in the neurogliovascular unit underlies the pathogenesis of ischemic cerebral edema. Transl Stroke Res 5:3–16
10. Ford AL, An H, Kong L, Zhu H, Vo KD, Powers WJ, Lin W, Lee JM (2014) Clinically relevant reperfusion in acute ischemic stroke: MTT performs better than Tmax and TTP. Transl Stroke Res 5:415–421
11. Sun D, Kahle KT (2014) Dysregulation of diverse ion transport pathways controlling cell volume homeostasis contribute to neuroglial cell injury following ischemic stroke. Transl Stroke Res 5:1–2
12. Song M, Yu SP (2014) Ionic regulation of cell volume changes and cell death after ischemic stroke. Transl Stroke Res 5:17–27
13. Betz AL, Keep RF, Beer ME, Ren XD (1994) Blood–brain barrier permeability and brain concentration of sodium, potassium, and chloride during focal ischemia. J Cereb Blood Flow Metab 14:29–37
14. Adachi M, Feigin I (1966) Cerebral oedema and the water content of normal white matter. J Neurol Neurosurg Psychiatry 29:446–450
15. Minamisawa H, Terashi A, Katayama Y, Kanda Y, Shimizu J, Shiratori T, Inamura K, Kaseki H, Yoshino Y (1988) Brain eicosanoid levels in spontaneously hypertensive rats after ischemia with reperfusion: leukotriene C4 as a possible cause of cerebral edema. Stroke 19:372–377
16. Yang GY, Betz AL, Chenevert TL, Brunberg JA, Hoff JT (1994) Experimental intracerebral hemorrhage: relationship between brain edema, blood flow, and blood- brain barrier permeability in rats. J Neurosurg 81:93–102
17. Faas FH, Ommaya AK (1968) Brain tissue electrolytes and water content in experimental concussion in the monkey. J Neurosurg 28:137–144
18. Gerriets T, Stolz E, Walberer M, Muller C, Kluge A, Bachmann A, Fisher M, Kaps M, Bachmann G (2004) Noninvasive quantification of brain edema and the space-occupying effect in rat stroke models using magnetic resonance imaging. Stroke 35:566–571
19. Marmarou A, Poll W, Shulman K, Bhagavan H (1978) A simple gravimetric technique for measurement of cerebral edema. J Neurosurg 49:530–537
20. Marshall LF, Bruce DA, Graham DI, Langfitt TW (1976) Alterations in behavior, brain electrical activity, cerebral blood flow, and intracranial pressure produced by triethyl tin sulfate induced cerebral edema. Stroke 7:21–25
21. Nelson SR, Mantz ML, Maxwell JA (1971) Use of specific gravity in the measurement of cerebral edema. J Appl Physiol 30:268–271
22. Tengvar C, Forssen M, Hultstrom D, Olsson Y, Pertoft H, Pettersson A (1982) Measurement of edema in the nervous system. Use of Percoll density gradients for determination of specific gravity in cerebral cortex and white matter under normal conditions and in experimental cytotoxic brain edema. Acta Neuropathol 57:143–150
23. Shohami E, Novikov M, Mechoulam R (1993) A nonpsychotropic cannabinoid, HU-211, has cerebroprotective effects after closed head injury in the rat. J Neurotrauma 10:109–119
24. Wagner KR, Xi G, Hua Y, Kleinholz M, de Courten-Myers GM, Myers RE, Broderick JP, Brott TG (1996) Lobar intracerebral hemorrhage model in pigs: rapid edema development in perihematomal white matter. Stroke 27:490–497
25. Sherchan P, Lekic T, Suzuki H, Hasegawa Y, Rolland W, Duris K, Zhan Y, Tang J, Zhang JH (2011) Minocycline improves functional outcomes, memory deficits, and histopathology after endovascular perforation-induced subarachnoid hemorrhage in rats. J Neurotrauma 28:2503–2512
26. Garcia JH, Wagner S, Liu KF, Hu XJ (1995) Neurological deficit and extent of neuronal necrosis attributable to middle cerebral artery occlusion in rats. Statistical validation. Stroke 26:627–634
27. Sugawara T, Jadhav V, Ayer R, Chen W, Suzuki H, Zhang JH (2009) Thrombin inhibition by argatroban ameliorates early brain injury and improves neurological outcomes after experimental subarachnoid hemorrhage in rats. Stroke 40:1530–1532
28. Lekic T, Hartman R, Rojas H, Manaenko A, Chen W, Ayer R, Tang J, Zhang JH (2010) Protective effect of melatonin upon neuropathology, striatal function, and memory ability after intracerebral hemorrhage in rats. J Neurotrauma 27:627–637
29. Lekic T, Rolland W, Manaenko A, Krafft PR, Kamper JE, Suzuki H, Hartman RE, Tang J, Zhang JH (2013) Evaluation of the hematoma consequences, neurobehavioral profiles, and histopathology in a rat model of pontine hemorrhage. J Neurosurg 118:465–477
30. Lekic T, Rolland W, Hartman R, Kamper J, Suzuki H, Tang J, Zhang JH (2011) Characterization of the brain injury, neurobehavioral profiles, and histopathology in a rat model of cerebellar hemorrhage. Exp Neurol 227:96–103
31. Tang J, Liu J, Zhou C, Ostanin D, Grisham MB, Neil Granger D, Zhang JH (2005) Role of NADPH oxidase in the brain injury of intracerebral hemorrhage. J Neurochem 94:1342–1350
32. Tso MK, Macdonald RL (2014) Subarachnoid hemorrhage: a review of experimental studies on the microcirculation and the neurovascular unit. Transl Stroke Res 5:174–189
33. Marbacher S, Nevzati E, Croci D, Erhardt S, Muroi C, Jakob SM, Fandino J (2014) The rabbit shunt model of subarachnoid haemorrhage. Transl Stroke Res 5:669–680
34. Pluta RM, Bacher J, Skopets B, Hoffmann V (2014) A non-human primate model of aneurismal subarachnoid hemorrhage (SAH). Transl Stroke Res 5:681–691
35. Zhang YP, Cai J, Shields LB, Liu N, Xu XM, Shields CB (2014) Traumatic brain injury using mouse models. Transl Stroke Res 5:454–471
36. Wada K, Makino H, Shimada K, Shikata F, Kuwabara A, Hashimoto T (2014) Translational research using a mouse model of intracranial aneurysm. Transl Stroke Res 5:248–251

Development of an Infarct Volume Algorithm to Correct for Brain Swelling After Ischemic Stroke in Rats

Devin W. McBride, Jiping Tang, and John H. Zhang

Introduction

A number of experimental ischemic stroke models are utilized to mimic human pathophysiology for the study of disease progression and underlying mechanisms, as well as to develop new therapeutics [11, 12, 15, 21, 26, 32, 33, 36, 37], all of which rely on infarct volume as the primary outcome measured. A variety of methods have been developed for evaluating the sizes of infarctions [1, 2, 6, 10, 17–19, 25, 28]; the most popular method is histological analysis, using triphenyl tetrazolium chloride (TTC) or Nissl stains, which require an algorithm to calculate infarct size.

The Algorithm of Lin et al. for Calculating Infarct Volume

Despite the vast amount of research on experimental models of ischemic stroke [16, 27, 31, 34], it was not until 1984 that an algorithm was developed for infarct quantification [19]. Jones and Coyle [19] developed the first algorithm that measured infarction of whole brains, utilizing curvature correction factors to compute the infarct surface area, but this method only lasted a few years [8, 9].

Simultaneous with the development of the Jones and Coyle model, Bederson et al. [1, 2] created an alternative algorithm that directly calculated infarct area by outlining the infarct in several brain slices and normalizing them to the area of the coronal section. This direct method of infarct size estimation was more widely accepted, leading to the direct method of infarct volume by Osborne et al. [29]. Although the direct infarct volume algorithm was used for several years, it did not yield a true measurement of infarct volume because of ipsilesional hemisphere swelling artifacts.

In 1990, Swanson et al. recognized that the direct method for infarct volume could be severely affected by brain swelling [1, 2, 29], thus the indirect infarct volume algorithm was developed [35]. Swanson et al. argued that brain swelling was corrected for when only gray matter was used for indirect infarction measurement. Shortly after, Lin et al. [24] modified Swanson's model to indirectly calculate infarct size of white and gray matter. Lin et al.'s algorithm was widely utilized and is now the gold standard algorithm for infarct quantification. Since the algorithm by Lin et al. was published, several additional algorithms have been developed [3, 23]. Lin et al.'s algorithm remains the gold standard for infarct volume.

The algorithm by Lin et al. utilizes the area of the contralesional hemisphere, C_i, the area of the nonischemic (healthy) tissue of the ipsilesional hemisphere, N_i, and the thickness of each brain slice, d. The infarct volume is expressed as a percentage of the contralesional hemisphere volume [24]. Herein we use a slight modification of Lin et al.'s algorithm to compare the infarct volume with the whole brain volume rather than a single hemisphere alone, or

$$\text{Infarct Volume}(\%) = \left(\frac{\sum_i (C_i - N_i)}{2\sum_i C_i} \right) 100. \qquad (1)$$

Assumptions of Lin et al.'s Algorithm

Lin et al. made several assumptions in their algorithm development. First, the contralesional hemisphere is unaffected by infarction and brain swelling. This implies that the measured volume of the contralesional hemisphere is the true volume and is typically a valid assumption. The second

D.W. McBride • J. Tang
Department of Physiology and Pharmacology, Loma Linda University School of Medicine, Loma Linda, CA 92350, USA

J.H. Zhang, MD, PhD (✉)
Department of Physiology and Pharmacology, Loma Linda University School of Medicine, Loma Linda, CA 92350, USA

Department of Neurosurgery, Loma Linda University School of Medicine, Loma Linda, CA, USA
e-mail: jhzhang@llu.edu

R.L. Applegate et al. (eds.), *Brain Edema XVI: Translate Basic Science into Clinical Practice*, Acta Neurochirurgica Supplement, Vol. 121,
DOI 10.1007/978-3-319-18497-5_18,

assumption is that swelling occurs only in the infarcted tissue, thus the area/volume of the nonischemic ipsilesional tissue is unaffected (i.e., the healthy ipsilesional tissue is its true size). This assumption makes Lin et al.'s algorithm vulnerable to artifacts caused by volume changes in the ipsilesional hemisphere, namely peri-infarct edema [4] and stunted brain growth.

Development of a New Algorithm for Calculating Infarct Volume

To better correct for the effects of brain hemisphere volume changes on infarct volume estimation, a new algorithm has been developed that relies on the ratio of the infarction to the whole ipsilesional hemisphere to estimate infarct area.

First, the infarct area is calculated by taking the difference in the area of the ipsilesional hemisphere and the noninfarcted ipsilesional hemisphere tissue, N_i, for slice i, or $(I_i - N_i)$. Taking this difference removes bias of the analyzer towards the infarct area. This difference (infarct area) is then normalized to the area of the ipsilesional hemisphere for slice i, yielding the fractional amount of the ipsilesional hemisphere that is infarcted per slice, or

$$\text{Fractional Amount of Infarcted Tissue per Slice} = \frac{I_i - N_i}{I_i}, \quad (2)$$

where I_i is the ipsilesional hemisphere for slice i, N_i is the noninfarcted ipsilesional tissue for slice i, and $(I_i - N_i)$ is the infarct area for slice i. To obtain the corrected area of the infarct, the fractional amount of infarcted tissue (Eq. 2) is multiplied by the area of the contralesional hemisphere for slice i (C_i), or

$$\text{Corrected Infarct Area per Slice} = \left(\frac{I_i - N_i}{I_i}\right)C_i. \quad (3)$$

The corrected infarct area is then summed over all slices and multiplied by the thickness of each slice, d. To determine the percentage of the whole brain that is infarcted, the infarct volume is divided by two times the volume of the contralesional hemisphere. Thus, the novel algorithm for computing infarct volume is

$$\text{Infarct Volume}(\%) = \left(\frac{d\sum_i\left(\left(\frac{I_i - N_i}{I_i}\right)C_i\right)}{2d\sum_i C_i}\right)100 \quad (4)$$

Assumptions of Our Algorithm

First, identical to the assumption made by Lin et al., the contralesional hemisphere is assumed to be unaffected by brain swelling, or the area of the contralesional hemisphere is the true area. Second, swelling occurs not only in the infarction but also in the peri-infarct region. This assumption relaxes the constraint of swelling only the infarct, made by Lin et al., which caused a majority of Lin et al.'s algorithm's artifacts to exist.

Methods

All experiments were approved by Loma Linda University Institutional Care and Use Committee. Fifty-one adult male Sprague-Dawley rats (270–290 g) were distributed into middle cerebral artery occlusion (MCAO) (n=24) or MCAO sham surgery groups (n=27). Forty-four postnatal day 10 (P10) Sprague-Dawley rat pups were distributed into hypoxia-ischemia (HI) (n=24) or HI sham surgery groups (n=20).

Middle Cerebral Artery Occlusion Model

Two hours of MCAO was performed as previously described [20]. Briefly, anesthetized animals (ketamine (80 mg/kg) and xylazine (20 mg/kg), intraperitoneally) had the right common, internal, and external carotid arteries isolated. The external carotid artery was ligated, leaving a 3–4 mm stump. A 4.0 monofilament nylon suture with a rounded tip was inserted into the external carotid artery stump, advanced up through the internal carotid artery, and stopped when resistance was felt. After 2 h of occlusion, the suture was removed, beginning reperfusion. Sham surgery involved all procedures except for suture insertion and occlusion. One day after reperfusion, deeply anesthetized animals were sacrificed. Brains were removed, sectioned into 2 mm thick slices, placed into 2 % 2,3,5-triphenyl-2H-tetrazolium chloride (TTC) for 15 min at room temperature, and then photographed.

Hypoxia-Ischemia Model

HI was performed as previously described [5, 7, 30]. Briefly, anesthetized P10 pups (isoflurane, 3 % induction, 2.5 % sustained, administered in a 100 % oxygen (0.3 mL/min)/medical gas (0.7 L/min) mixture), had the right common carotid

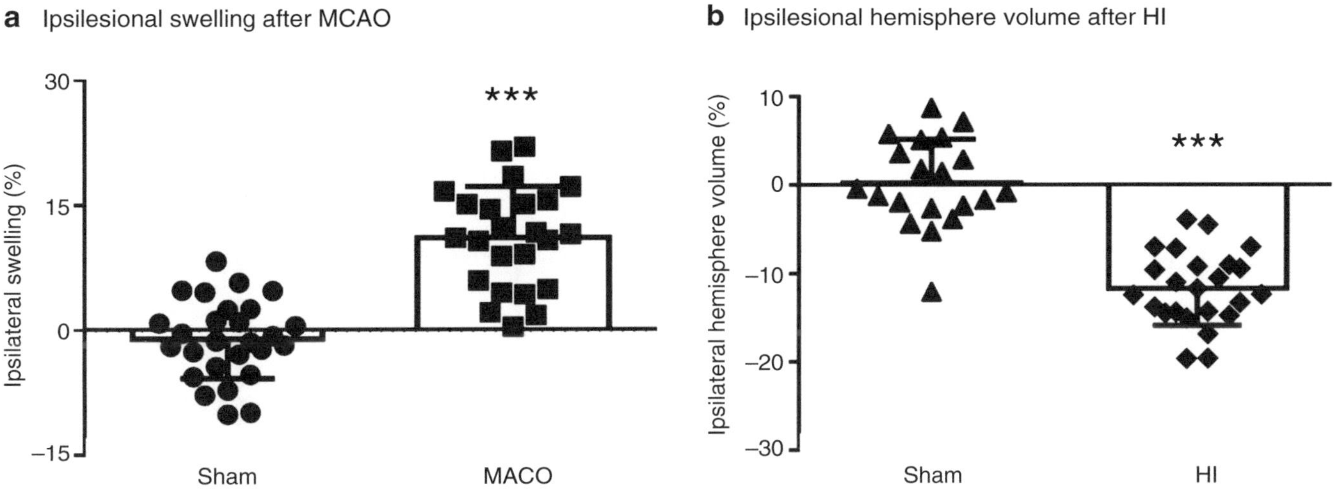

Fig. 1 Ipsilesional hemisphere volumes after ischemic stroke. (**a**) Ipsilesional swelling for animals subjected to MCAO ($n=24$) or MCAO sham surgery ($n=27$). (**b**) Ipsilesional hemisphere volume (%) for neonates subjected to HI ($n=24$) or HI sham surgery ($n=20$). *** $p<0.001$ vs sham

artery exposed, isolated, and ligated using 5–0 silk surgical suture. Surgery time was controlled to be less than 5 min [7]. One hour after surgery, animals were placed into a hypoxia chamber for 2.5 h (8 % O_2 and 92 % N_2, maintained at 37 °C using a temperature-controlled water bath). The gas was delivered at a flow rate of 93.82 mL/min for the first 1.25 h and 77.30 mL/min for the remaining 1.25 h. After 2.5 h in the hypoxia chamber, animals were returned to their dams. Sham animals underwent identical surgical procedures, except for artery ligation and hypoxia (animals were exposed to normoxic conditions for 2.5 h). Two days after HI, deeply anesthetized animals were sacrificed. Brains were removed, sectioned into 2 mm thick slices, and placed into 2 % TTC for 15 min at room temperature. Stained slices were photographed.

Ipsilesional Hemisphere Volume

Using ImageJ (ImageJ 1.48, NIH), the contralesional and ipsilesional hemispheres were outlined for images of TTC-stained brains. Ipsilesional hemisphere swelling was calculated as previously described [14, 22, 29].

Infarct Volume

ImageJ was used to trace the areas of the contralesional, ipsilesional, and nonischemic ipsilesional hemispheres. Infarct volume was calculated using Lin et al.'s algorithm (Eq. 1) and our algorithm (Eq. 1).

Statistical Analysis

Data is given as the mean ± standard deviation. Ipsilesional hemisphere volume data was analyzed using unpaired *t*-tests. Infarct volume data was analyzed using paired *t*-tests and *F*-tests.

Results

Ipsilesional Hemisphere Volumes

Animals subjected to MCAO presented with greater ipsilesional hemisphere volumes (ipsilesional hemisphere swelling) compared with that of sham animals ($p<0.001$) (Fig. 1a). Animals subjected to HI had significantly smaller ipsilesional hemisphere volumes than those of sham animals ($p<0.001$) (Fig. 1b).

Infarct Volume Comparison of Lin et al.'s Algorithm and Our Algorithm

Infarct volume computed using Lin et al.'s algorithm was statistically greater for MCAO animals than that of sham animals ($p<0.001$). Similarly, the infarct volume calculated using our algorithm was significantly greater for MCAO animals than that of sham animals ($p<0.001$). However, the infarct volumes of MCAO sham animals were significantly different between Lin et al.'s and our algorithms (*F*-test $p<0.001$) (Fig. 2a). Additionally, the infarct volumes of

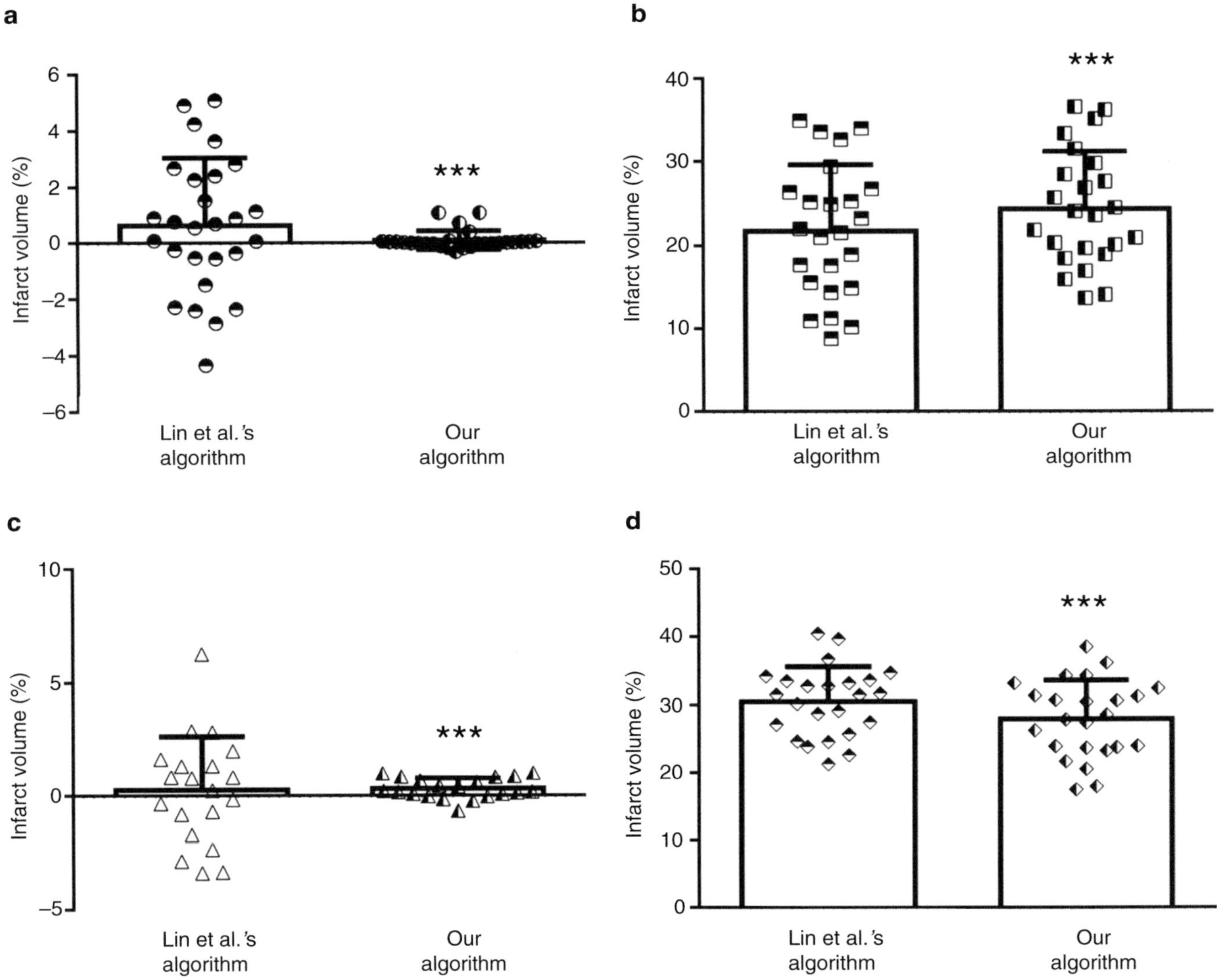

Fig. 2 Comparison of infarct volumes computed using Lin et al.'s algorithm and our algorithm. Infarct volumes of MCAO sham animals (**a**) ($n = 27$), animals subjected to MCAO (**b**) ($n = 24$), HI sham neonates (**c**) ($n = 20$), and neonates subjected to HI (**d**) ($n = 24$). ***$p < 0.001$ vs sham

MCAO animals were significantly different between the two algorithms (paired t-test $p < 0.001$) (Fig. 2b).

For the algorithm by Lin et al., the infarct volume was significantly greater for HI animals than that of sham animals ($p < 0.001$). Similarly, for our algorithm, the infarct volume was statistically greater for HI animals than that of sham animals ($p < 0.001$). The infarct volumes of HI sham animals were significantly different between Lin et al.'s and our algorithm (F-test $p < 0.001$) (Fig. 2c). The infarct volumes of HI animals were significantly different between the two algorithms (paired t-test $p < 0.001$) (Fig. 2d).

Discussion

Herein, a novel algorithm to compute infarct volume after experimental stroke is described. The new algorithm changes one of the assumptions made for Lin et al.'s algorithm, thus reducing the effects of several ipsilesional hemisphere volume artifacts that impact the infarction volume computed by Lin et al.'s algorithm. The infarct volumes obtained via Lin et al.'s algorithm and our algorithm were compared using data from two ischemic stroke models, and in both models, Lin et al.'s algorithm was more affected by brain hemisphere volume artifacts (Fig. 3).

Limitations of Lin et al.'s Algorithm

The major limitations of Lin et al.'s algorithm arise from the second assumption: only infarction swelling occurs. This makes their algorithm vulnerable to artifacts, the most influential of which is brain hemisphere volume changes. The two major causes of hemisphere volume changes in experimental stoke models are brain swelling and stunted brain growth; the former being primarily observed in adult experimental stroke models and the latter primarily observed in neonatal experimental stroke models.

Artifact 1: Negative Infarct Areas Caused by Brain Swelling

Adult rats subjected to MCAO are prone to hemispheric brain volume changes via brain swelling (Fig. 3a). While minimal swelling is corrected for in Lin et al.'s algorithm, severe brain swelling and peri-infarct swelling can result in altered infarct volume measurements, such that negative infarct areas can be obtained (Table 1). This occurs when the nonischemic ipsilesional area is greater than that of the contralesional area for slice *i* (i.e., $C_i < N_i$).

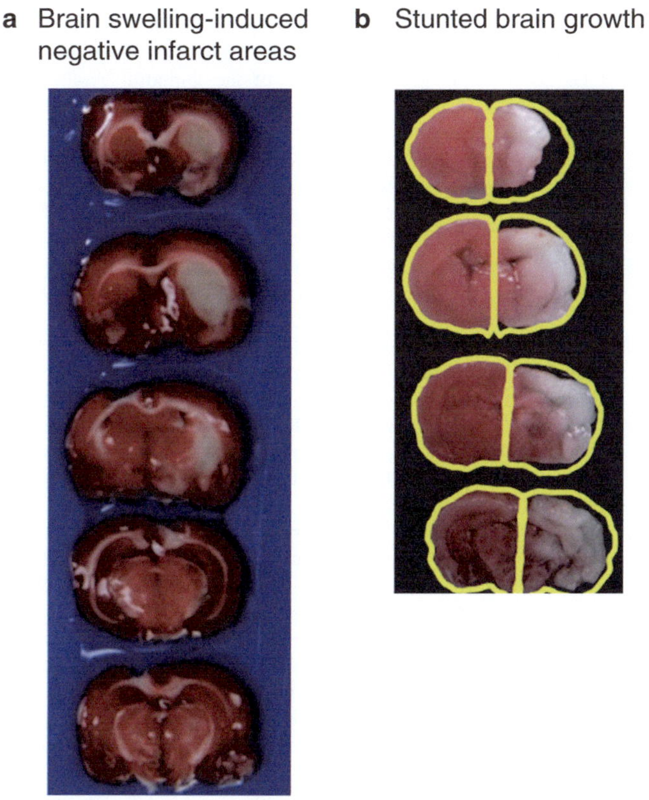

Fig. 3 Artifacts caused by changes in ipsilesional hemisphere volumes. (**a**) Representative MCAO brain for which brain swelling causes negative infarct areas. Table 1 contains the brain areas and the infarct areas for each slice. Ipsilesional swelling is 12 %. (**b**) Representative HI brain for which the ipsilesional hemisphere is smaller than that of the contralesional hemisphere. This difference leads to negative ipsilesional hemisphere brain volumes (ipsilesional hemisphere volume is −16 %)

Artifact 2: Overestimation of Infarct Volume

Neonatal rat pups subjected to HI are prone to reduced ipsilesional hemispheric brain volumes (Fig. 3b). This may be the result of stunted brain growth caused by severe tissue damage, altered growth rates of the ipsilesional hemisphere compared with that of the contralesional hemisphere, or a combination of both. Furthermore, brain swelling is also likely to be involved in this phenomenon, and thus contributions from all three mechanisms may yield the observed hemispheric brain volume changes. Regardless of mechanism, with a smaller ipsilesional hemisphere than the contralesional hemisphere (i.e., $I_i < C_i$), Lin et al.'s algorithm overestimates the infarct volume.

Limitations of Our Algorithm

The major limitations of our algorithm arise from the assumption that swelling is not confined to the infarction (contrary to Lin et al.'s algorithm). While our algorithm corrects for brain swelling artifacts on infarct volume estimation, our algorithm does not provide any information about the amount of peri-infarct swelling, nor does it uncouple peri-infarct swelling from that which is present in the infarction. While neither limitation creates artifacts for our algorithm, they remain to be studied to develop a more comprehensive infarct volume algorithm. The most probable scenario is that a gradient in brain swelling exists, for which the swelling is at a maximum within or near the infarction and at a minimum at or near the midline and/or the ipsilesional tissue that is farthest from the infarction. If a swelling gradient were to be incorporated into

Table 1 Brain swelling-induced negative infarct areas

			Infarct area (mm^2)	
	Contralesional area (mm^2)	Noninjured ipsilesional area (mm^2)	Lin et al.'s algorithm	Our algorithm
Slice 1	53.1	33.0	20.1	20.2
Slice 2	59.0	52.7	6.3	14.4
Slice 3	57.1	63.3	−6.2	6.9
Slice 4	63.9	64.2	−0.3	0.1
Slice 5	64.6	74.6	−10.0	0.2

Infarct area analysis of the representative MCAO brain in Fig. 3a. The infarct area for each slice is calculated (Lin et al.'s algorithm: numerator of Eq. 1 $(C_i - N_i)$, our algorithm: Eq. 3). Total infarct area is 9.9 mm^2 (infarct volume is 3.3 %) for Lin et al.'s algorithm and 41.8 mm^2 (infarct volume is 7.0 %) for our algorithm an infarct volume algorithm, then a unique algorithm for each animal would be required, greatly increasing the time for computing infarct volumes.

Towards an Algorithm that Calculates the True Infarct Volume

Since the 1980s, difficulties in infarction size calculation after ischemic stroke have been well documented [13] and various methods to identify true infarct volume have been pursued. However, no method has yet been successful.

Several algorithms have been developed for quantifying infarction volume in brain samples [1, 3, 23, 24, 35], with the most widely used algorithm being the indirect algorithm by Lin et al. [24]. Yet, despite the extensive use of Lin et al.'s algorithm, there remains a need for an infarct volume algorithm that can correct for the various anatomical, developmental, and pathophysiological artifacts. Such an algorithm will aid in a more comprehensive understanding of the true infarct size, as well as identify the degree to which various pathophysiologies affect infarct size, ultimately leading to better insight into injury mechanisms and therapeutic targets. Although our algorithm may not yield the true value of infarction size, it produces a more robust estimation of infarct volume than Lin et al.'s model.

Conclusions

Herein we developed a new algorithm for quantifying infarct volume that minimizes the effects of brain hemisphere volume changes. The new algorithm was validated using MCAO data, which had severe brain swelling, and HI data, which had smaller ipsilesional hemisphere volumes than those of the contralesional hemispheres. The assumption of peri-infarct swelling remains to be experimentally verified.

Acknowledgments This work was supported by NIH R01 NS043338 grant (J.H.Z.). The authors thank Xiping Liang and Brandon Dixon.

Disclosure The authors have no conflicts of interest.

References

1. Bederson JB, Pitts LH, Germano SM, Nishimura MC, Davis RL, Bartkowski HM (1986) Evaluation of 2,3,5-triphenyltetrazolium chloride as a stain for detection and quantification of experimental cerebral infarction in rats. Stroke 17:1304–1308
2. Bederson JB, Pitts LH, Tsuji M, Nishimura MC, Davis RL, Bartkowski H (1986) Rat middle cerebral artery occlusion: evaluation of the model and development of a neurologic examination. Stroke 17:472–476
3. Belayev L, Khoutorova L, Deisher TA, Belayev A, Busto R, Zhang Y, Zhao W, Ginsberg MD (2003) Neuroprotective effect of SolCD39, a novel platelet aggregation inhibitor, on transient middle cerebral artery occlusion in rats. Stroke 34:758–763
4. Bhattacharya P, Pandey AK, Paul S, Patnaik R, Yavagal DR (2013) Aquaporin-4 inhibition mediates piroxicam-induced neuroprotection against cerebral ischemia/reperfusion injury in rodents. PLoS One 8, e73481
5. Calvert JW, Cahill J, Yamaguchi-Okada M, Zhang JH (2006) Oxygen treatment after experimental hypoxia-ischemia in neonatal rats alters the expression of HIF-1 alpha and its downstream target genes. J Appl Physiol 101:853–865
6. Carano RA, Li F, Irie K, Helmer KG, Silva MD, Fisher M, Sotak CH (2000) Multispectral analysis of the temporal evolution of cerebral ischemia in the rat brain. J Magn Reson Imaging 12:842–858
7. Chen H, Burris M, Fajilan A, Spangnoli F, Tang J, Zhang JH (2011) Prolonged exposure to isoflurane ameliorates infarction severity in the rat pup model of neonatal hypoxia-ischemia. Transl Stroke Res 2011:382–390
8. Chen ST, Hsu CY, Hogan EL, Juan HY, Banik NL, Balentine JD (1987) Brain calcium content in ischemic infarction. Neurology 37:1227–1229
9. Chen ST, Hsu CY, Hogan EL, Maricq H, Balentine JD (1986) A model of focal ischemic stroke in the rat: reproducible extensive cortical infarction. Stroke 17:738–743
10. Duverger D, MacKenzie ET (1988) The quantification of cerebral infarction following focal ischemia in the rat: influence of strain, arterial pressure, blood glucose concentration, and age. J Cereb Blood Flow Metab 8:449–461
11. Fabian R, Kent T (2012) Hyperglycemia accentuates persistent "functional uncoupling" of cerebral microvascular nitric oxide and superoxide following focal ischemia/reperfusion in rats. Transl Stroke Res 3:482–490
12. Foley LM, Hitchens TK, Barbe B, Zhang F, Ho C, Rao GR, Nemoto EM (2010) Quantitative temporal profiles of penumbra and infarction during permanent middle cerebral artery occlusion in rats. Transl Stroke Res 1:220–229
13. Garcia JH (1984) Experimental ischemic stroke: a review. Stroke 15:5–14
14. Gartshore G, Patterson J, Macrae IM (1997) Influence of ischemia and reperfusion on the course of brain tissue swelling and blood–brain barrier permeability in a rodent model of transient focal cerebral ischemia. Exp Neurol 147:353–360
15. Hafez S, Coucha M, Bruno A, Fagan SC, Ergul A (2014) Hyperglycemia, acute ischemic stroke, and thrombolytic therapy. Transl Stroke Res 5:442–453
16. Harvey J, Rasmussen T (1951) Occlusion of the middle cerebral artery: an experimental study. Arch Neurol Psychiatry 66:20–29
17. Hoff JT, Nishimura M, Newfield P (1982) Pentobarbital protection from cerebral infarction without suppression of edema. Stroke 13:623–628
18. Jiang Q, Chopp M, Zhang ZG, Knight RA, Jacobs M, Windham JP, Peck D, Ewing JR, Welch KM (1997) The temporal evolution of MRI tissue signatures after transient middle cerebral artery occlusion in rat. J Neurol Sci 145:15–23
19. Jones PG, Coyle P (1984) Microcomputer assisted lesion size measurements in spontaneously hypertensive stroke-prone rats. J Electrophysiol Tech 11:71–78
20. Kawamura S, Yasui N, Shirasawa M, Fukasawa H (1991) Rat middle cerebral artery occlusion using an intraluminal thread technique. Acta Neurochir 109:126–132

21. Khanna A, Kahle KT, Walcott BP, Gerzanich V, Simard JM (2014) Disruption of ion homeostasis in the neurogliovascular unit underlies the pathogenesis of ischemic cerebral edema. Transl Stroke Res 5:3–16
22. Kondo T, Reaume AG, Huang TT, Carlson E, Murakami K, Chen SF, Hoffman EK, Scott RW, Epstein CJ, Chan PH (1997) Reduction of CuZn-superoxide dismutase activity exacerbates neuronal cell injury and edema formation after transient focal cerebral ischemia. J Neurosci 17:4180–4189
23. Lee J, Lee JK, Han K (2011) InfarctSizer: computing infarct volume from brain images of a stroke animal model. Comput Methods Biomech Biomed Engin 14:497–504
24. Lin TN, He YY, Wu G, Khan M, Hsu CY (1993) Effect of brain edema on infarct volume in a focal cerebral ischemia model in rats. Stroke 24:117–121
25. Lundy EF, Solik BS, Frank RS, Lacy PS, Combs DJ, Zelenock GB, D'Alecy LG (1986) Morphometric evaluation of brain infarcts in rats and gerbils. J Pharmacol Methods 16:201–214
26. Mandava P, Martini SR, Munoz M, Dalmeida W, Sarma AK, Anderson JA, Fabian RH, Kent TA (2014) Hyperglycemia worsens outcome after rt-PA primarily in the large-vessel occlusive stroke subtype. Transl Stroke Res 5:519–525
27. Meyer JS, Denny-Brown D (1957) The cerebral collateral circulation. I. Factors influencing collateral blood flow. Neurology 7:447–458
28. Nemoto E, Mendez O, Kerr M, Firlik A, Stevenson K, Jovin T, Yonas H (2012) CT density changes with rapid onset acute, severe, focal cerebral ischemia in monkeys. Transl Stroke Res 3:369–374
29. Osborne KA, Shigeno T, Balarsky AM, Ford I, McCulloch J, Teasdale GM, Graham DI (1987) Quantitative assessment of early brain damage in a rat model of focal cerebral ischaemia. J Neurol Neurosurg Psychiatry 50:402–410
30. Rice JE, Vannucci RC, Brierley JB (1981) The influence of immaturity on hypoxic-ischemic brain-damage in the rat. Ann Neurol 9:131–141
31. Robinson RG, Shoemaker WJ, Schlumpf M, Valk T, Bloom FE (1975) Effect of experimental cerebral infarction in rat brain on catecholamines and behaviour. Nature 255:332–334
32. Shimamura N, Matsuda N, Kakuta K, Narita A, Ohkuma H (2013) A model of rat embolic cerebral infarction with a quantifiable, autologous arterial blood clot. Transl Stroke Res 4:564–570
33. Song M, Yu SP (2014) Ionic regulation of cell volume changes and cell death after ischemic stroke. Transl Stroke Res 5:17–27
34. Sundt TM Jr, Waltz AG (1966) Experimental cerebral infarction: retro-orbital, extradural approach for occluding the middle cerebral artery. Mayo Clin Proc 41:159–168
35. Swanson RA, Morton MT, Tsao-Wu G, Savalos RA, Davidson C, Sharp FR (1990) A semiautomated method for measuring brain infarct volume. J Cereb Blood Flow Metab 10:290–293
36. Tajiri N, Dailey T, Metcalf C, Mosley Y, Lau T, Staples M, van Loveren H, Kim S, Yamashima T, Yasuhara T, Date I, Kaneko Y, Borlongan C (2013) In vivo animal stroke models. Transl Stroke Res 4:308–321
37. Watson BD, Dietrich WD, Busto R, Wachtel MS, Ginsberg MD (1985) Induction of reproducible brain infarction by photochemically initiated thrombosis. Ann Neurol 17:497–504

Changes in Brain Swelling and Infarction Volume over Four Days After Hypoxia Ischemia in Neonatal Rats

Devin W. McBride, Christine Jacob, Desislava Doycheva, Brandon J. Dixon, Jay Malaguit, Tim Lekic, Jiping Tang, and John H. Zhang

Introduction

Hypoxic-ischemic (HI) brain injury is a leading cause of mortality and morbidity in infants, affecting up to 0.4 % of full-term infants and up to 60 % of premature infants [22, 23]. In 20–40 % of HI cases, infants develop significant neurological impairments, including cerebral palsy, mental retardation, and epilepsy [21]. Following the primary HI insult, brain edema develops and is a major contributor to the overall deleterious effects of HI [5, 6, 10, 14, 17]. HI disruption of homeostasis leads to changes in the concentrations of metabolites, ions, and neurotransmitters, and as a result water accumulates in the brain tissue, inducing brain volume changes [10, 17, 18, 20].

A number of treatments have been identified and tested for reducing HI-induced sequelae, with only marginal success [11, 24]. One reason for the limited success and clinical translation of many promising therapeutics is the lack of a thorough mechanistic understanding in animal models. Herein, we observe the effect of post-HI sacrifice time on swelling of the ipsilateral hemisphere and infarct volume. We hypothesize that brain swelling and infarct volume will both reduce the longer the animal is allowed to survive post-HI.

D.W. McBride • C. Jacob • D. Doycheva • B.J. Dixon
J. Malaguit • T. Lekic • J. Tang
Department of Physiology and Pharmacology,
Loma Linda University School of Medicine,
Loma Linda, CA 92350, USA

J.H. Zhang, MD, PhD (✉)
Department of Physiology and Pharmacology,
Loma Linda University School of Medicine,
Loma Linda, CA 92350, USA

Department of Neurosurgery, Loma Linda
University School of Medicine, Loma Linda, CA, USA
e-mail: jhzhang@llu.edu

Materials and Methods

All experiments were approved by the Institutional Animal Care and Use Committee at Loma Linda University. Forty-four neonatal (P10) Sprague-Dawley rats (14–20 g) were used in all experiments. Animal groups were sham ($n=13$), HI sacrificed 2 days post-HI ($n=9$), HI sacrificed 3 days post-HI ($n=9$), and HI sacrificed 4 days post-HI ($n=13$).

Model of Hypoxia-Ischemia Injury

Hypoxia-ischemia was induced as previously described [3, 16] and surgery time was controlled to be less than 5 min [4]. Briefly, animals were anesthetized with isoflurane (3 % induction, 2.5 % sustained) delivered with medical gas. After animals reached an adequate level of anesthesia, by loss of paw pinch reflex, surgical procedures began. The right common carotid artery was exposed and isolated. A 5–0 silk surgical suture was used to ligate the right common carotid artery.

Animals were given 1 h of recovery after surgery, then placed in a hypoxia chamber (8 % O_2 and 92 % N_2), maintained at 37 °C using a water bath, for 2.5 h. Gas flow rate was 93.82 mL/min for 1.25 h and then 77.3 mL/min for the final 1.25 h. After 2.5 h, the animals were removed from the hypoxia chamber and returned to their dams. Sham surgery followed the same procedures with the exception of right common carotid artery ligation and hypoxia (normoxic conditions were used instead). Sham animals were sacrificed 2 days after surgery.

Histological Analysis

Animals were sacrificed at 2, 3, or 4, days after HI for histological analysis of hemispheric brain swelling and infarction volume. At the time of sacrifice, animals were

R.L. Applegate et al. (eds.), *Brain Edema XVI: Translate Basic Science into Clinical Practice*, Acta Neurochirurgica Supplement, Vol. 121,
DOI 10.1007/978-3-319-18497-5_19, © Springer International Publishing Switzerland 2016

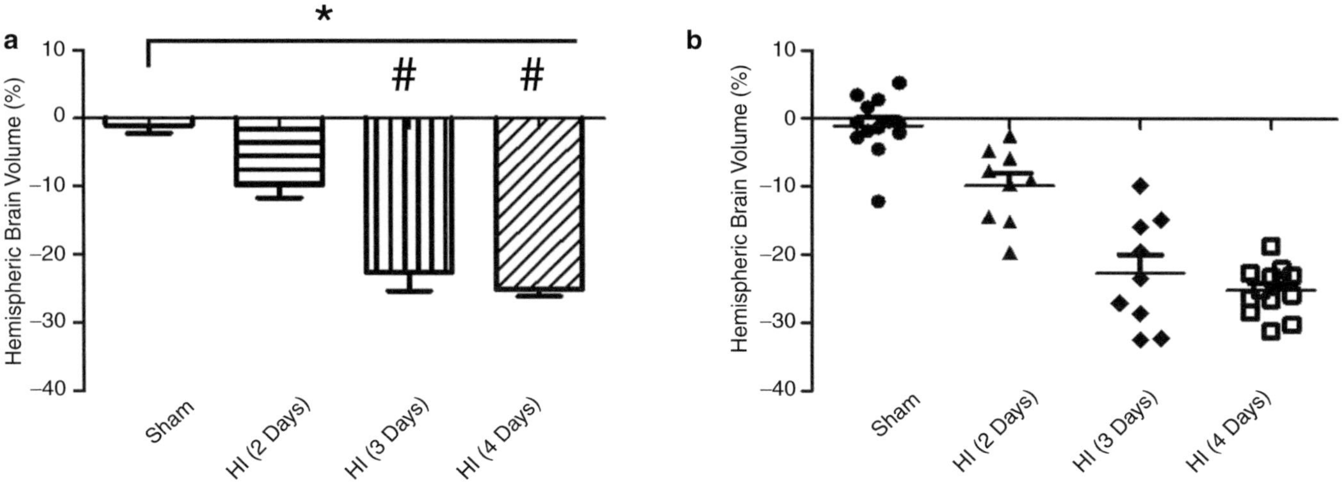

Fig. 1 Hemispheric Brain Volume after HI. Ipsilateral hemisphere brain volume (%) for HI animals is less than that of sham for all HI groups ($p<0.01$ for HI (2 days) vs. sham, $p<0.01$ for HI (3 days) vs. sham, $p<0.01$ for HI (4 days) vs. sham). The hemisphere brain volume for HI animals sacrificed at 3 and 4 days were indistinguishable ($p>0.05$) but both of these groups were significantly lower than that of 2 days post-HI ($p<0.01$ for HI (3 days) vs. HI (2 days), and $p<0.01$ for HI (4 days) vs. HI (2 days)). * $p<0.01$ vs. sham, # $p<0.01$ vs. HI (2 days). $n=9$–13/group. The same data shown as bar graphs (**a**) and as scatter plots (**b**)

deeply anesthetized, decapitated, their brains removed and sectioned into 2 mm thick slices, and then slices were stained using 2 % TTC (2,3,5-triphenyl-2H-tetrazolium chloride) for 30 min at room temperature. Brain slices were imaged. To determine the areas of the contralateral hemisphere (C_i), ipsilateral hemisphere (I_i), and the non-ischemic ipsilateral hemisphere (N_i), ImageJ (ImageJ, NIH) was used. The ipsilateral hemisphere volume was calculated using Eq. 1 [7, 12, 15] and infarct volume was calculated using Eq. 2 [19].

$$\text{Ipsilateral Hemisphere Volume }(\%)=\left(\frac{\sum_i (I_i - C_i)}{\left(\sum_i C_i\right)}\right)100 \tag{1}$$

$$\text{Infarct Volume}(\%)=\left(\frac{\sum_i (C_i - N_i)}{2\left(\sum_i C_i\right)}\right)100 \tag{2}$$

Data Analysis

Data are presented as the mean ± standard error of the mean (SEM). Data were analyzed using one-way analysis of variance (ANOVA) with Tukey *post-hoc* test. A $p<0.05$ was considered statistically significant.

Results

Ipsilateral Hemisphere Volume

Animals subjected to HI sacrificed at 2, 3, or 4 days after HI had significantly lower ipsilateral brain hemisphere volumes compared with sham animals (sham: −1.0 ± 1.20 %, $n=13$) ($p<0.01$ vs. sham for HI (2 days), HI (d Days), and HI (d Days)). Ipsilateral hemisphere volumes for the HI animals sacrificed at 2 days (HI (2 days): −9.8 ± 1.89 %, $n=9$) were significantly higher than those of animals sacrificed at either 3 days (HI (3 days): −22.6 ± 2.70 %, $n=9$) or 4 days (HI (d Days): −25.1 ± 0.97 %, $n=13$) ($p<0.01$ for HI (3 days) vs. HI (2 days) and $p<0.01$ for HI (4 days) vs. HI (2 days)). No statistical difference in hemispheric brain volume was observed between animals sacrificed at 3 days after HI compared with that of animals sacrificed at 4 days post-HI (Fig. 1).

Infarct Volume

Animals sacrificed at 2, 3, and 4 days after HI had significantly higher infarct volumes than those of sham animals (sham: 0.9 ± 0.52 %, $n=13$) ($p<0.001$ vs. sham for HI (48 h), HI (72 h), and HI (96 h)). The infarct volumes for HI animals sacrificed 2 days (HI (2 days): 35.8 ± 1.39 %, $n=9$) and 3 days (HI (3 days): 34.2 ± 1.09 %, $n=9$) were not significantly different from one another ($p>0.05$ HI (2 days) vs. HI (3 days)). However, 4 days post-HI, the infarct volume (HI (4days): 25.8 ± 1.28 %, $n=13$) was significantly lower than that of HI animals sacrificed at either 2 days or 3 days post-HI

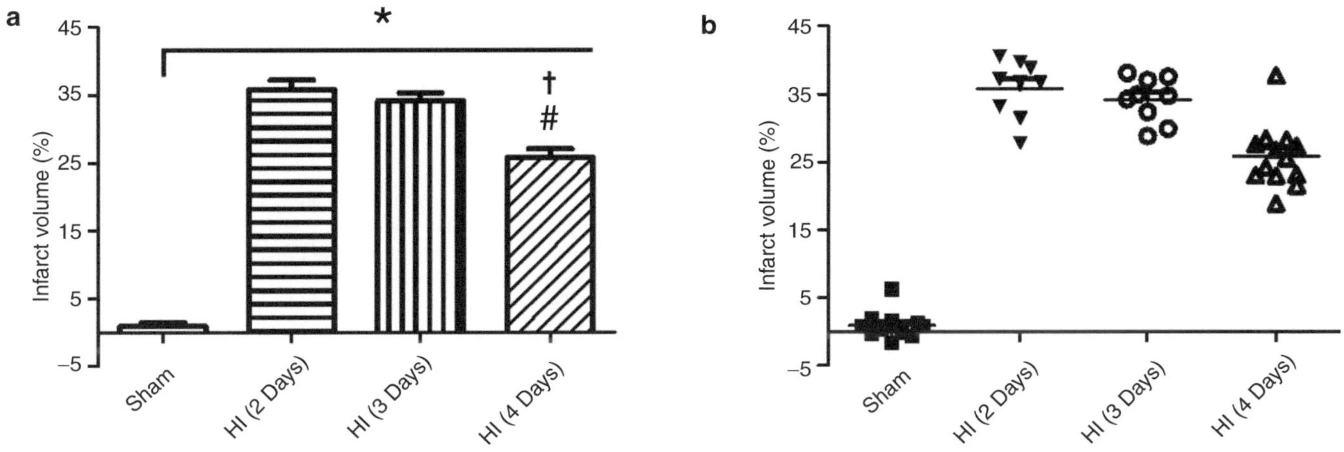

Fig. 2 Infarct volume after HI. Infarct volume (%) for HI animals is greater than that of sham for all HI groups ($p<0.01$ for HI (2 days) vs. sham, $p<0.01$ for HI (3 days) vs. sham, $p<0.01$ for HI (4 days) vs. sham). The infarct volume for HI animals sacrificed at 2 and 3 days were indistinguishable ($p>0.05$) but both of these groups were significantly higher than that of 4 days post-HI ($p<0.01$ for HI (4 days) vs. HI (2 days), and $p<0.01$ for HI (4 days) vs. HI (3 days)). * $p<0.01$ vs. sham, # $p<0.01$ vs. HI (2 days), † $p<0.01$ vs. HI (3 days). $n=9$–13/group. The same data shown as bar graphs (**a**) and as scatter plots (**b**)

($p<0.01$ for HI (4 days) vs. HI (2 days) and $p<0.01$ for HI (4 days) vs. HI (3 days)) (Fig. 2).

Discussion

Herein, we investigated the effect of post-HI sacrifice time on brain volume and infarction volume using a neonatal rat pup model of HI. To our knowledge, this is the first time the role of sacrifice time after HI has been investigated for both brain hemisphere volume and infarct volume.

Effect of Sacrifice Time on Ipsilateral Hemisphere Brain Volume after HI

Volume of the ipsilateral hemisphere is expected to decrease in the acute phase following HI [1, 9, 13], and this study supports the literature. The most plausible explanation for the smaller brain volume of the ipsilateral, injured hemisphere is that the brains of neonates are rapidly developing, gaining mass with each passing day. Any cerebral injury that causes tissue death will likely cause the ipsilateral brain volume to be smaller than the healthy, contralateral hemisphere. Additionally, tissue damage may retard growth in the ipsilateral hemisphere because of conflicting mechanisms of the injury (deleterious molecular mechanisms causing inflammation and/or cell death, and repair mechanisms) and developmental mechanisms.

However, the changes in brain volume over the days after HI have not been investigated in either patients or animal models. Herein we observed that the ipsilateral hemisphere brain volume decreases from day 2 to day 3 post-HI and seems to level at the third day following HI. While the reason for the decrease from 2 to 3 days after HI is unclear, it may include tissue growth and repair mechanism, but also may be a limitation of the current algorithm used for calculating ipsilateral hemisphere brain volume.

Effect of Sacrifice Time on Infarct Volume after HI

The infarction after HI includes a penumbra and a core in which the penumbra contains injured but salvageable tissue. The exact time in which cells transition from salvageable to irreversibly damaged is variable, but likely occurs over the first 5 days after HI [8]. Although the change from penumbra to core infarct may begin as early as a few hours after insult [2], Ghosh et al. [8] found that the overall infarct size is a maximum 2 days after HI and then decreases. One caveat of the study by Ghosh et al. is that the equation used to calculate infarct volume does not correct for swelling/volume changes. Regardless, the findings in this study agree with those of Ghosh et al. The changes in infarct volume are likely to the result of a combination of brain growth and repair mechanisms.

Conclusion

The changes in the brain hemisphere volume and infarction volume over the days following HI were examined. Although the causes of ipsilateral hemisphere brain volume decreasing over the days following HI, as well as the decrease in the infarct volume over this time period, are unknown, they will be investigated in future studies.

Acknowledgments This work was supported by NIH R01 NS043338 grant (J.H.Z.).

Disclosure The authors have no conflicts of interest to report.

References

1. Albertsson AM, Bi D, Duan L, Zhang X, Leavenworth JW, Qiao L, Zhu C, Cardell S, Cantor H, Hagberg H, Mallard C, Wang X (2014) The immune response after hypoxia-ischemia in a mouse model of preterm brain injury. J Neuroinflammation 11:153
2. Belayev L (2012) Overcoming barrier to translation from experimental stroke models. In: Lapchak PA, Zhang JH (eds) Translational stroke research: from target selection to clinical trials. Springer, New York, pp 471–492
3. Calvert JW, Cahill J, Yamaguchi-Okada M, Zhang JH (2006) Oxygen treatment after experimental hypoxia-ischemia in neonatal rats alters the expression of HIF-1 alpha and its downstream target genes. J Appl Physiol 101:853–865
4. Chen H, Burris M, Fajilan A, Spangnoli F, Tang J, Zhang JH (2011) Prolonged exposure to isoflurane ameliorates infarction severity in the rat pup model of neonatal hypoxia-ischemia. Transl Stroke Res 2011:382–390
5. Doycheva D, Shih G, Chen H, Applegate R, Zhang JH, Tang J (2013) Granulocyte-colony stimulating factor in combination with stem cell factor confers greater neuroprotection after hypoxic-ischemic brain damage in the neonatal rats than a solitary treatment. Transl Stroke Res 4:171–178
6. Ferrari DC, Nesic OB, Perez-Polo JR (2010) Oxygen resuscitation does not ameliorate neonatal hypoxia/ischemia-induced cerebral edema. J Neurosci Res 88:2056–2065
7. Gartshore G, Patterson J, Macrae IM (1997) Influence of ischemia and reperfusion on the course of brain tissue swelling and blood-brain barrier permeability in a rodent model of transient focal cerebral ischemia. Exp Neurol 147:353–360
8. Ghosh N, Yuan X, Turenius CI, Tone B, Ambadipudi K, Snyder EY, Obenaus A, Ashwal S (2012) Automated core-penumbra quantification in neonatal ischemic brain injury. J Cereb Blood Flow Metab 32:2161–2170
9. Inder TE, Huppi PS, Warfield S, Kikinis R, Zientara GP, Barnes PD, Jolesz F, Volpe JJ (1999) Periventricular white matter injury in the premature infant is followed by reduced cerebral cortical gray matter volume at term. Ann Neurol 46:755–760
10. Khanna A, Kahle KT, Walcott BP, Gerzanich V, Simard JM (2014) Disruption of ion homeostasis in the neurogliovascular unit underlies the pathogenesis of ischemic cerebral edema. Transl Stroke Res 5:3–16
11. Koenigsberger MR (2000) Advances in neonatal neurology 1950–2000. Rev Neurol 31:202–211
12. Kondo T, Reaume AG, Huang TT, Carlson E, Murakami K, Chen SF, Hoffman EK, Scott RW, Epstein CJ, Chan PH (1997) Reduction of CuZn-superoxide dismutase activity exacerbates neuronal cell injury and edema formation after transient focal cerebral ischemia. J Neurosci 17:4180–4189
13. Kumral A, Ozer E, Yilmaz O, Akhisaroglu M, Gokmen N, Duman N, Ulukus C, Genc S, Ozkan H (2003) Neuroprotective effect of erythropoietin on hypoxic-ischemic brain injury in neonatal rats. Biol Neonate 83:224–228
14. Nedelcu J, Klein MA, Aguzzi A, Boesiger P, Martin E (1999) Biphasic edema after hypoxic-ischemic brain injury in neonatal rats reflects early neuronal and late glial damage. Pediatr Res 46:297–304
15. Osborne KA, Shigeno T, Balarsky AM, Ford I, McCulloch J, Teasdale GM, Graham DI (1987) Quantitative assessment of early brain damage in a rat model of focal cerebral ischaemia. J Neurol Neurosurg Psychiatry 50:402–410
16. Rice JE, Vannucci RC, Brierley JB (1981) The influence of immaturity on hypoxic-ischemic brain-damage in the rat. Ann Neurol 9:131–141
17. Song M, Yu SP (2014) Ionic regulation of cell volume changes and cell death after ischemic stroke. Transl Stroke Res 5:17–27
18. Sun D, Kahle KT (2014) Dysregulation of diverse ion transport pathways controlling cell volume homeostasis contribute to neuroglial cell injury following ischemic stroke. Transl Stroke Res 5:1–2
19. Swanson RA, Morton MT, Tsao-Wu G, Savalos RA, Davidson C, Sharp FR (1990) A semiautomated method for measuring brain infarct volume. J Cereb Blood Flow Metab 10:290–293
20. Uria-Avellanal C, Robertson NJ (2014) Na(+)/H(+) exchangers and intracellular pH in perinatal brain injury. Transl Stroke Res 5:79–98
21. Vannucci RC, Connor JR, Mauger DT, Palmer C, Smith MB, Towfighi J, Vannucci SJ (1999) Rat model of perinatal hypoxic-ischemic brain damage. J Neurosci Res 55:158–163
22. Vannucci RC, Vannucci SJ (1997) A model of perinatal hypoxic-ischemic brain damage. In: Reis DJ, Posner JB (eds) Frontiers of neurology: a symposium in honor of Fred Plum, vol 835, Annals of the New York Academy of Sciences. New York Academy of Sciences, New York, pp 234–249
23. Volpe JJ (2001) Perinatal brain injury: from pathogenesis to neuroprotection. Ment Retard Dev Disabil Res Rev 7:56–64
24. Zanelli S, Naylor M, Kapur J (2009) Nitric oxide alters GABAergic synaptic transmission in cultured hippocampal neurons. Brain Res 1297:23–31

Zebrafish (*Danio rerio*) Developed as an Alternative Animal Model for Focal Ischemic Stroke

Xinge Yu and Yang V. Li

Introduction

Ischemic stroke induced by an acute cerebral artery occlusion has been reproduced by different methods. One of the methods is photothrombosis. This is induced by transcranial illumination of the brain after systemic delivery of Rose Bengal, a photosensitive dye [6, 10]. Rose Bengal releases singlet oxygen to injure endothelial cells of blood vessels under light exposure and triggers the coagulation pathway in the irradiated tissue. This model has the advantage of allowing the experimenter to predefine the ischemic region [1].

Alternative models such as mechanical occlusions of middle cerebral artery are often technically challenging. The use of invasive procedures as well as unstable effects from treatments are major limitations [13]. Although these limitations do not make the models less important or valuable, studies performed on alternative models are necessary to provide more objective results. The present work shows that a zebrafish model can be a choice that offers numerous advantages.

The zebrafish has been extensively explored as a research model using both embryos and adults. Our previous studies have shown that zebrafish can be used as a reproducible model of hypoxic-ischemic cerebral damage [14, 15]. In this study, we developed zebrafish as a focal cerebral ischemia model via the photothrombotic method. We evaluated ischemic brain injury of zebrafish by observing behavioral changes, mortality rate, and histological staining of the brain tissue. We also treated zebrafish with tissue plasminogen activator (Activase®, tPA), the only US Food and Drug Administration (FDA)-approved drug for thrombotic cerebral ischemia. We hypothesized that zebrafish are sensitive to photothrombosis-induced ischemic injury that would respond to tPA treatment. This would suggest that zebrafish can be used as an alternative model for studies of focal ischemic stroke.

X. Yu
Department of Biomedical Sciences, Ohio University, Athens, OH 45701, USA

Y.V. Li, PhD (✉)
Department of Biomedical Sciences, Ohio University, Athens, OH 45701, USA

Program in Biological Sciences, Ohio University, 346 Irvine Hall, Athens, OH 45701, USA
e-mail: Liy1@ohio.edu

Materials and Methods

Animals

All work in this study was conducted according to Ohio University Institutional Animal Care and Use Committee (IACUC) guidelines. Adult zebrafish (*Danio rerio*) were purchased from a local supplier and kept under a 12-h light/12-h dark cycle with tank water, which contained half deionized water plus half dechlorinated water at room temperature. The dechlorinated water was made with fresh tap water with 10–15 mg/L sodium thiosulfate [3]. Zebrafish were fed daily by commercial food flake. The average length of zebrafish used in this study was 3.82 ± 0.36 cm (mean ± SD).

Phototrombotic Treatment

Zebrafish were anesthetized by ethyl 3-aminobenzoate methanesulfonate (MS-222) (140 mg/l) and intraperitoneally injected with Rose Bengal dissolved in saline according to the body weight (100 μg/g). The total volume of injection was less than 0.1 ml. Then the zebrafish was placed into a Petri dish in the upright posture. The medium in the Petri dish was made of MS-222 (75 mg/l). The optic tectum region of the head was exposed under cold light at the light intensity of 800 μW/cm^2

R.L. Applegate et al. (eds.), *Brain Edema XVI: Translate Basic Science into Clinical Practice*, Acta Neurochirurgica Supplement, Vol. 121, DOI 10.1007/978-3-319-18497-5_20, © Springer International Publishing Switzerland 2016

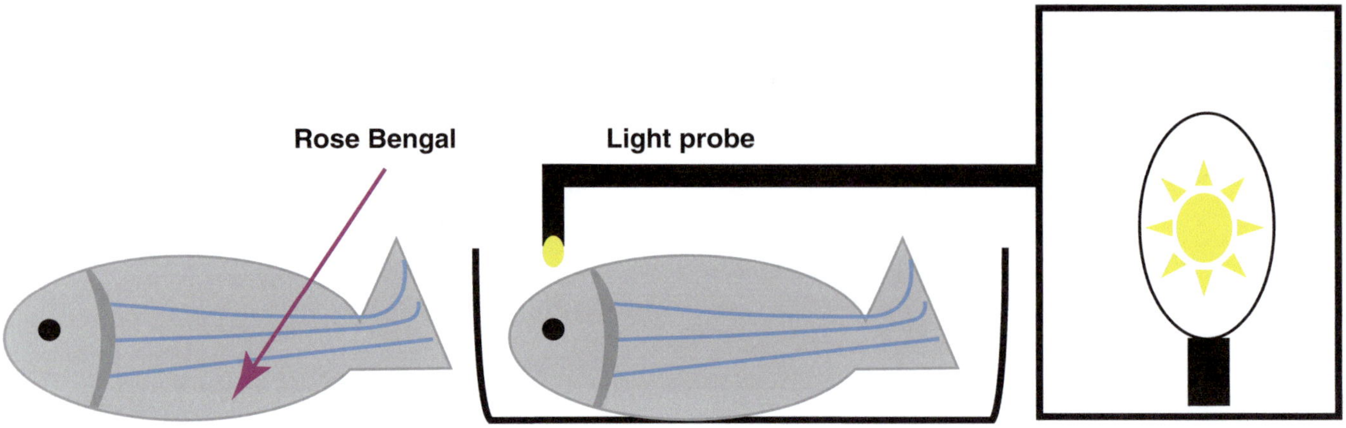

Fig. 1 Schematic diagram of the custom-designed restraint dish. Rose Bengal is intraperitoneally injected in zebrafish after anesthesia. The zebrafish is submerged in the Petri dish with MS-222 solution (75 mg/l) to maintain anesthesia. A rubber band (not shown here) is used to keep the zebrafish in upright position yet was loose enough to allow gill movement. Gentle perfusion of O_2 is provided during the process to ensure adequate O_2 supply

for 20 or 30 min according to design (Fig. 1). The illuminator and the light probe were purchased from Dolan Jenner (Boxborough, MA, USA). After photothrombotic treatment, the mortality rate of each group was measured, and recovery as well as behavioral changes were observed.

2,3,5-Triphenyltetrazolium Chloride (TTC) Staining and Quantification

The 2,3,5-triphenyltetrazolium chloride (TTC) staining method was adopted and modified from Preston et al. [9]. The brain slice was 1 mm thick of the optic lobe and was placed in TTC solution (2 % by weight) in the dark for 40 min at room temperature. After staining, the TTC solution was discarded and the slice was placed in a semi-micro cuvette with 400 μl DMSO/ethanol (1:1) solution in the dark for TTC extraction overnight. A spectrophotometer was used to measure TTC absorbance at 485 nm wavelength in each cuvette after slices were removed. Images of the brain slices were taken immediately after TTC staining and the volume of the brain slice was measured by software Motic plus 3.0.

Chemicals and Reagents

Ethyl 3-aminobenzoate methanesulfonate (MS-222), Rose Bengal, and 2,3,5-triphenyltetrazolium chloride (TTC) were purchased from Sigma Aldrich (St Louis, MO, USA). Activase®-tPA was purchased from Genentech (South San Francisco, CA, USA). All chemicals were dissolved in saline unless stated otherwise.

Statistical Analysis

Statistical analysis of percentage of recovery under different treatments was performed using Fisher's exact test with R program. Statistical analysis of TTC measurements was performed using two-tailed Student's *t*-test with Microsoft Excel. A value of $p < 0.05$ was considered significant.

Results

Zebrafish Exhibit Abnormal Behaviors after Photothrombotic Treatment

We placed the zebrafish in the Petri dish under anesthesia and placed the light probe on the skull in the region of optic tectum. The rest of the body was covered with aluminum foil. After 30 min of light exposure, the zebrafish was transferred to tank water to recover from anesthesia. Zebrafish regained normal swimming behavior after 15–30 min. We considered zebrafish managing normal and balanced swimming behavior as complete recovery from anesthesia. Zebrafish were kept in the dark. Only dim red light was used as necessary for observation, to prevent further excitation of Rose Bengal. We observed two types of abnormal swimming behavior by 24 h after photothrombotic treatment, rotating and circling (Fig. 2a, b). Rotating and circling were not observed in controls treated with Rose Bengal or light only. By 24 h after photothrombotic treatment, 96.8 % of zebrafish died or exhibited circling and rotating (Table 1). Our results indicate that photothrombosis produced delayed damage to zebrafish that was observed as behavioral change.

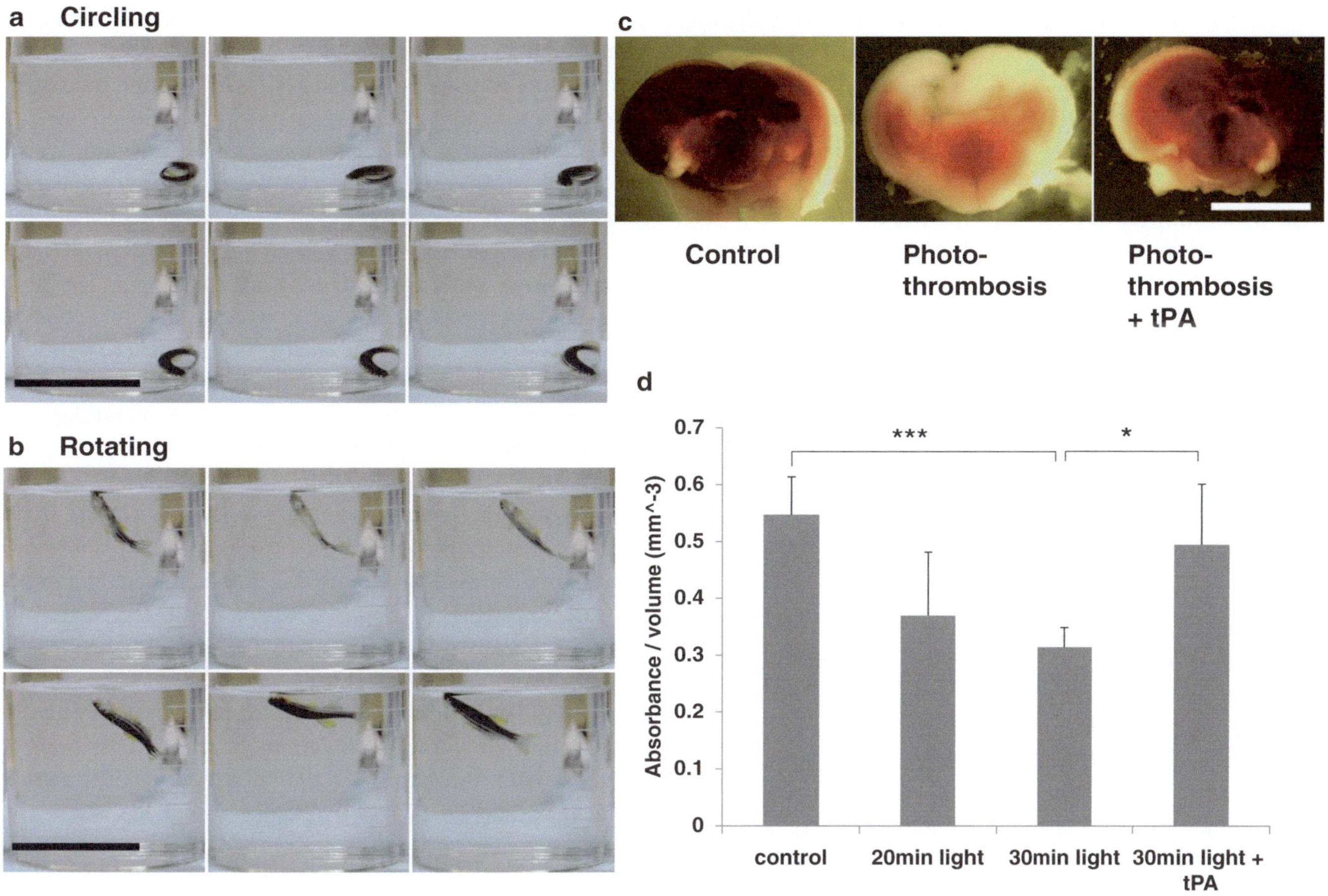

Fig. 2 Evaluation of brain damage after photo-thrombotic treatment. (**a**) Circling behavior after photothrombotic treatment. Scale bar: 5 cm. (**b**) Rotating behavior after photothrombotic treatment. Scale bar: 5 cm. Sequential images of zebrafish circling and rotating movements are acquired from 1 s of videos. (**c**) TTC staining of the zebrafish brain 24 h after photothrombotic treatment. Scale bar: 1 mm. (**d**) Spectrophotometric measurement shows that photothrombotic damage is light exposure dose-dependent, and treatment with tPA significantly improved TTC absorbance compared with the non-tPA treated group (* $p<0.05$, *** $p=4.36587e^{-05}$, $n=7$)

Table 1 Recovery rate between the tPA treated group and the non-tPA treated group after photothrombosis

	Non-tPA	tPA	Fisher test
Total number	31	20	
Number of death	17	6	0.0673
Number of behavior change	13	3	0.0642
Number of recovery	1	11	$3.359e^{-05}$

Photohrombotic Treatment Causes Quantitative Brain Damage

To confirm the brain damage, TTC staining was performed at 24 h after photothrombotic treatment. Zebrafish in the first control group were treated with Rose Bengal but not light exposed. The second control group was zebrafish receiving light exposure for 30 min, without Rose Bengal treatment. TTC staining and behavior observation indicated no brain damage from light exposure or Rose Bengal alone (data not shown). TTC staining of photothrombotic treated brain slices showed lack of staining in the area of light exposure, indicating ischemic cell death. Quantified measurement of TTC staining showed a significant reduction of brain cell viability with 20 min of light exposure, compared with the control group, and even greater reduction with 30 min of light exposure. Results also showed a strong correlation between abnormal swimming pattern and the extent of damage of the brain.

Photothrombosis-Induced Cerebral Damage Is Responsive to tPA Treatment

In a separate group (tPA group), we intraperitoneally injected tPA immediately after photothrombosis. TTC staining after 24 h showed that the application of tPA increased viability of brain tissue compared with photothrombosis without tPA. We also compared the 24-h recovery of zebrafish with and without tPA treatment. In non-tPA treated group, 41.9 % exhibited abnormal swimming, and 54.8 % zebrafish died by 24 h after photothrombosis. Only 3 % fully recovered without exhibiting behavioral changes. Treatment with tPA increased the recovery rate from 3 to 55 % at 24 h. The rate of abnormal swimming was decreased to 15 % and the mortality rate was reduced to 30 %. Detailed data are shown in Table 1. Treatment with tPA also improved brain viability after photothrombosis, quantified by TTC staining (Fig. 2c, d). Our results suggest that the zebrafish photothrombotic model is responsive to tPA treatment, which makes zebrafish a promising model for stroke studies and drug screening.

Discussion

In this study, we demonstrate that photothrombotic treatment effectively and reproducibly induces brain damage in zebrafish. Photothrombosis has been a well-accepted method to reproduce brain ischemia in rodent models. We are the first group to use zebrafish to develop a focal cerebral ischemia model.

To induce effective and reproducible brain damage via photothrombosis, both the dose of Rose Bengal and light exposure, as well as the time of exposure, have to be well controlled. The major finding of this study is that using adult zebrafish as a model of focal cerebral ischemia is feasible via the photothrombotic method. Brain injury of zebrafish can be observed as unbalanced swimming caused by the damage of optic tectum [5, 11]. We observed two characteristically abnormal swimming patterns of circling and rotating in zebrafish with brain injuries. TTC staining also showed significantly reduced staining compared with that of healthy controls. The lack of staining is closely correlated to the time of photothrombotic treatment (20 min versus 30 min of light exposure). The application of tPA resulted in both a significant increase of TTC staining and a significantly greater rate of recovery. Those results suggest that the brain damage was caused by occlusion of blood vessels in the zebrafish brain.

There are growing efforts to develop zebrafish as a model system in neurological studies ranging from genetic to behavioral evaluations [2, 4, 8]. Adult zebrafish as a model to study focal ischemic brain damage has not been extensively explored at the present. There are several reasons that the zebrafish model helps the research of thrombotic ischemic brain damage and ultimately contributes to the advancement of therapeutic drug development. First, the present study indicates that the brain of zebrafish is sensitive to thrombotic ischemic damage. As shown here (Fig. 2, Table 1), photothrombosis induced brain injury and death of zebrafish occurred in a short time. Second, the optic tectum of zebrafish communicates with the visual input and body movement [7] and is required for optomotor response while swimming [12]. As a result, consistent abnormal swimming patterns such as rotating and circling can be observed after local ischemia of the optic tectum, which makes zebrafish a reliable model for observing behavioral changes after brain damage. Delayed behavioral changes are observed in zebrafish 24 h after photothrombosis, which make the evaluation and measurements practical for delayed brain injury and recovery. Another advantage is that the zebrafish has a well-studied set of genes and a fully sequenced genome. Because of availability of well-characterized mutants, it is currently practical and convenient to use gene mutations and transgenic zebrafish for further studies.

Activase® (tPA) has been the only FDA approved drug for thrombotic cerebral ischemia. We suggest in this study that photothrombotic zebrafish respond well to tPA treatment. Application of tPA reduced brain damage and mortality rate, as well as improved behavioral recovery. We propose zebrafish as an alternative model for thrombotic stroke. This model can benefit the screening of neuroprotective candidates and studies to improve tPA efficacy. Considering the work on genetic modification in zebrafish, the zebrafish is thus a promising new animal model to study molecular mechanisms of ischemic stroke and ischemic neuronal death.

Acknowledgment We thank Dr. Christian J. Stork and Kira G. Slepchenko for constructive feedback.

Conflict of Interest Statement No competing financial interests exist.

References

1. Bacigaluppi M, Comi G, Hermann DM (2010) Animal models of ischemic stroke. Part two: Modeling cerebral ischemia. Open Neurol J 4:34–38
2. Carvan MJ, Sonntag DM, Cmar CB, Cook RS, Curran MA, Miller GL (2001) Oxidative stress in zebrafish cells: potential utility of transgenic zebrafish as a deployable sentinel for site hazard ranking. Sci Total Environ 274(1–3):183–196
3. Faulk CK, Holt GJ (2006) Responses of cobia *Rachycentron canadum* larvae to abrupt or gradual changes in salinity. Aquaculture 254(1–4):275–283
4. Hill AJ, Teraoka H, Heideman W, Peterson RE (2005) Zebrafish as a model vertebrate for investigating chemical toxicity. Toxicol Sci 86(1):6–19
5. Laale HW (1977) The biology and use of zebrafish, *Brachydanio rerio* in fisheries research. A literature review. J Fish Biol 10(2):121–173
6. Mosinger JL, Olney JW (1989) Photothrombosis-induced ischemic neuronal degeneration in the rat retina. Exp Neurol 113:110–113
7. Papoutsoglou SE (2012) The role of the brain in farmed fish. Rev Aquacult 4(1):1–10

8. Parng C, Ton C, Lin Y-X, Roy NM, McGrath P (2006) A zebrafish assay for identifying neuroprotectants in vivo. Neurotoxicol Teratol 28(4):509–516
9. Preston E, Webster J (2000) Spectrophotometric measurement of experimental brain injury. J Neurosci Methods 94(2):187–192
10. Schroeter M, Jander S, Stoll G (2002) Non-invasive induction of focal cerebral ischemia in mice by photothrombosis of cortical microvessels: characterization of inflammatory responses. J Neurosci Methods 117(1):43–49
11. Tanden KK, Sharma SC (1965) On the degeneration and regeneration of optic nerve fibers with return of vision in Danio rerio (Ham.). Proc Indian Acad Sci B 60:287–292
12. Springer AD, Easter SS Jr, Agranoff BW (1977) The role of the optic tectum in various visually mediated behaviors of goldfish. Brain Res 128:393–404
13. Traystman RJ (2003) Animal models of focal and global cerebral ischemia. ILAR J 44(2):85–95
14. Yu X, Li YV (2011) Zebrafish as an alternative model for hypoxic-ischemic brain damage. Int J Physiol Pathophysiol Pharmacol 3(2):88–96
15. Yu X, Li YV (2013) Neuroprotective effect of zinc chelator DEDTC in a zebrafish (*Danio rerio*) model of hypoxic brain injury. Zebrafish 10(1):30–35

Brain Hemorrhage Section

Signaling Pathway in Early Brain Injury after Subarachnoid Hemorrhage: News Update

Chengyuan Ji and Gang Chen

Introduction

Early brain injury (EBI) usually occurs within 72 h after SAH [2]. In 2004, Zhang et al. first defined EBI as the direct brain tissue damage that occurs within 72 h after spontaneous SAH and includes all of the pathophysiological processes that continue until the appearance of delayed cerebral vasospasm (CVS) (normally 3 days to 2 weeks). The mechanisms underlying early brain damage are complex and are summarized below.

Pathophysiological Mechanisms

Global Cerebral Ischemia

Intracranial arterial aneurysm rupture leads to a large volume of blood released into the subarachnoid space, resulting in a sharp increase in intracranial pressure. This causes a reduction in cerebrospinal fluid and a significantly lower intracranial perfusion pressure (CPP), leading to cerebral ischemia, swelling, and edema, which ultimately damages nerve cells [17].

Apoptosis

Apoptosis plays an important role in post-SAH EBI and disease prognosis. When the aneurysm ruptures, a sharp increase in intracranial pressure in conjunction with toxic components released from blood and elevated radicals caused by ischemia cause neuronal apoptosis.

C. Ji • G. Chen (✉)
Department of Neurosurgery, The First Affiliated Hospital of Soochow University, 188 Shizi Street, Suzhou 215006, P. R. China
e-mail: nju_neurosurgery@163.com

Damage to the Blood-Brain Barrier and Brain Edema

The collective effects of global cerebral ischemia, neuronal apoptosis, and neuronal necrosis induce blood-brain barrier damage, further causing vasogenic cerebral edema.

Molecular Mechanisms

Ischemic Pathways

Subarachnoid blood can decrease CBF and blood hemoglobin, and endothelin- 1 (ET-1) can reduce the activity of Na/K-ATPase, leading to disorders in cerebrovascular depolarization, thus affecting vasodilatation.

Apoptotic Pathways

1. Death receptor-mediated apoptosis pathway—SAH can activate p53, FAS, BCL-2, and NF-κB to activate caspase-8, resulting in the activation of caspase-3. The effector caspases, including caspases 3, 6, and 7, can activate endonucleases, leading to DNA fragmentation, ultimately resulting in destruction of the whole cell structures [14].
2. Mitochondrial apoptosis pathway—SAH promotes the release of cytochrome *c* from mitochondria into the cytosol to form a complex with apoptotic protease activating factor-1 (APAF-1) and procaspase-9. This Cyt-c-Apaf-1-Procaspase-9 complex further activates downstream effector molecules to trigger apoptosis.
3. Caspase-independent pathways—Apoptosis-inducing factor (AIF) is a mitochondrial intermembrane protein. In the absence of APAF-I, p53 can regulate the release of AIF, thereby activating caspase-independent pathways.
4. p53—p53 is a transcription factor that functions as the central regulator of the apoptotic cascade.

R.L. Applegate et al. (eds.), *Brain Edema XVI: Translate Basic Science into Clinical Practice*, Acta Neurochirurgica Supplement, Vol. 121,
DOI 10.1007/978-3-319-18497-5_21, © Springer International Publishing Switzerland 2016

Inflammatory Pathways

After SAH, the level of heat shock proteins in cerebrospinal fluid or brain tissue is increased, leading to the activation of TLR4 receptors. Some studies have shown that TLR4 is the key receptor involved in LPS-induced damage to the central nervous system [10], which causes brain damage.

Signaling Pathways in EBI

mTOR Pathway

Mammalian target of rapamycin (mTOR) is a serine/threonine protein kinase that belongs to the phosphoinositide kinase-related kinase family (PIKK family) and is a downstream effector of the PI3K/PKB (protein kinase B) signaling pathway. mTOR plays important roles in transcription, protein translation, apoptosis, and actin cytoskeleton organization.

The interaction of mitogens with their receptors leads to activation of PI3K, which converts PIP2 into PIP3. PIP3 directly interacts with the PH domain of AKT, thus leading to its membrane translocation and activation. Tuberin, the heterodimer consisting of tuberous sclerosis complex 1 and 2 (TSC1/2), is a substrate of AKT and a negative regulator of the mTOR signaling pathway. Tuberin converts the active GTP-bound Rheb into the inactive GDP-bound form of Rheb. Rheb is an upstream regulator of mTOR that directly binds to the mTOR kinase domain and changes the conformation of mTOR-Raptor complex to activate mTOR kinase activity [21].

Studies have shown that the mTOR pathway plays an important role in cerebral ischemia and also in neuronal autophagy and apoptosis. Currently, mTOR is believed to play a dual role in post-SAH EBI. Zhang et al. [24] found that the mTOR signaling pathway also plays an important role in cerebral vasospasm after SAH. They examined expression levels of several important components of the mTOR signaling pathway after SAH, including mTOR and P70S6K1. In addition, they also investigated the effects of the mTOR inhibitors rapamycin and AZD8055 on basilar artery after SAH and on the expression levels of mTOR and P70S6K1. Their results showed that, after SAH, activation of the mTOR pathway may promote proliferation of vascular smooth muscle, and thus is involved in the regulation of vasospasm of the basilar artery. The application of the mTOR inhibitors rapamycin and AZD8055 can significantly relieve arterial spasticity.

The mTOR pathway and mTOR inhibitors have become the focus of intensive research. These studies will likely help us to better understand EBI and CVS after SAH and could provide new ideas for intervention in the progression of EBI after SAH.

Toll-Like Receptors/MAPK/NF-κB Signaling Pathway

Toll-like receptors (TLRs) are a class of innate immune receptors initially discovered in *Drosophila.* TLRs are expressed in many immune cells, including macrophages, dendritic cells, lymphocytes, and natural killer cells. They play a key role in the immune response. At least 12 TLR receptors have been identified, among which TLR4 is the main receptor for endotoxin/LPS (lipopolysaccharide) [18].

Ligand binding triggers signal transduction of the TIR region of TLR4 and activation of the nuclear factor κB (NF-κB) pathway and mitogen-activated protein kinase (MAPK) signaling pathway, thereby promoting the expression of various inflammatory cytokines. NF-κB can be activated by a variety of inflammatory substances and also by oxidative stress to promote transcription of a plethora of genes that play important roles in the immune response and tissue damage response.

Toll receptors act through an intracellular signaling cascade to activate the inflammation-related MAPK pathway and NF-κB signaling pathway. Activated NF-κB enters the nucleus to promote the transcription of inflammatory cytokines, including IL-1β, TNF-α, IL-6, ICAM-1, and MCP-1. Furthermore, NF-κB is closely related to apoptosis pathways; NF-κB can inhibit the caspase family, therefore inhibiting neuronal apoptosis after EBI. However, NF-κB also stimulates the expression of TNF-α, thus inducing apoptosis. Thus, NF-κB is a key factor in regulating post-EBI inflammation and neuronal apoptosis. Caspase signaling and MAPK signaling pathways are also important to EBI after SAH, as treatment with the caspase inhibitor z-VAD-FMK or MAPK inhibitor PP1 can significantly mitigate symptoms of EBI [12].

Sun et al. [20] showed that the TLR/NF-κB signaling pathway is involved in the inflammatory response in EBI after SAH and that tamoxifen can protect the brain from EBI after SAH by effectively inhibiting the expression of TLR4, NF-κB, and some other downstream inflammatory mediators (IL-1β, TNF-α, IL-6, etc.). They further confirmed that the use of tamoxifen can improve neurological cognition of SAH patients. Wang et al. [23] also confirmed the important role of the TLR4 pathway in post-SAH EBI and further showed that melatonin treatment can protect the brain and improve cognitive function of patients.

Studies on Toll receptor and its downstream MAPK/NF-κB signaling pathway have been summarized [1]. Progesterone has also been shown to function through the TLR pathway to play a protective role in EBI after SAH [4]. Taken together, these findings will provide new ideas for clinical intervention in EBI after SAH.

Autophagy

Autophagy is a conserved mechanism in all eukaryotic cells whereby excessive or aberrant proteins and damaged organelles are degraded to maintain normal cell function. With autophagy, substrates are recognized and then encapsulated in autophagic vesicles, and these vesicles then fuse with and release their content to lysosomes. This process leads to the digestion of damaged organelles and aberrant proteins by the lysosome. Autophagy is also an important mechanism to supply nutrients when cells are starved. Thus, autophagy plays an important role in growth, development, and metabolism [15]. In recent years, many studies have shown that autophagy is important to a variety of brain injuries.

The mTOR pathway and PI3K pathway are two major pathways regulating autophagy. In the mTOR-dependent autophagy pathway, mTOR complex 1 (mTORC1) is a major regulator of autophagy that may act through two mechanisms to control autophagy. The first mechanism involves direct phosphorylation of ATG by mTORC1. The second involves signal transduction to control autophagy-related gene transcription and translation. (2) PI3K-dependent autophagy pathway: PI3K catalyzes the generation of phosphatidylinositol 3-phosphate (PI3P) to promote autophagy. It also can prevent apoptosis and necrosis [3].

A growing number of studies have found that in SAH or ICH models, autophagy is activated and may function as a protective mechanism. Lee et al. [13] found in a rat model of SAH that the levels of LC3-II and Beclin-1 were increased significantly, indicating that autophagy persists in post-SAH EBI. Wang et al. found that in a rat model of SAH, LC3 and Beclin-1 levels in the cerebral cortex of SAH rat were increased and that the autophagy activator rapamycin (RAP) could further increase the expression of LC3 and Beclin-1 and mitigate early brain damage. In addition, the autophagy inhibitor 3-MA reduced LC3 and Beclin-1 expression and aggravated brain injury. These results support a protective role of autophagy in EBI of rats [22]. Further research has found that autophagy may protect the brain by reducing apoptosis, in which the mitochondrial apoptotic pathway may play a key role.

Numerous studies have confirmed that autophagy is activated and plays an important role in EBI after SAH. However, its role in neuroprotection needs further investigation, as autophagy is a double-edged sword that removes intracellular toxic substances to protect nerve cells but can cause degeneration of nerve cells and possibly apoptosis.

Keap1-Nrf2-ARE Pathway

A large number of studies have found that the Keap1-Nrf2-ARE pathway plays an important role in many diseases. Activation of this signaling pathway can induce expression of a variety of antioxidant and detoxification enzymes, raise the levels of glutathione and superoxide dismutase, and scavenge free radicals and other oxidizing substances, thus playing a protective role for the cell [11].

In the resting state, Keap1 and Nrf2 form a cytosolic complex [8]. After SAH, Nrf2 dissociates from Keap1 and enters into the nucleus. In the nucleus, Nrf2 binds to the ARE (antioxidant response element) of the genes of some enzymes involved in detoxification and antioxidant properties to promote their expression. These enzymes include heme oxygenase 1 (HO-1), glutathione-S-transferase a1 (GST-a1), and NAD(P)H: quinone oxidoreductase 1 (NQO1). They act collectively to confer antioxidant and detoxification capabilities that protect the nervous system.

HO-1 is a downstream target gene of the Nrf2-ARE pathway, and its transcription level is upregulated in EBI after SAH. In post-EBI SAH, GST maintains redox homeostasis and plays a role in anti-apoptosis [7]. NQO1 is a free riboflavin dimeric protein that is ubiquitously distributed in tissues. The role of NQO1 in oxidative stress has been extensively studied, and the results reveal differences in its activity among individuals and between normal tissues and tumor tissues of the same individual [19]. Both basal and induced expression by EBI after SAH of NQO1 are mediated by ARE.

Studies have shown that Keap1-Nrf2-ARE pathway plays important roles in apoptosis, stress response, inflammation, cardiovascular regulation, and neuroprotection to protect cells. Targeting the Keap1-Nrf2-ARE pathway has become an effective way to treat a variety of diseases caused by oxidative stress [9].

Adenosine A3 Receptors Pathway

Adenosine is a metabolite of adenine nucleotide metabolism and functions as an important CNS neuromodulator in a variety of biological processes by binding to different adenosine receptors (AR). Human A3AR gene (ADORA3) is located on chromosome 1p13.3 and encodes a protein of 318 amino acids. The levels of A3AR are high in the hippocampus, cerebellum, hypothalamus, thalamus, olfactory nerves, and auditory nerves, but low in the cortex and amygdala [5].

Currently, at least four pathways have been found to act downstream of A3AR: (1) A3AR activation can inhibit adenylate cyclase (AC) activity to decrease intracellular cAMP levels, therefore playing a regulatory role in the growth and differentiation of cells [6]. (2) A3AR activation can activate phospholipase C (PLC) to release Ca^{2+}. Ca^{2+} acts as a second messenger to elicit various cell responses. (3) A3AR can regulate the PI3K-AKT signaling pathway. (4) Ras-Raf-MAPK (mitogen-activated protein kinase) pathway is also involved in signal transduction mediated by A3AR.

Luo et al. [16] found that in EBI after SAH, A3R receptor activation can alleviate inflammation and that administration of an A3R agonist (CL-IB-MECA) has marked effects. They found that after CL-IB-MECA intervention, mortality rate, nerve injury, and brain edema are all remarkably decreased in patients with post-SAH EBI. Moreover, CL-IB-MECA intervention was found to inhibit the proliferation of microglia, thereby reducing expression of pro-inflammatory cytokines, such as tumor necrosis factor-α and interleukin-1β. The importance of A3R in EBI after SAH is emerging, and further studies will provide new ideas for the treatment of cerebrovascular disease like aneurysm, traumatic brain injury, and other central nervous system diseases.

Conclusion

There is evidence showing that EBI is the leading cause of death in patients with SAH, but the underlying mechanism is complicated. Currently, there is no medicine or treatment that can target the signaling pathways involved in the pathology. Thus, to prevent or mitigate harm caused by post-SAH EBI, a goal of future studies is to understand the molecular mechanisms of EBI and to inhibit the process of EBI.

References

1. Akira S, Takeda K (2004) Toll-like receptor signalling. Nat Rev Immunol 4:499–511
2. Cahill J, Calvert JW, Zhang JH (2006) Mechanisms of early brain injury after subarachnoid hemorrhage. J Cereb Blood Flow Metab 26:1341–1353
3. Castino R, Bellio N, Follo C, Murphy D, Isidoro C (2010) Inhibition of PI3k class III-dependent autophagy prevents apoptosis and necrosis by oxidative stress in dopaminergic neuroblastoma cells. Toxicol Sci 117:152–162
4. Chen G, Shi J, Jin W, Wang L, Xie W, Sun J, Hang C (2008) Progesterone administration modulates TLRs/NF-kappaB signaling pathway in rat brain after cortical contusion. Ann Clin Lab Sci 38:65–74
5. Dixon AK, Gubitz AK, Sirinathsinghji DJ, Richardson PJ, Freeman TC (1996) Tissue distribution of adenosine receptor mRNAs in the rat. Br J Pharmacol 118:1461–1468
6. Fishman P, Madi L, Bar-Yehuda S, Barer F, Del Valle L, Khalili K (2002) Evidence for involvement of Wnt signaling pathway in IB-MECA mediated suppression of melanoma cells. Oncogene 21:4060–4064
7. Guney O, Erdi F, Esen H, Kiyici A, Kocaogullar Y (2010) N-acetylcysteine prevents vasospasm after subarachnoid hemorrhage. World Neurosurg 73:42–49; discussion e43
8. Itoh K, Wakabayashi N, Katoh Y, Ishii T, Igarashi K, Engel JD, Yamamoto M (1999) Keap1 represses nuclear activation of antioxidant responsive elements by Nrf2 through binding to the amino-terminal Neh2 domain. Genes Dev 13:76–86
9. Jeong WS, Jun M, Kong AN (2006) Nrf2: a potential molecular target for cancer chemoprevention by natural compounds. Antioxid Redox Signal 8:99–106
10. Kariko K, Weissman D, Welsh FA (2004) Inhibition of toll-like receptor and cytokine signaling–a unifying theme in ischemic tolerance. J Cereb Blood Flow Metab 24:1288–1304
11. Kobayashi M, Yamamoto M (2005) Molecular mechanisms activating the Nrf2-Keap1 pathway of antioxidant gene regulation. Antioxid Redox Signal 7:385–394
12. Kusaka G, Ishikawa M, Nanda A, Granger DN, Zhang JH (2004) Signaling pathways for early brain injury after subarachnoid hemorrhage. J Cereb Blood Flow Metab 24:916–925
13. Lee JY, He Y, Sagher O, Keep R, Hua Y, Xi G (2009) Activated autophagy pathway in experimental subarachnoid hemorrhage. Brain Res 1287:126–135
14. Leist M, Jaattela M (2001) Four deaths and a funeral: from caspases to alternative mechanisms. Nat Rev Mol Cell Biol 2: 589–598
15. Li J, Ni M, Lee B, Barron E, Hinton DR, Lee AS (2008) The unfolded protein response regulator GRP78/BiP is required for endoplasmic reticulum integrity and stress-induced autophagy in mammalian cells. Cell Death Differ 15:1460–1471
16. Luo C, Yi B, Tao G, Li M, Chen Z, Tang W, Zhang JH, Feng H (2010) Adenosine A3 receptor agonist reduces early brain injury in subarachnoid haemorrhage. Neuroreport 21:892–896
17. Ostrowski RP, Colohan AR, Zhang JH (2006) Molecular mechanisms of early brain injury after subarachnoid hemorrhage. Neurol Res 28:399–414
18. Poltorak A, He X, Smirnova I, Liu MY, Van Huffel C, Du X, Birdwell D, Alejos E, Silva M, Galanos C, Freudenberg M, Ricciardi-Castagnoli P, Layton B, Beutler B (1998) Defective LPS signaling in C3H/HeJ and C57BL/10ScCr mice: mutations in Tlr4 gene. Science 282:2085–2088
19. Riley RJ, Workman P (1992) DT-diaphorase and cancer chemotherapy. Biochem Pharmacol 43:1657–1669
20. Sun X, Ji C, Hu T, Wang Z, Chen G (2013) Tamoxifen as an effective neuroprotectant against early brain injury and learning deficits induced by subarachnoid hemorrhage: possible involvement of inflammatory signaling. J Neuroinflammation 10:157
21. Swiech L, Perycz M, Malik A, Jaworski J (2008) Role of mTOR in physiology and pathology of the nervous system. Biochim Biophys Acta 1784:116–132
22. Wang Z, Shi XY, Yin J, Zuo G, Zhang J, Chen G (2012) Role of autophagy in early brain injury after experimental subarachnoid hemorrhage. J Mol Neurosci 46:192–202
23. Wang Z, Wu L, You W, Ji C, Chen G (2013) Melatonin alleviates secondary brain damage and neurobehavioral dysfunction after experimental subarachnoid hemorrhage: possible involvement of TLR4-mediated inflammatory pathway. J Pineal Res 55: 399–408
24. Zhang W, Khatibi NH, Yamaguchi-Okada M, Yan J, Chen C, Hu Q, Meng H, Han H, Liu S, Zhou C (2012) Mammalian target of rapamycin (mTOR) inhibition reduces cerebral vasospasm following a subarachnoid hemorrhage injury in canines. Exp Neurol 233:799–806

Effects of Low-Dose Unfractionated Heparin Pretreatment on Early Brain Injury after Subarachnoid Hemorrhage in Mice

Orhan Altay, Hidenori Suzuki, Yu Hasegawa, Mehmet Sorar, Han Chen, Jiping Tang, and John H. Zhang

Introduction

Subarachnoid hemorrhage (SAH) is a life-threatening disease with a 12.4 % risk for sudden death before receiving medical intervention [13]; a majority of deaths occur within the first 48 h post ictus owing to the impact of the initial bleeding [5]. Subarachnoid blood clot, elevation of intracranial pressure, and reduced cerebral perfusion initiate an acute injury cascade such as microvascular disturbance and inflammatory reaction, leading to early brain injury (EBI), one of the important causes of unfavorable outcomes after SAH [8]. SAH is caused by rupture of an intracranial aneurysm in approximately 85 % patients, accounting for 5 % of strokes but associated with a case fatality rate of around 50 % [23].

Thrombin is a multifunctional serine protease coagulation protein [17], and acts through protease-activated receptors (PARs), which are expressed on the surface of various cell types, including endothelial, epithelial, neuronal, and glial cells [18]. Thrombin has been implicated in blood-brain barrier (BBB) disruption, brain edema, inflammation, and apoptosis [18]. However, it has been reported that activation of PAR1 [7], the principle thrombin receptor, induces or inhibits apoptosis, depending on the dosage of thrombin in human endothelial cells [26].

Heparin, a glycosaminoglycan, inhibits the coagulation process by inhibiting the action of thrombin, and therefore may have neuroprotective effects [12]. However, the clinical use of heparin as a protective or anti-inflammatory agent has been held back by the fear of bleeding. The aim of this study was to test the hypothesis that two doses of unfractionated heparin can be used safely as pretreatment at the SAH occurrence in mice.

Materials and Methods

Experimental Design and Animal Groups

The animal and ethics review committee at Loma Linda University approved all protocols. Forty-five 8-week-old male CD-1 mice (30–38 g; Charles River, Wilmington, MA, USA) were used for the study. Animals were randomly divided into 4 groups and evaluated at 24 h after surgery: sham-operated ($n=8$), SAH + vehicle ($n=12$), SAH + 10 U heparin pretreatment ($n=11$), and SAH + 30 U heparin pretreatment ($n=14$). SAH severity and neurological scores were evaluated by experienced researchers who were kept blinded to the animal's experimental group assignment.

Mouse SAH Model

The SAH endovascular monofilament perforation model was produced as described previously [1]. Briefly, animals were anesthetized with an intraperitoneal injection of ketamine/xylazine (100/10 mg/kg). A sharpened 4–0 monofilament

O. Altay, MD • H. Suzuki, MD, PhD • Y. Hasegawa, MD, PhD
H. Chen, MD • J. Tang, MD
Departments of Physiology, Loma Linda University
School of Medicine, Risley Hall, Room 223,
Loma Linda, CA 92354, USA

M. Sorar, MD
Department of Neurosurgery, Ankara Diskapi
Training and Research Hospital, Ankara, Turkey

J.H. Zhang, MD, PhD (✉)
Departments of Physiology, Loma Linda University
School of Medicine, Risley Hall, Room 223,
Loma Linda, CA 92354, USA

Departments of Neurosurgery, Loma Linda University
School of Medicine, Loma Linda, CA, USA
e-mail: johnzhang3910@yahoo.com

R.L. Applegate et al. (eds.), *Brain Edema XVI: Translate Basic Science into Clinical Practice*, Acta Neurochirurgica Supplement, Vol. 121,
DOI 10.1007/978-3-319-18497-5_22,

nylon suture was advanced through the internal carotid artery (ICA) to perforate the anterior cerebral artery. In the sham surgery, the filament was advanced 5 mm through the ICA without perforating the artery. Body temperature was kept constant (37.5 ± 0.5 °C) during the operation.

Drug Administration

It was reported that daily subcutaneous injections (SCs) of unfractionated porcine heparin of 20 U per mouse (average body weight, 33 g), which is comparable to 600 U/kg/d and within the human therapeutic dose range, has been given safely [20]. Based on this reference, at 2 h before SAH induction, either 10 U or 30 U heparin (McGuff Co., Inc., Santa Ana, CA, USA) was subcutaneously administered.

Severity of SAH

The severity of SAH was evaluated using the SAH grading scale with high-resolution photographs at the time of sacrifice [1]. The SAH grading system was as follows: the basal cistern was divided into six segments, and each segment was allotted a grade from 0 to 3 depending on the amount of subarachnoid blood clot in the segment; grade 0, no subarachnoid blood; grade 1, minimal subarachnoid blood; grade 2, moderate blood clot with recognizable arteries; and grade 3, blood clot obliterating all arteries within the segment. The animals received a total score ranging from 0 to 18 after adding the scores from all six segments.

Mortality and Neurological Scores

The neurological score was evaluated at 24 h after SAH as previously described [1, 2]. The evaluation consists of six tests that can be scored 0–3 or 1–3. The six tests are spontaneous activity, symmetry in the movement of all four limbs, forelimbs outstretching, climbing, side stroking, and response to vibrissae (whisker stimulation). Animals were given a score of 3–18 in 1-number steps (higher scores indicate greater function). Mortality was calculated at 24 h after SAH.

Brain Water Content (BWC)

Brains were quickly removed and separated into the left and right cerebral hemispheres and weighed (wet weight) at 24 h ($n=8$ per group) after surgery. Next, brain specimens were dried in an oven at 105 °C for 72 h and weighed again (dry weight). The percentage of BWC was calculated as ([wet weight – dry weight]/wet weight) ×100 % [1].

Statistics

All values were expressed as the mean ± SD and were analyzed using one-way analysis of variance (ANOVA) with Tukey-Kramer post hoc tests. Differences of $p<0.05$ were considered significant.

Results

Mortality and SAH Grade

The mortality rate was not significantly different among the vehicle, 10 U, and 30 U heparin pretreatment groups of SAH mice (33.3 %, 4 of 12 mice; 27.3 %, 3 of 11 mice; 42.9 %, 6 of 14 mice, respectively). No sham-operated mice died. There was no significant difference in SAH grade between the vehicle and treatment groups, although the SAH + 30 U heparin pretreatment group had more severe SAH compared with the SAH + 10 U heparin pretreatment group ($p=0.037$, Fig. 1).

Neurological Score and BWC

Neurological score was significantly worse after SAH, and a significant improvement was observed only in the 10 U

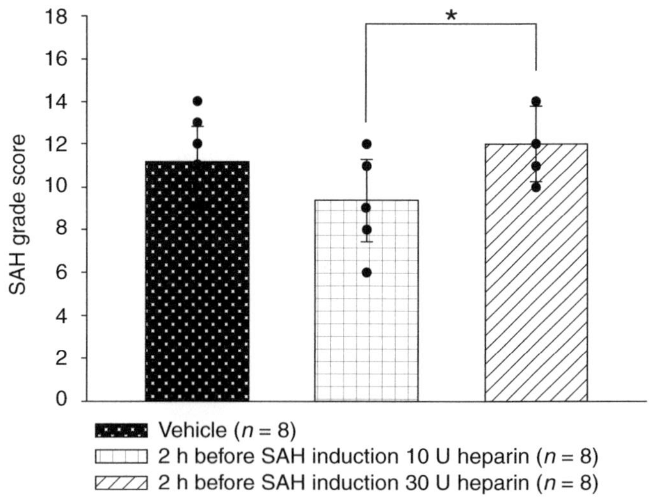

Fig. 1 Subarachnoid hemorrhage (*SAH*) grade at 24 h post-SAH. Values, mean ± SD; *$p<0.05$, ANOVA

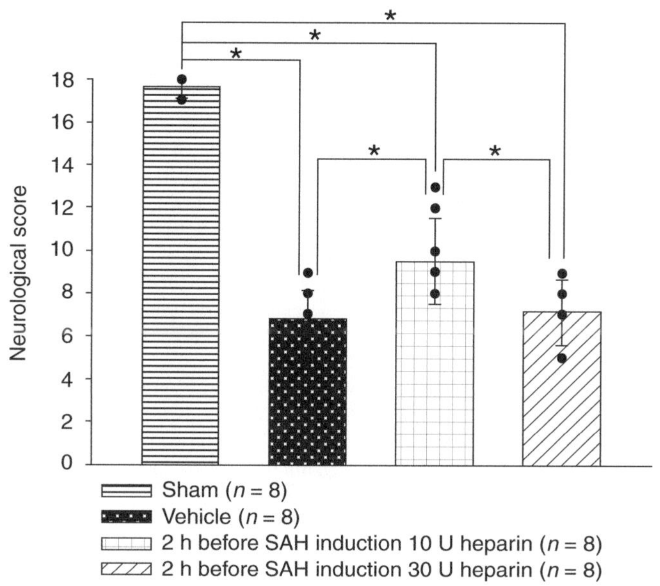

Fig. 2 Neurological score at 24 h after subarachnoid hemorrhage (*SAH*). Values, mean ± SD; *$p < 0.05$, ANOVA

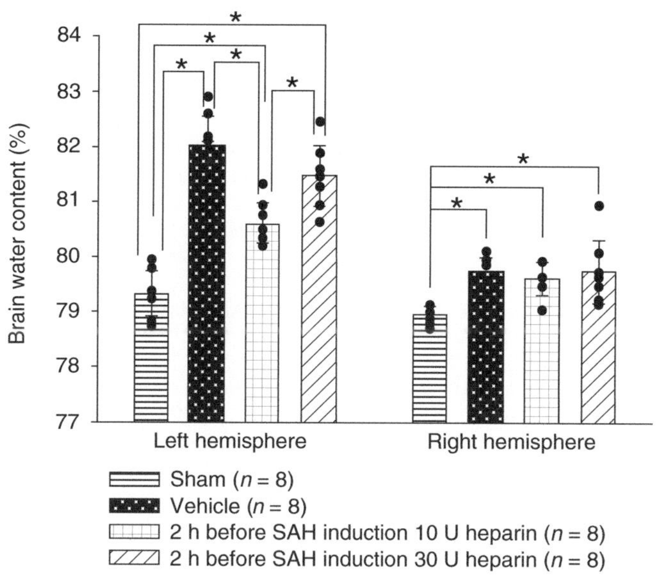

Fig. 3 Brain water content at 24 h after subarachnoid hemorrhage (*SAH*). Values, mean ± SD; *$p < 0.05$, ANOVA

heparin pretreatment group compared with the vehicle group at 24 h after SAH (Fig. 2). BWC in the left cerebral hemisphere was significantly suppressed in the SAH + 10 U heparin pretreatment group but not in the 30 U heparin pretreatment group compared with the vehicle group (Fig. 3). Heparin pretreatment had no effects on post-SAH BWC in the right cerebral hemisphere.

Discussion

The present study showed that low-dose heparin pretreatment attenuated EBI at 24 h after SAH. Deleterious effects from SAH include disruption of the BBB, amplification of inflammatory infiltrates, and possibly disruption of cell-cell and cell-matrix interactions, which may trigger cell death. Under such a situation, thrombin is produced and dramatically upregulated immediately at sites of cerebrovascular injury and may persist for days after injury [22]. At concentrations below 100 pM, the PAR1-dependent signaling activity of thrombin is protective, but at concentrations of higher than 100 pM, thrombin produces a pro-inflammatory response through the activation of PAR1 in endothelial cells [3] or thrombin-induced PAR1 activation engages multiple signaling mechanisms in multiple cell types, leading to neuronal injury [9, 11].

In 1954, Korn [15] established that the lipolytic activity of the lipoprotein lipase enzyme is heparin dependent. The disappearance of lipoprotein lipase activity appears to parallel the circulating heparin level [15]. Endothelial lipase (EL) is a member of the triglyceride lipase family, which includes lipoprotein lipase and hepatic lipase. EL is principally a phospholipase, with nominal triglyceride lipase activity [14]. EL is synthesized principally by endothelial cells [25] and hydrolyzes high-density lipoprotein (HDL) much more efficiently than other lipoproteins [16]. HDL particles represent the predominant sphingosine 1 phosphate (S1P)-carrier in plasma [6, 21]. Free S1P is also protective at low concentrations [4] but proinflammatory and harmful at high or excessive concentrations [24].

Approximately one-third of an administered dose of heparin binds to antithrombin III, and this fraction is responsible for most of the anticoagulant effect or antithrombin effect [9], possibly causing increased sphingosine kinase (SphK)1 and S1P, and therefore the antiapoptotic effects [19]. The remaining two-thirds has minimal anticoagulant activity at therapeutic concentrations, but at concentrations greater than those usually obtained clinically it possibly promotes HDL hydrolysis. The resultant over physiological levels of free S1P may antagonize heparin's protective effects [11, 6, 24]. In addition, 30 U heparin showed a tendency to increase SAH, which potentially causes more severe brain injury associated with a decrease in SphK1 expression [10]. Thus, it is suggested that 10 U heparin was protective, but 30 U heparin lost the protective effects, as this study demonstrated.

Conflict of Interest The authors report no conflicts of interest.

References

1. Altay O, Hasegawa Y, Sherchan P, Suzuki H, Khatibi NH, Tang J, Zhang JH (2012) Isoflurane delays the development of early brain injury after subarachnoid hemorrhage through sphingosine-related pathway activation in mice. Crit Care Med 40:1908–1913
2. Altay O, Suzuki H, Hasegawa Y, Caner B, Krafft PR, Fujii M, Tang J, Zhang JH (2012) Isoflurane attenuates blood-brain barrier disruption in ipsilateral hemisphere after subarachnoid hemorrhage in mice. Stroke 43:2513–2516
3. Bae JS, Kim YU, Park MK, Rezaie AR (2009) Concentration dependent dual effect of thrombin in endothelial cells via Par-1 and Pi3 kinase. J Cell Physiol 219:744–751
4. Bolick DT, Srinivasan S, Kim KW, Hatley ME, Clemens JJ, Whetzel A, Ferger N, Macdonald TL, Davis MD, Tsao PS, Lynch KR, Hedrick CC (2005) Sphingosine-1-phosphate prevents tumor necrosis factor-{alpha}-mediated monocyte adhesion to aortic endothelium in mice. Arterioscler Thromb Vasc Biol 25:976–981
5. Broderick JP, Brott TG, Duldner JE, Tomsick T, Leach A (1994) Initial and recurrent bleeding are the major causes of death following subarachnoid hemorrhage. Stroke 25:1342–1347
6. Christoffersen C, Obinata H, Kumaraswamy SB, Galvani S, Ahnström J, Sevvana M, Egerer-Sieber C, Muller YA, Hla T, Nielsen LB, Dahlbäck B (2011) Endothelium-protective sphingosine-1-phosphate provided by HDL-associated apolipoprotein M. Proc Natl Acad Sci U S A 108:9613–9618
7. Flynn AN, Buret AG (2004) Proteinase-activated receptor 1 (PAR-1) and cell apoptosis. Apoptosis 9:729–737
8. Fujii M, Yan J, Rolland WB, Soejima Y, Caner B, Zhang JH (2013) Early brain injury, an evolving frontier in subarachnoid hemorrhage research. Transl Stroke Res 4:432–446
9. Gingrich MB, Junge CE, Lyuboslavsky P, Traynelis SF (2000) Potentiation of NMDA receptor function by the serine protease thrombin. J Neurosci 20:4582–4595
10. Hasegawa Y, Suzuki H, Altay O, Rolland W, Zhang JH (2013) Role of the sphingosine metabolism pathway on neurons against experimental cerebral ischemia in rats. Transl Stroke Res 4:524–532
11. Henrich-Noack P, Riek-Burchardt M, Baldauf K, Reiser G, Reymann KG (2006) Focal ischemia induces expression of protease-activated receptor1 (PAR1) and PAR3 on microglia and enhances PAR4 labeling in the penumbra. Brain Res 1070: 232–241
12. Hirsh J, Anand SS, Halperin JL, Fuster V, American Heart Association (2001) Guide to anticoagulant therapy: heparin: a statement for healthcare professionals from the American Heart Association. Circulation 103:2994–3018
13. Huang J, van Gelder JM (2002) The probability of sudden death from rupture of intracranial aneurysms: a meta-analysis. Neurosurgery 51:1101–1105
14. Jaye M, Lynch KJ, Krawiec J, Marchadier D, Maugeais C, Doan K, South V, Amin D, Perrone M, Rader DJ (1999) A novel endothelial-derived lipase that modulates HDL metabolism. Nat Genet 21:424–428
15. Korn ED (1955) Clearing factor, a heparin-activated lipoprotein lipase. I. Isolation and characterization of the enzyme from normal rat heart. J Biol Chem 215:1–14
16. McCoy MG, Sun GS, Marchadier D, Maugeais C, Glick JM, Rader DJ (2002) Characterization of the lipolytic activity of endothelial lipase. J Lipid Res 43:921–929
17. Ohyama H, Hosomi N, Takahashi T, Mizushige K, Kohno M (2001) Thrombin inhibition attenuates neurodegeneration and cerebral edema formation following transient forebrain ischemia. Brain Res 902:264–271
18. Ossovskaya VS, Bunnett NW, de Garavilla L, Vergnolle N, Young SH, Ennes H, Steinhoff M, D'Andrea MR, Mayer EA, Wallace JL, Hollenberg MD, Andrade-Gordon P (2004) Protease-activated receptors: contribution to physiology and disease. Physiol Rev 84:579–621
19. Pchejetski F, Kunduzova O, Dayon A, Calise D, Seguelas M, Leducq N, Seif I, Parini A, Cuvillier O (2007) Oxidative stress-dependent sphingosine kinase-1 inhibition mediates MAO-A-associated cardiac cell apoptosis. Circ Res 100:41–49
20. Reilly MP, Taylor SM, Hartman NK, Arepally GM, Sachais BS, Cines DB, Poncz M, McKenzie SE (2001) Heparin-induced thrombocytopenia/thrombosis in a transgenic mouse model requires human platelet factor 4 and platelet activation through FcgammaRIIA. Blood 98:2442–2447
21. Sevvana M, Ahnstrom J, Egerer-Sieber C, Lange HA, Dahlbäck B, Muller YA (2009) Serendipitous fatty acid binding reveals the structural determinants for ligand recognition in apolipoprotein M. J Mol Biol 393:920–936
22. Smirnova IV, Jianxin YM, Citron BA, Ratzlaff KT, Gregory EJ, Akaaboune M, Festoff BW (1996) Neural thrombin and protease nexin I kinetics after murine peripheral nerve injury. J Neurochem 67:2188–2199
23. van Gijn J, Kerr RS, Rinkel GJ (2007) Subarachnoid hemorrhage. Lancet 369:306–318
24. Xia P, Gamble JR, Rye KA, Wang L, Hii CS, Cockerill P, Khew-Goodall Y, Bert AG, Barter PJ, Vadas MA (1998) Tumor necrosis factor-alpha induces adhesion molecule expression through the sphingosine kinase pathway. Proc Natl Acad Sci U S A 95:14196–14201
25. Yu KCW, David C, Kadambi S, Stahl A, Hirata K, Ishida T, Quertermous T, Cooper AD, Choi SY (2004) Endothelial lipase is synthesized by hepatic and aorta endothelial cells and its expression is altered in apoE deficient mice. J Lipid Res 45:1614–1623
26. Zania P, Papaconstantinou M, Flordellis CS, Maragoudakis ME, Tsopanoglou NE (2008) Thrombin mediates mitogenesis and survival of human endothelial cells through distinct mechanisms. Am J Physiol Cell Physiol 294:C1215–C1226

Lipocalin 2 and Blood-Brain Barrier Disruption in White Matter after Experimental Subarachnoid Hemorrhage

Yusuke Egashira, Ya Hua, Richard F. Keep, Toru Iwama, and Guohua Xi

Introduction

We previously reported that subarachnoid hemorrhage (SAH) causes acute white matter injury in mice and lipocalin 2 (LCN2) plays an important role in this injury [4]. However, the mechanisms of white matter injury and the detailed role in LCN2 in that injury still remain uncertain. Blood-brain barrier (BBB) disruption occurs in a wide variety of central nervous system diseases, including ischemic stroke, traumatic brain injury, and hemorrhagic stroke [9]. BBB disruption is also a key mechanism of SAH-induced white matter injury. In this study, we investigated the role of LCN2 in acute BBB disruption in the white matter after SAH.

Materials and Methods

Animal Preparation and SAH Induction

All animal protocols were approved by the University of Michigan Committee on the Use and Care of Animals. A total of 17 male C57BL/6 mice (Charles River Laboratories, Portage, MI, USA) weighing 22–30 g and 6 male LCN2 knockout ($LCN2^{-/-}$) mice with C57BL/6 background (University of Michigan Breeding Core, gift from Dr. Xiaoli Chen, University of Minnesota) were used. Food and water were available to all animals ad libitum before and after surgery. SAH was induced, as previously described, by a single surgeon (YE) [8]. In brief, anesthesia was induced by inhalation of 4 % isoflurane and maintained by 2 % isoflurane administered through a facemask. A midline skin incision was made to expose the left common carotid artery. The external carotid artery (ECA) was isolated and cut; thereafter, a heat-blunted 5-0 nylon suture was introduced into the left internal carotid artery through the ECA stump until resistance was felt. Then the suture was advanced 3 mm further to perforate the artery and was immediately withdrawn, allowing reperfusion and producing SAH. Sham control mice underwent the same surgical procedure without perforation. Body temperature of all mice was maintained at 37.5 °C with a feedback-controlled heating pad throughout the procedures. After the surgery, mice were housed in heated cages until recovery.

Magnetic Resonance Imaging Technique and Measurement of the Lesion

MRI was performed at 24 h after SAH using a 7.0-T Varian MR scanner (Varian Inc., Palo Alto, CA, USA) with acquisition of T2 fast spin-echo and T2* gradient-echo sequences using a field of view of 20 × 20 mm, matrix of 256 × 256 mm, and 25 coronal slices (0.5 mm thick) [1]. The areas of hyperintensity of T2 (T2-hyperintensity) in the white matter were measured as previously described [4].

Severity of SAH

After MRI, animals were euthanized and their brains were examined. The severity of SAH was assessed using a modified grading system [10]. The basal brain including brainstem

Y. Egashira, MD, PhD
Department of Neurosurgery, University of Michigan, 5018 BSRB, 109 Zina Pitcher Place, Ann Arbor, MI 48109-2200, USA

Department of Neurosurgery, Gifu University Graduate School of Medicine, Gifu, Japan

Y. Hua, MD • R.F. Keep, PhD • G. Xi, MD (✉)
Department of Neurosurgery, University of Michigan, 5018 BSRB, 109 Zina Pitcher Place, Ann Arbor, MI 48109-2200, USA
e-mail: guohuaxi@umich.edu

T. Iwama, MD, PhD
Department of Neurosurgery, Gifu University Graduate School of Medicine, Gifu, Japan

R.L. Applegate et al. (eds.), *Brain Edema XVI: Translate Basic Science into Clinical Practice*, Acta Neurochirurgica Supplement, Vol. 121,
DOI 10.1007/978-3-319-18497-5_23,

was divided into six segments. Each segment was assigned a grade from 0 to 3, depending on the amount of SAH, as follows: Grade 0 – no SAH; Grade 1 – minimal SAH; Grade 2 – moderate SAH with recognizable arteries; and Grade 3 – SAH covering the cerebral arteries.

Western Blot Analysis

Western blot analysis was performed as previously described [6]. Brain tissues ($n=3$ for each group) were collected and the brains were cut into 1-mm-thick coronal sections between 1 and 2 mm posterior to the bregma, and the white matter was carefully separated. Brain tissues were homogenized in Western blot sample buffer. Equivalent amounts of total protein were separated by sodium dodecyl sulfate-polyacrylamide gel electrophoresis and then transferred to nitrocellulose membrane. Membranes were probed with the following antibodies: goat anti-LCN2 (R&D Systems, Minneapolis, MN, USA; 1:1,000) and rabbit anti-β-actin (Cell Signaling Technology, Danvers, MA, USA; 1:5,000). Antigen-antibody complexes were visualized with chemiluminescence detection reagent and exposed to an autoradiography film. Signal intensity was measured by Image-J (National Institutes of Health, Bethesda, MD, USA), and normalized to the β-actin signal intensity.

Immunohistochemistry

Mice underwent lethal anesthesia and were perfused transcardially by 4 % paraformaldehyde in 0.1 mol/L phosphate-buffered saline (PBS; pH 7.4). The forebrains were removed, fixed in 4 % paraformaldehyde for 48 h, immersed in 30 % sucrose for 48 h at 4 °C, and then frozen. Fresh frozen forebrains were sliced into 10-μm-thick coronal sections using a cryostat, and sectioned tissues were placed onto individual slides [13]. An anti-albumin antibody (Bethyl Laboratories, Inc., Montgomery, TX, USA; 1:1,000) was used to assess BBB disruption.

Immunofluorescence Double Labeling

For immunofluorescent double labeling, the primary antibodies were rabbit anti-24p3R (LCN2 receptor; Abcam, Cambridge, MA, USA; 1:50), mouse anti-GST-π (mature oligodendrocyte; BD Biosciences, San Jose, CA, USA; 1:200), mouse anti-glial fibrillary acid protein (GFAP; Millipore, Billerica, MA, USA; 1:400), rat anti-CD-31 (endothelial cell; BD Biosciences), and mouse anti-α-smooth muscle actin (smooth muscle/pericyte; α-SMA; Abcam; 1:100). The appropriate Alexa-Flour conjugated antibodies (Molecular Probes, Eugene, OR, USA; 1:400) were used as secondary antibodies. The slides were covered with Prolong Gold reagent with DAPI (Molecular Probes), and were observed underneath a fluorescence microscope (Olympus BX51; Olympus, Tokyo, Japan).

Quantification of Immunostaining

Quantification of immunostaining was performed by a blinded investigator. For analysis, 10-μm-thick coronal sections (bregma −1.5 mm to −2.1 mm) were used. For quantitative measurements of albumin staining, two brain sections were digitized under a 10x magnification using Olympus BX-51 microscope. Albumin-positive areas in the white matter tract were marked and calculated using Image-J.

Statistics

Data are expressed as the mean ± SD. Commercially available software (JMP 7; SAS Institute Inc., Cary, NC, USA) was used for all statistical analysis. Statistical differences among the groups were analyzed using one-way ANOVA and Fisher exact test. A post hoc Bonferroni correction was used for multiple comparisons. $p<0.05$ was considered statistically significant.

Results

The mortality rates were 20 % (2 of 10) and 16.7 % (1 of 6) at 24 h after SAH induction in WT and $LCN2^{-/-}$ animals, respectively ($p=0.62$; Fisher exact test). No sham animals died ($n=7$). SAH severity scores were equivalent in WT and in $LCN2^{-/-}$ animals (9.5 ± 3.2 and 9.2 ± 5.6, respectively; $p=0.90$).

LCN2 Expression in White Matter after SAH

Our previous data showed that LCN2 expression was prominently observed in the white matter at 24 h after SAH [4]. This was confirmed in the current study by Western blot. LCN2 expression in the white matter was significantly increased after SAH in WT mice compared with sham-operated animals ($p<0.05$; $n=3$ each; Fig. 1).

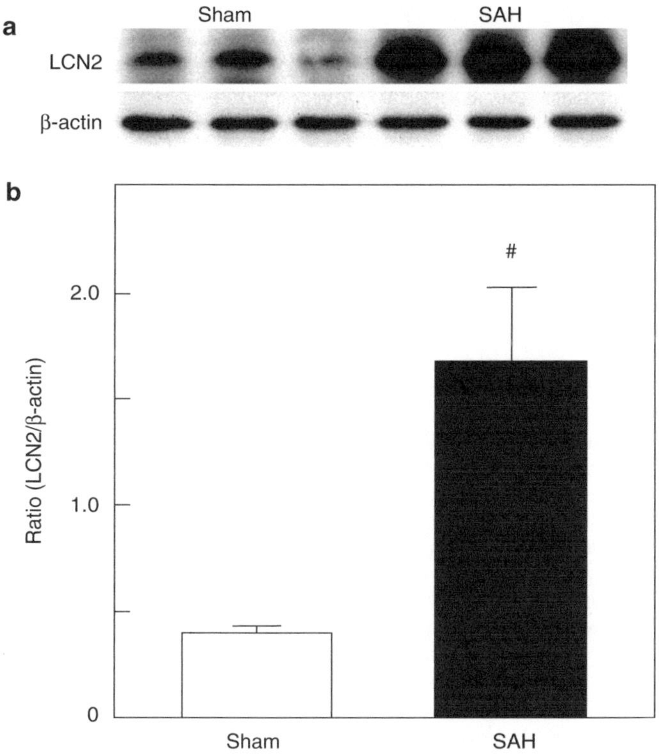

Fig. 1 LCN2 expression was significantly increased in the white matter at 24 h after subarachnoid hemorrhage (SAH). (**a**) Representative bands of Western blotting of the expression of lipocalin-2 (LCN2). (**b**) Optical densitometry quantification for the expression of LCN2, normalized to β-actin. Values are expressed as mean ± SD; # $p<0.05$ vs. sham group; ANOVA; $n=3$

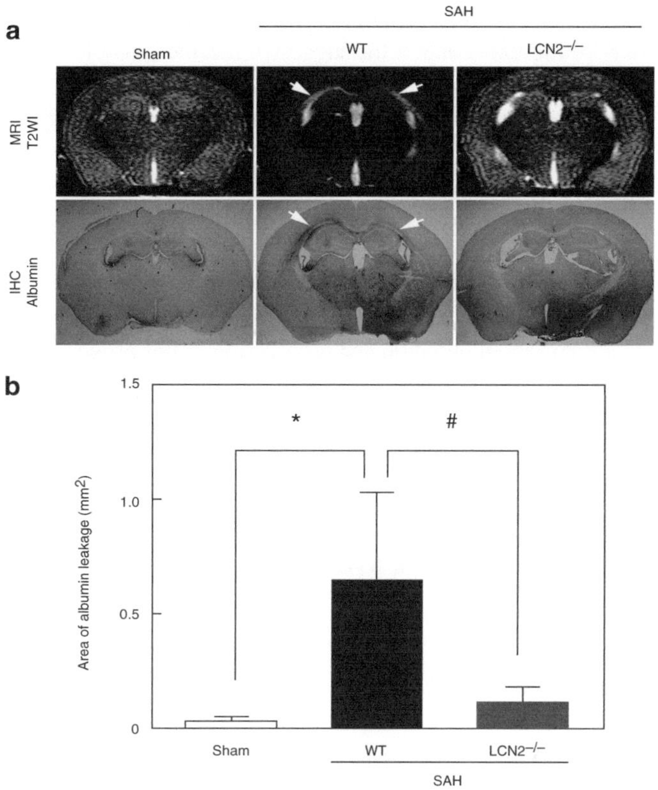

Fig. 2 (**a**) White matter injury detected by T2-weighted images (T2WI) and albumin immunohistochemistry (IHC) at 24 h after subarachnoid hemorrhage (SAH) in wild-type (WT) sham, WT with SAH, and lipocalin-2-knockout ($LCN2^{-/-}$) with SAH mice. *Arrows* indicate white matter lesion. (**b**) Quantification of the areas of albumin leakage in each group. * $p<0.05$ vs. WT sham, and # $p<0.05$ vs. WT + SAH mice; Values are expressed as mean ± SD; ANOVA with Bonferroni; $n=4$–5

LCN2 Receptor, 24p3R Expression in White Matter after SAH

Next, we investigated the expression of the known LCN2 receptor 24p3R in the white matter after SAH using immunofluorescence double labeling. Diffuse expression of 24p3R was observed in the white matter at 24 h after SAH induction. LCN2 receptor 24p3R expressing cells were merged to GST-π (mature oligodendrocyte marker), GFAP (astrocyte marker), CD-31 (endothelial marker), and α-SMA (pericyte/smooth muscle marker) expressing cells.

LCN2 Deletion Ameliorates Albumin Leakage in White Matter after SAH

Mice that underwent endovascular perforation (SAH) but not a sham operation developed white matter T2-hyperintensity at 24 h, whereas $LCN2^{-/-}$ mice developed less of this T2-hyperintensity, as also shown in our previous study [4]. Immunohistochemistry revealed that SAH also induced albumin leakage (BBB disruption) along the white matter in WT mice, and the area of albumin leakage correlated with the T2-hyperintensity on MRI (Fig. 2a). The area of albumin leakage was significantly larger in SAH- than in sham-operated mice (0.65 ± 0.38 vs. 0.03 ± 0.02 mm^2; $p<0.05$; $n=4$–5). This albumin leakage was much less evident in $LCN2^{-/-}$ mice (0.12 ± 0.06; $p<0.05$ vs. WT + SAH; $n=5$; Fig. 2b).

Discussion

Accumulated evidence suggests that LCN2 is implicated in various neuronal injuries [3, 7, 11]. We recently reported that LCN2 plays an important role in SAH-induced acute white matter injury [4]. However, the detailed role of LCN2 in that injury remains uncertain. In this study, a significant increase of LCN2 expression in the white matter at 24 h after SAH was confirmed, and LCN2 receptor 24p3R was expressed in oligodendrocytes and BBB components. These results suggest that LCN2 might exert effects on these cells through its receptor.

LCN2-24p3R-mediated apoptosis via the regulation of intracellular iron levels is one of the suggested mechanisms of LCN2-mediated cell death [2]. In this study, we demonstrated that LCN2 deletion attenuated acute BBB leakage after SAH. BBB disruption is recognized as a key mechanism of white matter injury in various central nervous system diseases that often occur early in the disease and contribute to promoting consequent white matter injury at a later time point [5, 12]. It is possible that acute BBB disruption is also involved in the pathology of SAH-induced white matter injury, and LCN2 might play an important role in initiation and progression of this process.

In summary, it was suggested that BBB leakage occurs in white matter after SAH, and it is one of the major mechanisms of LCN2-mediated white matter injury.

Acknowledgment This study was supported by grants NS-073595, NS-079157, and NS-084049 from the National Institutes of Health (NIH), 973 Program-2014CB541600, and Japan Heart Foundation/Bayer Yakuhin Research Grant Abroad.

References

1. Cheng Y, Xi G, Jin H, Keep RF, Feng J, Hua Y (2014) Thrombin-induced cerebral hemorrhage: role of protease-activated receptor-1. Transl Stroke Res 5:472–475
2. Devireddy LR, Gazin C, Zhu X, Green MR (2005) A cell-surface receptor for lipocalin 24p3 selectively mediates apoptosis and iron uptake. Cell 123:1293–1305
3. Dong M, Xi G, Keep RF, Hua Y (2013) Role of iron in brain lipocalin 2 upregulation after intracerebral hemorrhage in rats. Brain Res 1505:86–92
4. Egashira Y, Hua Y, Keep RF, Xi G (2014) Acute white matter injury after experimental subarachnoid hemorrhage: potential role of lipocalin 2. Stroke 45:2141–2143
5. Glushakova OY, Johnson D, Hayes RL (2014) Delayed increases in microvascular pathology after experimental traumatic brain injury are associated with prolonged inflammation, blood-brain barrier disruption, and progressive white matter damage. J Neurotrauma 31:1180–1193
6. Jin H, Xi G, Keep RF, Wu J, Hua Y (2013) DARPP-32 to quantify intracerebral hemorrhage-induced neuronal death in basal ganglia. Transl Stroke Res 4:130–134
7. Jin M, Kim JH, Jang E, Lee YM, Soo Han H, Woo DK, Park DH, Kook H, Suk K (2014) Lipocalin-2 deficiency attenuates neuroinflammation and brain injury after transient middle cerebral artery occlusion in mice. J Cereb Blood Flow Metab 34:1306–1314
8. Kamii H, Kato I, Kinouchi H, Chan PH, Epstein CJ, Akabane A, Okamoto H, Yoshimoto T (1999) Amelioration of vasospasm after subarachnoid hemorrhage in transgenic mice overexpressing CuZn-superoxide dismutase. Stroke 30:867–871; discussion 872
9. Keep RF, Xiang J, Ennis SR, Andjelkovic A, Hua Y, Xi G, Hoff JT (2008) Blood-brain barrier function in intracerebral hemorrhage. Acta Neurochir Suppl 105:73–77
10. Lee JY, Keep RF, He Y, Sagher O, Hua Y, Xi G (2010) Hemoglobin and iron handling in brain after subarachnoid hemorrhage and the effect of deferoxamine on early brain injury. J Cereb Blood Flow Metab 30:1793–1803
11. Rathore KI, Berard JL, Redensek A, Chierzi S, Lopez-Vales R, Santos M, Akira S, David S (2011) Lipocalin 2 plays an immunomodulatory role and has detrimental effects after spinal cord injury. J Neurosci 31:13412–13419
12. Seo JH, Miyamoto N, Hayakawa K, Pham LD, Maki T, Ayata C, Kim KW, Lo EH, Arai K (2013) Oligodendrocyte precursors induce early blood-brain barrier opening after white matter injury. J Clin Invest 123:782–786
13. Zhao J, Chen Z, Xi G, Keep RF, Hua Y (2014) Deferoxamine attenuates acute hydrocephalus after traumatic brain injury in rats. Transl Stroke Res 5:586–594

Cannabinoid Receptor Type 2 Agonist Attenuates Acute Neurogenic Pulmonary Edema by Preventing Neutrophil Migration after Subarachnoid Hemorrhage in Rats

Mutsumi Fujii, Prativa Sherchan, Yoshiteru Soejima, Desislava Doycheva, Diana Zhao, and John H. Zhang

Abbreviations

NPE	neurogenic pulmonary edema
SAH	subarachnoid hemorrhage
CB2R	Cannabinoid type 2 receptor
MPO	myeloperoxidase
JAM	junctional adhesion molecule
EBI	early brain injury
IP	intraperitoneal administration
TJs	tight junctions
PBS	phosphate-buffered saline
ANOVA	analysis of variance.

Introduction

In spite of dramatic improvements in surgical repair of aneurysms, aneurysmal subarachnoid hemorrhage (SAH) is associated with high mortality and permanent functional deficit [2, 10]. Neurogenic pulmonary edema (NPE), an increase of interstitial and alveolar fluid, is one of the most severe and life-threatening complications after SAH [7, 9]. Clinical-pathological analysis of fatal SAH showed that 70–90 % of deaths were associated with NPE [12, 17], whereas only 31 % had clinically diagnosed NPE [17]. However, NPE after SAH continues to be a prevalent clinical problem with few efficient pharmacological treatment options. Some studies have indicated that cannabinoid receptor type 2 (CB2R) activation plays important roles in preventing septic lung injury by attenuating neutrophil recruitment [16]. Since the influx of neutrophils can aggravate lung damage, inhibiting infiltration of neutrophils by CB2R agonist may reduce NPE after SAH.

Material and Methods

The animal and ethics review committee at Loma Linda University evaluated and approved all protocols. The endovascular perforation model of SAH was produced in adult male Sprague–Dawley rats (Harlan, Indianapolis, IN, USA) weighing 226–311 g, as previously described [3, 6, 13]. The SAH rats received vehicle (0.2 ml of ethanol with 1.8 ml of 0.9 % saline) or the selective CB2R agonist JWH133 (0.3, 1.0, or 3.0 mg/kg, Tocris Bioscience, Minneapolis, MN, USA) by intraperitoneal administration (IP) 1 h after surgery. The selective CB2R antagonist SR144528 (3.0 mg/kg, Cayman Chemicals, Ann Arbor, MI, USA) was administered IP at 15 min before JWH133 administration. The dosage of JWH133 and SR144528 was selected based on previous publications [4, 5]. Rats received two more doses of vehicle or JWH133 at 24 and 48 h after surgery if they were to be sacrificed at 72 h. At each sacrifice time, rats were deeply anesthetized with 5 % isoflurane. Both lungs were harvested through a midline sternotomy and brains were harvested through a midline craniotomy. The surviving rats were randomly assigned to the following groups: sham-operated (sham), SAH+vehicle (vehicle), SAH+JWH133 (0.3) (low-JWH), SAH+JWH133 (1.0) (JWH), SAH+JWH133 (3.0) (high-

M. Fujii
Department of Physiology, Loma Linda University, Loma Linda, CA, USA

Department of Neurosurgery, Tsuchiura Kyodo General Hospital, Ibaraki, Japan

P. Sherchan • Y. Soejima • D. Doycheva • D. Zhao
Department of Physiology, Loma Linda University, Loma Linda, CA, USA

J.H. Zhang (✉)
Department of Physiology, Neurosurgery, and Anesthesiology, Loma Linda University, 11234 Anderson Street, Room 2562B, Loma Linda, CA 92354, USA
e-mail: johnzhang3910@yahoo.com

R.L. Applegate et al. (eds.), *Brain Edema XVI: Translate Basic Science into Clinical Practice*, Acta Neurochirurgica Supplement, Vol. 121,
DOI 10.1007/978-3-319-18497-5_24,

JWH), or SAH+SR144528 (3.0)+JWH133 (1.0) (SR-JWH). The severity of SAH was evaluated in a blinded manner using the SAH grade, as previously described [4, 5]. Briefly, SAH rats received a total score ranging from 0 (no SAH) to 18 (most severe SAH). Animals with SAH grade 7 or less were excluded from the study for low SAH grade.

Pulmonary Wet-to-Dry Weight Ratio

We evaluated NPE by measuring lung water content. The left lung lobe was removed 24 or 72 h after surgery and weighed immediately after removal (wet weight) and again after drying in 100 °C for 72 h (dry weight). The ratio of water content was calculated as wet/dry weight.

Western Blot Analyses

Protein homogenates from right lung lobe were obtained from the same animals whose left lobe was used to measure lung water content at 24 h after SAH Protein levels of myeloperoxidase (MPO, 1:200), junctional adhesion molecule (JAM)-A (1:200), and actin (1:2,000; all from Santa Cruz Biotechnology, Dallas, TX, USA) was measured by Western blot analysis, as previously described [4, 5]. Results are expressed as relative density to actin and subsequently normalized to the mean value of the sham group.

Immunohistochemistry

At 24 h after SAH, the left lung tissue was fixed by cardiovascular perfusion with phosphate-buffered saline (PBS) and 10 % paraformaldehyde at 4 °C. The tissue was incubated in 30 % sucrose for 3 days at 4 °C and embedded in OCT. Ten-micron-thick coronal sections around the level of the hilar region were cut on a cryostat (LM3050S: Leica Microsystems, Bannockburn, IL, USA) and mounted on poly-L-lysine-coated slides. We immunostained lung sections with rabbit polyclonal primary antibody for anti-MPO (1:100, Dako North America, Inc., Carpinteria, CA, USA) overnight at 4 °C. The slides were then rinsed three times in PBS and incubated with FITC (fluorescein isothiocyanate)-labeled anti-rabbit IgG (1:100, Jackson Laboratory, Bar Harbor, ME, USA) for 60 min. The stained sections were processed using a fluorescent microscope and Manga Fire SP system (Olympus, Melville, NY, USA).

Statistics

SAH grade was expressed as median and 25th to 75th percentiles and was analyzed by Kruskal-Wallis test or Mann–Whitney *U* test. Other values were expressed as mean ± standard deviation. Mortality was analyzed by Fischer exact test. All other values were analyzed by one-way analysis of variance (ANOVA) followed by Tukey post hoc analysis. $p<0.05$ was considered statistically significant.

Results

After performing 119 surgeries, 20 rats having mild SAH were excluded (4 rats in vehicle sacrificed at 24 h, 5 in JWH at 24 h, 2 in SR-JWH at 24 h, 4 in vehicle at 72 h, and 5 in JWH at 72 h). In 33 rats that died because of severe SAH, 15 SAH rats (12 rats allocated to be sacrificed at 24 h and 3 rats at 72 h) died within 1 h. The rats that died after 1 h were included in mortality statistics. The mortality rates between the groups did not show statistical differences at 24 or 72 h (p = not significant (N.S.), Fig. 1a). For the 24 or 72 h outcome study, there was no significant difference in SAH grade (p = N.S., Fig. 1b). Wet-to-dry weight ratio in vehicle was significantly higher compared with sham and both low-JWH and JWH at 24 h (Fig. 1c). Although it was not statistically significant, the JWH group showed lower mortality and more severe SAH grade than the low-JWH group. Because the effect of low- and middle-dose treatment seemed equivalent, we regarded the most effective dosage as the JWH133 (1.0 mg/kg) and continued to use this dosage as a treatment. SR-JWH also showed significantly worse lung edema compared with sham, low-JWH, and JWH groups. For the 72 h outcome study, wet-to-dry weight ratio in vehicle was not higher compared with the JWH or sham groups (p = N.S., Fig. 1d).

MPO is a major component of azurophilic granules of neutrophils and polymorphonuclear leukocytes. The levels of MPO were significantly higher in vehicle compared with sham and JWH groups (Fig. 2a). The levels of JAM-A were significantly lower in vehicle compared with sham and JWH groups (Fig. 2b). The levels of MPO or JAM-A in SR-JWH showed the reverse tendency compared with that in JWH group. We also performed immunofluorescent staining of MPO after cardiac perfusion to further determine MPO existence in the alveolar and interstitial spaces, not in the vessels (Fig. 3). Sham did not demonstrate MPO positive cells. On the other hand, vehicle showed several MPO-positive cells. JWH133 treatment reduced the number of MPO-positive cells in the lung.

a Mortality rate

	Sham	SAH vehicle	SAH low-JWH	SAH JWH	SAH high-JWH	SAH SR-JWH
24 h group	0.0 % (0/7)	27.3 % (3/11)	25.0 % (2/8)	11.1 % (1/9)	22.2 % (2/9)	11.1 % (1/9)
72 h group	0.0 % (0/7)	38.5 % (5/13)		36.4 % (4/11)		

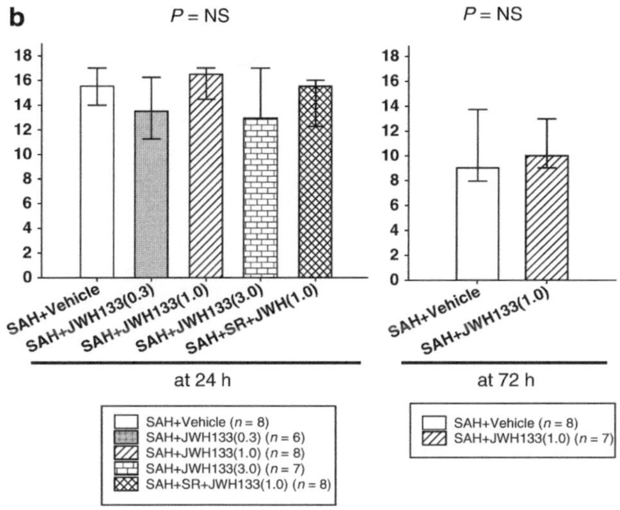

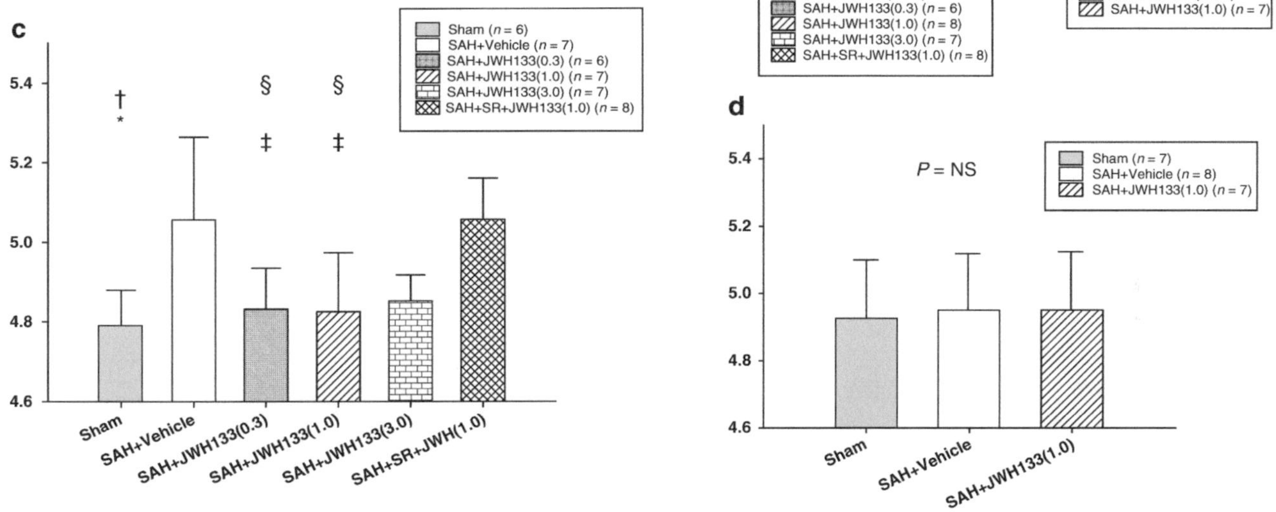

Fig. 1 Mortality rate in this study (**a**). Grading score of subarachnoid hemorrhage (SAH) results at 24 and 72 h (B). Wet-to-dry weight ratio at 24 h after SAH (**c**). In the wet-to-dry weight ratio at 24 h, the low- and middle-dose treatment ameliorated the lung edema compared with the vehicle group. Administration of both the middle dose of JWH133 and the CB2R antagonist, SR144528, reversed the protective effect of JWH133 (SR+JWH(1.0)). *: $p<0.01$ vs. vehicle, †: $p<0.01$ vs. SR+JWH(1.0), ‡: $p<0.05$ vs. vehicle, §: $p<0.05$ vs. SR+JWH(1.0) (**b**). In the wet-to-dry weight ratio at 72 h, no differences could be seen among the groups (**d**). Values are expressed as median and 25th to 75th percentiles (**b**) and mean ± SD (**c**, **d**)

Discussion

In this study, we demonstrated that SAH-triggered NPE was ameliorated by JWH133. JWH133 attenuated NPE induced lung edema and neutrophil infiltration into the lungs, which was associated with increased JAM-A expression in the lung 24 h after SAH. However, NPE no longer occurred at 72 h, suggesting that NPE is not frequent after 72 h. To the best of our knowledge, this is the first report to describe the protective effects of CB2R agonist on NPE immediately after SAH.

One putative mechanism of NPE is that increased intracranial pressure causes excessive release of catecholamine, resulting in high permeability. Meanwhile, SAH can cause a systemic inflammatory response, which activates capillary leakage permeability. Norepinephrine also causes activation of cytokines and inflammatory reactions associated with recruitment of neutrophils [15], which result in NPE by damaging the alveolar capillary barrier [11].

In this study, the exposure of rats to SAH increased MPO activity and lung edema in the tissue, indicating the infiltration of polymorphonuclear neutrophils and the development of increased capillary permeability. Immunohistochemical assessment also confirmed that leukocytes infiltrated from vessels substantially in the model of SAH. JAM is a small immunoglobulin family and one of the main constituents of TJs that are important for lung defense [14]. JAM-A is expressed by endothelial and epithelial cells and can mediate leukocyte diapedesis; however, reported roles of JAM-A in leukocyte mediation are not consistent [8]. In the context of

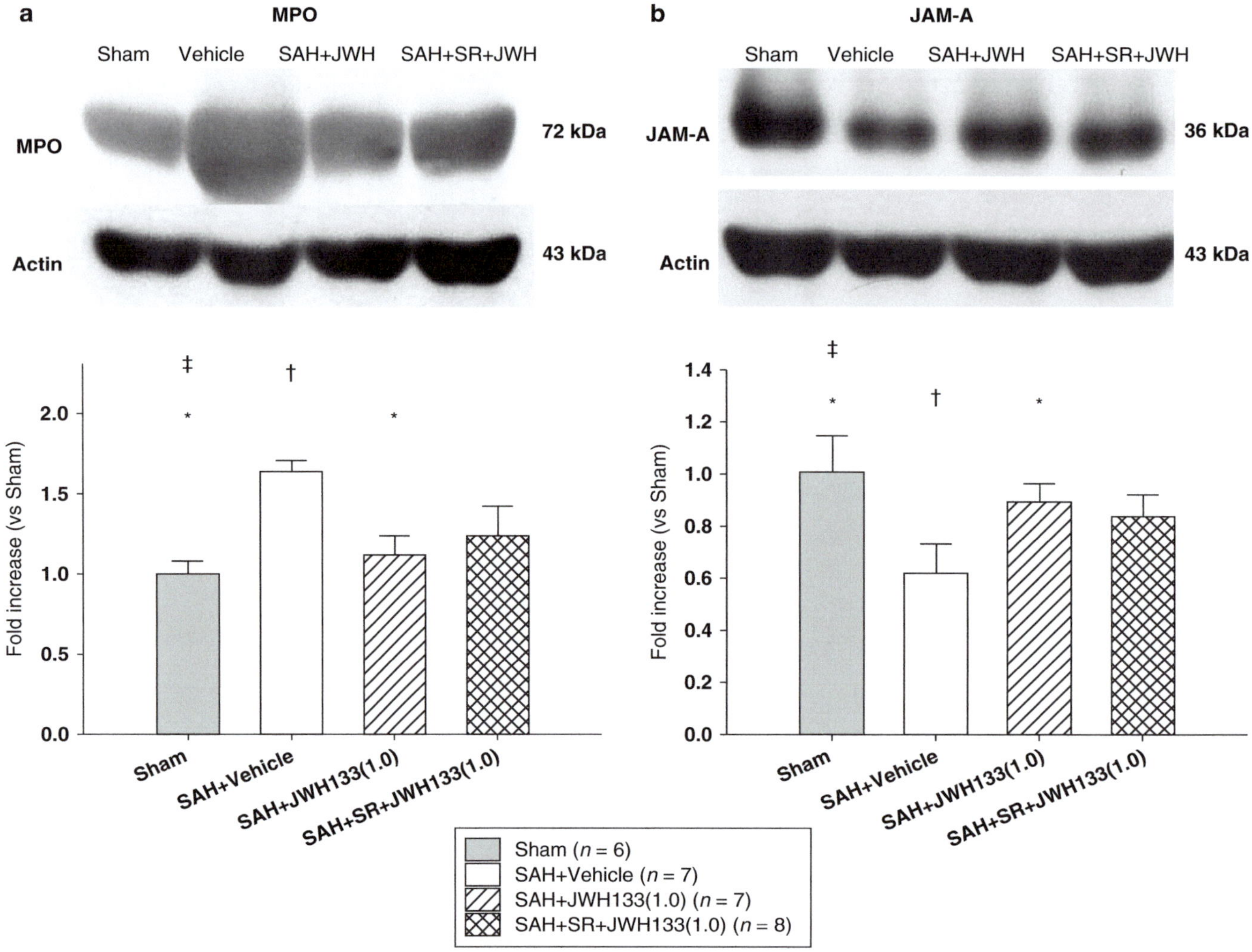

Fig. 2 Representative Western blots and quantitative analysis after SAH. Myeloperoxidase (MPO) (**a**) and junctional adhesion molecule – A (JAM-A) (**b**) in the right lung lobes were evaluated 24 h after SAH. Expression levels of each protein in Western blot are expressed as a ratio of actin levels for normalization. Values are mean ± SD. *: $p<0.01$ vs. vehicle, †: $p<0.01$ vs. SR + JWH(1.0), ‡: $p<0.05$ vs. SR + JWH(1.0)

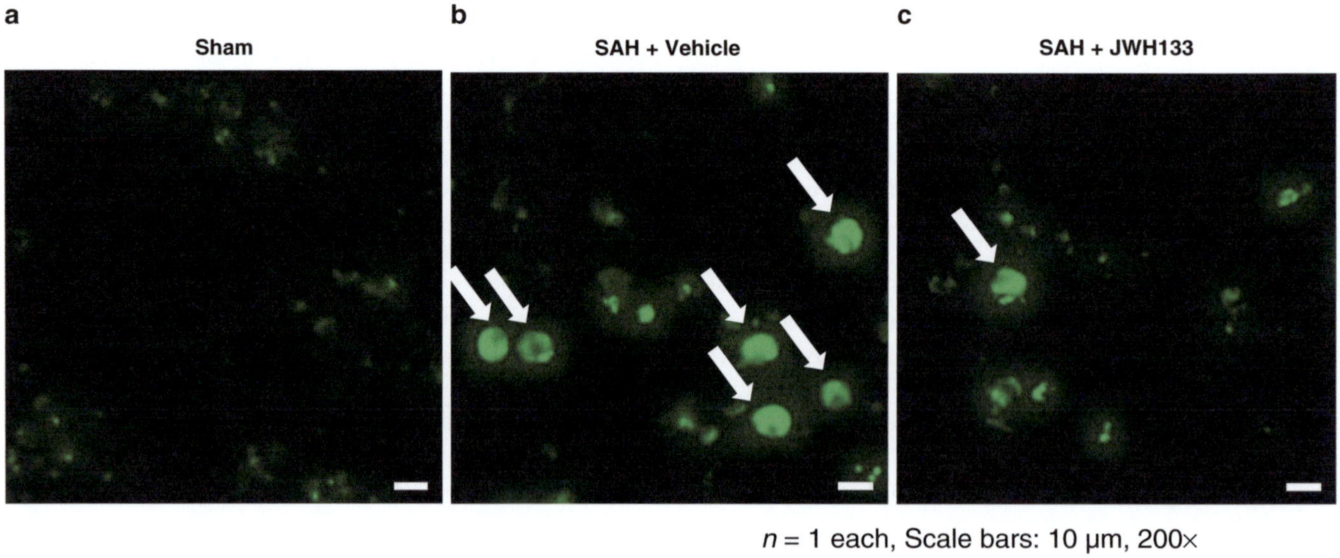

Fig. 3 Representative pictures of immunofluorescent staining with MPO. FITC signals (*arrows*) indicate MPO-positive cells expressing infiltrated neutrophils in the alveolar and interstitial spaces in the left lung tissues. Sham (**a**), SAH + vehicle (**b**), and SAH + the middle dose of JWH133 treatment (**c**)

acute NPE after SAH, we demonstrated that JAM-A was damaged in the lung, which is consistent with damage in the brain at the same time point (24 h) of SAH [1]. Finally, CB2R activation may represent a potent target for the future development of novel therapies in NPE after SAH through attenuation of TJ disruption and preventing neutrophil infiltration. Further studies are necessary for clinical translation.

Acknowledgments This study is partially supported by National Institutes of Health grant NS081740 to JHZ.

Conflict of Interest The authors declare no conflicts of interest.

References

1. Altay O, Suzuki H, Hasegawa Y, Caner B, Krafft PR, Fujii M, Tang J, Zhang JH (2012) Isoflurane attenuates blood–brain barrier disruption in ipsilateral hemisphere after subarachnoid hemorrhage in mice. Stroke 43:2513–2516
2. Brathwaite S, Macdonald RL (2014) Current management of delayed cerebral ischemia: update from results of recent clinical trials. Transl Stroke Res 5:207–226
3. Bühler D, Schüller K, Plesnila N (2014) Protocol for the induction of subarachnoid hemorrhage in mice by perforation of the circle of Willis with an endovascular filament. Transl Stroke Res 5: 653–659
4. Fujii M, Sherchan P, Krafft PR, Rolland WB, Soejima Y, Zhang JH (2014) Cannabinoid type 2 receptor stimulation attenuates brain edema by reducing cerebral leukocyte infiltration following subarachnoid hemorrhage in rats. J Neurol Sci 342:101–106
5. Fujii M, Sherchan P, Soejima Y, Hasegawa Y, Flores J, Doycheva D, Zhang JH (2014) Cannabinoid receptor type 2 agonist attenuates apoptosis by activation of phosphorylated CREB-Bcl-2 pathway after subarachnoid hemorrhage in rats. Exp Neurol 261: 396–403
6. Fujii M, Yan J, Rolland WB, Soejima Y, Caner B, Zhang JH (2013) Early brain injury, an evolving frontier in subarachnoid hemorrhage research. Transl Stroke Res 4:432–446
7. Macmillan CS, Grant IS, Andrews PJ (2002) Pulmonary and cardiac sequelae of subarachnoid haemorrhage: time for active management? Intensive Care Med 28:1012–1023
8. Nourshargh S, Krombach F, Dejana E (2006) The role of JAM-A and PECAM-1 in modulating leukocyte infiltration in inflamed and ischemic tissues. J Leukoc Biol 80:714–718
9. Piazza O, Venditto A, Tufano R (2011) Neurogenic pulmonary edema in subarachnoid hemorrhage. Panminerva Med 53: 203–2101
10. Pluta RM, Bacher J, Skopets B, Hoffmann V (2014) A non-human primate model of aneurismal subarachnoid hemorrhage (SAH). Transl Stroke Res 5:681–691
11. Rassler B, Reissig C, Briest W, Tannapfel A, Zimmer HG (2003) Pulmonary edema and pleural effusion in norepinephrine-stimulated rats–hemodynamic or inflammatory effect? Mol Cell Biochem 250:55–63
12. Schievink WI, Wijdicks EF, Parisi JE, Piepgras DG, Whisnant JP (1995) Sudden death from aneurysmal subarachnoid hemorrhage. Neurology 45:871–874
13. Sehba FA (2014) Rat endovascular perforation model. Transl Stroke Res 5:660–668
14. Soini Y (2011) Claudins in lung diseases. Respir Res 12:70
15. Steinberg J, Halter J, Schiller H, Gatto L, Carney D, Lee HM, Golub L, Nieman G (2005) Chemically modified tetracycline prevents the development of septic shock and acute respiratory distress syndrome in a clinically applicable porcine model. Shock 24:348–356
16. Tschöp J, Kasten KR, Nogueiras R, Goetzman HS, Cave CM, England LG, Dattilo J, Lentsch AB, Tschöp MH, Caldwell CC (2009) The cannabinoid receptor 2 is critical for the host response to sepsis. J Immunol 183:499–505
17. Weir BK (1978) Pulmonary edema following fatal aneurysm rupture. J Neurosurg 49:502–507

Basal Ganglia Damage in Experimental Subarachnoid Hemorrhage

Haining Zhang, Shuichi Okubo, Ya Hua, Richard F. Keep, and Guohua Xi

Introduction

Aneurysmal subarachnoid hemorrhage (SAH) is a devastating form of stroke associated with high mortality and disability rates [6]. Although there are important longer-term sequelae, early brain injury is a significant cause of mortality and disability and a primary therapeutic target [1, 9, 11, 13].

Although basal ganglia hematoma has been reported in a traumatic SAH case [2], SAH-induced basal ganglia injury is not well studied. The present study examined the occurrence of basal ganglia injury in a rat model of SAH using magnetic resonance imaging (MRI). Basal ganglia albumin levels were also used to assess blood-brain barrier disruption, and dopamine- and cAMP-regulated phosphoprotein, Mr 32 kDa (DARPP-32), levels were used to assess neuronal injury. DARPP-32 is a cytosolic protein highly expressed in medium-sized spiny neurons of the striatum and has been used as a neuronal marker in the striatum [14]. In an intracerebral hemorrhage model, DARPP-32 can be used as a simple and reliable marker of neuronal injury in basal ganglia [5].

Materials and Methods

Animal preparation and use protocols were approved by the University of Michigan Committee on the Use and Care of Animals. Adults male Sprague-Dawley rats ($n=78$) weighing 275–300 g underwent endovascular perforation [7] to mimic aneurysmal SAH. Sham rats ($n=12$) underwent the same procedure but without perforation.

Twenty-four hours after surgery, Garcia behavior scores were assessed [4]. The animals then underwent MRI (T2 fast spin-echo), using a field of view of 35×35 mm, matrix of 256×256 mm, and 25 coronal slices (0.5 mm thick) in a 7.0-T Varian MR scanner (Varian Inc.). Ventricle and brain T2 lesion volumes were measured. The frontal horn of lateral ventricle to the foramen of Luschka was included when setting the scanning area. Ventricular and basal ganglia lesion volumes were determined by multiplying the total area over all slices by the section thickness [8, 12].

For immunohistochemistry, rats underwent transcardiac perfusion with 4 % paraformaldehyde (pH 7.4) under pentobarbital anesthesia. Brains were kept in 4 % paraformaldehyde for 12 h and then immersed in 30 % sucrose for 3–4 days at 4 °C. Brains were then embedded and sectioned on a cryostat (18 μm). Immunofluorescent staining was performed as described previously [5]. Briefly, coronal sections from basal ganglia were stained for DARPP-32 immunoreactivity. The primary antibody was rabbit anti-DARPP-32 antibody (Cell Signaling Technology, 1:800 dilution). Alexa Fluro 488-conjugated donkey anti-rabbit antibody (Invitrogen, 1:500 dilution) was used as the secondary antibody.

Western blotting analysis was performed as previously described [10]. A 3-mm-thick coronal brain slice 5 mm apart from the frontal pole was obtained. The basal ganglia were sonicated in sample buffer and protein concentration was measured by Bio-Rad protein assay kit. From each sample, 40 μg of protein was separated by sodium dodecyl sulfate-polyacrylamide gel electrophoresis and transferred to a Hybond-C pure nitrocellulose membrane (Amersham). The membranes were probed with DARPP-32 (Cell Signaling; 1:10,000 dilution) primary antibody followed by a goat anti-rabbit IgG (Bio-Rad; 1:2,000 dilution) secondary antibody, and albumin (Sigma; 1:50,000 dilution) primary antibody followed by a rabbit anti-sheep IgG (Millipore; 1:2,000 dilution)

H. Zhang
Department of Neurosurgery, University of Michigan, 5018 BSRB, 109 Zina Pitcher Place, Ann Arbor, MI 48109-2200, USA

Department of Neurology, The First Hospital of Jilin University, Changchun, Jilin, China

S. Okubo • Y. Hua • R.F. Keep • G. Xi, MD (✉)
Department of Neurosurgery, University of Michigan, 5018 BSRB, 109 Zina Pitcher Place, Ann Arbor, MI 48109-2200, USA
e-mail: guohuaxi@umich.edu

R.L. Applegate et al. (eds.), *Brain Edema XVI: Translate Basic Science into Clinical Practice*, Acta Neurochirurgica Supplement, Vol. 121,
DOI 10.1007/978-3-319-18497-5_25,

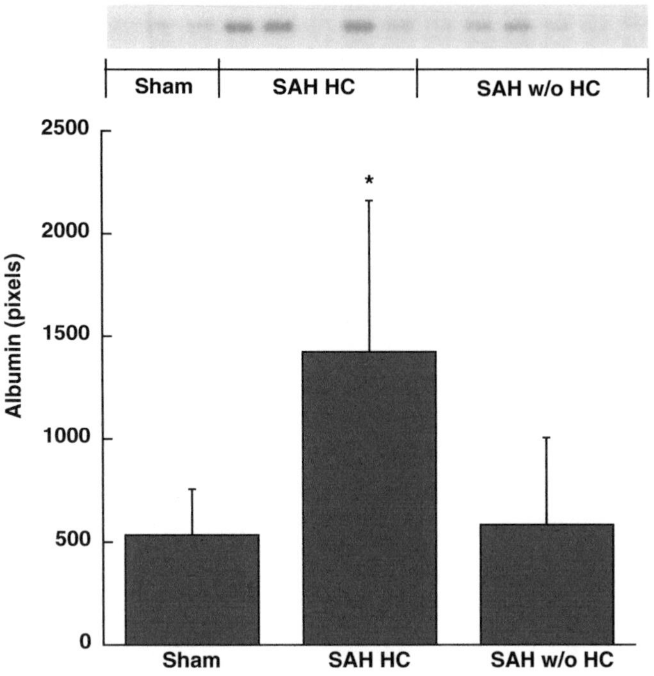

Fig. 1 Albumin levels in the basal ganglia at 24 h after a sham operation or endovascular perforation. Data are mean ± SD, $n=3–6$ in sham, SAH with hydrocephalus (SAH HC), and SAH without hydrocephalus (SAH w/o HC), $*p<0.05$ vs. the other groups

secondary antibody. The relative densities of the Western blotting bands were analyzed using NIH Image 1.62.

All data in this study are presented as mean ± standard deviation (SD). Statistical comparisons were conducted using unpaired Student's *t*-test or analysis of variance (ANOVA). Significance levels were measured at $p<0.05$.

Results

The mortality rate after SAH in the present study was 23 % at 24 h and 27 % at 8 days after surgery. Sixty rats survived, and 40 % of those animals had T2 lesions in the basal ganglia. The basal ganglia lesion volume in SAH animals correlated with behavioral deficits (Garcia scores; $r=-0.69$, $p<0.01$). Twenty-six SAH rats developed hydrocephalus and 34 rats did not (ventricular volumes: 28.0 ± 6.0 vs. 15.1 ± 3.3 mm^3, respectively; $p<0.01$). Rats with hydrocephalus had higher incidence of basal ganglia lesions on 24-h MRIs (69 % vs. 18 % in rats without hydrocephalus, $p<0.01$). All sham animals did not have T2 lesions in the brain.

To assess blood-brain barrier disruption, albumin levels in the basal ganglia were examined by Western blot at 24 h after SAH. Albumin levels in SAH animals with hydrocephalus were higher compared with SAH without hydrocephalus (1,426 ± 732 vs. 583 ± 425 pixels in SAH without hydrocephalus, $p<0.05$; Fig. 1).

Dopamine- and cAMP-regulated phosphoprotein, Mr 32 kDa (DARPP-32) levels were utilized to quantify basal ganglia neuronal injury at 8 days after surgery. We found that rats with hydrocephalus had more severe basal ganglia injury (DARPP-32/beta-actin: 0.38 ± 0.32 vs. 0.86 ± 0.45 in rats without hydrocephalus, $p<0.05$; Fig. 2).

Discussion

In the present study, we found SAH resulted in basal ganglia damage, which is associated with neurological deficits, hydrocephalus, and blood-brain barrier disruption after SAH. SAH-induced basal ganglia injury is not well studied, although basal ganglia hematoma has been reported in a traumatic SAH case [2].

We found that the incidence rate of basal ganglia (T2) lesions after endovascular perforation SAH in rats was 40 %. The size of the basal ganglia lesion correlated with the degree of behavioral deficit as assessed by the Garcia score. These results suggest that basal ganglia injury is common in the endovascular perforation SAH rat model and has an important role in SAH-induced neurological deficits. Attenuating basal ganglia damage may be an important target for improving functional outcome following SAH.

In rats that had a basal ganglia lesion after SAH, there was a marked increase (~4-fold) in the occurrence of hydrocephalus. In animals with SAH-induced hydrocephalus, there was also more neuronal death in the basal ganglia as shown by DARPP-32 levels. DARPP-32 is a reliable marker to quantify basal ganglia neuronal injury [5, 14]. The nature of the link between a basal ganglia lesion and hydrocephalus development is still unclear; for example, does a basal ganglia lesion induce hydrocephalus or vice versa, or are they independent events induced by another factor such as intraventricular blood? This needs further investigation. Our data did show that rats with hydrocephalus had greater blood-brain barrier disruption in the basal ganglia following SAH. It has been suggested that some cerebrospinal fluid absorption may occur across the blood-brain barrier [3], but this is controversial. Future studies need to determine the role of basal ganglia blood-brain barrier permeability in hydrocephalus development after SAH.

In conclusion, SAH caused severe basal ganglia damage in the rat. The occurrence of basal ganglia damage is associated with hydrocephalus development and blood-brain barrier disruption.

Acknowledgment This study was supported by grants NS-073595, NS-079157, and NS-084049 from the National Institutes of Health (NIH), 973 Program-2014CB541600.

Fig. 2 DARPP-32 immunoreactivity (**a**) and protein levels (**b**) in the basal ganglia at day 8 after a sham operation or SAH. Data are mean ± SD, $n=3–6$ SAH with hydrocephalus (SAH HC) and SAH without hydrocephalus (SAH w/o HC), #$p<0.05$ vs. the other groups

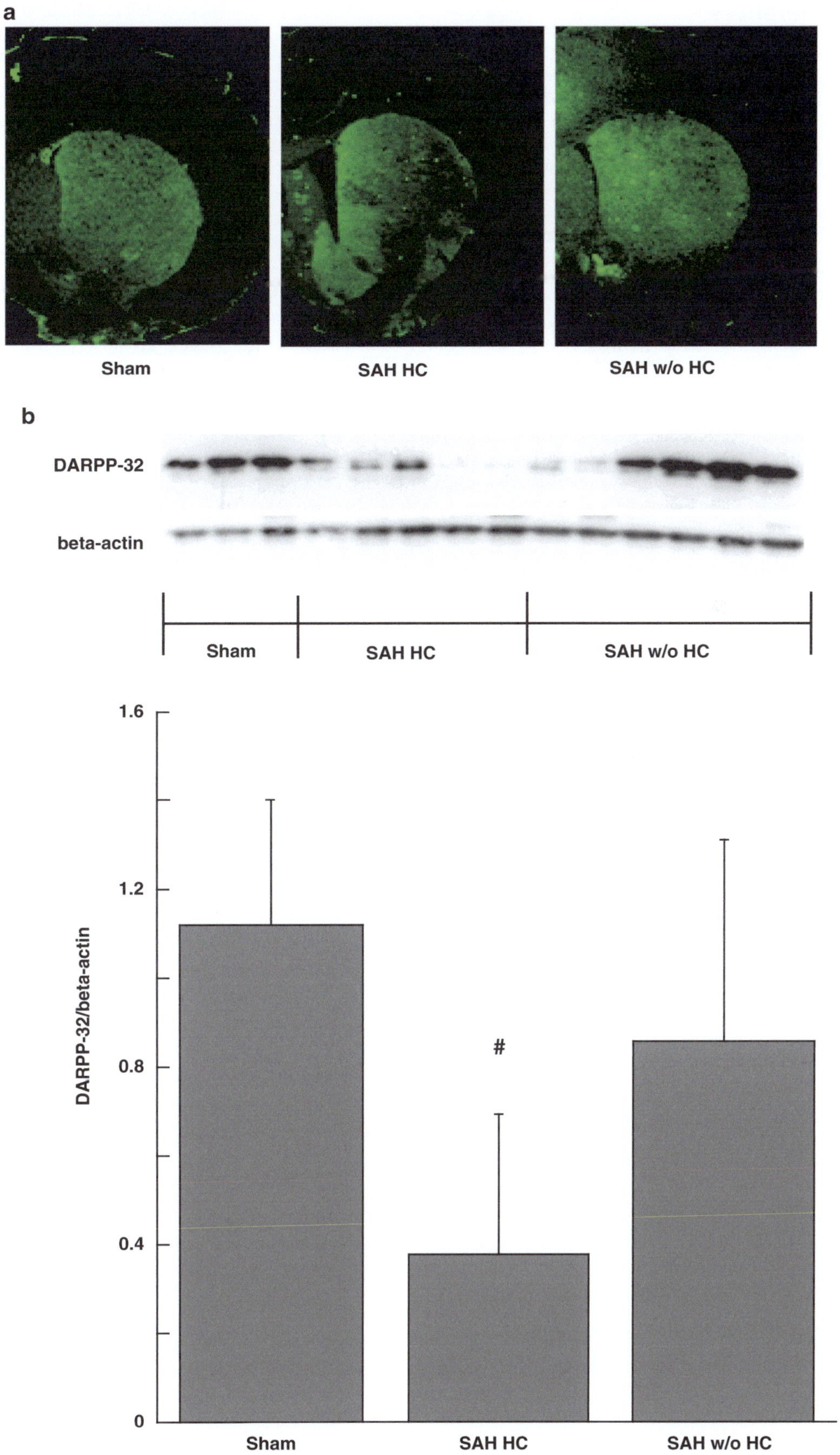

References

1. Cahill J, Zhang JH (2009) Subarachnoid hemorrhage: is it time for a new direction? Stroke 40:S86–S87
2. Fung C, Z'Graggen WJ, Beck J, Gralla J, Jakob SM, Schucht P, Raabe A (2012) Traumatic subarachnoid hemorrhage, basal ganglia hematoma and ischemic stroke caused by a torn lenticulostriate artery. Acta Neurochir 154:59–62
3. Greitz D (2004) Radiological assessment of hydrocephalus: new theories and implications for therapy. Neurosurg Rev 27:145–165; discussion 166–167
4. Jeon H, Ai J, Sabri M, Tariq A, Shang X, Chen G, Macdonald RL (2009) Neurological and neurobehavioral assessment of experimental subarachnoid hemorrhage. BMC Neurosci 10:103
5. Jin H, Xi G, Keep RF, Wu J, Hua Y (2013) DARPP-32 to quantify intracerebral hemorrhage-induced neuronal death in basal ganglia. Transl Stroke Res 4:130–134
6. le Roux AA, Wallace MC (2010) Outcome and cost of aneurysmal subarachnoid hemorrhage. Neurosurg Clin N Am 21:235–246
7. Lee JY, Keep RF, He Y, Sagher O, Hua Y, Xi G (2010) Hemoglobin and iron handling in brain after subarachnoid hemorrhage and the effect of deferoxamine on early brain injury. J Cereb Blood Flow Metab 30:1793–1803
8. Okubo S, Strahle J, Keep RF, Hua Y, Xi G (2013) Subarachnoid hemorrhage-induced hydrocephalus in rats. Stroke 44:547–550
9. Sabri M, Lass E, Macdonald RL (2013) Early brain injury: a common mechanism in subarachnoid hemorrhage and global cerebral ischemia. Stroke Res Treat 2013:394036
10. Wu J, Hua Y, Keep RF, Nakamura T, Hoff JT, Xi G (2003) Iron and iron-handling proteins in the brain after intracerebral hemorrhage. Stroke 34:2964–2969
11. Zhang JH (2014) Vascular neural network in subarachnoid hemorrhage. Transl Stroke Res 5:423–428
12. Zhao J, Chen Z, Xi G, Keep RF, Hua Y (2014) Deferoxamine attenuates acute hydrocephalus after traumatic brain injury in rats. Transl Stroke Res 5:586–594
13. Zhou Y, Martin RD, Zhang JH (2011) Advances in experimental subarachnoid hemorrhage. Acta Neurochir Suppl 110:15–21
14. Zhu JP, Xu W, Angulo JA (2006) Methamphetamine-induced cell death: selective vulnerability in neuronal subpopulations of the striatum in mice. Neuroscience 140:607–622

Subarachnoid Hemorrhage-Triggered Acute Hypotension Is Associated with Left Ventricular Cardiomyocyte Apoptosis in a Rat Model

Mutsumi Fujii, Prativa Sherchan, Yoshiteru Soejima, Desislava Doycheva, and John H. Zhang

Introduction

Myocardial "stunning" is a term that has been applied to sudden and sometimes unexpected ventricular hypokinesis [10]. Subarachnoid hemorrhage (SAH)-induced cardiac dysfunction, which is often labeled neurogenic stunned myocardium, is one of the most frequently associated complications after aneurysmal SAH [9, 11]. Hypotension related to neurogenic stunned myocardium has a great impact on mortality and functional outcome after SAH [17]. The most widely accepted theory for SAH-induced neurogenic myocardial stunning is the "catecholamine hypothesis" that plasma catecholamine levels increase in the acute stage after SAH [9, 11–13]. Although high levels of catecholamine have been shown to cause apoptotic as well as necrotic myocytes [7], it remains unknown whether heart failure after SAH is associated with apoptotic cell death in the heart. We hypothesized that (1) SAH induces acute apoptotic cell death in the heart and (2) SAH-induced hypotension is associated with apoptotic cell death of the cardiomyocyte in the left ventricle.

M. Fujii
Department of Physiology, Loma Linda University, Loma Linda, CA, USA

Department of Neurosurgery, Tsuchiura Kyodo General Hospital, Ibaraki, Japan

P. Sherchan • Y. Soejima • D. Doycheva
Department of Physiology, Loma Linda University, Loma Linda, CA, USA

J.H. Zhang (✉)
Department of Physiology, Neurosurgery, and Anesthesiology, Loma Linda University Medical Center, 11234 Anderson Street, Room 2562B, Loma Linda, CA 92354, USA
e-mail: johnzhang3910@yahoo.com

Materials and Methods

Experimental Model of SAH and Study Protocol

All protocols were approved by the Institutional Animal Care and Use Committee of Loma Linda University. The endovascular perforation model of SAH was produced in adult male Sprague–Dawley rats (Harlan, Indianapolis, IN, USA) weighing 239–308 g, as previously described [2, 6, 15]. Mean arterial pressure (MAP) and heart rate were measured via the cannulated right femoral artery. Both parameters were measured 15 min before, immediately after, and at 30, 60, 90, and 120 min after SAH. All animals were then euthanized at 2 h after the surgical procedure.

We used 18 rats; 5 sham and 13 SAH rats. Two SAH rats had mild SAH and 1 SAH rat died 20 min after puncture because of severe SAH. Thus, 15 rats were enrolled for this study: sham ($n=5$) and SAH rats ($n=10$). SAH rats were separated into two groups based on blood pressure (BP) measurements: SAH followed by hypotension (SAH hypotension group; $n=5$) and SAH with BP preservation (SAH BP preservation group; $n=5$). The rats in the hypotension group had a MAP <60 mmHg at 1 h after SAH, and the rats in the BP preservation group did not have hypotension but maintained BP after SAH. Four rats from each group were designated for Western blot analysis and one rat from each group was designated for immunofluorescence staining.

Severity of SAH

The severity of SAH was evaluated in a blinded manner using the SAH grade as previously described [4, 5]. Briefly, rats were sacrificed by decapitation under deep general anesthesia and the brain was removed. SAH rats received a total

R.L. Applegate et al. (eds.), *Brain Edema XVI: Translate Basic Science into Clinical Practice*, Acta Neurochirurgica Supplement, Vol. 121, DOI 10.1007/978-3-319-18497-5_26, © Springer International Publishing Switzerland 2016

score ranging from 0 (no SAH) to 18 (most severe SAH). Animals with SAH grade 7 or less were excluded from the study for low SAH grade.

Western Blot Analyses

The heart was exposed through a midline sternotomy and then removed. The heart was cut halfway between the base and apex transversely and only the apex part was used for further study. Protein extraction of the samples was performed by homogenizing in RIPA buffer (Santa Cruz Biotechnology, Santa Cruz, CA, USA) supplemented with a protease and phosphatase inhibitor cocktail (Sigma-Aldrich, St. Louis, MO, USA) followed by centrifugation at 14,000 g at 4 °C for 20 min. The protein concentration was determined using a detergent-compatible assay (Bio-Rad, DC protein assay, Philadelphia, PA, USA). The supernatants were used for performing Western blot analysis as previously described [4, 5]. Equal amounts of protein (40 μg) were loaded. Primary antibodies were rabbit polyclonal anti-caspase-3 (1:1000, Cell Signaling Technology, Danvers, MA, USA) to detect endogenous levels of full-length caspase-3 (35 kDa) and the large fragment of cleaved caspase-3 (17 kDa). The membranes were incubated with the appropriate secondary antibody (1:2000). Immunoblots were then probed with an ECL Plus chemiluminescence reagent kit (Amersham Bioscience, Arlington Heights, IL, USA). Blot bands were quantified by densitometry using Image J software (Image J, National Institutes of Health, Bethesda, MD, USA). Results are expressed as a ratio of cleaved caspase-3/caspase-3 and normalized to mean value of sham, as previously described [3].

Immunofluorescence and Terminal Deoxynucleotidyl Transferase-Mediated Uridine 5′-Triphosphate-Biotin Nick End-Labeling Staining

The heart was infused retrogradely, via aortic cannulation, with 100 ml of phosphate-buffered saline, followed by 100 ml of 10 % paraformaldehyde for approximately 10 min, as previously described with modification [18]. The samples were then fixed in 10 % paraformaldehyde at 4 °C for 3 days. The tissues were incubated in 30 % sucrose for 3 days at 4 °C and embedded in OCT. Using a cryostat (LM3050S; Leica Microsystems, Bannockburn, IL, USA), 5-μ-thick coronal sections were cut at the level of apex of the heart region. The sections were mounted on poly-L-lysine-coated slides. Double-fluorescence labeling was performed using the primary antibody, anti-α-Actinin (Sarcomeric) (1:100, Sigma-Aldrich, St. Louis, MO, USA) and then subjected to terminal deoxynucleotidyl transferase-deoxyuridine triphosphate nick end labeling (TUNEL) using an in situ cell death detection kit (Roche, Diagnostics, Berlin, Germany). The stained sections were processed using a fluorescent microscope and Manga Fire SP system (Olympus, Center Valley, PA, USA). One rat from each group was used to show representative pictures in the sham, SAH hypotension, and SAH BP preservation group.

Statistical Analysis

Data for the SAH grade and Western blot analysis were analyzed by Mann-Whitney U test or Kruskal-Wallis analysis of variance (ANOVA) on ranks followed by Student-Neuman-Keuls post hoc analysis. Heart rate and MAP were expressed as mean ± standard deviation (SD) and analyzed by two-way repeated measures ANOVA. A p-value of <0.05 was considered statistically significant.

Results

Physiological Parameters and SAH Grade

The SAH hypotension group ($n=5$) had a significantly lower heart rate and BP compared with the SAH BP preservation group ($n=5$) (Fig. 1a, $p<0.001$). There was no significant difference in overall SAH grade between the SAH hypotension group ($n=5$) (median [25-75th percentiles], 18.00 [16.75–18.00]) and the SAH BP preservation group (16.00 [16.00–16.50]) (Fig. 1b, p = not significant (N.S.)).

Quantification of Cleaved Caspase-3/Caspase-3 Ratio at the Apex of Heart

Western blot analysis was used to quantify the levels of cleaved caspase-3/caspase-3 (CC3/C3) ratio in the sham ($n=4$) and SAH rats ($n=8$), including both the SAH hypotension and SAH BP preservation groups. The levels of CC3/C3 ratio in SAH group were 4.9 times higher at the apex of the heart compared with the sham group (Fig. 2a, b, $p<0.05$). Next, the levels of CC3/C3 ratio were quantified in the sham ($n=4$), SAH hypotension group ($n=4$), and SAH BP preservation group ($n=4$). The SAH hypotension group had significantly higher CC3/C3 ratio compared with the sham as well as the SAH BP preservation groups (Fig. 2a, c, $p<0.05$).

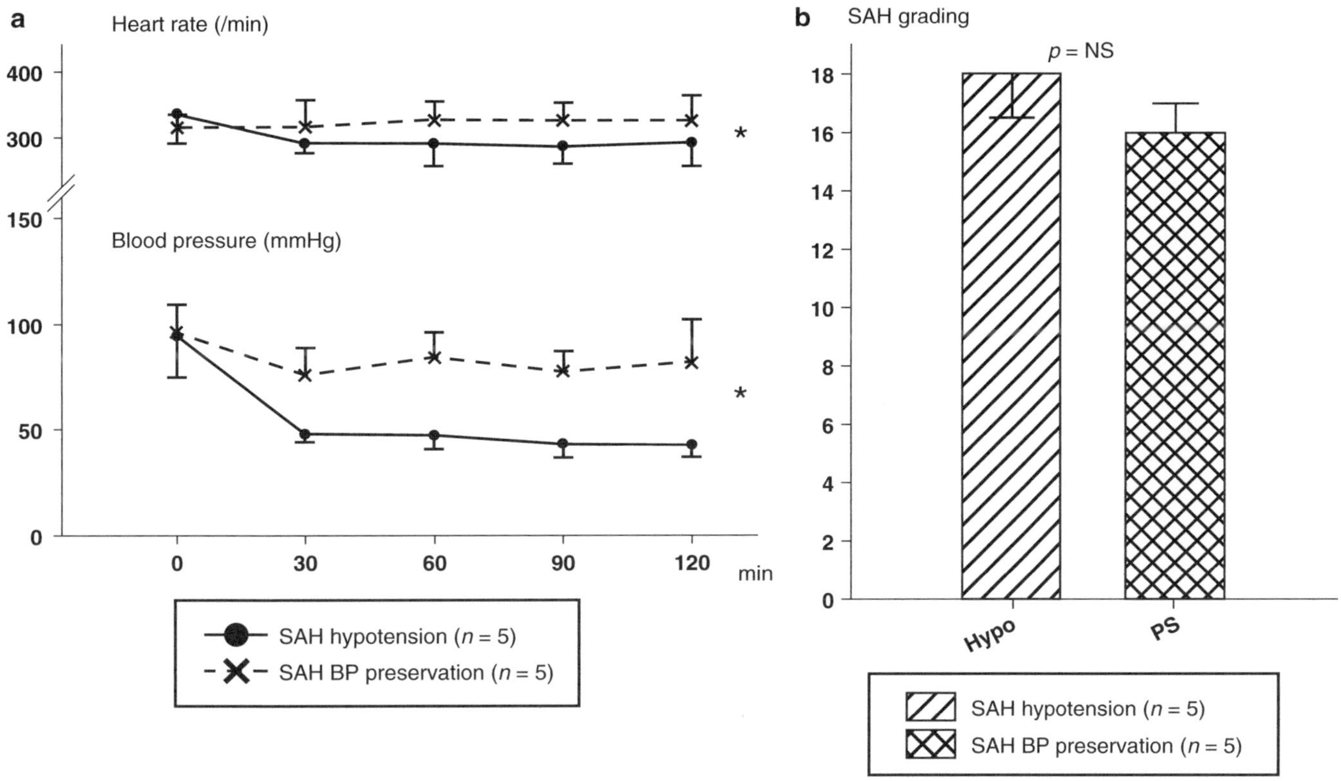

Fig. 1 Physiological parameters after surgical procedures up to 120 min after SAH (**a**). The data before SAH are not shown. There are significant differences between the SAH hypotension and SAH BP preservation groups in heart rate and mean arterial blood pressure after SAH (* $p<0.001$). Values are mean ± SD. Severity of SAH scores demonstrated equivalent SAH severity between SAH hypotension and SAH BP preservation groups (**b**). Values are expressed as median and 25th to 75th percentiles

Immunofluorescence Localization of Cardiomyocyte Apoptosis at the Apex of the Heart after SAH

Immunofluorescence staining was performed in the sham, SAH hypotension, and SAH BP preservation groups to localize apoptotic cell death at the apex of the heart using antibody specific to the cardiomyocyte. α-Actinin is one of the essential structural proteins required for establishing cardiomyocyte elongation and coordinated muscle contraction [14]. TUNEL-positive cells were detected in the heart tissue, which co-localized with the α-Actinin-positive cells in the SAH groups (Fig. 3). In the left ventricular (LV) wall, SAH with hypotension increased the number of TUNEL-positive cardiomyocytes, which were relatively fewer in the SAH BP preservation group.

Discussion

Our results demonstrate that apoptotic cell death was detected in the heart at 2 h after SAH, and there was more apoptotic cell death in the SAH hypotension group than in the SAH BP preservation group, located on the cardiomyocyte in the LV wall.

Neurogenic stunned myocardium is the most severe form of cardiac injury after SAH [17]. Explosive increases in intracranial pressure can cause catecholamine release at the nerve terminal of the cardiac myocytes. As the heart muscles contract, adenosine triphosphate is depleted, which causes mitochondrial dysfunction and resultant myocardial cell death [11]. Although high levels of catecholamine have been shown to cause apoptotic and necrotic myocytes [7], it remains unknown whether heart failure after SAH is associated with apoptotic cell death in the heart. An intriguing syndrome that overlaps substantially with SAH-related cardiac dysfunction is tako-tsubo cardiomyopathy, also known as apical ballooning syndrome, stress cardiomyopathy, or “broken heart” syndrome [9]. Because we wanted to elucidate whether cardiomyocyte apoptosis is involved in acute heart failure after SAH, we measured BP and regarded the hypotension as a result of LV dyskinesis after SAH in this study. We detected cardiomyocyte apoptosis as a ratio of caspase-3 activation by taking the ratio of cleaved caspase-3 to caspase-3 because cleaved caspase-3 is the

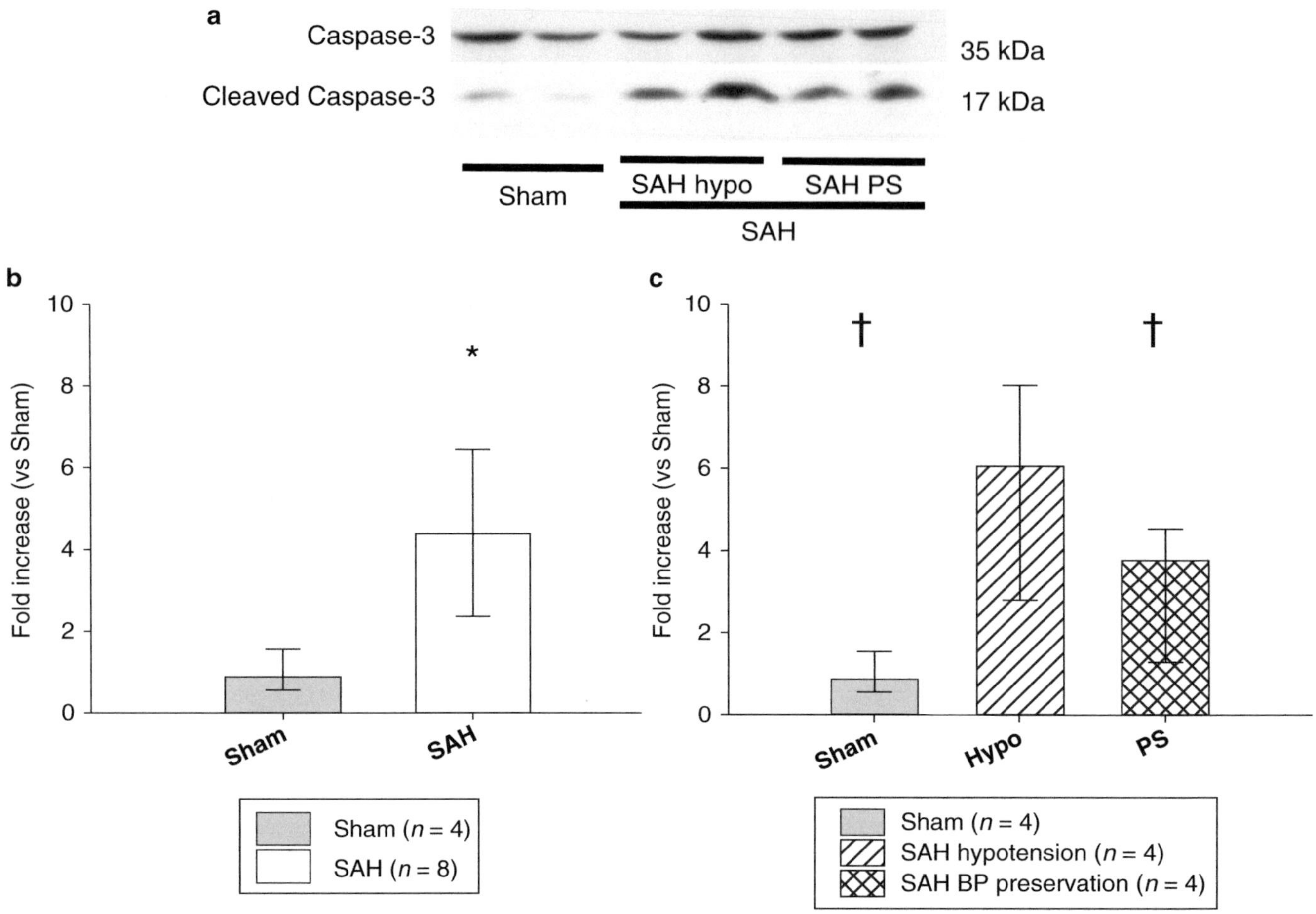

Fig. 2 Representative Western blots analysis 2 h after the surgical procedure in sham, SAH hypotension (hypo), and SAH BP preservation groups (PS) (**a**). In quantitative Western blot analysis, the SAH groups, including SAH hypotension (hypo) and SAH BP preservation groups, induced significantly higher cleaved caspase-3/ caspase-3 ratio than sham (**b**). The SAH hypotension group had significantly higher cleaved caspase-3/caspase-3 ratio compared with the SAH BP preservation group (**c**). Values are expressed as median and 25th to 75th percentiles. * $p<0.05$ vs. sham, † $p<0.05$ vs. SAH hypotension group

active form of the pro-apoptotic caspase-3 [3]. Our results suggest for the first time that cardiomyocyte apoptosis in the LV wall may cause the acute heart failure sometimes seen after SAH. Further studies are necessary for clinical translation in humans [1, 8, 16].

Conflict of Interest Authors declare no conflicts of interest.

Funding Source

This study is partially supported by National Institutes of Health grant NS081740 to JHZ.

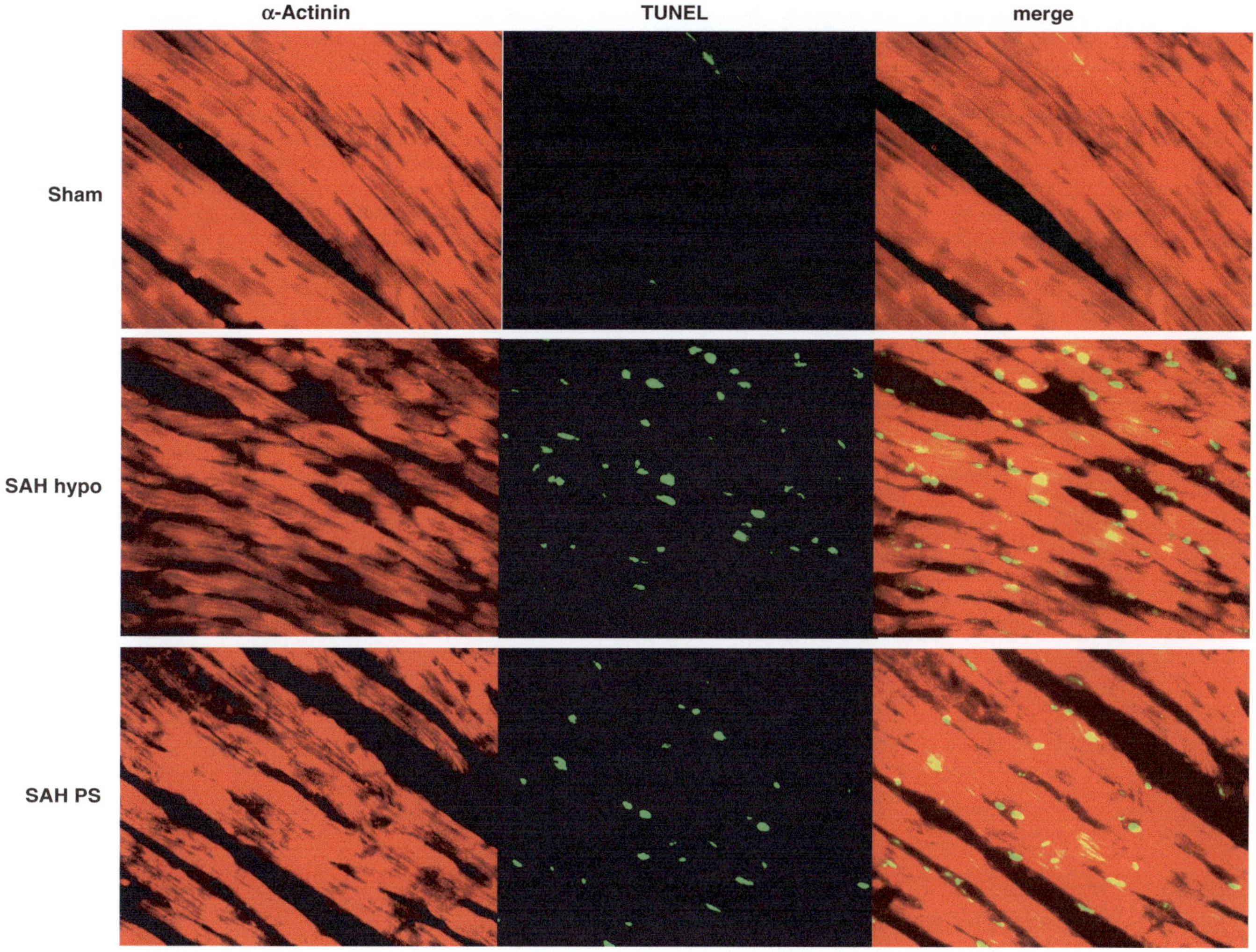

Fig. 3 Representative immunofluorescence of α-Actinin and transferase-mediated uridine 5′-triphosphate-biotin nick end-labeling (*TUNEL*) staining in sham, SAH hypotension, and SAH BP preservation groups in the left ventricle. SAH with hypotension had more TUNEL-positive cardiomyocytes than SAH BP preservation

References

1. Bahjat FR, Gesuete R, Stenzel-Poore MP (2013) Steps to translate preconditioning from basic research to the clinic. Transl Stroke Res 4:89–103
2. Bühler D, Schüller K, Plesnila N (2014) Protocol for the induction of subarachnoid hemorrhage in mice by perforation of the circle of Willis with an endovascular filament. Transl Stroke Res 5: 653–659
3. Fortress AM, Buhusi M, Helke KL, Granholm AC (2011) Cholinergic degeneration and alterations in the TrkA and p75NTR balance as a result of Pro-NGF injection into aged rats. J Aging Res 2011:460543
4. Fujii M, Sherchan P, Krafft PR, Rolland WB, Soejima Y, Zhang JH (2014) Cannabinoid type 2 receptor stimulation attenuates brain edema by reducing cerebral leukocyte infiltration following subarachnoid hemorrhage in rats. J Neurol Sci 342:101–106
5. Fujii M, Sherchan P, Soejima Y, Hasegawa Y, Flores J, Doycheva D, Zhang JH (2014) Cannabinoid receptor type 2 agonist attenuates apoptosis by activation of phosphorylated CREB-Bcl-2 pathway after subarachnoid hemorrhage in rats. Exp Neurol 261:396–403
6. Fujii M, Yan J, Rolland WB, Soejima Y, Caner B, Zhang JH (2013) Early brain injury, an evolving frontier in subarachnoid hemorrhage research. Transl Stroke Res 4:432–446
7. Goldspink DF, Burniston JG, Ellison GM, Clark WA, Tan LB (2004) Catecholamine-induced apoptosis and necrosis in cardiac and skeletal myocytes of the rat in vivo: the same or separate death pathways? Exp Physiol 89:407–416
8. Lapchak PA (2013) Drug-like property profiling of novel neuroprotective compounds to treat acute ischemic stroke: guidelines to develop pleiotropic molecules. Transl Stroke Res 4:328–342
9. Lee VH, Oh JK, Mulvagh SL, Wijdicks EF (2006) Mechanisms in neurogenic stress cardiomyopathy after aneurysmal subarachnoid hemorrhage. Neurocrit Care 5:243–249
10. Macmillan CS, Grant IS, Andrews PJ (2002) Pulmonary and cardiac sequelae of subarachnoid haemorrhage: time for active management? Intensive Care Med 28:1012–1023
11. Mashaly HA, Provencio JJ (2008) Inflammation as a link between brain injury and heart damage: the model of subarachnoid hemorrhage. Cleve Clin J Med 75(Suppl 2):S26–S30

12. Masuda T, Sato K, Yamamoto S, Matsuyama N, Shimohama T, Matsunaga A, Obuchi S, Shiba Y, Shimizu S, Izumi T (2002) Sympathetic nervous activity and myocardial damage immediately after subarachnoid hemorrhage in a unique animal model. Stroke 33:1671–1676
13. Naredi S, Lambert G, Edén E, Zäll S, Runnerstam M, Rydenhag B, Friberg P (2000) Increased sympathetic nervous activity in patients with nontraumatic subarachnoid hemorrhage. Stroke 31:901–906
14. Risebro CA, Searles RG, Melville AA, Ehler E, Jina N, Shah S, Pallas J, Hubank M, Dillard M, Harvey NL, Schwartz RJ, Chien KR, Oliver G, Riley PR (2009) Prox1 maintains muscle structure and growth in the developing heart. Development 136:495–505
15. Sehba FA (2014) Rat endovascular perforation model. Transl Stroke Res 5:660–668
16. Tajiri N, Dailey T, Metcalf C, Mosley YI, Lau T, Staples M, van Loveren H, Kim SU, Yamashima T, Yasuhara T, Date I, Kaneko Y, Borlongan CV (2013) In vivo animal stroke models: a rationale for rodent and non-human primate models. Transl Stroke Res 4:308–321
17. Wartenberg KE, Mayer SA (2006) Medical complications after subarachnoid hemorrhage: new strategies for prevention and management. Curr Opin Crit Care 12:78–84
18. Zhang DX, Zhao PT, Xia L, Liu LL, Liang J, Zhai HH, Zhang HB, Guo XG, Wu KC, Xu YM, Jia LT, Yang AG, Chen SY, Fan DM (2010) Potent inhibition of human gastric cancer by HER2-directed induction of apoptosis with anti-HER2 antibody and caspase-3 fusion protein. Gut 59:292–299

The Role of Matricellular Proteins in Brain Edema after Subarachnoid Hemorrhage

Hidenori Suzuki, Masashi Fujimoto, Masato Shiba, Fumihiro Kawakita, Lei Liu, Naoki Ichikawa, Kenji Kanamaru, Kyoko Imanaka-Yoshida, and Toshimichi Yoshida

Introduction

A key pathologic manifestation of early brain injury after aneurysmal subarachnoid hemorrhage (SAH) is an increase in blood-brain barrier (BBB) permeability, which leads to vasogenic brain edema. Global cerebral edema has been reported in approximately 20–40 % of aneurysmal SAH patients who receive medical attention, and has been described as an independent risk factor for poor outcome after SAH [2]. BBB dysfunction may allow greater influx of blood-borne cells and substances into brain parenchyma, thus amplifying inflammation, leading to further parenchymal damage and edema formation [13, 15]. The BBB is formed by specialized brain endothelial cells that are interconnected by tight junctions, surrounded by a highly specialized basal membrane, a large number of pericytes embedded in the basal membrane, and astrocytic perivascular end-feet. An understanding of how BBB is disturbed in SAH could lead to the development of new protective and restorative therapies.

The components of extracellular matrix (ECM) include basic structural proteins such as collagen, elastin and specialized proteins such as fibronectin, proteoglycans, and matricellular proteins (MCPs). MCPs are a class of inducible nonstructural and secreted ECM proteins that exert diverse functions through direct binding to cell surface receptors, other matrix proteins, and soluble extracellular factors such as growth factors and cytokines [1, 21]. The term was introduced in 1995 to explain the unusual diversity of functions [21], and the number of MCPs is still increasing. MCPs include osteopontin (OPN); tenascin-C (TNC); thrombospondin-1; thrombospondin-2; secreted protein, acidic and rich in cystein (osteonectin); members of the cysteine-rich 61/connective growth factor/nephroblastoma overexpressed family; galectin; periostin; and so on [24]. MCPs are different from classical ECM proteins in the following ways: (1) MCPs induce cell motility (tissue remodeling), rather than providing scaffolds for stable cell adhesion (structural organization); (2) their levels are generally low in steady-state condition in adult tissues but are readily and transiently upregulated during specific developmental stages and in pathological conditions rather than constitutively expressed; (3) MCPs can be present as soluble proteins rather than present as structural components; (4) MCPs can associate with various biological active molecules, including growth factors, chemokines, cytokines, and proteases, modulating their functions and acting as reservoirs of those molecules; and (5) MCPs do not produce apparent phenotypes after targeted gene disruption in mice, however, they do exhibit various phenotypes in response to various insults [1, 24]. It becomes clear that MCPs are key mediators of various physiological and pathological conditions [1, 24].

Among MCPs, OPN and TNC have been reported to be involved in post-SAH brain injury, although the information is still limited. In this chapter, we review the possible role of OPN and TNC in post-SAH pathology, especially focusing on BBB disruption and brain edema formation.

H. Suzuki, MD, PhD (✉) • M. Fujimoto, MD, PhD
M. Shiba, MD, PhD • F. Kawakita, MD • L. Liu, MD
N. Ichikawa, MD
Department of Neurosurgery, Mie University Graduate School of Medicine, 2-174 Edobashi, Tsu, Mie 514-8507, Japan
e-mail: suzuki02@clin.medic.mie-u.ac.jp

K. Kanamaru, MD, PhD
Department of Neurosurgery, Suzuka Kaisei Hospital, Suzuka, Mie, Japan

K. Imanaka-Yoshida, MD, PhD • T. Yoshida, MD, PhD
Department of Pathology and Matrix Biology,
Mie University Graduate School of Medicine, Tsu, Mie, Japan

OPN

Expression of OPN in SAH Brain

Expression of OPN has never been investigated in aneurysmal SAH patients. However, in an endovascular puncture model of SAH in rats, the natural course of OPN induction was examined

R.L. Applegate et al. (eds.), *Brain Edema XVI: Translate Basic Science into Clinical Practice*, Acta Neurochirurgica Supplement, Vol. 121,
DOI 10.1007/978-3-319-18497-5_27, © Springer International Publishing Switzerland 2016

in brain related to BBB disruption [15]. Expression levels of OPN were very low in brains of healthy adult rats. SAH caused a significant loss in body weight, sensorimotor disturbance, BBB disruption, and brain edema formation, which peaked at 24 or 48 h post-SAH, and significantly improved at 72 h post-SAH. OPN induction was observed in all brain regions studied, that is, bilateral cerebral hemispheres, cerebellum, and brainstem, with a peak at 72 h post-SAH, corresponding with the animal's recovery of body weight losses and neurological impairments as well as BBB disruption. Immunohistochemistry showed that reactive astrocytosis and angiogenesis occurred predominantly in the basal cortex covered with thick SAH at 72 h post-SAH, where OPN was induced in the reactive astrocytes and capillary endothelial cells [15].

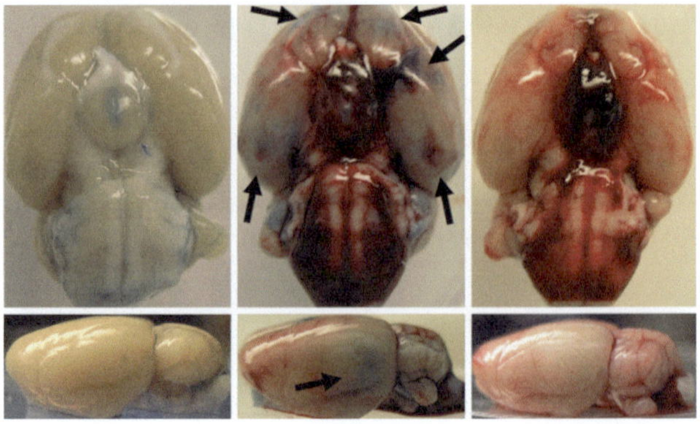

Fig. 1 Preventive effects of intracerebroventricular injection of r-OPN on Evans blue dye extravasation (*arrow*, meaning BBB disruption) at 24 h after SAH by endovascular puncture. Sham, sham-operated rats treated with phosphate-buffered saline (PBS) vehicle; SAH or SAH-OPN, SAH rats treated with PBS or 0.1 μg of r-OPN

Role of Endogenous OPN Induction in BBB Disruption after SAH

OPN small interfering RNA (siRNA) was intracerebroventricularly injected to block endogenous OPN induction in SAH brain by endovascular puncture in rats, and the effects were studied at 72 h post-SAH when brain OPN induction peaked [15]. OPN siRNA treatment resulted in significantly increased BBB permeability and aggravated neurological impairments compared with the control SAH rats. The blockage of endogenous OPN induction suppressed post-SAH induction of an endogenous mitogen-activated protein kinase (MAPK) inhibitor, MAPK phosphatase (MKP)-1, and activated MAPKs including c-Jun N-terminal kinase (JNK), p38, and extracellular signal-regulated kinase (ERK)1/2, which act both upstream and downstream of vascular endothelial growth factor (VEGF)-A, a potent inducer of BBB disruption [7, 10], causing VEGF-A upregulation. Because blockage of endogenous OPN also decreased angiopoietin (Ang)-1 which has a potent anti-permeability property and blocks the effect of VEGF-A [5], endogenous OPN induction may play a role in keeping Ang-1 levels within a normal range and restoring the BBB at 72 h post-SAH. Neither SAH nor OPN siRNA affected levels of VEGF-B, which may maintain the BBB in steady states, and Ang-2, an inhibitor of Ang-1 activity [10]. These findings suggest that OPN represents a naturally occurring protective factor against BBB disruption after SAH.

Exogenous OPN Treatment Prevents Post-SAH BBB Disruption

Pre-SAH intracerebroventricular injection of recombinant OPN (r-OPN) prevented a loss in body weight, neurological impairments, BBB disruption, and brain edema formation at 24–72 h after SAH by endovascular puncture in rats (Fig. 1) [13, 15], whereas r-OPN had no effects on sham-operated rats [13]. r-OPN's neuroprotective effects were associated with deactivation of nuclear factor (NF)-κB activity, leading to inhibition of proteolytic matrix metalloproteinase (MMP)-9 induction, the maintenance of a matrix stabilizing factor tissue inhibitor of MMP (TIMP)-1, and the consequent preservation of substrates of MMP-9, the cerebral microvessel basal lamina protein laminin, and the inter-endothelial tight junction protein zona occludens-1 [13]. SAH also activated interleukin (IL)-1β, but r-OPN did not suppress IL-1β activation [13]. The findings may be explained by IL-1β induction via NF-κB-independent mechanisms such as post-SAH sympathetic activation or catecholamine release [22]. Although OPN regulates the bioavailability of MMPs depending on cell types, receptor interactions, post-translational modifications, and the phosphorylation state of OPN [6], the inhibitory effects of OPN on MMP-9 and NF-κB activities may be observed only in the presence of proinflammatory cytokines such as IL-1β elevation following SAH. It is also possible but unproven that OPN might inactivate NF-κB and thereby inhibit MMP-9 induction by reducing oxidative stress [8]. r-OPN also induced MKP-1, resulting in inhibition of post-SAH JNK activation and VEGF-A upregulation, whereas these effects of r-OPN were blocked by a L-arginyl-glycyl-L-aspartate (RGD)-dependent integrin receptor antagonist, GRGDSP [15]. Neither SAH nor r-OPN affected Ang-1, activated p38, and ERK1/2 levels in brain.

Nasal administration of r-OPN also decreased neuronal cell death and brain edema, and improved the neurological status in SAH rats by endovascular puncture, possibly through focal adhesion kinase-phosphatidylinositol 3-kinase-Akt-induced inhibition of capase-3 cleavage [23]. This study did not examine anti-apoptotic effects of r-OPN on capillary endothelial cells, which can potentially explain r-OPN's inhibition of brain edema formation after SAH.

On the other hand, r-OPN suppressed post-SAH endogenous OPN induction in brain, although r-OPN had no effects on endogenous OPN levels in the sham-operated rats [13]. These findings may reflect the decreased brain damage by r-OPN, because OPN is induced in response to tissue injuries or inflammation and may play a role in the maintenance of tissue homeostasis and the induction of tissue repair in a variety of situations [3].

TNC

Expression of TNC in SAH Brain

In a clinical setting, TNC levels were increased in both serum and cerebrospinal fluid (CSF) after aneurysmal SAH [16–20]. CSF TNC levels peaked immediately after SAH and decreased with time, whereas serum TNC levels increased transiently and peaked on Days 4–6 [19]. Serum TNC levels were greater in patients with subsequent angiographic vasospasm; the peak occurred 2.4 days before an increase in the mean transcranial Doppler velocity to ≥120 cm/s and 3.6 days before the onset of delayed cerebral ischemia [18]. In contrast, CSF TNC levels were below the diagnostic threshold level in control patients and markedly increased after SAH [20]. Higher CSF TNC levels were observed in patients with worse admission clinical grade, more severe SAH on admission computed tomography, acute obstructive hydrocephalus, subsequent angiographic vasospasm, delayed cerebral ischemia, chronic shunt-dependent hydrocephalus, and a worse outcome [16, 17, 20]. To predict the onset of delayed cerebral ischemia, 16.2 ng/mL was considered as an appropriate cut-off value for CSF TNC on Days 1–6, giving a sensitivity of 81.0 % and a specificity of 79.5 % [16]. Clinical findings suggest that more severe SAH or initial brain injury may induce more TNC, which may cause angiographic vasospasm and delayed cerebral ischemia separately or simultaneously; that is, delayed cerebral ischemia may occur by severe angiographic vasospasm with more TNC induction, and/or by vasospasm-unrelated causes with TNC induction, which is thought to be early brain injury [17].

TNC is induced in both cerebral arterial wall [12] and brain parenchyma after experimental SAH by endovascular puncture in rats [11]. TNC induction in the cerebral artery caused vasospasm [4, 12]. On the other hand, TNC was increased in neuropil mainly in the brain surface of the cerebral cortex irrespective of cerebral vasospasm development at both 24 and 72 h after SAH [11]. It was considered that astrocytes, neurons, and capillary endothelial cells produced TNC [11].

Role of Endogenous TNC Induction in BBB Disruption after SAH

Because there are neither inhibitors nor neutralizing antibodies specific for TNC, a previous study used imatinib mesylate (a selective inhibitor of the tyrosine kinases of platelet-derived growth factor [PDGF] receptors [PDGFRs]) to block endogenous TNC induction and to examine the effects on brain injury after SAH by endovascular puncture in rats [11]. PDGF is well known to be a potent inducer of TNC [12]. Actually, imatinib mesylate, a PDGFR inhibitor, prevented brain PDGFR activation, TNC upregulation, MAPK activation, neuronal apoptosis, and neurological impairments after SAH in rats (Fig. 2), although the effects on endothelial cell apoptosis or brain edema formation were not examined [11]. Another study reported that imatinib mesylate prevented post-SAH BBB disruption and brain edema formation by inhibiting JNK-mediated MMP-9 activation in rats [26]. In a clinical setting, TNC was observed around hyperplastic blood vessels of astrocytomas, regardless of their grade, as well as around newly formed vascular channels of inflammatory, ischemic, and traumatic diseases of the brain, suggesting the role of TNC in angiogenesis [25]. Taken together, TNC induction in SAH brain may cause BBB disruption and brain edema formation, although the possibility that imatinib mesylate exerts neuroprotective effects by TNC-unrelated mechanisms cannot be excluded. Our preliminary study also showed that TNC-knockout mice had a significant decrease in post-SAH BBB disruption and brain edema formation associated with MMP-9 inhibition (unpublished data).

Effects of Exogenous TNC on BBB Disruption after SAH

A cisternal injection of intact (full-length) TNC induced prolonged cerebral arterial constriction but did not cause neurological impairments in healthy rats [4], whereas a cisternal injection of recombinant TNC (r-TNC; murine myeloma cell line, NS0-derived, Gly23–Pro625, with a C-terminal 6-His tag) caused vasospasm, neuronal apoptosis, and neurological impairments in imatinib mesylate-treated filament puncture SAH rats [11, 12]. Exogenous TNC activated MAPKs in the cerebral artery and caused cerebral arterial contraction in both healthy rats and imatinib mesylate-treated SAH rats [4, 11, 12]. However, effects of exogenous TNC on brain may be different between healthy and SAH rats, because SAH may induce MMPs, which can cleave TNC. Cleaved TNC may activate different signaling and exert diverse cell responses depending on domains of TNC [9]. Our recent

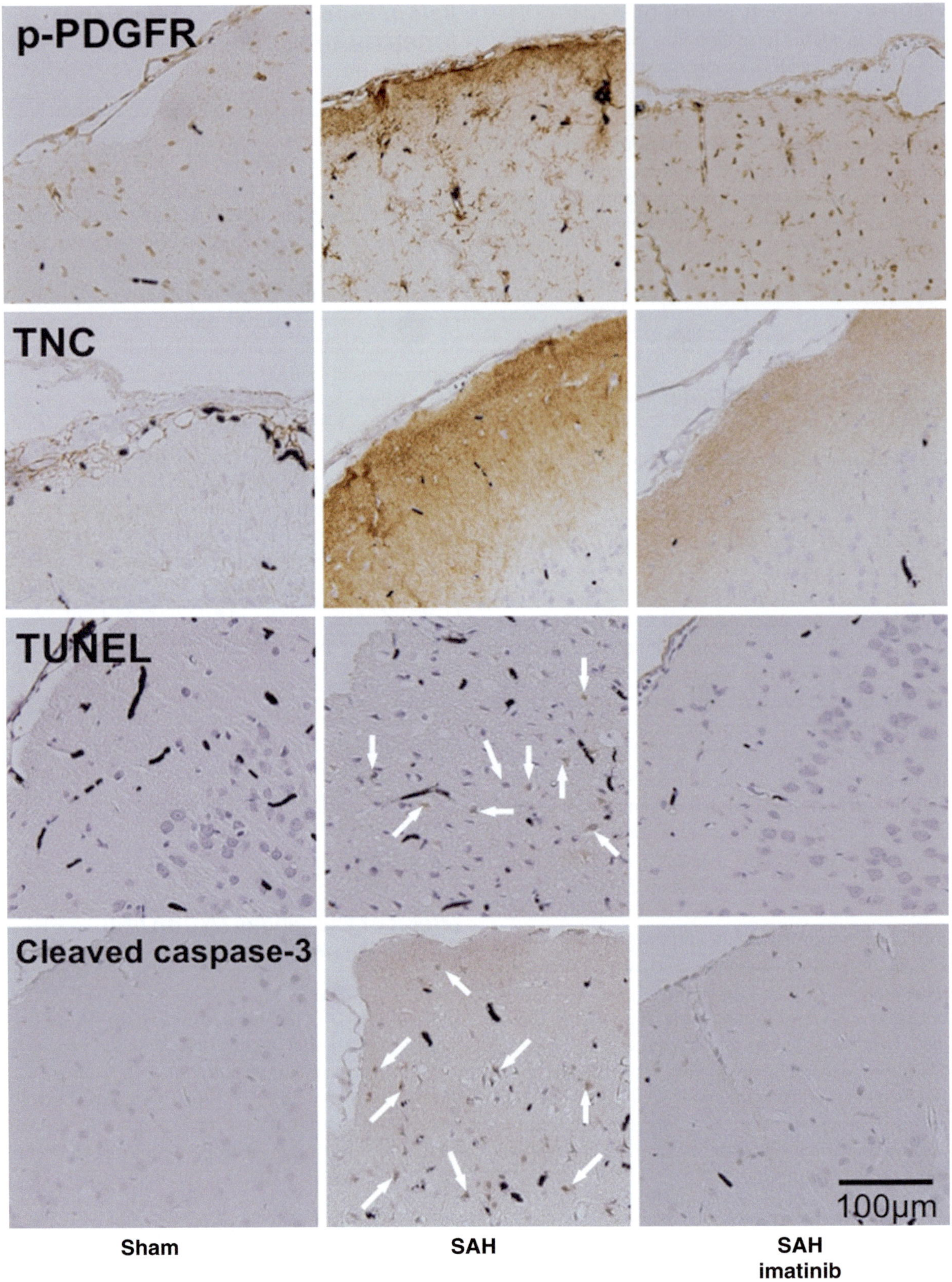

Fig. 2 Inhibitory effects of intraperitoneal injection of imatinib mesylate on expression of phosphorylated PDGFR (p-PDGFR), TNC, and cleaved caspase-3, or terminal deoxynucleotidyltransferase-mediated dUTP nick end labeling (TUNEL) staining in brain at 24 h after SAH by endovascular puncture. *Arrow*, apoptotic neuron; SAH-imatinib, SAH rats treated with imatinib mesylate (50 mg/kg body weight). Black stains depict India ink, because specimens were harvested after India ink angiography

preliminary study showed that a cisternal injection of intact TNC aggravated BBB disruption and brain edema in TNC-knockout filament puncture SAH mice (unpublished data).

An interesting feature of TNC is the existence of positive feedback mechanisms to augment TNC's actions [4, 11, 12]. A r-TNC injection induced TNC itself in the cerebral artery and brain after SAH, which may internally augment vasospasm and neuronal apoptosis [11, 12]. After SAH, PDGF may induce endogenous TNC, and r-TNC also induced both PDGFR-β upregulation and PDGFR activation [12]. These findings suggest that PDGF-induced TNC may positively feed back on PDGFR activation via PDGFR upregulation and crosstalk signaling between receptors as well as upregulation of TNC, leading to more MAPK activation and therefore cerebral vasospasm or neurological impairments in SAH rats [12]. Another study using healthy rats showed that a cisternal intact TNC injection induced prolonged cerebral arterial constriction via toll-like receptor 4 (TLR4) and activation of MAPKs, and suggested that TLR4 activation may have positive feedback on TLR4 activation via MAPK-mediated upregulation of TNC and TLR4 in cerebral arteries, causing more activation of MAPKs and more prolongation of vasoconstriction, even though post-injection TNC concentration in CSF decreases over time [4].

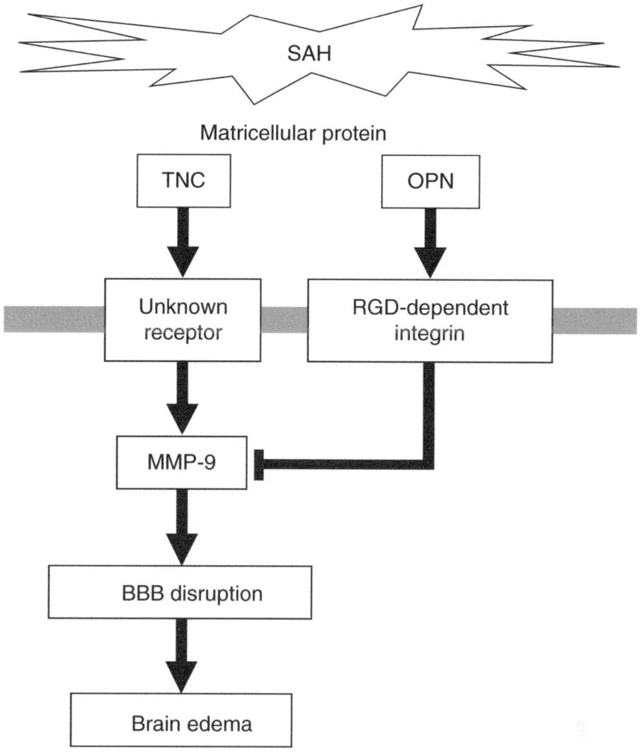

Fig. 3 Possible mechanisms for TNC and OPN to control brain edema formation after SAH

Discussion

The biological functions of MCPs are highly variable and often seemingly contradictory, depending on the biological scenario surrounding their induction [13]. However, OPN is consistently protective [13, 15], whereas TNC is deleterious for brain or BBB after SAH [11, 17, 20]. It is notable that the function of OPN and TNC, representatives of MCPs, is conflicting in the setting of SAH. As to cerebral vasospasm after SAH, r-OPN activated the protective pathways including MKP-1, an endogenous MAPK inhibitor, via binding to RGD-dependent integrins [14]. In contrast, exogenous TNC activated MAPKs via binding to TLR4 and caused cerebral vasospasm or prolonged cerebral artery contraction [4, 12]. Although the mechanisms of how OPN antagonizes TNC's effect remain unclear in cerebral vasospasm after SAH, another possibility is that OPN may inhibit TNC's binding to its receptor competitively, because they share some receptors [21]. TNC signaling may positively feed back on upregulation of TNC itself in an acute phase, leading to more activation of the signaling transduction and the development of cerebral vasospasm [12], while OPN has no such action and seems to be induced in a delayed fashion in response to tissue injuries or inflammation [3, 13].

This review shows that TNC and OPN may be efficient modulators of BBB disruption and brain edema formation, as well as cerebral vasospasm, after SAH at several different levels. There is compelling evidence that OPN can protect the BBB after SAH [13, 15, 23]. Post-SAH BBB breakdown is a transient phenomenon and a functional recovery may ensue. A clarification of the intrinsic mechanisms to reverse BBB disruption may lead to a novel therapeutic approach for the treatment of early brain injury after SAH, and OPN-mediated pathways are good candidates [13, 15, 23]. Multiple independent or interconnected signaling pathways may be involved in the protective effects of OPN against BBB disruption. r-OPN is promising for the treatment of post-SAH BBB disruption that has complex pathogenesis. On the other hand, TNC may be an important inducer of post-SAH BBB disruption, although accumulated evidence suggests that many molecules are involved, acting simultaneously or at different stages during BBB disruption [11, 26]. It is unknown whether the signaling of TNC and OPN in the setting of BBB disruption is identical to or different from that observed in cerebral vasospasm after SAH, but it may include MMP-9 as a key player (Fig. 3).

There are many other known MCPs that have been never investigated in the context of BBB disruption or brain edema formation. Future studies will determine how MCPs including TNC and OPN are involved in the pathophysiology of BBB disruption and brain edema formation after SAH. It is hoped that this review provides valuable information that

MCPs such as OPN and TNC potentially play a key role in the development of BBB disruption and brain edema and can be future therapeutic targets after SAH.

Acknowledgments This work was supported in part by a grant-in-aid for scientific research from the Japan Society for the Promotion of Science to Drs. Suzuki and Shiba.

Conflict of Interest Statement The authors declare that they have no conflicts of interest.

References

1. Chiodoni C, Colombo MP, Sangaletti S (2010) Matricellular proteins: from homeostasis to inflammation, cancer, and metastasis. Cancer Metastasis Rev 29:295–307
2. Claassen J, Carhuapoma JR, Kreiter KT, Du EY, Connolly ES, Mayer SA (2002) Global cerebral edema after subarachnoid hemorrhage: frequency, predictors, and impact on outcome. Stroke 33:1225–1232
3. Denhardt DT, Noda M, O'Regan AW, Pavlin D, Berman JS (2001) Osteopontin as a means to cope with environmental insults: regulation of inflammation, tissue remodeling, and cell survival. J Clin Invest 107:1055–1061
4. Fujimoto M, Suzuki H, Shiba M, Shimojo N, Imanaka-Yoshida K, Yoshida T, Kanamaru K, Matsushima S, Taki W (2013) Tenascin-C induces prolonged constriction of cerebral arteries in rats. Neurobiol Dis 55:104–109
5. Gavard J, Patel V, Gutkind JS (2008) Angiopoietin-1 prevents VEGF-induced endothelial permeability by sequestering Src through mDia. Dev Cell 14:25–36
6. Kazanecki CC, Uzwiak DJ, Denhardt DT (2007) Control of osteopontin signaling and function by post-translational phosphorylation and protein folding. J Cell Biochem 102:912–924
7. Kusaka G, Ishikawa M, Nanda A, Granger DN, Zhang JH (2004) Signaling pathways for early brain injury after subarachnoid hemorrhage. J Cereb Blood Flow Metab 24:916–925
8. Mazzali M, Kipari T, Ophascharoensuk V, Wesson JA, Johnson R, Hughes J (2002) Osteopontin. A molecule for all seasons. Q J Med 95:3–13
9. Midwood KS, Orend G (2009) The role of tenascin-C in tissue injury and tumorigenesis. J Cell Commun Signal 3:287–310
10. Nag S, Manias JL, Stewart DJ (2009) Pathology and new players in the pathogenesis of brain edema. Acta Neuropathol 118: 197–217
11. Shiba M, Fujimoto M, Imanaka-Yoshida K, Yoshida T, Taki W, Suzuki H (2014) Tenascin-C causes neuronal apoptosis after subarachnoid hemorrhage in rats. Transl Stroke Res 5:238–247
12. Shiba M, Suzuki H, Fujimoto M, Shimojo N, Imanaka-Yoshida K, Yoshida T, Kanamaru K, Matsushima S, Taki W (2012) Imatinib mesylate prevents cerebral vasospasm after subarachnoid hemorrhage via inhibiting tenascin-C expression in rats. Neurobiol Dis 46:172–179
13. Suzuki H, Ayer R, Sugawara T, Chen W, Sozen T, Hasegawa Y, Kanamaru K, Zhang JH (2010) Protective effects of recombinant osteopontin on early brain injury after subarachnoid hemorrhage in rats. Crit Care Med 38:612–618
14. Suzuki H, Hasegawa Y, Chen W, Kanamaru K, Zhang JH (2010) Recombinant osteopontin in cerebral vasospasm after subarachnoid hemorrhage. Ann Neurol 68:650–660
15. Suzuki H, Hasegawa Y, Kanamaru K, Zhang JH (2010) Mechanisms of osteopontin-induced stabilization of blood-brain barrier disruption after subarachnoid hemorrhage in rats. Stroke 41:1783–1790
16. Suzuki H, Kanamaru K, Shiba M, Fujimoto M, Imanaka-Yoshida K, Yoshida T, Taki W (2011) Cerebrospinal fluid tenascin-C in cerebral vasospasm after aneurysmal subarachnoid hemorrhage. J Neurosurg Anesthesiol 23:310–317
17. Suzuki H, Kanamaru K, Shiba M, Fujimoto M, Kawakita F, Imanaka-Yoshida K, Yoshida T, Taki W (2015) Tenascin-C is a possible mediator between initial brain injury and vasospasm-related and -unrelated delayed cerebral ischemia after aneurysmal subarachnoid hemorrhage. Acta Neurochir Suppl 120:117–121
18. Suzuki H, Kanamaru K, Suzuki Y, Aimi Y, Matsubara N, Araki T, Takayasu M, Kinoshita N, Imanaka-Yoshida K, Yoshida T, Taki W (2010) Tenascin-C is induced in cerebral vasospasm after subarachnoid hemorrhage in rats and humans: a pilot study. Neurol Res 32:179–184
19. Suzuki H, Kanamaru K, Suzuki Y, Aimi Y, Matsubara N, Araki T, Takayasu M, Takeuchi T, Okada K, Kinoshita N, Imanaka-Yoshida K, Yoshida T, Taki W (2008) Possible role of tenascin-C in cerebral vasospasm after aneurysmal subarachnoid hemorrhage. Acta Neurochir Suppl 104:179–182
20. Suzuki H, Kinoshita N, Imanaka-Yoshida K, Yoshida T, Taki W (2008) Cerebrospinal fluid tenascin-C increases preceding the development of chronic shunt-dependent hydrocephalus after subarachnoid hemorrhage. Stroke 39:1610–1612
21. Suzuki H, Shiba M, Fujimoto M, Kawamura K, Nanpei M, Tekeuchi E, Matsushima S, Kanamaru K, Imanaka-Yoshida K, Yoshida T, Taki W (2013) Matricellular protein: a new player in cerebral vasospasm following subarachnoid hemorrhage. Acta Neurochir Suppl 115:213–218
22. Tan KS, Nackley AG, Satterfield K, Maixner W, Diatchenko L, Flood PM (2007) β2 adrenergic receptor activation stimulates pro-inflammatory cytokine production in macrophages via PKA- and NF-κB-independent mechanisms. Cell Signal 19:251–260
23. Topkoru BC, Altay O, Duris K, Krafft PR, Yan J, Zhang JH (2013) Nasal administration of recombinant osteopontin attenuates early brain injury after subarachnoid hemorrhage. Stroke 44: 3189–3194
24. Uede T (2011) Osteopontin, intrinsic tissue regulator of intractable inflammatory diseases. Pathol Int 61:265–280
25. Zagzag D, Capo V (2002) Angiogenesis in the central nervous system: a role for vascular endothelial growth factor/vascular permeability factor and tenascin-C. Common molecular effectors in cerebral neoplastic and non-neoplastic "angiogenic diseases". Histol Histopathol 17:301–321
26. Zhan Y, Krafft PR, Lekic T, Ma Q, Souvenir R, Zhang JH, Tang J (2014) Imatinib preserves blood-brain barrier integrity following experimental subarachnoid hemorrhage in rats. J Neurosci Res. doi:10.1002/jnr.23475

Early Cerebral Infarction after Aneurysmal Subarachnoid Hemorrhage

George Kwok Chu Wong, Joyce Hoi Ying Leung, Janice Wong Li Yu, Sandy Wai Lam, Emily Kit Ying Chan, Wai Sang Poon, Jill Abrigo, and Deyond Yun Woon Siu

Introduction

Aneurysmal subarachnoid hemorrhage (SAH) is a serious disease with high case fatality and morbidity [9, 15–17]. A high rate of hypodense lesions consistent with cerebral infarctions has been evident on follow-up CT scanning among survivors at 3 months [4, 20]. In a post hoc path analysis, cerebral infarction also had a direct effect on outcome independent of angiographic vasospasm [19]. One study suggested that high SAH grade (using the Fisher scale) was related to cerebral infarction [3]. Early cerebral infarction has been recognized as a risk factor for poor outcome at 3 months according to the Glasgow Outcome Scale [3]. In this study, we aimed to assess the pattern of early and delayed cerebral infarction after aneurysmal subarachnoid hemorrhage.

G.K.C. Wong, MD (✉)
Division of Neurosurgery, Department of Surgery, Prince of Wales Hospital, The Chinese University of Hong Kong, Hong Kong, China

Department of Surgery, Prince of Wales Hospital, 4/F Clinical Science Building, 30-32 Ngan Shing Street, Shatin, New Territories, Hong Kong, SAR, China
e-mail: georgewong@surgery.cuhk.edu.hk

J.H.Y. Leung, MBChB • J.W.L. Yu, MBBS • J. Abrigo, FRCR
D.Y.W. Siu, FRCR
Department of Diagnostic Radiology and Organ Imaging, Prince of Wales Hospital, The Chinese University of Hong Kong, Hong Kong, China

S.W. Lam, BSocSc • E.K.Y. Chan, FRCS • W.S. Poon, FRCS
Division of Neurosurgery, Department of Surgery, Prince of Wales Hospital, The Chinese University of Hong Kong, Hong Kong, China

Materials and Methods

We prospectively enrolled consecutive aneurysmal SAH patients presenting to an academic neurosurgical referral center (Prince of Wales Hospital, the Chinese University of Hong Kong) in Hong Kong. The study was approved by the Joint CUHK-NTEC Clinical Research Ethics Committee. This study conformed to the Declaration of Helsinki, and written informed consent was obtained from all of the participants or their next of kin.

The patient inclusion criteria were as follows: (1) spontaneous SAH with angiography-confirmed etiology of intracranial aneurysms; (2) hospital admission within 96 h after ictus; (3) between 21 and 75 years of age; (4) a speaker of Chinese (Cantonese); and (5) informed consent from the patients or their next of kin. The patient exclusion criteria were a history of previous cerebrovascular or neurological disease other than unruptured intracranial aneurysm, a history of neurosurgery before ictus, or inability to cooperate in cognitive assessments (not obeying commands).

All the computed tomography (CT) scans were done on 64-slice scanners and reformatted into 5 mm thicknesses. CT films were categorized into early and delayed. Early CT was defined as post-treatment (clipping or coiling) Day 1 scan. Delayed CT was defined as 4–6 weeks post-treatment. Early cerebral infarction was defined as new parenchymal hypoattenuation on early CT; all cerebral infarction was defined as new parenchymal hypoattenuation on delayed CT; delayed cerebral infarction was defined as new parenchymal hypoattenuation on delayed CT, which was not present in early CT.

Modified Rankin Scale (mRS) [13, 18]

The mRS is a valid and clinically relevant disability scale to assess recovery and is commonly used in stroke trials. mRS

R.L. Applegate et al. (eds.), *Brain Edema XVI: Translate Basic Science into Clinical Practice*, Acta Neurochirurgica Supplement, Vol. 121,
DOI 10.1007/978-3-319-18497-5_28, © Springer International Publishing Switzerland 2016

identifies activity limitation and does not identify deficits. It ranges from 0 (no symptoms) to 6 (death).

Chinese Lawton Instrumental Activity of Daily Living (IADL) Scale

The Lawton IADL Scale is an appropriate instrument to assess independent living skills [6, 14]. Items assessed include ability to use the telephone, go shopping, prepare food, do the housekeeping, do the laundry, use transportation, be responsible for one's own medications, and handle finances. The Chinese version has been validated and used previously [14].

Statistical Analysis

The trial data were collected on printed forms and entered into a computer using Access 2003 software (Microsoft Inc., Redmond, WA, USA). Statistical analyses were generated using SPSS for Windows Version 15.0 (SPSS Inc., Chicago, IL, USA) [10]. Categorical data are given as numbers (percentages), unless otherwise specified; numerical data are given as means and standard deviations (SD); and ordinal data are given as medians and interquartile ranges. A difference with a *p*-value less than 0.05 was regarded as statistically significant (two-tailed test). Categorical data were analyzed using the Fisher's exact test or Chi-square test, with odds ratios and 95 % confidence intervals (CI) as appropriate. Correlations between numerical or ordinal data were assessed using Kendall's rank correlation (Kendall's tau-b coefficient).

Results

Fifty-two consecutive eligible aneurysmal SAH patients were recruited and 2 patients were excluded due to lack of delayed CT. Age was 53±10 years and 32 (62 %) were female. Twenty-two (42 %) patients were hypertensive and 18 (35 %) were smokers. Years of formal education were 9±4 years. World Federation of Neurosurgical Societies (WFNS) Grade was I in 25 (48 %), II in 14 (27 %), III in 3 (6 %), IV in 6 (12 %), and V in 4 (8 %). Clinical rebleeding before aneurysm treatment occurred in 1 (2 %) patient. Aneurysm location was posterior circulation in 11 (22 %) patients with the rest located in anterior circulation: anterior communicating artery: 12 (24 %); internal carotid artery communicating segment or posterior communicating artery: 10 (20 %); internal carotid artery, other segment: 14 (28 %); middle cerebral artery: 9 (18 %). Coiling was performed in 30 (58 %) patients and clipping was performed in 20 (40 %) patients. An external ventricular drain was inserted in 20 (40 %) patients and ventriculoperitoneal shunts were eventually required in 8 (16 %) patients.

Median CT Hijdra SAH score was 17 and interquartile range was 17–21.75. Intraventricular hemorrhage (IVH) occurred in 24 (48 %) patients. Median CT Graeb score for IVH was 0 and interquartile range was 0–2.75. CT Fisher scale was II in 1 (2 %), III in 22 (44 %), and IV in 29 (58 %). At 3 months, median mRS was 2 and interquartile range was 2–5; median Lawton Instrumental Activity of Daily Living (LIADL) was 15 and interquartile range was 0–18.

Out of the 50 patients with early and delayed CT, cerebral infarction occurred in 24 (48 %) patients, in which anterior circulation cerebral infarction occurred in 22 (44 %), and posterior circulation cerebral infarction occurred in 7 (14 %). Anterior cerebral infarction occurred in a similar proportion of anterior and posterior circulation aneurysms (46 % vs. 39 %, OR 1.4, 95 % CI: 0.4–4.9, $p=0.640$), whereas posterior circulation aneurysm patients had a higher proportion of early posterior cerebral infarction compared with anterior circulation aneurysm patients (23 % vs. 11 %, OR 2.5, 95 % CI: 0.5–12.9, $p=0.357$).

Early cerebral infarction occurred in 14 (27 %) patients, in which anterior circulation cerebral infarction occurred in 12 (24 %), and posterior circulation cerebral infarction occurred in 3 (6 %). Early anterior cerebral infarction occurred in a similar proportion of anterior and posterior circulation aneurysms (24 % vs. 21 %, OR 1.1, 95 % CI: 0.3–5.0, $p=1.000$), whereas posterior circulation aneurysm patients had a higher proportion of early posterior cerebral infarction compared with anterior circulation aneurysm patients (18 % vs. 2 %, OR not available, $p=0.110$).

Delayed cerebral infarction occurred in 14 (28 %) patients, in whom anterior circulation cerebral infarction occurred in 14 (28 %), and posterior circulation cerebral infarction occurred in 2 (4 %). Delayed anterior cerebral infarction occurred more frequently in anterior circulation than posterior circulation aneurysms (32 % vs. 15 %, OR 2.6, 95 % CI: 0.5–13.8, $p=0.239$), whereas delayed posterior cerebral infarction occurred in a similar proportion of anterior and posterior circulation aneurysms (5 % vs. 0 %, OR not available, $p=1.000$). In multivariable analysis, occurrence of delayed cerebral infarction correlated with occurrence of early cerebral infarction (Kendall's tau-b coefficient 0.617, $p<0.001$).

Discussion

Nimodipine was shown to reduce incidence of delayed cerebral infarction by one third, with a similar improvement in outcome [11]. However, subsequent clinical trials failed to find a second magic bullet to further improve the clinical outcome after SAH [2, 7, 8, 11, 12, 17]. There was a suggestion that earlier events such as early brain injury and early cerebral infarction should be the new target for future research and treatment.

Our study found that anterior circulation infarction was equally common for ruptured anterior and posterior circulation aneurysms, in contrast to posterior circulation infarction, which was more common in ruptured posterior circulation aneurysm. The results seemed to suggest that raised intracranial pressure and cerebral ischemia related to aneurysm rupture had a more unified effect supratentorially than infratentorially. This finding should be further confirmed in future studies.

There are several weaknesses in the current study. Hypodense lesion on CT at 4–6 weeks post-treatment may not be accurately detected in all early cerebral infarctions. Metallic artifacts from clips and coils used to secure the ruptured aneurysm may have interfered with the precise interpretation of CT findings, especially in the posterior fossa [5]. CT diagnosis of delayed cerebral infarction is less sensitive than magnetic resonance imaging (MRI). The sample size did not allow subgroup analyses by aneurysm locations.

Because of the prognostic significance of early cerebral infarction, a routine early CT brain at Day 1 after aneurysm treatment should be performed, especially with clinical deterioration or after microsurgical clipping performed later than 3 days after SAH. Causes of ischemia may be difficult to diagnose in plain CT; CT angiography and perfusion can be helpful to identify potential ischemic penumbra for aggressive treatment [1].

Conclusions

Early cerebral infarction was common and different from delayed cerebral infarction. Posterior circulation infarction occurred mainly in patients with ruptured posterior circulation aneurysm.

References

1. Binaghi S, Colleoni ML, Maeder P, Uske A, Regli L, Dehdashti AR, Schnyder P, Meuli R (2007) CT angiography and perfusion CT in cerebral vasospasm after subarachnoid hemorrhage. AJNR Am J Neuroradiol 28:750–758
2. Dorhout Mees SM, Algra A, Vandertop WP, van Kooten F, Kuijsten HA, Boiten J, van Oostenbrugge RJ, Al-Shahi Salman R, Lavados PM, Rinkel GJ, van den Bergh WM (2012) Magnesium for aneurysmal subarachnoid haemorrhage (MASH-2): a randomised placebo-controlled trial. Lancet 380:44–49
3. Juvela S, Siironen J (2012) Early cerebral infarction as a risk factor for poor outcome after aneurysmal subarachnoid haemorrhage. Eur J Neurol 19:332–339
4. Juvela S, Siironen J, Varis J, Poussa K, Porras M (2005) Risk factors for ischemic lesions following aneurysmal subarachnoid hemorrhage. J Neurosurg 102:194–201
5. Kivisaari RP, Salonen O, Servo A, Autti T, Hernesniemi J, Ohman J (2001) MR imaging after aneurysmal subarachnoid hemorrhage and surgery: a long-term follow-up study. AJNR Am J Neuroradiol 21:1143–1148
6. Lawton MP, Brody EM (1969) Assessment of older people: self-maintaining and instrumental activities of daily living. Gerontologist 9:179–186
7. Macdonald RL, Higashida RT, Keller E, Mayer SA, Molyneux A, Raabe A, Vajkoczy P, Wanke I, Bach D, Frey A, Marr A, Roux S, Kassell N (2011) Clazosentan, an endothelial receptor antagonist, in patients with aneurysmal subarachnoid haemorrhage undergoing surgical clipping: a randomised, double-blind, placebo-controlled phase 3 trial (CONSCIOUS-2). Lancet Neurol 10:618–625
8. Macdonald RL, Higashida RT, Keller E, Mayer SA, Molyneux A, Raabe A, Vajkoczy P, Wanke I, Bach D, Frey A, Nowbakht P, Roux S, Kassell N (2012) Randomized trial of clazosentan in patients with aneurysmal subarachnoid hemorrhage undergoing endovascular coiling. Stroke 43:1463–1469
9. Nieuwkamp DJ, Setz LE, ALgra A, Linn FHH, de Rooij NK, Rinkel GJ (2009) Changes in case fatality of aneurysmal subarachnoid haemorrhage over time, according to age, sex, and region: a meta-analysis. Lancet Neurol 8:635–642
10. Pallant J (2007) SPSS survival manual: a step by step guide to data analysis using SPSS for windows, 3rd edn. Open University Press/McGraw-Hill Education, Maidenhead/Berkshire
11. Pickard JD, Murray GD, Illingworth R, Shaw MD, Teasdale GM, Foy PM, Humphrey PR, Lang DA, Nelson R, Richards P, Sinar J, Bailey S, Skene A (1989) Effect of oral nimodipine on cerebral infarction and outcome after subarachnoid haemorrhage: British aneurysm nimodipine trial. Br Med J 298:636–642
12. Rabinstein AA, Friedman JA, Weignan SD, McClelland RL, Fulgham JR, Manno EM, Atkinson JL, Wijdicks EF (2004) Predictors of cerebral infarction in aneurysmal subarachnoid hemorrhage. Stroke 35:1862–1866
13. Rankin L (1957) Cerebral vascular accidents in patients over the age of 60. II. Prognosis. Scott Med J 2:200–215
14. Tong A, Man DW (2002) The validation of the Hong Kong Chinese version of the Lawton instrumental activities of daily living scale for institutionalized elderly persons. OTJR Occup Particip Health 22:132–142
15. Wong GK, Lam S, Ngai K, Wong A, Mok V, Poon WS, Cognitive Dysfunction after Aneurysmal Subarachnoid Haemorrhage Investigators (2012) Evaluation of cognitive impairment by the Montreal Cognitive Assessment in patients with aneurysmal subarachnoid haemorrhage: prevalence, risk factors, and correlations with 3 month outcome. J Neurol Neurosurg Psychiatry 83:1112 1117
16. Wong GK, Poon WS, Boet R, Chan MT, Gin T, Ng SC, Zee BC (2011) Health-related quality of life after aneurysmal subarachnoid hemorrhage: profile and clinical factors. Neurosurgery 68:1556–1561
17. Wong GK, Poon WS, Chan MT, Boet R, Gin T, Ng SC, Zee BC, Investigators IMASH (2010) Intravenous magnesium sulphate for aneurysmal subarachnoid hemorrhage (IMASH): a randomized, double-blinded, placebo-controlled, multicenter phase III trial. Stroke 41:921–926
18. van Sieten JC, Koudstaal PJ, Visser MC, Schouten HJ, van Gijn GJ (1988) Interobserver agreement for the assessment of handicap in stroke patients. Stroke 19:604–607
19. Vilkki JS, Juvela S, Siironen J, Ilvoen T, Varis J, Porras M (2004) Relationship of local infarctions to cognitive and psychosocial impairment after aneurysmal subarachnoid hemorrhage. Neurosurgery 55:790–803
20. Vergouwen MD, Ilodigwe D, Macdonald RL (2011) Cerebral infarction after subarachnoid hemorrhage contributes to poor outcome by vasospasm-dependent and -independent effects. Stroke 42:924–929

Signaling Pathway in Cerebral Vasospasm After Subarachnoid Hemorrhage: News Update

Lingyun Wu and Gang Chen

Introduction

Cerebral vasospasm (CVS) after subarachnoid hemorrhage (SAH) caused by ruptured intracranial aneurysms is a major cause of death and disability [12]. After SAH, signs of CVS can be revealed in the angiograms of 70 % of patients, whereas the remaining 30 % of patients show clear clinical manifestations and symptoms of CVS [8]. With the rapid development of molecular biology and molecular immunology techniques, studies on CVS have gradually moved to the level of molecules and genes, and the importance of deciphering the relevant signal transduction pathways for understanding the mechanisms of CVS has become clear [20]. This chapter briefly reviews current progress in the studies of the different signal transduction pathways relevant to CVS after SAH.

Mitogen-Activated Protein Kinase (MAPK) Signaling Pathway and Its Regulation

MAPKs are a group of intracellular serine (Ser)/threonine (Thr) protein kinases commonly found in a variety of organisms. MAPKs maintain their active and inactive states typically via the phosphorylation and dephosphorylation of specific sites [17]. Human MAPKs are divided into three subfamilies: ERK, JNK, and p38 MAPK.

L. Wu • G. Chen (✉)
Department of Neurosurgery, The First Affiliated Hospital of Soochow University, 188 Shizi Street, Suzhou 215006, P.R.China
e-mail: nju_neurosurgery@163.com

JNK/SAPK Pathway

C-Jun N-terminal kinases (JNKs) can be divided into three subtypes: JNK1, JNK2, and JNK3. The MAPK kinases MKK4 and MKK7 are the kinases upstream of JNK. MKK7 activates JNK specifically [26], whereas MKK4 can activate JNK1 and p38.

p38 MAPK Pathway

MKK3, MKK4, and MKK6 are the kinases upstream from p38 MAPK. The observation that MKK3 and MKK4 are upstream activators of both the p38 and JNK pathways suggests that there may be crosstalk between these two pathways. p38 MAPK is also involved in the activation of NF-κB activation.

Raf/MEK/ERK Signaling Pathway

Raf Kinase Family

The mammalian Raf family contains predominantly proteins (A-Raf, B-Raf, and C-Raf [Raf-1]). Raf-1 is expressed in almost all tissues, A-Raf is expressed mainly in the genitourinary tissues, and B-Raf is expressed in the nerves, testis, spleen, and hematopoietic tissues.

Downstream Regulation of Raf Kinases

Ras kinases are activated mainly by Ras and other small GTPases. All Ras subtypes can interact with Raf [21]. Activated Raf transduces the activation signal mainly via the phosphorylation of two dual specificity MAPKKs: MEK1 (MKK1) and MEK2 (MKK2) [13].

R.L. Applegate et al. (eds.), *Brain Edema XVI: Translate Basic Science into Clinical Practice*, Acta Neurochirurgica Supplement, Vol. 121,
DOI 10.1007/978-3-319-18497-5_29,

Raf/ERK1/2 Pathway

The substrates of MEK1 and MEK2 are ERK (p44 MAPK) and ERK2 (p42 MAPK), respectively. After activation, ERK1 and ERK2 are translocated from the cytoplasm to the nucleus, where they directly phosphorylate and activate transcription factors to induce the transcription of a series of cytoplasmic and nuclear proteins [1].

Raf/NF-κB Pathway

Raf-1 can stimulate the NF-κB pathway in two ways: (1) a direct and rapid pathway via the phosphorylation and activation of MEKK1 and I kappa B kinase p (IKKp), which stimulates the degradation of IκB via phosphorylation; and (2) in some cell lines, the activation may be achieved via an autocrine loop [18].

Relationship Between the MAPK Signaling Pathway and CVS after SAH

MAPK may be involved in the occurrence of CVS via the following mechanisms:

1. Proliferation of vascular wall cells. Borel et al. [5] demonstrated that, after SAH, cerebral vascular walls exposed to the blood clot showed substantially increased cell proliferation and wall thickening, suggesting that these processes might participate in CVS.
2. Sustained contraction of vascular smooth muscle. After SAH, increased intracellular Ca^{2+} concentrations in cerebral vascular cells activate calmodulin-dependent myosin light-chain kinase (MLCK), which leads to smooth muscle contraction [11].
3. Immune and inflammatory responses.
4. Apoptosis of vascular endothelial cells. Elevated expression of JNK and p38 MAPK is associated with endothelial cell apoptosis in brain vessels [3]. However, the mechanism by which MAPK modulates vascular endothelial cell apoptosis requires additional clarification in future studies.

PKC-Mediated Pathways

Structure and Biological Properties of PKC

PKC is a calcium/phospholipid-dependent protein kinase that regulates cell metabolism, growth, proliferation, and differentiation by catalyzing the Ser/Thr phosphorylation of many different proteins [25]. All PKC subtypes are composed of a single peptide chain, which is divided into four conserved domains, C1–C4 (in nPKC and aPKC the C2 domain is missing), and five variable regions, V1–V5 [14]. Based on their structures and activators, PKC isoforms are divided into three related families: groups A, B, and C.

PKC Activation

The pathways of PKC activation after SAH include the following:

1. Increased endothelin (ET) expression. Studies have suggested that after SAH, high concentrations of OxyHb can directly stimulate ET expression in vascular endothelial cells, which catalyzes phosphatidylinositol bisphosphate (PIP2) decomposition to generate diacylglycerol (DAG). DAG then activates PKC [7].
2. Decreased nitric oxide (NO). NO enters adjacent SMCs after its release from endothelial cells, where it activates soluble guanylate cyclase (GC) to produce cyclic guanosine monophosphate (cGMP). cGMP activates the intracellular calcium pump driving free calcium into the cell, relaxing smooth muscles.
3. Formation of the "complement membrane attack complex."

Relation Between PKC and CVS

Increasing evidence supports essential roles for PKC in delayed CVS. After SAH, sustained DAG increase activates PKC, which maintains sustained vascular SMC [7]. PKC inhibits the activation of potassium channels in vascular SMCs. This depolarizes vascular SMCs, leading to contraction. Adhesion of extracellular collagen matrix in the cerebral arteries after SAH affects the vessel diameter. PKC can activate protein tyrosine kinase (PTK), which activates Ras. PKC may also directly activate Raf-1 and thus activate MAPK, which results in sustained vascular SMC contraction.

Rho/Rho Signaling Pathway

Structure and Biological Properties of Rho Molecules

Rho proteins are small GTPases. Based on their primary structure, Rho proteins can be divided into at least five families: the Ras, Rho, Rab, Sarl/Arf, and Ran families. RhoA regulates the assembly of actin stress fibers, whereas Rac and Cdc42 regulate actin polymerization to form specific peripheral structures. Rho proteins also participate in the regulation of many basic cellular functions, including contraction, movement, adhesion, the maintenance of cell shape and polarity, gene transcription, and apoptosis [9].

Regulation of Rho Protein Activity

During cell metabolism, Rho proteins act as molecular switches and exist in the GTP-bound state (active state) or GDP-bound state (inactive state). Three major proteins regulate the activation of Rho: (1) GTP exchange factor, which promotes the phosphorylation of GDP and its exchange with GTP; (2) GTPase-activating protein, which activates the endogenous GTPase activity of Rho protein, hydrolyzing GTP into GDP; and (3) GDP dissociation inhibitor, which inhibits the conversion between GDP and GTP [27].

Relationship Between Rho-Related Signaling Pathways and CVS

After SAH, spasm-inducing substances in the blood can activate cell surface receptors and the downstream Rho/Rho kinase signaling pathway, resulting in increased MLC phosphorylation and SMC contraction. OxyHb and ET-1 are the two spasm-inducing substances that are well understood. In SAH, OxyHb released from self-dissolved red blood cells can cause persistent contraction of cerebral arteries in vitro. Studies suggest that activation of the OxyHb-dependent Rho/Rho kinase pathway is one step in the signaling cascade that leads to CVS [28]. ET-1 is another main cause of CVS after SAH. In the blood-containing CSF of SAH patients, ET-1 levels are elevated compared with control patients. In addition, cisternal injection of ET-1 in vivo produced CVS similar to that observed in humans. Lan et al. [15] examined rabbit basilar arteries with endothelial cells removed and found that ET-1 could significantly increase the amplitude of OxyHb-induced vasoconstriction. Importantly, the Rho kinase inhibitors Y-27632 and fasudil could reduce this effect.

JAK/STAT Signaling Pathway

Composition and Biological Properties of the JAK/STAT Signaling Pathway

JAKs are a class of soluble cytoplasmic PTKs with a molecular weight of 120–130 kDa and are an important component of various signaling pathways that regulate cell proliferation, differentiation, and apoptosis [19]. STATs are a cytoplasmic protein family that can bind to the regulatory domains of target genes. Their activity is coupled with the tyrosine phosphorylation signal to regulate transcription. A variety of cytokines can activate different STAT family members via JAK activation [10].

JAK/STAT Signal Regulation

After cytokine receptors on the cell membrane bind with the corresponding ligands, homo- or hetero-dimers are formed, which orients cytoplasmic JAKs to enable them to phosphorylate each other. Activated JAKs then phosphorylate the Tyr residue on receptor molecules. STAT then positions in proximity to the phosphorylated Tyr via the SH2 domain. JAK then phosphorylates one hydroxyl Tyr on STAT, causing its activation [4].

Relationship Between JAK/STAT and CVS

After SAH, a large number of cytokines and growth factors are released. These factors can lead to local brain ischemia caused by CVS and can also activate the JAK/STAT signaling pathway. Takagi et al. [24] assessed STAT1 phosphorylation and nuclear translocation after cerebral ischemia. This suggests that cerebral ischemia can induce the phosphorylation, activation, and nuclear translocation of STAT1, which plays a role in ischemic brain damage by regulating the transcription and phosphorylation of caspase-3.

AKT Signaling Pathway

Akt Structure

Akt is a proto-oncogene and serine/threonine kinase with a molecular weight of 60 kDa. Currently, three forms of Akt have been shown to exist in mammals: Akt1, Akt2, and Akt3. Akt1 is expressed widely in various tissues, whereas Akt2 is expressed predominantly in the liver, kidney, heart, skeletal muscle, and other insulin-responsive tissues, and Akt3 is expressed in the testis and brain.

Akt Signaling Pathway and Its Regulation

There are two main pathways that regulate Akt activation. One is the PI3K-dependent pathway, which is the major upstream pathway regulating Akt that has been studied extensively. The other pathway that regulates Akt activation is non-PI3K-dependent. There are a relatively large number of Akt substrates, including BCL-2 antagonist of cell death (BAD), forkhead box (FOX) family, glycogen synthase kinase (GSK3), Iκ-B kinase (IKK), and caspase 9. Akt phosphorylates these substrates to regulate metabolism of blood sugar, lipids, and proteins, and plays important roles in cell proliferation, differentiation, and survival.

Relationship Between AKT Signaling Pathways and CVS

PI3K/ATK/mTOR Signaling Pathway and mTOR/HIF-1α/VGEF Signaling Pathways

Mammalian target of rapamycin (mTOR) is a Ser/Thr kinase that was first discovered in yeast. In the steady state, mTOR is located mainly in the cytoplasm; when activated, it enters the nucleus where it regulates the downstream target proteins 4E-BPl and S6K. In particular, the mTOR/P70S6K1/4E-BP1 signaling pathway may be associated with the proliferation of vascular SMCs [16]. In addition, a study demonstrated that an mTOR inhibitor can also reduce the expression of hypoxia-inducible factor 1α (HIF-1α) [29]. The above studies demonstrate that mTOR inhibitors likely inhibit the HIF-1α/vascular endothelial growth factor (VEGF) signaling pathway, thereby improving the pathological development of CVS after SAH.

Phenotype Transformation of Vascular Smooth Muscle Cells (SMCs)

Studies have suggested that the AKT signaling pathway maintains the differentiated phenotype of vascular SMCs. Song et al. reported that on days 1–14 after SAH, the expression of upstream PCNA and downstream SMα-actin in SMCs of the basilar arteries were both upregulated significantly compared with control. However, the levels of AKT precursor protein (pAKT) before day four was not changed significantly, suggesting that the AKT signaling pathway does not stimulate the transformation of vascular SMC phenotypes, but rather maintains and promotes the contractile phenotype of vascular SMCs [22].

AKT/eNOS Signaling Pathway

The PI3K/AKT/eNOS pathway regulates the angiogenesis promoted by many angiogenic factors [2]. Nitric oxide synthase (NOS) can be divided into structural (eNOS, nNOS) and inducible (iNOS) isoforms. Santhanam et al. [23] reported that the mechanism underlying the effect of recombinant EPO (AdEPO) on CVS after SAH treatment was via the AKT/eNOS signaling pathway. Specifically, AdEPO increased NO production in the basilar arteries and also enhanced the diameter of the basilar arteries after CVS, thereby reversing the effect of cerebral vasospasm.

Nrf-ARE Signaling Pathway

Molecular Structures of Proteins in the Nrf2-ARE Signaling Pathway

Nuclear factor erythroid-derived factor 2-related factor (Nrf2) is a redox-sensitive transcription factor. Together with antioxidant response element (ARE) it forms the Nrf2-ARE pathway. Nrf2 belongs to the Drosophila transcription factor Cap'n'Collar (CNC) family. ARE is a cis-acting regulatory element or enhancer sequence that occurs mainly in the promoter region of genes encoding phase II detoxification enzymes and antioxidant proteins.

Regulation of the Nrf2-ARE Signaling Pathway

The Nrf2-Keap1 pathway is regulated by three main mechanisms. One is direct phosphorylation of Nrf2, which is the major mechanism by which protein kinases regulate the Nrf2-Keapl pathway. In previous studies, PKC, protein kinase RNA-like endoplasmic reticulum kinase, ERK1, and p38 MAPK have all been used to directly phosphorylate and activate Nrf2, causing increased expression of ARE. The other mechanisms are ubiquitination and Keap1 regulation.

Role of Nrf2-ARE Signaling Pathway in CVS after SAH

Activation of the Nrf2-ARE pathway can effectively block neurotoxicity caused by glutathione (GSH) deficiency, lipid peroxidation, intracellular calcium overload, and destruction of mitochondrial electron transport chain [6]. Reactive oxygen species (ROS) play a key role in the pathogenesis of CVS. ROS can cause a variety of damage to DNA in neural tissues. In addition, oxidative stress can also trigger transcription of genes related to the redox-sensitive NF-κB-mediated pro-inflammatory response, and thus indirectly affect the inflammatory response in neural tissues and cause damage. Activation of the Nrf2-ARE pathway, which results in a clear protective effect of antioxidant inflammation in the brain, can improve CVS, possibly through this mechanism.

Prospect

CVS after SAH involves many signaling pathways, and those discussed above are only some of these pathways. Studies on the various signaling pathways provide a solid basis for developing future clinical treatments for CVS and shed new light on current clinical treatments. Continued efforts must be made in this research field.

References

1. Araki E, Forster C, Dubinsky JM, Ross ME, Iadecola C (2001) Cyclooxygenase-2 inhibitor ns-398 protects neuronal cultures from lipopolysaccharide-induced neurotoxicity. Stroke 32:2370–2375
2. Babaei S, Teichert-Kuliszewska K, Zhang Q, Jones N, Dumont DJ, Stewart DJ (2003) Angiogenic actions of angiopoietin-1 require endothelium-derived nitric oxide. Am J Pathol 162:1927–1936
3. Behrens A, Sibilia M, Wagner EF (1999) Amino-terminal phosphorylation of c-Jun regulates stress-induced apoptosis and cellular proliferation. Nat Genet 21:326–329
4. Best SM, Morris KL, Shannon JG, Robertson SJ, Mitzel DN, Park GS, Boer E, Wolfinbarger JB, Bloom ME (2005) Inhibition of interferon-stimulated JAK-STAT signaling by a tick-borne flavivirus and identification of NS5 as an interferon antagonist. J Virol 79:12828–12839
5. Borel CO, McKee A, Parra A, Haglund MM, Solan A, Prabhakar V, Sheng H, Warner DS, Niklason L (2003) Possible role for vascular cell proliferation in cerebral vasospasm after subarachnoid hemorrhage. Stroke 34:427–433
6. Calkins MJ, Jakel RJ, Johnson DA, Chan K, Kan YW, Johnson JA (2005) Protection from mitochondrial complex II inhibition in vitro and in vivo by Nrf2-mediated transcription. Proc Natl Acad Sci U S A 102:244–249
7. Dietrich HH, Dacey RG Jr (2000) Molecular keys to the problems of cerebral vasospasm. Neurosurgery 46:517–530
8. Dorsch NW (1995) Cerebral arterial spasm–a clinical review. Br J Neurosurg 9:403–412
9. Etienne-Manneville S, Hall A (2002) Rho GTPases in cell biology. Nature 420:629–635
10. Hou XS, Melnick MB, Perrimon N (1996) Marelle acts downstream of the Drosophila HOP/JAK kinase and encodes a protein similar to the mammalian STATs. Cell 84:411–419
11. Kilic U, Kilic E, Reiter RJ, Bassetti CL, Hermann DM (2005) Signal transduction pathways involved in melatonin-induced neuroprotection after focal cerebral ischemia in mice. J Pineal Res 38:67–71
12. Kolias AG, Sen J, Belli A (2009) Pathogenesis of cerebral vasospasm following aneurysmal subarachnoid hemorrhage: putative mechanisms and novel approaches. J Neurosci Res 87:1–11
13. Kumar A, Takada Y, Boriek AM, Aggarwal BB (2004) Nuclear factor-kappaB: its role in health and disease. J Mol Med (Berl) 82:434–448
14. Laher I, Zhang JH (2001) Protein kinase C and cerebral vasospasm. J Cereb Blood Flow Metab 21:887–906
15. Lan C, Das D, Wloskowicz A, Vollrath B (2004) Endothelin-1 modulates hemoglobin-mediated signaling in cerebrovascular smooth muscle via RhoA/Rho kinase and protein kinase C. Am J Physiol Heart Circ Physiol 286:H165–H173
16. Liao Q, Shi DH, Zheng W, Xu XJ, Yu YH (2010) Antiproliferation of cardamonin is involved in mTOR on aortic smooth muscle cells in high fructose-induced insulin resistance rats. Eur J Pharmacol 641:179–186
17. Liebmann C (2001) Regulation of MAP kinase activity by peptide receptor signalling pathway: paradigms of multiplicity. Cell Signal 13:777–785
18. Liptay S, Weber CK, Ludwig L, Wagner M, Adler G, Schmid RM (2003) Mitogenic and antiapoptotic role of constitutive NF-kappaB/Rel activity in pancreatic cancer. Int J Cancer 105:735–746
19. Nicholson SE, Novak U, Ziegler SF, Layton JE (1995) Distinct regions of the granulocyte colony-stimulating factor receptor are required for tyrosine phosphorylation of the signaling molecules JAK2, Stat3, and p42, p44MAPK. Blood 86:3698–3704
20. Nishziawa S (2011) Roles of signal transduction mechanisms in cerebral vasospasm following subarachnoid hemorrhage: overview. Acta Neurochir Suppl 110:27–30
21. Ogunshola OO, Antic A, Donoghue MJ, Fan SY, Kim H, Stewart WB, Madri JA, Ment LR (2002) Paracrine and autocrine functions of neuronal vascular endothelial growth factor (VEGF) in the central nervous system. J Biol Chem 277:11410–11415
22. Paravicini TM, Yogi A, Mazur A, Touyz RM (2009) Dysregulation of vascular TRPM7 and annexin-1 is associated with endothelial dysfunction in inherited hypomagnesemia. Hypertension 53: 423–429
23. Santhanam AV, Smith LA, Akiyama M, Rosales AG, Bailey KR, Katusic ZS (2005) Role of endothelial NO synthase phosphorylation in cerebrovascular protective effect of recombinant erythropoietin during subarachnoid hemorrhage-induced cerebral vasospasm. Stroke 36:2731–2737
24. Takagi Y, Harada J, Chiarugi A, Moskowitz MA (2002) STAT1 is activated in neurons after ischemia and contributes to ischemic brain injury. J Cereb Blood Flow Metab 22:1311–1318
25. Takai Y, Kishimoto A, Inoue M, Nishizuka Y (1977) Studies on a cyclic nucleotide-independent protein kinase and its proenzyme in mammalian tissues. I. Purification and characterization of an active enzyme from bovine cerebellum. J Biol Chem 252:7603–7609
26. Tournier C, Whitmarsh AJ, Cavanagh J, Barrett T, Davis RJ (1997) Mitogen activated protein kinase kinase 7 is an activator of the c-Jun NH2-terminal kinase. Proc Natl Acad Sci U S A 94: 7337–7342
27. Van Aelst L, D'Souza-Schorey C (1997) Rho GTPases and signaling networks. Genes Dev 11:2295–2322
28. Wickman G, Lan C, Vollrath B (2003) Functional roles of the rho/rho kinase pathway and protein kinase C in the regulation of cerebrovascular constriction mediated by hemoglobin: relevance to subarachnoid hemorrhage and vasospasm. Circ Res 92:809–816
29. Zhou C, Yamaguchi M, Kusaka G, Schonholz C, Nanda A, Zhang JH (2004) Caspase inhibitors prevent endothelial apoptosis and cerebral vasospasm in dog model of experimental subarachnoid hemorrhage. J Cereb Blood Flow Metab 24:419–431

Cerebral Infarction After Aneurysmal Subarachnoid Hemorrhage

Kenji Kanamaru, Hidenori Suzuki, and Waro Taki

Introduction

Outcome of aneurysmal subarachnoid hemorrhage (SAH) remains poor [1]. The most important determinant of poor outcome is the initial brain injury caused by an aneurysmal rupture or acute SAH, and therefore early aneurysmal obliteration is recommended to prevent aneurysm rebleeding [1]. However, early aneurysm obliteration may cause a complication of cerebral infarction [13]. Cerebral infarction also occurs as a result of treatment failure for delayed cerebral ischemia, another important determinant of poor outcome after SAH [16]. It has been shown that early brain injury, as well as cerebral vasospasm, causes delayed cerebral infarction [5]. Because cerebral infarction has the strongest association with poor outcomes in clinical trials of SAH patients with early coiling or clipping of a ruptured aneurysm, multidisciplinary research groups recommend use of cerebral infarction as the primary outcome measure in SAH clinical trials [16]. However, only limited studies have investigated predictors for vasospasm-induced or vasospasm-unrelated cerebral infarction [7], although many predictors have been reported for the occurrence of cerebral vasospasm [2, 6]. Thus, the aim of this study was to examine factors for the development of all kinds of cerebral infarction after aneurysmal SAH.

K. Kanamaru, MD, PhD
Department of Neurosurgery, Suzuka Kaisei Hospital, Suzuka, Japan

H. Suzuki, MD, PhD (✉)
Department of Neurosurgery, Mie University Graduate School of Medicine, 2-174 Edobashi, Tsu, Mie 514-8507, Japan
e-mail: suzuki02@clin.medic.mie-u.ac.jp

W. Taki, MD, PhD
Department of Neurosurgery, Mie University Graduate School of Medicine, Tsu, Mie, Japan

Materials and Methods

Patient and Clinical Variables

This study used data from a prospective cohort study (Prospective Registry of Subarachnoid Aneurysms Treatment) performed at 29 Japanese tertiary referral centers in 2006–2007 [7, 12–15]. The Institutional Ethics Committee approved the study. Inclusion criteria were as follows: ≥20 years of age at onset, SAH on computed tomography (CT) scans, saccular aneurysm as the cause of SAH, and aneurysmal obliteration by clipping or coiling within 14 days of onset. Excluded from the study were patients who were treated using medical instruments or drugs that were not approved by the Japanese Ministry of Health, Labor and Welfare. Thus, no patients were treated with nimodipine, surface-modified or bio-active coils, or intracranial stents. There were 588 patients registered, but 9 cases of missing data of vasospasm were excluded. Thus, 579 cases were eligible for this study. Timing of aneurysmal obliteration, selection of clipping or coiling, and other medical management or treatment were decided by site investigators and not limited.

Demographic and clinical data included age, gender, pre-SAH modified Rankin Scale (mRS), World Federation of Neurosurgical Societies (WFNS) grade on admission, Fisher CT group on admission, interval from ictus to aneurysmal obliteration, pretreatment rebleeding (in-hospital), modality used for aneurysmal obliteration, location and size of the ruptured aneurysm, cerebrospinal fluid (CSF) drainage, antiplatelet administration, intra- or post-procedure (clipping or coiling) rebleeding, endovascular therapy for vasospasm, symptomatic vasospasm, noninfectious cardiopulmonary complication, infection, epilepsy, and shunt-dependent hydrocephalus. The aneurysms were classified into four groups: small size (<10 mm)/small neck (<4 mm), small size/wide neck (≥4 mm), large (≥10 mm but <25 mm), and giant (≥25 mm) [13]. Ventricular, cisternal, or spinal CSF

R.L. Applegate et al. (eds.), *Brain Edema XVI: Translate Basic Science into Clinical Practice*, Acta Neurochirurgica Supplement, Vol. 121,
DOI 10.1007/978-3-319-18497-5_30, © Springer International Publishing Switzerland 2016

drainage was established to control acute hydrocephalus or to promote subarachnoid blood clearance. Antiplatelet medications were administered to prevent over-thrombosis after coiling or symptomatic vasospasm. Procedure-related cerebral infarction was defined as a new infarct on CT or magnetic resonance images on the first postoperative day that was not visible on admission. Symptomatic vasospasm was defined as otherwise unexplained clinical deterioration (i.e., a new focal deficit, decrease in the level of consciousness, or both) or a new infarct on CT that was not visible on immediate postoperative scan, or both. Others were diagnosed as previously reported [13]. Outcome was blindly assessed using mRS at 3 and 12 months post-SAH.

Statistics

Categorical variables were reported as a proportion and percentile and were analyzed using chi-square or Fisher's exact test, as appropriate. Continuous variables were reported as a mean ± standard deviation and compared using unpaired *t*-test. The impact of each variable on cerebral infarction was determined by multivariate unconditional logistic regression analyses using the dichotomous status (presence or absence) as the dependent variable. All variables were considered independent variables irrespective of the significance on univariate analysis, although only the variable with the smallest probability value was used as a candidate variable among similar clinical variables that were intercorrelated. Adjusted odds ratios (ORs) with 95 % confidence intervals were calculated and independence of variables was tested using the likelihood ratio test on reduced models. Two-tailed probability values <0.05 were considered significant.

Results

Characteristics of Patients Who Had Cerebral Infarction

Ruptured aneurysms were clipped in 282 patients and coiled in 297 patients, when patients were treated with either treatment modality judged by the attending neurosurgeon to be appropriate for the individual patient. New cerebral infarction occurred in 162 patients (28.0 %): 34 patients on neuroimages on the first post-clipping day, 33 patients on neuroimages on the first post-coiling day, and 101 patients in the so-called "period of cerebral vasospasm occurrence." Univariate analyses showed that significant factors associated with cerebral infarction development were Fisher CT group 3 on admission, premature aneurysm rupture during clipping procedure, CSF drainage, symptomatic vasospasm, endovascular treatment for vasospasm, and shunt-dependent hydrocephalus. Fisher CT group 2 on admission was associated with significantly less occurrence of cerebral infarction (Table 1). Patients with cerebral infarction had a significantly worse outcome compared with those without infarction (Table 2).

Independent Variables for Cerebral Infarction Occurrence

Multivariate logistic regression analyses showed that Fisher CT group 3 on admission, larger aneurysm dome size, ruptured posterior circulation aneurysms, premature aneurysm rupture during clipping procedure, symptomatic vasospasm, and infection were significant factors for cerebral infarction occurrence (Table 3). Among these factors, symptomatic vasospasm had the greatest OR and the lowest probability value, whereas endovascular treatment for vasospasm significantly decreased the development of cerebral infarction (Table 3).

Discussion

This prospective registry study showed that Fisher CT group 3 on admission, larger aneurysm dome size, ruptured posterior circulation aneurysms, premature aneurysm rupture during clipping procedure, symptomatic vasospasm, and infection were associated with increased cerebral infarction occurrence, whereas endovascular treatment for vasospasm was associated with decreased cerebral infarction occurrence. Larger aneurysm dome size, ruptured posterior circulation aneurysms, and premature aneurysm rupture during clipping procedure seem to increase the risk of cerebral infarction as a complication by treatment modalities. Among these factors, however, symptomatic vasospasm had the greatest impact on cerebral infarction, and to be the most important treatable factor against it.

Siironen et al. [11] reported that a new hypodense lesion (possibly treatment complications) on the first postoperative day CT might be a more important predictor for poor outcome than late ischemic lesions possibly caused by vasospasm. Taki et al. [13] reported that factors including both post-coiling and vasospasm-induced cerebral infarctions significantly caused poor outcome. Fu et al. [3] reported that early cerebral infarction within 3 days after SAH occurred in 26.7 %, and that surgical treatment, acute hydrocephalus, and high admission plasma glucose level were the independent predictors. Early cerebral infarction was associated with delayed cerebral infarction and poor outcome [3].

Table 1 Summary of patient characteristics stratified by cerebral infarction occurrence after subarachnoid hemorrhage (SAH)

Characteristics	Presence ($n=162$)	Absence ($n=417$)	p Value
Age, y	60.6 ± 13.1	61.6 ± 13.9	ns[a]
Sex			ns[b]
Female	110 (67.9 %)	284 (68.1 %)	
Male	52 (32.1)	133 (31.9)	
Pre-SAH morbidity			ns[b]
mRS 0-1	156 (96.3)	395 (94.7)	
mRS 2-4	6 (3.7)	22 (5.3)	
WFNS grade			
I	40 (24.7)	129 (30.9)	ns[b]
II	37 (22.8)	120 (28.8)	ns[b]
III	18 (11.1)	41 (9.8)	ns[b]
IV	43 (26.5)	80 (19.2)	ns[b]
V	24 (14.8)	47 (11.3)	ns[b]
Fisher CT group			
1	0 (0)	7 (1.7)	ns[c]
2	23 (14.2)	94 (22.5)	<0.05[b]
3	122 (75.3)	251 (60.2)	<0.001[b]
4	17 (10.5)	65 (15.6)	ns[b]
Aneurysm dome, mm	6.6 ± 3.8	6.4 ± 3.4	ns[a]
neck, mm	3.5 ± 1.7	3.4 ± 1.5	ns[a]
Aneurysm classification			
Small size/small neck	77 (47.5)	212 (50.8)	ns[b]
Small size/wide neck	57 (35.2)	151 (36.2)	ns[b]
Large	28 (17.3)	52 (12.5)	ns[b]
Giant	0 (0)	1 (0.2)	ns[c]
Aneurysm location			
Internal carotid artery	42 (25.9)	133 (31.9)	ns[b]
Middle cerebral artery	41 (25.3)	90 (21.6)	ns[b]
Anterior communicating artery	47 (29.0)	115 (27.6)	ns[b]
Distal anterior cerebral artery	5 (3.1)	23 (5.5)	ns[c]
Posterior circulation	25 (15.4)	52 (12.5)	ns[b]
Other	2 (1.2)	4 (1.0)	ns[c]
Date of aneurysm obliteration			ns[b]
Days 0–3	152 (93.8)	385 (92.3)	
Days 4–12	10 (6.2)	32 (7.7)	
Treatment modality			ns[b]
Clip	89 (54.9)	193 (46.3)	
Coil	73 (45.1)	224 (53.7)	
Pretreatment re-rupture	15 (9.3)	28 (6.7)	ns[b]
Intratreatment re-rupture: Clip	26 (16.0)	36 (8.6)	<0.025[b]
Coil	5 (3.1)	15 (3.6)	ns[c]
Post-treatment re-rupture	2 (1.2)	10 (2.4)	ns[c]
Cerebrospinal fluid drainage	119 (73.5)	263 (63.1)	<0.025[b]

(continued)

Table 1 (continued)

Characteristics	Presence ($n = 162$)	Absence ($n = 417$)	p Value
Antiplatelet therapy	38 (23.5)	104 (24.9)	ns[b]
Symptomatic vasospasm	103 (63.6)	23 (5.5)	<0.001[b]
Endovascular treatment for vasospasm	48 (29.6)	17 (4.1)	<0.001[b]
Infection	19 (11.7)	31 (7.4)	ns[b]
Noninfectious cardiopulmonary complication	8 (4.9)	29 (7.0)	ns[c]
Epilepsy	7 (4.3)	21 (5.0)	ns[c]
Shunt-dependent hydrocephalus	43 (26.5)	68 (16.3)	<0.005[b]

Data, mean ± standard deviation; number of cases (%)
CT computed tomography, *mRS* modified Rankin Scale, *WFNS* World Federation of Neurosurgical Societies; day 0 refers to the calendar day of SAH onset, *ns* not significant
[a]unpaired *t*-test
[b]chi-square test
[c]Fisher's exact test

Table 2 Modified Rankin Scale (mRS) at 3 and 12 months in patients with or without cerebral infarction after subarachnoid hemorrhage

Variable	Presence ($n = 162$)	Absence ($n = 417$)	p Value[a]
mRS at 3 months	$n = 161$	$n = 414$	
0	34 (21.1)	207 (50.0)	<0.001
1	18 (11.2)	48 (11.6)	ns
2	24 (14.9)	43 (10.4)	ns
3	15 (9.3)	19 (4.6)	<0.05
4	34 (21.1)	34 (8.2)	<0.001
5	20 (12.4)	27 (6.5)	<0.05
6	16 (9.9)	36 (8.7)	ns
0-1	52 (32.3)	255 (61.6)	<0.001
0-2	76 (47.2)	298 (72.0)	<0.001
mRS at 12 months	$n = 160$	$n = 400$	
0	43 (26.9)	230 (57.5)	<0.001
1	25 (15.6)	40 (10.0)	ns
2	16 (10.0)	35 (8.8)	ns
3	18 (11.3)	19 (4.75)	<0.01
4	24 (15.0)	21 (5.3)	<0.001
5	15 (9.4)	14 (3.5)	<0.005
6	19 (11.9)	41 (10.3)	ns
0-1	68 (42.5)	270 (67.5)	<0.001
0-2	84 (52.5)	305 (76.3)	<0.001

Number of cases (%)
ns not significant
[a]chi-square test

Kumar et al. [8] reported that more than 24 % of patients had almost equally early (≤48 h post-surgery) and/or delayed infarctions visible on CT: early infarctions were more likely deep in location and delayed infarctions more likely cortical. Larger infarction volume caused worse outcome in both early and delayed infarctions [8]. Factors associated with early infarctions were clipping, whereas those with delayed infarctions were smoking and angiographic vasospasm [8]. Using magnetic resonance imaging, however, a study of aneurysms treated by coiling revealed a high rate of asymptomatic (and often small) infarction [4]. It is possible that some of the higher incidence of early infarctions in those

Table 3 Significant variables in multivariate logistic regression with cerebral infarction occurrence after subarachnoid hemorrhage (SAH) as a binary outcome

Variable	Odds Ratio	95 % Confidence Interval	*p* Value
Fisher CT group 3 (versus group 4)	3.806	1.473–9.830	0.006
Aneurysm dome size	1.143	1.041–1.254	0.005
Posterior circulation (versus internal carotid artery)	2.619	1.138–6.028	0.024
Intra-clipping aneurysm re-rupture	2.701	1.191–6.127	0.017
Symptomatic vasospasm	125.535	43.717–360.480	<0.001
Endovascular treatment for vasospasm	0.259	0.082–0.814	0.021
Infection	2.873	1.152–7.164	0.024

Age, sex, pre-SAH modified Rankin scale, World Federation of Neurosurgical Societies grade on admission, Fisher computed tomography (CT) group, dome size, neck size, aneurysm location, date of aneurysm obliteration, treatment modality, pretreatment aneurysm re-rupture (in-hospital), intra-treatment aneurysm re-rupture, post-treatment aneurysm re-rupture, cerebrospinal fluid drainage (with/without irrigation), antiplatelet therapy, symptomatic vasospasm, endovascular treatment for vasospasm, infection, noninfectious cardiopulmonary complications, epilepsy and shunt-dependent hydrocephalus are used in multivariate logistic regression. Age and size are used as a continuous variable

clipped represents bias toward more frequent repeat imaging of surgical patients in the postoperative period, whereas those treated by endovascular means may still be at risk of early infarction that is either not captured on CT or when imaging is not performed. It is important to select the treatment modality that minimizes the procedural risks based on the integration of information about the patient's medical condition, the aneurysm characteristics, available techniques and equipment, and the surgeon's skills and experience.

Early brain injury has attracted considerable attention as a cause of delayed cerebral infarction after SAH, other than vasospasm [5]. Naidech et al. [9] reported that some cerebral infarction occurred by day 2 or associated with no angiographic vasospasm. According to Shimoda et al. [10], early asymptomatic infarction was detected in 8 % of pretreatment aneurysmal SAH patients on diffusion-weighted images at the time of admission. The occurrence of early infarction on admission was significantly correlated with delayed angiographic vasospasm, delayed cerebral ischemia, CT-detected delayed extensive infarction, and unfavorable outcome [10]. Thus, causes of a new infarction on CT or magnetic resonance images on the first postoperative day in this study might include early brain injury, in addition to procedural complications. Naidech et al. [9] suggested that physiological derangement and cerebral edema might be clinical indicators of early brain injury and worthwhile targets for intervention to decrease the occurrence and clinical impact of cerebral infarction after SAH.

The term "symptomatic vasospasm" in this study, if described precisely, means delayed cerebral ischemia by both cerebral vasospasm and vasospasm-unrelated causes. However, it is unchangeable that cerebral vasospasm is the most important treatable factor to prevent cerebral infarction, because endovascular treatment for vasospasm independently decreased cerebral infarction occurrence in this study. Jabbarli et al. [6] reported that significant predictors for severe vasospasm were younger age (<51 years of age) and early onset of mean flow velocities >160 cm/s on transcranial Doppler ultrasound, most of which were treated endovascularly. Fergusen et al. [2] reported that predictors associated with cerebral infarction in the tirilazad data set, in which all ruptured aneurysms were treated by clipping, were increasing age, history of hypertension or diabetes mellitus, worse WFNS grade, larger aneurysm size, symptomatic vasospasm, temperature greater than 38 °C at 8 days after SAH, and use of prophylactically or therapeutically induced hypertension. Cerebral infarction was strongly associated with poor outcome, and the most important potentially treatable factor associated with infarction was symptomatic vasospasm [2]. In our previous study using the same registry as this study [7], admission WFNS grade IV-V, Fisher CT group 3–4, and ruptured middle cerebral artery aneurysms were independent factors for the development of vasospasm-induced cerebral infarction.

In summary, this study showed that cerebral infarction has a significant impact on poor outcome after SAH irrespective of the causes, and that cerebral vasospasm is still the most important potentially treatable factor against it.

Conflict of Interest Statement The authors declare that they have no conflict of interest.

References

1. Connolly ES Jr, Rabinstein AA, Carhuapoma JR, Derdeyn CP, Dion J, Higashida RT, Hoh BL, Kirkness CJ, Naidech AM, Ogilvy CS, Patel AB, Thompson BG, Vespa P, American Heart Association Stroke Council; Council on Cardiovascular Radiology and Intervention; Council on Cardiovascular Nursing; Council on Cardiovascular Surgery and Anesthesia; Council on Clinical Cardiology (2012) Guidelines for the management of aneurysmal subarachnoid hemorrhage: a guideline for healthcare professionals from the American Heart Association/American Stroke Association. Stroke 43:1711–1737

2. Fergusen S, Macdonald RL (2007) Predictors of cerebral infarction in patients with aneurysmal subarachnoid hemorrhage. Neurosurgery 60:658–667
3. Fu C, Yu W, Sun L, Li D, Zhao C (2013) Early cerebral infarction following aneurysmal subarachnoid hemorrhage: frequency, risk factors, patterns, and prognosis. Curr Neurovasc Res 10:316–324
4. Hill MD, Martin RH, Mikulis D, Wong JH, Silver FL, Terbrugge KG, Milot G, Clark WM, Macdonald RL, Kelly ME, Boulton M, Fleetwood I, McDougall C, Gunnarsson T, Chow M, Lum C, Dodd R, Poublanc J, Krings T, Demchuk AM, Goyal M, Anderson R, Bishop J, Garman D, Tymianski M, ENACT trial investigators (2012) Safety and efficacy of NA-1 in patients with iatrogenic stroke after endovascular aneurysm repair (ENACT): a phase 2, randomised, double-blind, placebo-controlled trial. Lancet Neurol 11:942–950
5. Hou J, Zhang JH (2013) Does prevention of vasospasm in subarachnoid hemorrhage improve clinical outcome? No. Stroke 44(Suppl 1):S34–S36
6. Jabbarli R, Gläsker S, Weber J, Taschner C, Olschewski M, Van Velthoven V (2013) Predictors of severity of cerebral vasospasm caused by aneurysmal subarachnoid hemorrhage. J Stroke Cerebrovasc Dis 22:1332–1339
7. Kanamaru K, Suzuki H, Taki W (2015) Risk factors for vasospasm-induced cerebral infarct when both clipping and coiling are equally available. Acta Neurochir Suppl 120:291–295
8. Kumar A, Brown R, Dhar R, Sampson T, Derdeyn CP, Moran CJ, Diringer MN (2013) Early vs. delayed cerebral infarction after aneurysm repair after subarachnoid hemorrhage. Neurosurgery 73:617–623
9. Naidech AM, Drescher J, Tamul P, Shaibani A, Batjer HH, Alberts MJ (2006) Acute physiological derangement is associated with early radiographic cerebral infarction after subarachnoid haemorrhage. J Neurol Neurosurg Psychiatry 77:1340–1344
10. Shimoda M, Hoshikawa K, Shiramizu H, Oda S, Yoshiyama M, Osada T, Matsumae M (2010) Early infarction detected by diffusion-weighted imaging in patients with subarachnoid hemorrhage. Acta Neurochir (Wien) 152:1197–1205
11. Siironen J, Porras M, Varis J, Poussa K, Hernesniemi J, Juvela S (2007) Early ischemic lesion on computed tomography: predictor of poor outcome among survivors of aneurysmal subarachnoid hemorrhage. J Neurosurg 107:1074–1079
12. Suzuki H, Taki W, Prospective Registry of Subarachnoid Aneurysms Treatment (PRESAT) group (2013) Effect of aneurysm treatment modalities on cerebral vasospasm after aneurysmal subarachnoid hemorrhage. Acta Neurochir Suppl 115:99–105
13. Taki W, Sakai N, Suzuki H, Prospective Registry of Subarachnoid Aneurysms Treatment (PRESAT) group (2011) Determinants of poor outcome following aneurysmal subarachnoid hemorrhage when both clipping and coiling are available: PRESAT in Japan. World Neurosurg 76:437–445
14. Taki W, Sakai N, Suzuki H, Prospective Registry of Subarachnoid Aneurysms Treatment (PRESAT) group (2012) Factors predicting retreatment and residual aneurysms at 1 year after endovascular coiling for ruptured cerebral aneurysms: PRESAT in Japan. Neuroradiology 54:597–606
15. Taki W, Sakai N, Suzuki H, Prospective Registry of Subarachnoid Aneurysms Treatment (PRESAT) group (2013) Importance of independently evaluated initial anatomic result after endovascular coiling for ruptured cerebral aneurysms. J Clin Neurosci 20:527–531
16. Vergouwen MDI, Vermeulen M, van Gijn J, Rinkel GJE, Wijdicks EF, Muizelaar JP, Mendelow AD, Juvela S, Yonas H, Terbrugge KG, Macdonald RL, Diringer MN, Broderick JP, Dreier JP, Roos YB (2010) Definition of delayed cerebral ischemia after aneurysmal subarachnoid hemorrhage as an outcome event in clinical trials and observational studies. Proposal of a Multidisciplinary Research Group. Stroke 41:2391–2395

Vascular Endothelial Growth Factor in Brain Edema Formation After Subarachnoid Hemorrhage

Lei Liu, Masashi Fujimoto, Fumihiro Kawakita, Naoki Ichikawa, and Hidenori Suzuki

Introduction

Subarachnoid hemorrhage (SAH) is one of the most life-threatening diseases of the central nervous system, with high rates of mortality and morbidity [1]. Blood-brain barrier (BBB) disruption is an important pathological process during SAH and causes brain edema. The detailed mechanisms of BBB disruption are still indistinct, though many researchers suggest that the permeability of the BBB is induced by many different molecules [2].

Vascular endothelial growth factor (VEGF) is a specific cytokine with multiple functions related to its mitogenic and permeability properties. The effects are mediated by VEGF receptor-2, which is present in vascular endothelial cells [3, 4]. Some studies have demonstrated that the expression of VEGF was upregulated and might be responsible for increased permeability of BBB after SAH or inflammatory disease [5–7], but it remains unknown whether blockage of VEGF upregulation prevents post-SAH BBB disruption. In this study, we administrated anti-VEGF antibody to neutralize VEGF protein and evaluated the effect on brain edema formation after experimental SAH in mice.

Materials and Methods

All procedures were approved by the Animal Ethics Review Committee of Mie University and were carried out according to the institution's Guidelines for Animal Experiments.

L. Liu, MD (✉) • M. Fujimoto, MD, PhD • F. Kawakita, MD
N. Ichikawa, MD • H. Suzuki, MD, PhD
Department of Neurosurgery, Mie University Graduate School of Medicine, 2-174 Edobashi, Tsu, Mie 514-8507, Japan
e-mail: liulei715127@gmail.com

Experimental Model of SAH and Study Protocol

The endovascular filament puncture SAH model and sham-operated model were produced in adult, male C57BL/6 mice (25–30 g), as previously described [8]. Briefly, mice were anesthetized with an intraperitoneal injection of tribromoethanol (0.25 g/g body weight) and fixed on an operation table supinely. After exposing and separating the left common carotid artery, left external carotid artery, and left internal carotid artery, a sharpened 4–0 monofilament nylon suture was advanced rostrally into the left internal carotid artery about 1.8 cm from the external carotid artery stump to perforate the bifurcation of the anterior and middle cerebral arteries. The filament was advanced only 0.5 cm into the internal carotid artery for sham operation. The blood pressure and heart rate were noninvasively monitored before and after operation from a mouse's tail. Animals had free access to feed and water until sacrifice.

To evaluate whether anti-VEGF antibody ameliorates brain edema, mice were randomly divided into three groups: sham, SAH + vehicle (phosphate-buffered saline [PBS], 2 μl), and SAH + anti-VEGF antibody (0.5 μg/μl, 2 μl) groups. The vehicle or anti-VEGF antibody was administrated by an intracerebroventricular injection after 30 min of operation. Randomization terminated at a sample size ≥4 in each group for statistical analysis. Neurological score was recorded 24 h later with the modified Garcia's neurological score system. Mice were then sacrificed, brains were harvested, and brain water content was measured.

To assess the protective effects of anti-VEGF antibody on BBB disruption, mice were divided into three groups randomly and underwent SAH or sham operation as above. Either 2 μl anti-VEGF antibody (0.5 μg/μl) or 2 μl vehicle (PBS) was administrated by an intracerebroventricular injection after 30 min of operation. Randomization also terminated at a sample size ≥4 in each group. Neurological score

R.L. Applegate et al. (eds.), *Brain Edema XVI: Translate Basic Science into Clinical Practice*, Acta Neurochirurgica Supplement, Vol. 121,
DOI 10.1007/978-3-319-18497-5_31,

was recorded at 24 h post-operation. Mice were then deeply anesthetized and the brain was fixed by intracardiac perfusion with formalin, and immunoglobulin (Ig) G staining was performed.

Intracerebroventricular Injection of Anti-VEGF Antibody or Vehicle

The intracerebroventricular (icv) injection was performed with modifications, as previously described [9]. Mice were placed in a stereotactic head holder and the needle of a 2-μl Hamilton syringe (Hamilton Company) was inserted through a burr hole perforated on the skull into the left lateral ventricle using the following coordinates relative to the bregma: 1 mm lateral, 0.2 mm posterior, and 2.2 mm below the horizontal plane of cortex. Sterile PBS (2 μl) or anti-VEGF antibody (R&D Systems; 0.5 μg/μl, 2 μl) was injected at a rate of 1 μl/min after 30 min of surgery. The needle was slowly removed after 5 min of injection and the wound was quickly sutured.

Neurobehavioral Test

Neurobehavioral impairments were blindly assessed at 24 h after SAH as previously described [8, 10]. Neurological score was tested by six tests: spontaneous activity, spontaneous movement of four limbs, forepaw outstretching, climbing, body proprioception, and response to whisker stimulation. Animals were given a score of 3–18, and higher scores indicated better function.

Severity of SAH

The severity of SAH was blindly evaluated using the SAH grading scale at each sacrifice [8]. High-resolution pictures of the base of the brain depicting the circle of Willis and basilar artery were taken after the brain was harvested. In the photographs, the basal and pre-brain stem cisterns were divided into six segments and each segment was allotted a grade from 0 to 3 depending on the amount of SAH clot in the segment: grade 0, no subarachnoid blood; grade 1, minimal subarachnoid blood; grade 2, moderate blood clot with recognizable arteries; and grade 3, blood clot obliterating all arteries within the segment. The animals received a total score ranging from 0 to 18 after adding the scores from all six segments. The mice with SAH grading scores ≤7, which had no significant brain injury, were excluded.

Brain Water Content

Brain water content was calculated to assess the level of brain edema using the wet/dry method as previously described [9]. After mice were sacrificed under deep anesthesia, the brain was rapidly removed and separated into the left and right cerebral hemispheres, cerebellum, and brain stem. These segments were each weighed and recorded as wet weight, and then the brain tissues were dried in an oven at 105 °C for 72 h and weighed again as dry weight. The percentage of water content was calculated according to the following formula: [(wet weight − dry weight)/wet weight] × 100 %.

BBB Permeability

IgG staining was performed to evaluate the BBB permeability by a modification of a previously reported method [11]. After dewaxing and rehydration, 4 μm formalin-fixed paraffin-embedded coronal sections were rinsed in distilled water twice, placed in 1 mM ethylenediaminetetraacetic acid (EDTA; pH 8.0), and heated in a water bath for 20 min to retrieve the antigen. The sections were rinsed in Tris-buffered saline and Tween 20 (TBS-T) twice and incubated in 1 % hydrogen peroxide (H_2O_2) in TBS-T for 10 min to quench any endogenous peroxidase activity, and then rinsed again twice in TBS-T. The sections were then blocked in 10 % horse serum-containing TBS-T for another 1 h at room temperature followed by overnight incubation at 4 °C with biotinylated horse anti-mouse polyclonal IgG antibody (1:100, Vector Laboratories). After rinsing with TBS-T, sections were incubated with avidin-biotin-horseradish peroxidase (HRP) complex (Vectastain ABC Kit, Vector Laboratories) for 1 h at room temperature. All sections were rinsed in TBS-T and the color reaction product was visualized using 0.2 mg/ml 3, 3′-diaminobenzidine in the presence of 0.02 % H_2O_2 and lightly counterstained with hematoxylin. The left temporal cortex was photographed using microscopy and evaluated.

Statistics

Neurological scores were expressed as median ± 25th–75th percentiles and were analyzed using Mann-Whitney *U* test or Kruskal-Wallis test, followed by Steel-Dwass multiple comparisons. Other values were expressed as mean ± standard deviation and one-way analysis of variance (ANOVA) with Bonferroni post hoc test. All analyses were performed using the SPSS 20.0 statistical package (IBM SPSS Inc.) and differences were considered significant at $p < 0.05$.

Results

Anti-VEGF Antibody Ameliorates Neurobehavior after 24 h of SAH

Comparisons of physiological parameters revealed no significant differences among the groups (data not shown). None of the 8 sham-operated mice died within the 24-h observation period. The mortality of SAH mice was 11 % (1 of 9 mice) in the SAH + vehicle group and 20 % (2 of 10 mice) in the SAH + anti-VEGF antibody group. There was no significant difference in SAH severity between SAH + vehicle and SAH + anti-VEGF antibody groups after 24 h of surgery (Fig. 1a).

Neurological score in the SAH + vehicle group was significantly impaired compared with the sham group after 24 h of surgery. In the SAH mice treated with anti-VEGF antibody, neurological score (Fig. 1b) was significantly improved compared with the SAH + vehicle group ($p<0.05$, Mann-Whitney *U* or Kruskal–Wallis test).

Anti-VEGF Antibody Alleviates Brain Edema after 24 h of SAH

Brain water content analysis showed that the brain edema that was caused by SAH occurred only in the left cerebral hemisphere and was significantly alleviated after treated with anti-VEGF antibody compared with the SAH + vehicle group ($p<0.05$, ANOVA, Fig. 2).

IgG Extravasation in Brain Tissue Is Inhibited by Anti-VEGF Antibody

Based on the result of brain water content analyses, anti-VEGF antibody was administered using an icv injection, and BBB permeability of the left cerebral hemisphere was evaluated by IgG immunohistochemistry. IgG immunohistochemistry analysis showed that BBB disruption markedly occurred in the left cerebral cortex, especially the temporal cortex, in the SAH + vehicle group compared with the sham-operated group. After treatment with anti-VEGF antibody, the IgG extravasation was markedly suppressed compared with the SAH + vehicle group (Fig. 3).

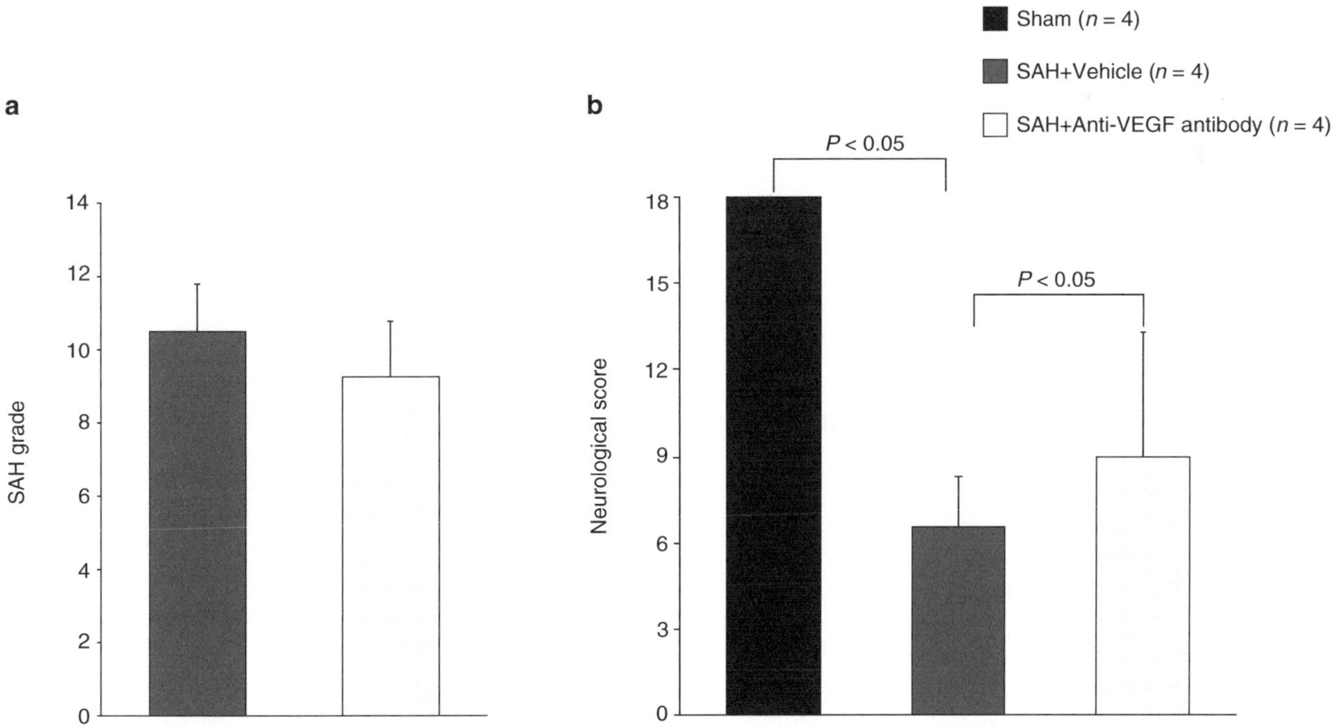

Fig. 1 (**a**) SAH grade in the SAH + vehicle and the SAH + anti-VEGF antibody groups. Data were expressed as mean ± standard deviation. No significant difference between the groups. Mann-Whitney *U* tests. (**b**) Neurological score in the sham, SAH + vehicle and SAH + anti-VEGF antibody groups. Data were expressed as median ± 25th–75th percentiles. *p* Value, Kruskal-Wallis test

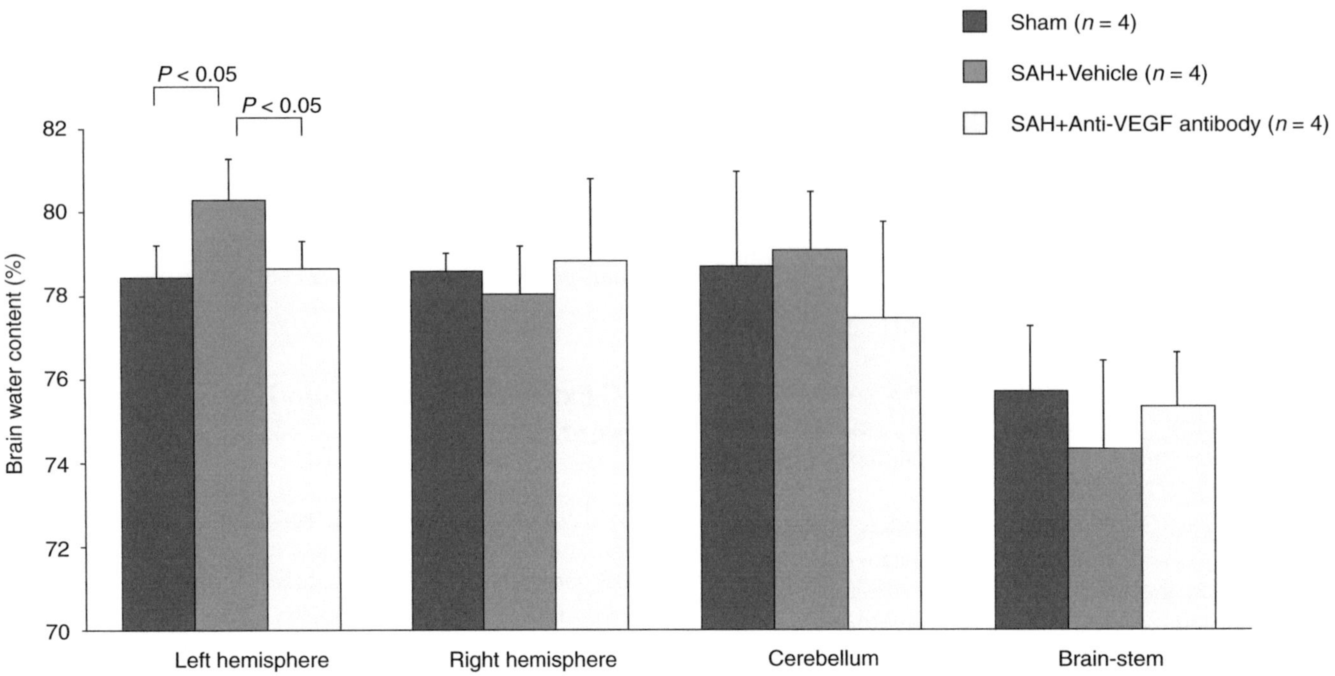

Fig. 2 Brain water content in the left cerebral hemisphere, right cerebral hemisphere, cerebellum, and brain stem in the sham, SAH + vehicle, and SAH + anti-VEGF antibody groups. Data were expressed as mean ± standard deviation. *p* Value, ANOVA

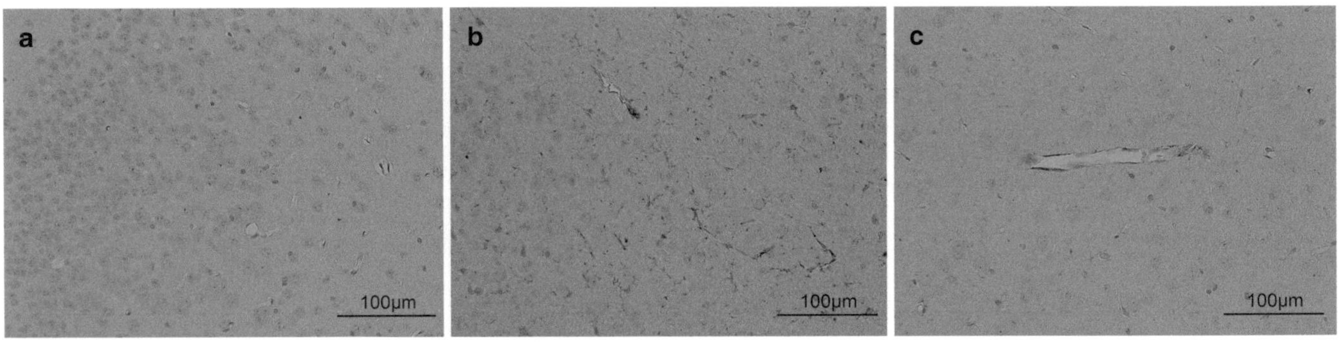

Fig. 3 IgG immunohistochemistry in the sham (**a**), SAH + vehicle (**b**), and SAH + anti-VEGF antibody (**c**) groups

Discussion

In this study, we investigated the protective effect of anti-VEGF antibody on brain edema formation after SAH. The findings indicated that VEGF is involved in brain edema formation after SAH, and that anti-VEGF antibody can improve neurobehavioral outcome, decrease BBB permeability and ameliorate brain edema after 24 h of SAH in mice.

BBB is the basic unit between the peripheral circulation and central nervous system and regulates the homeostasis of brain [12]. Some researchers have demonstrated that the BBB disruption was a critical pathologic manifestation that occurred in an early stage of SAH and allowed numerous inflammatory mediators to transfer into brain parenchyma, leading to brain edema formation and further brain parenchymal damage [13]. The mechanisms of brain edema formation are complex and still indistinct, though many specific molecules have been identified during the pathological procedure of SAH.

VEGF is a pivotal regulator of angiogenesis that controls vascular growth under physiological and pathological conditions and, meanwhile, promotes vascular permeability [3]. It has been reported that the expression of VEGF was upregulated after ischemic or hemorrhagic brain injury and responsible for increased BBB permeability [7, 14, 15]. One report stated that application of appropriate dosages of exogenous human VEGF165 increased BBB permeability in normal mice [5]. Some researchers also have demonstrated that inhibition of endogenous VEGF with topical application of anti-VEGF antibody attenuated BBB disruption in focal cerebral ischemia [16]. However, there is no previous study on experimental SAH in which the effects of inhibition of VEGF on BBB disruption were investigated.

In the present study, we demonstrated our hypothesis that VEGF is a key molecule that causes BBB disruption and induces brain edema formation, and thus, that suppressing VEGF after SAH is a possible way to protect BBB and to reduce brain edema. It is suggested that neutralization of VEGF protein using anti-VEGF antibody may be a prospect for SAH therapy, though the detailed mechanisms responsible for the attenuated brain edema formation remain unclear.

Conflict of Interest Statement We declare that we have no conflicts of interest.

References

1. Fujii M, Yan J, Rolland WB, Soejima Y, Caner B, Zhang JH (2013) Early brain injury, an evolving frontier in subarachnoid hemorrhage research. Transl Stroke Res 4:432–446
2. Easton AS (2012) Regulation of permeability across the blood–brain barrier. Adv Exp Med Biol 763:1–19
3. Ferrara N, Gerber HP, LeCouter J (2003) The biology of VEGF and its receptors. Nat Med 9:669–676
4. Roy H, Bhardwaj S, Yla-Herttuala S (2006) Biology of vascular endothelial growth factors. FEBS Lett 580:2879–2887
5. Jiang S, Xia R, Jiang Y, Wang L, Gao F (2014) Vascular endothelial growth factors enhance the permeability of the mouse blood–brain barrier. PLoS One 9, e86407
6. Argaw AT, Asp L, Zhang J, Navrazhina K, Pham T, Mariani JN, Mahase S, Dutta DJ, Seto J, Kramer EG, Ferrara N, Sofroniew MV, John GR (2012) Astrocyte-derived VEGF-A drives blood–brain barrier disruption in CNS inflammatory disease. J Clin Invest 122:2454–2468
7. Suzuki H, Hasegawa Y, Kanamaru K, Zhang JH (2010) Mechanisms of osteopontin-induced stabilization of blood–brain barrier disruption after subarachnoid hemorrhage in rats. Stroke 41:1783–1790
8. Sugawara T, Ayer R, Jadhav V, Zhang JH (2008) A new grading system evaluating bleeding scale in filament perforation subarachnoid hemorrhage rat model. J Neurosci Methods 167:327–334
9. Altay O, Suzuki H, Hasegawa Y, Caner B, Krafft PR, Fujii M, Tang J, Zhang JH (2012) Isoflurane attenuates blood–brain barrier disruption in ipsilateral hemisphere after subarachnoid hemorrhage in mice. Stroke 43:2513–2516
10. Suzuki H, Zhang JH (2012) Neurobehavioral assessments of subarachnoid hemorrhage. In: Chen J, Xu X-M, Xu ZC, Zhang JH (eds) Animal models of acute neurological injuries II, Springer protocols handbooks. Humana Press, New York, pp 435–440
11. Richmon JD, Fukuda K, Maida N, Sato M, Bergeron M, Sharp FR, Panter SS, Noble LJ (1998) Induction of heme oxygenase-1 after hyperosmotic opening of the blood–brain barrier. Brain Res 780:108–118
12. Obermeier B, Daneman R, Ransohoff RM (2013) Development, maintenance and disruption of the blood–brain barrier. Nat Med 19:1584–1596
13. Doczi T (1985) The pathogenetic and prognostic significance of blood–brain barrier damage at the acute stage of aneurysmal subarachnoid haemorrhage. Clinical and experimental studies. Acta Neurochir (Wien) 77:110–132
14. Yatsushige H, Ostrowski RP, Tsubokawa T, Colohan A, Zhang JH (2007) Role of c-Jun N-terminal kinase in early brain injury after subarachnoid hemorrhage. J Neurosci Res 85:1436–1448
15. Zhao Y, Li Z, Wang R, Wei J, Li G, Zhao H (2010) Angiopoietin 1 counteracts vascular endothelial growth factor-induced blood–brain barrier permeability and alleviates ischemic injury in the early stages of transient focal cerebral ischemia in rats. Neurol Res 32:748–755
16. Chi OZ, Hunter C, Liu X, Weiss HR (2007) Effects of anti-VEGF antibody on blood–brain barrier disruption in focal cerebral ischemia. Exp Neurol 204:283–287

Perihematomal Cerebral Tissue Iron Quantification on MRI Following Intracerebral Hemorrhage in Two Human Subjects: Proof of Principle

Neeraj Chaudhary, Aditya S. Pandey, Kevin Merchak, Joseph J. Gemmete, Tom Chenevert, and Guohua Xi

Introduction

Each year, approximately 800,000 people suffer a stroke in the United States. The causes of stroke are, in general, either hemorrhagic or nonhemorrhagic. Intracranial hemorrhage (ICH) is a common and often fatal stroke subtype [1, 2]. More than 30,000 patients die from spontaneous ICH annually. Iron has a major role in ICH-induced brain injury [1, 3, 4]. There is a progressive accumulation of iron in the cerebral tissue surrounding a hematoma from hemoglobin degradation within the hematoma as it resolves. The high level of non-heme iron remains in the brain for at least 1 month [5]. By enhanced Perls' reaction, iron-positive cells are found in the perihematomal zone as early as the first day [5]. Our studies also have shown that free iron levels in cerebrospinal fluid (CSF) increase almost 14-fold after ICH on the third day and remain high for at least 28 days after experimental ICH [7]. Increases of brain iron levels cause brain edema, oxidative stress, brain atrophy, and neurological deficits following ICH [1, 6, 8].

If the patient survives the ictus, the resulting hematoma within brain parenchyma triggers a series of events leading to secondary insults and severe neurological deficits [9]. There is currently no proven therapy for ICH other than supportive care [10, 11]. Although the hematoma in humans gradually resolves, neurological deficits in ICH patients are usually permanent and disabling. Iron has a major role in brain damage following ICH [1, 11]. Brain injury after ICH appears to involve several phases [1]. These include an early phase involving the clotting cascade activation and thrombin production [10–16] and a later phase involving erythrocyte lysis and iron toxicity [2–4, 17–19]. After erythrocyte lysis within the hematoma, iron concentrations in surrounding brain can reach very high levels. Studies have shown that high levels of serum ferritin, an iron-binding protein, are independently associated with poor outcome and severe brain edema in ICH patients [16, 17].

It is well known that iron has a key role in brain edema formation following ICH [1, 19]. Perihematomal brain edema develops immediately after ICH and peaks several days later [6, 19]. Edema formation following ICH elevates intracranial pressure and may result in herniation [20]. In experimental ICH models, brain edema peaks around the third or fourth day after the hemorrhage then declines slowly [10, 21–23]. In species with significant white matter, perihematomal edema is mainly located within that tissue [22]. In humans, perihematomal edema develops within 3 h of symptom onset and peaks between 10 and 20 days after the ictus [23]. Several studies show that the degree of brain edema around the hematoma correlates with poor outcome in patients [20, 24, 25]. We have shown that desferoxamine, an iron chelate, reduces brain edema and hemorrhagic brain injury in aged rats and pigs [26–28]. Deferoxamine has been examined by a phase I trial in human subjects [29]. The promise it has shown in these trials has led to a further phase II trial, which was approved by the NIH.

Although there is a growing body of evidence for the role of iron in neuronal damage following parenchymal hemorrhage, there is a conspicuous lack of a reliable paradigm for accurate quantification of the tissue iron load. Interest in

N. Chaudhary, MD, MRCS, FRCR (✉)
Neurointerventional Radiology, Departments of Radiology & Neurosurgery, University of Michigan, Ann Arbor, MI, USA
e-mail: neerajc@med.umich.edu

A.S. Pandey, MD • J.J. Gemmete, MD FACR FSIR
Departments of Neurosurgery and Radiology, University of Michigan, Ann Arbor, MI, USA

K. Merchak
Department of Biomed Engineering, University of Michigan, Ann Arbor, MI, USA

T. Chenevert, PhD
Department of Radiology, University of Michigan, Ann Arbor, MI, USA

G. Xi, MD
Department of Neurosurgery, University of Michigan, Ann Arbor, MI, USA

R.L. Applegate et al. (eds.), *Brain Edema XVI: Translate Basic Science into Clinical Practice*, Acta Neurochirurgica Supplement, Vol. 121,
DOI 10.1007/978-3-319-18497-5_32,

noninvasive quantification of tissue iron has resurged with development of effective iron chelate therapy in prevention of iron toxicity [30]. Existing noninvasive modalities such as magnetic resonance imaging (MRI) have been utilized to develop iron measurement algorithms in the heart [31]. Traumatic brain injury is another condition where MRI-based estimation of iron deposition in the cerebral tissue has been explored [32, 33]. Human physiology is incapable of excreting excess iron. Iron is deposited in various tissues in the body in clinical conditions that require repeated blood transfusions. Paramagnetic effects of tissue-deposited iron, causing signal inhomogeneity on MRI, have been exploited to estimate tissue iron levels in human visceral tissue [30, 31, 34]. Although some advances have been made in quantifying iron in the human liver by MRI, a robust technique has not been developed yet [35, 36]. Bilgic et al. [37] have demonstrated feasibility of detection of iron levels in brain tissue of normal aging population by quantitative susceptibility mapping (QSM). They demonstrated specificity of the field-dependent relaxation rate (FDRI) technique in detection of minute concentrations of iron in the brain tissue with age. Preliminary clinical studies have demonstrated the ability to detect cerebral tissue iron in traumatic brain injury by utilizing T2* magnetic field correlation on MRI [32]. Liu et al. [38], utilizing a porcine model, demonstrated the ability of R2 (1/T2) relaxivity maps in detecting superparamagnetic iron oxide (SPIO) nanoparticles in the brain tissue following disruption of blood brain barrier (BBB) by low-frequency ultrasound. Sammet et al. [39] showed the importance of multiple spin echo sequences on MRI for reliable correlation with iron levels and developed a mathematical model to differentiate between ferritin and hemosiderin on MRI using an agarose-phantom. In a porcine ICH model, utilizing 7 T MRI, Wu et al. [40] demonstrated the application of T2* sequences to correlate with hematoma size and histopathological evidence of tissue iron. A study from Wang et al. [41] showed the reliability of QSM on T2* MRI scan in patients with ICH. They utilized the application of R2* (1/T2*) relaxivity maps to obtain a reliable calculation of hematoma volume.

At the time of this writing, there have been no studies performed to ascertain accurate tissue iron levels at the periphery of the hematoma in patients with ICH. Our hypothesis is that MRI is sensitive enough to pick up field inhomogeneity due to the presence of excess brain tissue iron. A reliable MR-based iron quantification algorithm can be beneficial in management of patients with ICH. It can serve as a surrogate marker of severity of neurotoxicity. Once validated, it can serve to monitor efficacy of the iron-chelating agents like deferoxamine currently being tested in this patient population. Above all, it may possibly enable prediction of ICH in patients if correlation of brain tissue iron levels can be demonstrated with functional outcome in the future.

Materials and Methods

MRI Phantom Construction

Institutional Review Board approval was obtained to perform MRI scans on selected patients with ICH. Initially, we constructed a phantom with varying concentrations of iron and then scanned the phantom in a 3 T MRI. The phantom was constructed with a cylindrical container made out of material that would not cause signal aberration on MRI; a plastic cylindrical container was utilized. A liquid iron preparation, ferumoxytol (Feraheme®, AMAG Pharmaceuticals, Waltham, MA, USA), which is used for intravenous ferrous sulfate therapy, was selected as the appropriate liquid preparation. It is a non-stoichiometric magnetite (superparamagnetic iron oxide) coated with polyglucose sorbitol carboxymethylether.

We then prepared serial dilutions of the ferumoxytol in seven different reducing dilutions, commencing with 6 mg/ml and ending with 0.0047 mg/ml. Each subsequent concentration was 50 % less than the prior. The above concentrations were chosen as the iron concentrations in the published literature lie in the middle of the above distribution. Four milliliters of each concentration was placed in a 4-ml glass vial, avoiding any air bubbles. Seven glass vials were then attached to the undersurface of the lid of the plastic container selected for the phantom (Fig 1a), which was then filled with sterile water to replace any air bubbles in the container. The phantom was scanned in a 3 T MRI with the following susceptibility weighted sequences: 3D TR = 40 ms, TE = 6.5, 11, 15.5, 20, 24.5, 29, 33.5, 38 ms, 1.5 mm slice-to-slice, acquired as 3 mm, acquired resolution matrix = 240 × 240, FOV – 240 mm × 240 mm (Fig 1b). T2* signal magnitude measurements were then obtained corresponding to these concentrations (Table 1).

Human Subjects Scanned

ICH patients, age 18–85 years, with brain parenchymal hemorrhage, no previous ICH, and no evidence of physiological calcification on noncontrast CT of the head were included in the study. One control and two human subjects who met the inclusion criteria for the study were scanned with the same MRI protocol utilized on the phantom. The two human subjects had spontaneous basal ganglia hemorrhage and were scanned on day 7 of their hemorrhage. In the control human brain, MRI regions of interest (ROIs) were drawn in the basal ganglia region on both hemispheres. Calculations were performed on R2* maps generated from the MRI sequences (Fig. 2a). In the two human subjects, regions of interest were

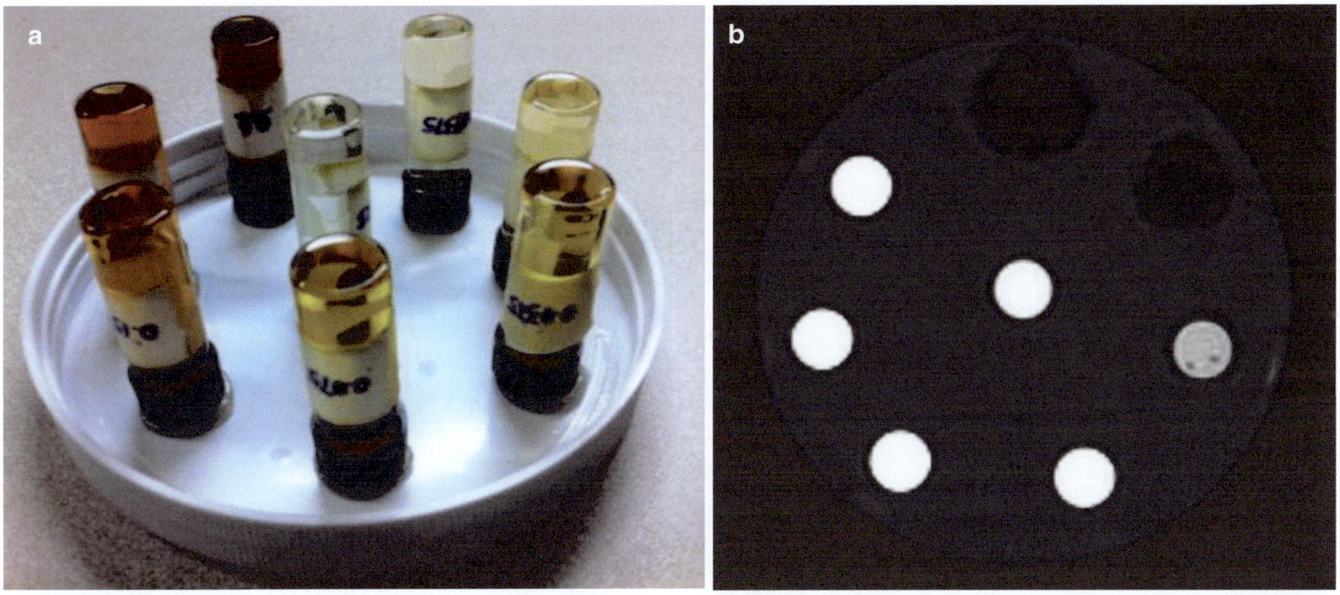

Fig. 1 (**a**) Image of the lid of the phantom with seven 4-cc vials containing serial dilutions of iron concentration in sterile water stuck to the undersurface. (**b**) MRI of the phantom on a 3 T scanner with following sequence specifications: 3D TR=40 ms, TE=6.5, 11, 15.5, 20, 24.5, 29, 33.5, 38 ms, 1.5 mm slice-to-slice, acquired as 3 mm, acquired resolution matrix=240×240, FOV – 240 mm×240 mm

Table 1 Seven serial dilutions scanned in the MRI phantom with T2* signal measurements corresponding to each concentration

Iron concentration in the vial (mg/ml)	Corresponding MR signal magnitude ± SD
0.6	NA
0.3	2.33 ± 0.46
0.15	3.83 ± 0.14
0.075	7.99 ± 0.12
0.0375	15.15 ± 0.29
0.01875	29.65 ± 0.91
0.009375	54.77 ± 3.85
0.0046875	98.23 ± 3.27

drawn on the periphery of the hematoma in the left basal ganglia (Fig. 2b, c). Region of interest measurements were also performed on the contralateral normal hemisphere in an identical anatomical location.

Results

Control Human Subject

In the right basal ganglia, the T2* average of three ROIs measured 44.3. In the left basal ganglia in the same control human subject, the average of three ROIs measured 53.2. Both of these measurements correspond to an iron concentration of 0.01 mg/ml.

First Human Subject with ICH

Perihematomal measurements performed with three ROIs in the left basal ganglia showed T2* values of 15.3. This corresponds to an iron concentration of 0.04 mg/ml. An average of three ROIs in the contralateral normal brain in an identical anatomical location measured 49.5. This corresponds to 0.01 mg/ml of iron concentration.

Second Human Subject with ICH

Perihematomal measurements performed with three ROIs in the left basal ganglia showed T2* values of 18.97. This corresponds to an iron concentration of 0.04 mg/ml. An average of three ROIs in the contralateral normal brain in an identical anatomical location measured 53.3. This corresponds to 0.01 mg/ml of iron concentration.

The above measurements demonstrate consistently that the detection of an iron concentration in the periphery of the hematoma of an ICH in the left basal ganglia on day 7 following the ictus are 4 times higher than the normal baseline concentration.

Conclusion

Our experiment demonstrates proof of principle of MRI being able to detect a 4 times increase in tissue iron levels in the periphery of the hematoma in comparison to baseline.

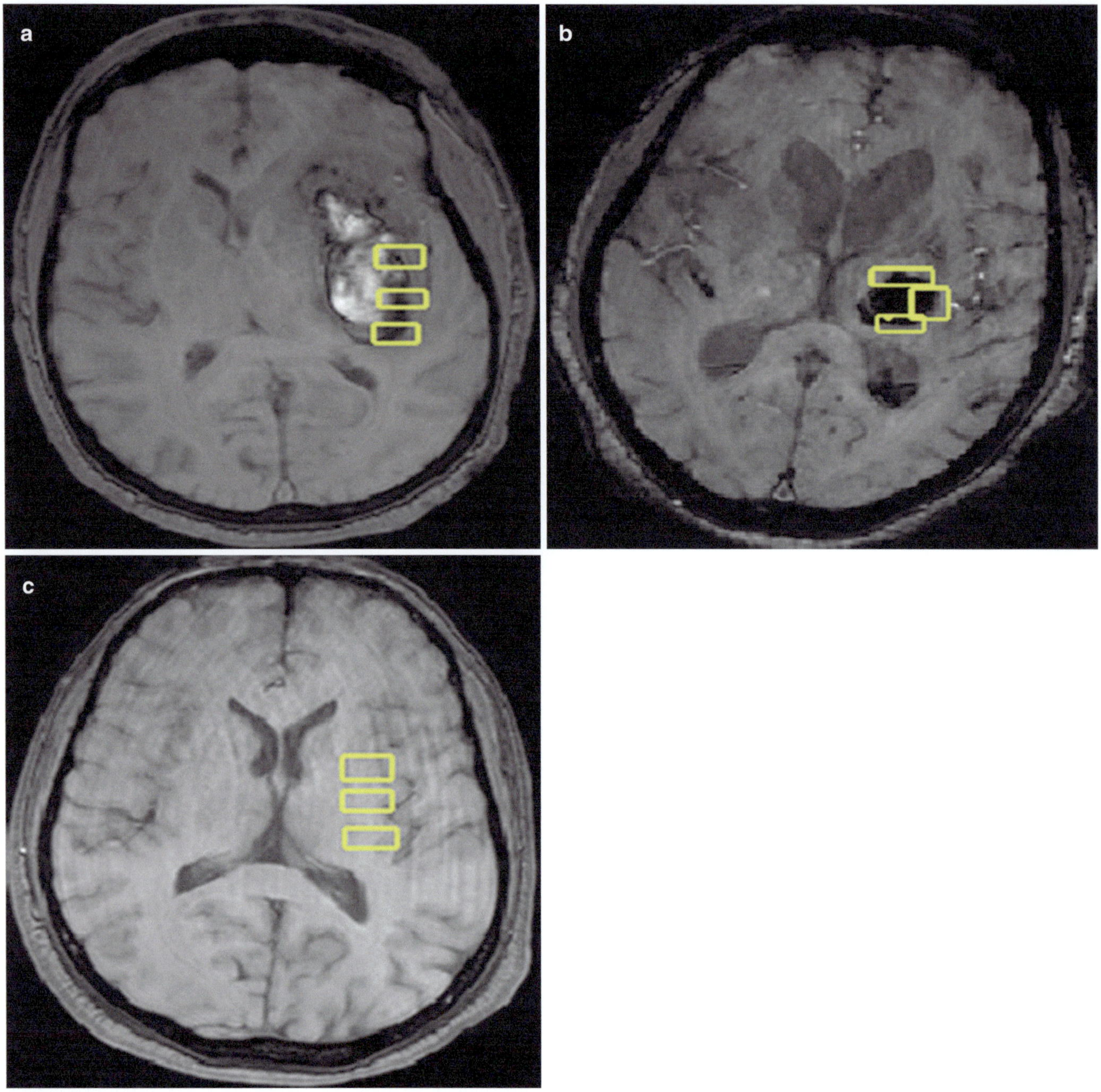

Fig. 2 (**a**) A 70-year-old male patient with axial MRI brain showing left basal ganglia hemorrhage with regions of interest drawn for measurement of the R2* magnitude. (**b**) A 68-year-old male patient with axial MRI brain showing left basal ganglia hemorrhage with regions of interest drawn for measurement of the R2* magnitude. (**c**) A 45-year-old male subject utilized as control showing axial MRI with regions of interest drawn for baseline R2* magnitude measurement

The initial translation from bench to bedside of iron-chelating therapy with deferoxamine being investigated by a phase II trial holds promise. Our hypothesis, once validated in a larger study, can provide a surrogate marker of severity of neurotoxicity following an ICH. Moreover, an MRI-based brain tissue iron quantification may provide a more objective way of monitoring therapy with iron chelates. Furthermore, the correlation of tissue iron quantification with functional outcome following an ICH needs to be studied in a large-scale prospective analysis involving human subjects.

References

1. Xi G, Keep RF, Hoff JT (2006) Mechanisms of brain injury after intracerebral haemorrhage. Lancet Neurol 5(1):53–63, PubMed Epub 2005/12/20
2. Morgenstern LB, Hemphill JC 3rd, Anderson C, Becker K, Broderick JP, Connolly ES Jr et al (2010) Guidelines for the management of spontaneous intracerebral hemorrhage: a guideline for healthcare professionals from the American Heart Association/American Stroke Association. Stroke 41(9):2108–2129, PubMed

3. Perez de la Ossa N, Sobrino T, Silva Y, Blanco M, Millan M, Gomis M et al (2010) Iron-related brain damage in patients with intracerebral hemorrhage. Stroke 41(4):810–813, PubMed
4. Selim M (2009) Deferoxamine mesylate: a new hope for intracerebral hemorrhage: from bench to clinical trials. Stroke 40(3 Suppl):S90–S91, PubMed
5. Wu J, Hua Y, Keep RF, Nakamura T, Hoff JT, Xi G (2003) Iron and iron-handling proteins in the brain after intracerebral hemorrhage. Stroke 34(12):2964–2969, PubMed
6. Nakamura T, Keep RF, Hua Y, Schallert T, Hoff JT, Xi G (2004) Deferoxamine-induced attenuation of brain edema and neurological deficits in a rat model of intracerebral hemorrhage. J Neurosurg 100(4):672–678, PubMed PMID: 15070122
7. Wan S, Hua Y, Keep RF, Hoff JT, Xi G (2006) Deferoxamine reduces CSF free iron levels following intracerebral hemorrhage. Acta Neurochir Suppl 96:199–202, PubMed PMID: 16671454
8. Hua Y, Nakamura T, Keep RF, Wu J, Schallert T, Hoff JT et al (2006) Long-term effects of experimental intracerebral hemorrhage: the role of iron. J Neurosurg 104(2):305–312, PubMed PMID: 16509506
9. Qureshi AI, Mendelow AD, Hanley DF (2009) Intracerebral haemorrhage. Lancet 373(9675):1632–1644, PubMed
10. Wagner KR, Sharp FR, Ardizzone TD, Lu A, Clark JF (2003) Heme and iron metabolism: role in cerebral hemorrhage. J Cereb Blood Flow Metab 23(6):629–652, PubMed
11. Pandey AS, Xi G (2014) Intracerebral hemorrhage: a multimodality approach to improving outcome. Transl Stroke Res 5(3):313–315. doi:10.1007/s12975-014-0344-z, Epub 2014 Apr 26
12. Lee KR, Colon GP, Betz AL, Keep RF, Kim S, Hoff JT (1996) Edema from intracerebral hemorrhage: the role of thrombin. J Neurosurg 84(1):91–96, PubMed
13. Xi G, Wagner KR, Keep RF, Hua Y, de Courten-Myers GM, Broderick JP et al (1998) Role of blood clot formation on early edema development after experimental intracerebral hemorrhage. Stroke 29(12):2580–2586, PubMed
14. Lee KR, Kawai N, Kim S, Sagher O, Hoff JT (1997) Mechanisms of edema formation after intracerebral hemorrhage: effects of thrombin on cerebral blood flow, blood-brain barrier permeability, and cell survival in a rat model. J Neurosurg 86(2):272–278, PubMed
15. Gebel JM, Sila CA, Sloan MA, Granger CB, Mahaffey KW, Weisenberger J et al (1998) Thrombolysis-related intracranial hemorrhage: a radiographic analysis of 244 cases from the GUSTO-1 trial with clinical correlation. Global Utilization of Streptokinase and Tissue Plasminogen Activator for Occluded Coronary Arteries. Stroke 29(3):563–569, PubMed
16. Wagner KR, Xi G, Hua Y, Kleinholz M, de Courten-Myers GM, Myers RE et al (1996) Lobar intracerebral hemorrhage model in pigs: rapid edema development in perihematomal white matter. Stroke 27(3):490–497, PubMed
17. Xi G, Keep RF, Hoff JT (1998) Erythrocytes and delayed brain edema formation following intracerebral hemorrhage in rats. J Neurosurg 89(6):991–996, PubMed
18. Huang FP, Xi G, Keep RF, Hua Y, Nemoianu A, Hoff JT (2002) Brain edema after experimental intracerebral hemorrhage: role of hemoglobin degradation products. J Neurosurg 96(2):287–293, PubMed
19. Xi G, Keep RF, Hoff JT (2002) Pathophysiology of brain edema formation. Neurosurg Clin N Am 13(3):371–383, PubMed
20. Ropper AH (1986) Lateral displacement of the brain and level of consciousness in patients with an acute hemispheral mass. N Engl J Med 314(15):953–958, PubMed
21. Enzmann DR, Britt RH, Lyons BE, Buxton JL, Wilson DA (1981) Natural history of experimental intracerebral hemorrhage: sonography, computed tomography and neuropathology. AJNR Am J Neuroradiol 2(6):517–526, PubMed
22. Tomita H, Ito U, Ohno K, Hirakawa K (1994) Chronological changes in brain edema induced by experimental intracerebral hematoma in cats. Acta Neurochir Suppl (Wien) 60:558–560, PubMed PMID: 7976649
23. Yang GY, Betz AL, Chenevert TL, Brunberg JA, Hoff JT (1994) Experimental intracerebral hemorrhage: relationship between brain edema, blood flow, and blood-brain barrier permeability in rats. J Neurosurg 81(1):93–102, PubMed PMID: 82075
24. Zazulia AR, Diringer MN, Derdeyn CP, Powers WJ (1999) Progression of mass effect after intracerebral hemorrhage. Stroke 30(6):1167–1173, PubMed
25. Ropper AH, King RB (1984) Intracranial pressure monitoring in comatose patients with cerebral hemorrhage. Arch Neurol 41(7):725–728, PubMed
26. Okauchi M, Hua Y, Keep RF, Morgenstern LB, Xi G (2009) Effects of deferoxamine on intracerebral hemorrhage-induced brain injury in aged rats. Stroke 40(5):1858–1863, PubMed Pubmed Central PMCID: 2674519
27. Okauchi M, Hua Y, Keep RF, Morgenstern LB, Schallert T, Xi G (2010) Deferoxamine treatment for intracerebral hemorrhage in aged rats: therapeutic time window and optimal duration. Stroke 41(2):375–382, PubMed PMID: 20044521
28. Gu Y, Hua Y, Keep RF, Morgenstern LB, Xi G (2009) Deferoxamine reduces intracerebral hematoma-induced iron accumulation and neuronal death in piglets. Stroke 40(6):2241–2243, PubMed Pubmed Central PMCID: 2693321
29. Selim M, Yeatts S, Goldstein JN, Gomes J, Greenberg S, Morgenstern LB et al (2011) Safety and tolerability of deferoxamine mesylate in patients with acute intracerebral hemorrhage. Stroke 42(11):3067–3074, PubMed Pubmed Central PMCID: 3202043
30. Brittenham GM, Badman DG (2003) Noninvasive measurement of iron: report of an NIDDK workshop. Blood 101(1):15–19, PubMed
31. He T, Gatehouse PD, Anderson LJ, Tanner M, Keegan J, Pennell DJ et al (2006) Development of a novel optimized breathhold technique for myocardial T2 measurement in thalassemia. J Magn Reson Imaging 24(3):580–585, PubMed
32. Raz E, Jensen JH, Ge Y, Babb JS, Miles L, Reaume J et al (2011) Brain iron quantification in mild traumatic brain injury: a magnetic field correlation study. AJNR Am J Neuroradiol 32(10):1851–1856, PubMed
33. Jensen JH, Chandra R, Ramani A, Lu H, Johnson G, Lee SP et al (2006) Magnetic field correlation imaging. Magn Reson Med 55(6):1350–1361, PubMed PMID:16700026
34. Jensen PD (2004) Evaluation of iron overload. Br J Haematol 124(6):697–711, PubMed
35. St Pierre TG, Clark PR, Chua-Anusorn W (2004) Single spin-echo proton transverse relaxometry of iron-loaded liver. NMR Biomed 17(7):446–458, PubMed
36. Jensen JH, Chandra R (2002) Theory of nonexponential NMR signal decay in liver with iron overload or superparamagnetic iron oxide particles. Magn Reson Med 47(6):1131–1138, PubMed PMID: 12111959
37. Bilgic B, Pfefferbaum A, Rohlfing T, Sullivan EV, Adalsteinsson E (2012) MRI estimates of brain iron concentration in normal aging using quantitative susceptibility mapping. Neuroimage 59(3):2625–2635, PubMed Pubmed Central PMCID: 3254708
38. Liu HL, Chen PY, Yang HW, Wu JS, Tseng IC, Ma YJ et al (2011) In vivo MR quantification of superparamagnetic iron oxide nanoparticle leakage during low-frequency-ultrasound-induced blood-brain barrier opening in swine. J Magn Reson Imaging 34(6):1313–1324, PubMed
39. Sammet CL, Swaminathan SV, Tang H, Sheth S, Jensen JH, Nunez A et al (2013) Measurement and correction of stimulated echo contamination in T2-based iron quantification. Magn Reson Imaging 31(5):664–668, PubMed
40. Wu G, Xi G, Hua Y, Sagher O (2010) T2* magnetic resonance imaging sequences reflect brain tissue iron deposition following intracerebral hemorrhage. Transl Stroke Res 1(1):31–34, PubMed
41. Wang S, Lou M, Liu T, Cui D, Chen X, Wang Y (2013) Hematoma volume measurement in gradient echo MRI using quantitative susceptibility mapping. Stroke 44(8):2315–2317. doi:10.1161/STROKEAHA.113.001638

Src Family Kinases in Brain Edema After Acute Brain Injury

DaZhi Liu, Xiong Zhang, BeiLei Hu, and Bradley P. Ander

Introduction

Brain edema occurs when a cerebral blood vessel is blocked or ruptured following ischemic stroke, intracerebral hemorrhage (ICH), traumatic brain injury (TBI), or other neurological diseases [1–3]. There are two main categories of brain edema, cytotoxic (cellular) and vasogenic (extracellular) [4]. In cytotoxic edema, the blood-brain barrier (BBB) remains intact, but there is essentially a shift of water from the extracellular to the intracellular compartment, with no increase of brain water content or rise in intracranial pressure (ICP). Though it does not require BBB disruption, cytotoxic brain edema changes cellular metabolism and eventually damages BBB after brain injury. By contrast, vasogenic edema requires BBB disruption, allowing fluid (i.e., circulating blood) to accumulate in the extracellular space in brain parenchyma, and will increase ICP [4]. It is generally thought that cytotoxic edema is dominant immediately following ischemic stroke [5], whereas vasogenic edema is dominant at the acute stage after TBI [4]. However, cytotoxic and vasogenic edema usually combine when brain injury progresses into the chronic phase in which a characteristic breakdown of the BBB occurs no matter what type of edema was first in the acute stage after brain injury [6]. Therefore, maintenance of BBB integrity has become a focus of recent research to prevent brain edema and improve outcomes of acute brain injury.

Brain edema has been associated with high mortality, mostly because it can induce rapid increase in ICP, which leads to compression of blood vessels, reduced tissue blood flow, and reduced oxygenation and shifts tissue down pressure gradients (herniations) that may crush vital brain centers and eventually cause respiratory or heart failure [4]. An aggressive treatment for raised ICP can reduce mortality and improve outcome [7, 8], although ICP control alone (i.e., osmotherapy) may be insufficient to benefit long-term recovery after brain injury [9]. This is probably because osmotherapy is unable to block the release of many toxic molecules that follow acute brain injury, such as glutamate, adenosine, oxyhemoglobin, thrombin, cytokines, reactive oxygen species (ROS), damage associated molecular pattern molecules (DAMPs), and others [10–40]. These molecules mediate BBB disruption and brain edema through multiple ligand-receptor pathways. Because brain edema might occur via many parallel pathways, blocking just one or two of these pathways may not be clinically effective in treating human brain injury [16].

Src family kinases (SFKs), a family of proto-oncogenic, non-receptor tyrosine kinases, include nine family members: c-Src, Fyn, Yes, Yrk, Lyn, Fgr, Hck, Blk, and Lck [41–43]. They can be activated by many trans-membrane receptors, such as adhesion receptors, tyrosine kinase receptors, G protein-coupled receptors, cytokine receptors, and others [44]. This makes SFKs a point of convergence for many molecules, and targeting SFKs has potential to prevent disruption of BBB components (i.e., endothelial cells, astrocytes, pericytes, neurons, tight junctions, and others) and block brain edema by modulating their multiple downstream targets, such as NMDA receptors [45–50], mitogen-activated protein kinases (MAPKs) [51–57], and cyclin-dependent kinases (Cdks) [58–62]. Many studies have demonstrated that acute administration of SFK inhibitors (e.g., PP1, PP2) attenuates BBB breakdown and prevents brain edema after acute brain injury [18–20, 63–66]. However, delayed and chronic administration of PP2 prevents BBB self-repair and lengthens the period to resolve the edema in the recovery stage after brain injury [20]. These findings suggest SFKs

D. Liu (✉) • B.P. Ander
Department of Neurology, M.I.N.D. Institute,
University of California at Davis Medical Center,
2805 50th Street, Sacramento, CA 95817, USA
e-mail: dzliu@ucdavis.edu

X. Zhang • B. Hu
Department of Neurology, The Second Affiliated Hospital,
Wenzhou Medical University, Wenzhou, China

R.L. Applegate et al. (eds.), *Brain Edema XVI: Translate Basic Science into Clinical Practice*, Acta Neurochirurgica Supplement, Vol. 121,
DOI 10.1007/978-3-319-18497-5_33, © Springer International Publishing Switzerland 2016

may play dual roles in both brain edema formation and resolution during different stages following acute brain injury (Fig. 1).

Tissue Specificity, Structure, Activity, and Functions of SFKs

Several SFK family members (c-Src, Fyn, Yes, Yrk) are ubiquitously expressed, whereas others (Lyn, Fgr, Hck, Blk, Lck) are generally found in brain and hematopoietic cells [47, 67–72]. In adult mice, Fyn and c-Src mRNA expression is highest in hippocampal neurons [73, 74]. Importantly, one tissue can express multiple SFK members, for example, Src, Fyn, Yes, and Lck have been examined in brain [47, 67–72], and the different SFK family members are often found to compensate for one another [75].

Structurally, SFK family members share a conserved domain structure consisting of consecutive SH3 (polyproline type II helix for protein-protein interaction), SH2 (phosphotyrosine recognition), and SH1 (tyrosine kinase catalytic activity) [43]. They also contain a membrane-targeting region at their N-terminus that is followed by a unique domain of 50–70 residues, which is divergent among family members [43]. Although still incompletely clear, Src activity is regulated by tyrosine phosphorylation at two sites (one is at Tyr416 in the SH1 domain, the other at Tyr527 in the short C-terminal tail), but with opposing effects. Whereas phosphorylation at Tyr416 activates Src, phosphorylation at Tyr527 results in inactivation [72, 76].

Under normal physiological conditions, SFKs are implicated in the regulation of embryonic development, cell growth, cellular differentiation, and inflammatory responses [74, 77–79]. SFKs can initiate negative feedback to prevent their sustained activation via recruitment of inhibitory factor C-terminal Src (Csk) [80]. The feedback loop consists of SFK activation leading to phosphorylation of Csk binding protein (Cbp), and the phosphorylated Cbp targets Csk to SFKs and promotes inhibitory Csk phosphorylation of SFKs [81].

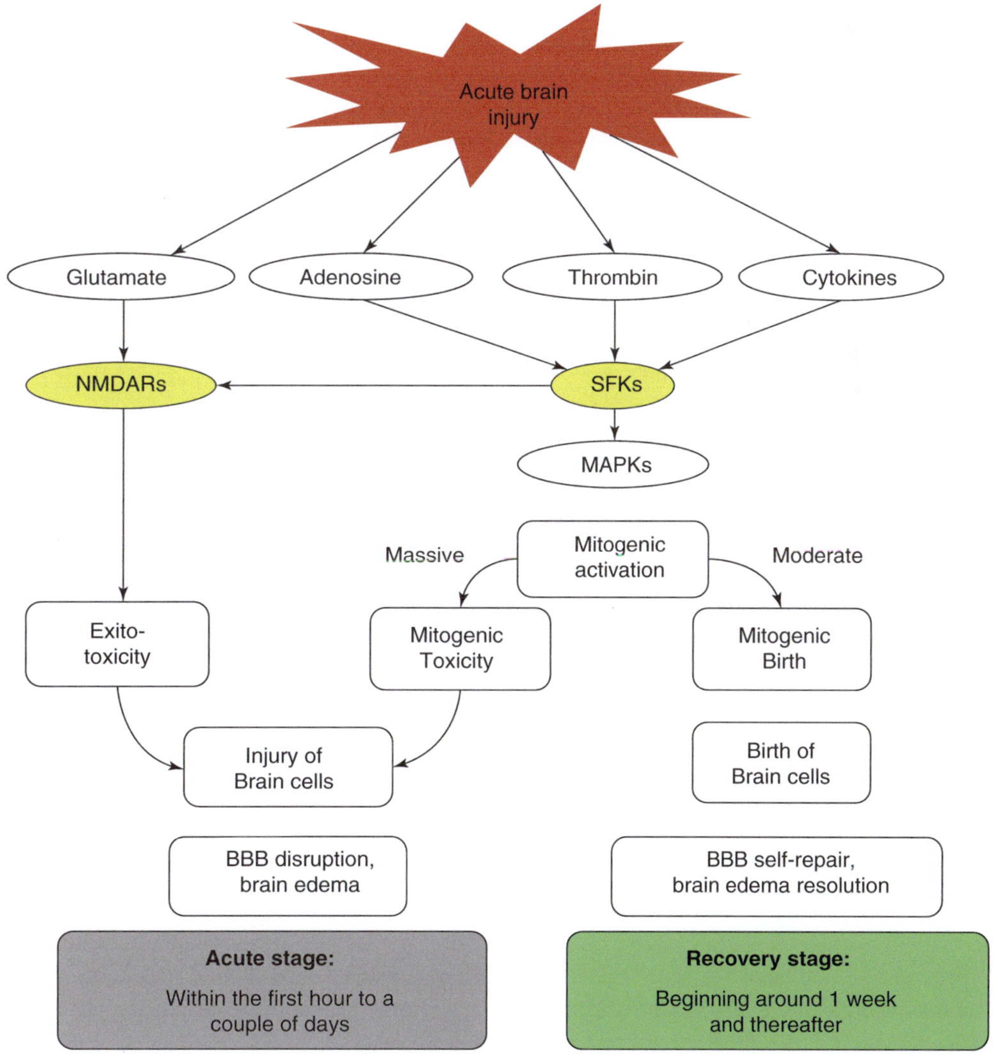

Fig. 1 Activation of SFKs results in BBB disruption and brain edema formation in the acute stage, but leads to BBB self-repair and brain edema resolution in the recovery stage after acute brain injury, such as ICH, TBI, and ischemic stroke

Because of mutations in SFKs or Csk, aberrant activation of SFKs can occur in cancers, and the abnormal SFK signaling contributes to many aspects of tumor development, including proliferation, survival, adhesion, migration, and invasion, as well as metastasis [82–84]. Thus, it is likely that targeting SFKs may be a promising therapeutic approach for cancer, as SFK antagonists have been tested and well tolerated in cancer clinical trials [85–88].

We and others have demonstrated a new function of SFKs in acute brain injury, that is, transient activation of SFKs associated with BBB disruption, brain edema, and spatial memory deficits after experimental ICH (intracerebroventricular fresh blood or thrombin model), TBI (lateral fluid percussion (LFP) model), and stroke (middle cerebral artery occlusion (MCAO) model) [18, 19, 63–66].

SFK Activation, Excitotoxicity, BBB Disruption, and Brain Edema

After acute brain injury (i.e., ICH, TBI, ischemic stroke), there occurs a transient increase of glucose utilization and local cerebral blood flow [53, 89, 90], presumably because of the actions of glutamate in blood at the time of brain injury. This was supported by findings that glucose hypermetabolism could be blocked by antagonists of NMDA and AMPA receptors [53, 90]. However, glutamate alone could not explain the hypermetabolism, inasmuch as glutamate injected directly into brain does not produce hypermetabolism [53]. This suggests that acute brain injury affects NMDA receptors in some way to make them more sensitive to glutamate so as to mediate brain injury and/or hypermetabolism.

A large number of studies have revealed that the molecules released after acute brain injury (e.g., adenosine, thrombin, cytokines) can activate SFKs [10–32], and SFKs directly bind NMDA receptors and modulate their activity [45–50]. Our data show that either an NMDA receptor inhibitor (MK801) or an SFK inhibitor (PP2) is able to prevent brain edema and improve behavioral outcomes after intracerebroventricular injection of thrombin in rats [19]. Therefore, it is plausible that SFKs and NMDA receptors are coupling to mediate calcium overload, glucose hypermetabolism, and brain edema after acute brain injury.

SFK Activation, Mitogenic Signaling, Brain Edema Formation, and Resolution

SFKs can be activated by many trans-membrane receptors, such as adhesion receptors, tyrosine kinase receptors, G protein-coupled receptors, cytokine receptors, and others [44]. This unique feature of SFKs makes them a point of convergence for many toxic molecules that are released after brain injury [10–40]. Most of these molecules are abruptly released and reach peak concentrations within a couple of hours to a day after brain injury. In the acute stage, overactivated SFK mitogenic signaling causes neurons to enter the cell cycle and die, and damages astroctyes and endothelial cells via MAPKs or CdKs [14, 19, 20, 51–62]. The disruption of BBB components increases BBB permeability, resulting in brain edema after acute brain injury.

Within about a day after acute brain injury, the molecules resolve gradually, and the disease progresses to a recovery stage of brain injury. The restored moderate SFK/mitogenic signaling leads to birth of new endothelial cells, astrocytes, and other cells that mediate BBB self-repair and brain edema resolution. Recent studies suggest that a number of stem cells exist throughout the mammalian brain, and some of these are associated with vascular niches [91]. Such stem cells could serve as a source of newborn endothelial cells, astrocytes, and other cells of the neurovascular unit that would play a major role in reestablishing the BBB after brain injury [92].

Although SFK inhibitors prevent toxicity signaling at the acute phase after ICH, they also block cellular proliferation of stem cells to delay and prolong BBB self-repair [55, 56, 93, 94]. This may provide at least a partial explanation for the findings that (1) acute single administration of SFK inhibitors (PP2, 1mg/kg, i.p. (intraperitoneally) immediately after ICH) can attenuate the BBB disruption and brain edema induced by intracerebroventricular injection of thrombin [20, 52] and (2) that delayed and chronic administration of SFK inhibitor (PP2, 1 mg/kg, i.p. daily, days 2 through 6) prevents thrombin-induced BBB repair and brain edema resolution in rats [20, 52].

Additionally, SFKs also activate hypoxia-inducible factors (HIFs) that can increase BBB permeability for brain edema formation or promote angiogenesis for brain edema resolution after brain injury through expression of aquaporins (AQPs), matrix metalloproteinases (MMPs), vascular endothelial growth factor (VEGF), BBB proteins (i.e., occluding), and others [95–97]. Interactions and cross-talk with these and other molecules and pathways add complexity to timing and development of appropriate treatment strategies involving the SFKs.

Future Directions

Future studies need to address exactly which specific SFK members found in brain (e.g., Src, Fyn, Lck, and Yrk) mediate edema after acute brain injury. In view of findings that SFKs also play critical roles in brain edema resolution, the therapeutic time window of SFK inhibition should be studied for treating edema following acute brain injury while avoiding the possible side effects caused by chronic inhibition of SFKs. A nanoparticle-based siRNA transfection system can be used for knockdown of individual SFK genes, as it allows transient knockdown of target genes, high efficiency of *in vivo* siRNA delivery, high specificity for gene targets, low cytotoxicity [98, 99], and is approved by the FDA for human use [100–103].

Disclosure The authors acknowledge the support of AHA Beginning Grant-in-Aid 12BGIA12060381 (DZL) and National Institutes of Health grant RO1NS089901 (DZL).

References

1. Marmarou A (2003) Pathophysiology of traumatic brain edema: current concepts. Acta Neurochir Suppl 86:7–10
2. Thiex R, Tsirka SE (2007) Brain edema after intracerebral hemorrhage: mechanisms, treatment options, management strategies, and operative indications. Neurosurg Focus 22, E6
3. Kasner SE, Demchuk AM, Berrouschot J, Schmutzhard E, Harms L et al (2001) Predictors of fatal brain edema in massive hemispheric ischemic stroke. Stroke 32:2117–2123
4. Donkin JJ, Vink R (2010) Mechanisms of cerebral edema in traumatic brain injury: therapeutic developments. Curr Opin Neurol 23:293–299
5. Rosenberg GA (1999) Ischemic brain edema. Prog Cardiovasc Dis 42:209–216
6. Iencean SM (2003) Brain edema – a new classification. Med Hypotheses 61:106–109
7. Sadaka F, Veremakis C (2012) Therapeutic hypothermia for the management of intracranial hypertension in severe traumatic brain injury: a systematic review. Brain Inj 26:899–908
8. Pitfield AF, Carroll AB, Kissoon N (2012) Emergency management of increased intracranial pressure. Pediatr Emerg Care 28:200–204; quiz 205–207
9. Sandsmark DK, Sheth KN (2014) Management of increased intracranial pressure. Curr Treat Options Neurol 16:272
10. Prins M, Greco T, Alexander D, Giza CC (2013) The pathophysiology of traumatic brain injury at a glance. Dis Model Mech 6:1307–1315
11. Namjoshi DR, Good C, Cheng WH, Panenka W, Richards D et al (2013) Towards clinical management of traumatic brain injury: a review of models and mechanisms from a biomechanical perspective. Dis Model Mech 6:1325–1338
12. Gaetz M (2004) The neurophysiology of brain injury. Clin Neurophysiol 115:4–18
13. Perel P, Roberts I, Bouamra O, Woodford M, Mooney J et al (2009) Intracranial bleeding in patients with traumatic brain injury: a prognostic study. BMC Emerg Med 9:15
14. Liu D, Sharp FR, Van KC, Ander BP, Ghiasvand R et al (2014) Inhibition of Src family kinases protects hippocampal neurons and improves cognitive function after traumatic brain injury. J Neurotrauma 31:1268–1276
15. NINDS (2013) Traumatic brain injury: hope through research. http://www.nindsnihgov/disorders/tbi/detail_tbihtm
16. Ray SK, Dixon CE, Banik NL (2002) Molecular mechanisms in the pathogenesis of traumatic brain injury. Histol Histopathol 17:1137–1152
17. Xi G, Reiser G, Keep RF (2003) The role of thrombin and thrombin receptors in ischemic, hemorrhagic and traumatic brain injury: deleterious or protective? J Neurochem 84:3–9
18. Sharp F, Liu DZ, Zhan X, Ander BP (2008) Intracerebral hemorrhage injury mechanisms: glutamate neurotoxicity, thrombin, and Src. Acta Neurochir Suppl 105:43–46
19. Liu DZ, Cheng XY, Ander BP, Xu H, Davis RR et al (2008) Src kinase inhibition decreases thrombin-induced injury and cell cycle re-entry in striatal neurons. Neurobiol Dis 30:201–211
20. Liu DZ, Ander BP, Xu H, Shen Y, Kaur P et al (2010) Blood-brain barrier breakdown and repair by Src after thrombin-induced injury. Ann Neurol 67:526–533
21. Keep RF, Hua Y, Xi G (2012) Intracerebral haemorrhage: mechanisms of injury and therapeutic targets. Lancet Neurol 11:720–731
22. Yao X, Balamurugan P, Arvey A, Leslie C, Zhang L (2010) Heme controls the regulation of protein tyrosine kinases Jak2 and Src. Biochem Biophys Res Commun 403:30–35
23. Corcoran A, Cotter TG (2013) Redox regulation of protein kinases. FEBS J 280:1944–1965
24. Giannoni E, Chiarugi P (2014) Redox circuitries driving Src regulation. Antioxid Redox Signal 20(13):2011–2025
25. Johnson P, Cross JL (2009) Tyrosine phosphorylation in immune cells: direct and indirect effects on toll-like receptor-induced proinflammatory cytokine production. Crit Rev Immunol 29:347–367
26. Cabodi S, Di Stefano P, Leal Mdel P, Tinnirello A, Bisaro B et al (2010) Integrins and signal transduction. Adv Exp Med Biol 674:43–54
27. Page TH, Smolinska M, Gillespie J, Urbaniak AM, Foxwell BM (2009) Tyrosine kinases and inflammatory signalling. Curr Mol Med 9:69–85
28. Hou CH, Fong YC, Tang CH (2011) HMGB-1 induces IL-6 production in human synovial fibroblasts through c-Src, Akt and NF-kappaB pathways. J Cell Physiol 226:2006–2015
29. Banerjee S, de Freitas A, Friggeri A, Zmijewski JW, Liu G et al (2011) Intracellular HMGB1 negatively regulates efferocytosis. J Immunol 187:4686–4694
30. Musumeci D, Roviello GN, Montesarchio D (2014) An overview on HMGB1 inhibitors as potential therapeutic agents in HMGB1-related pathologies. Pharmacol Ther 141:347–357
31. Ibrahim ZA, Armour CL, Phipps S, Sukkar MB (2013) RAGE and TLRs: relatives, friends or neighbours? Mol Immunol 56:739–744
32. Zhong C, Zhao X, Van KC, Bzdega T, Smyth A et al (2006) NAAG peptidase inhibitor increases dialysate NAAG and reduces glutamate, aspartate and GABA levels in the dorsal hippocampus following fluid percussion injury in the rat. J Neurochem 97:1015–1025
33. Hua Y, Keep RF, Hoff JT, Xi G (2007) Brain injury after intracerebral hemorrhage: the role of thrombin and iron. Stroke 38:759–762
34. Matz PG, Fujimura M, Lewen A, Morita-Fujimura Y, Chan PH (2001) Increased cytochrome c-mediated DNA fragmentation and cell death in manganese-superoxide dismutase-deficient mice after exposure to subarachnoid hemolysate. Stroke 32:506–515
35. Wu J, Hua Y, Keep RF, Schallert T, Hoff JT et al (2002) Oxidative brain injury from extravasated erythrocytes after intracerebral hemorrhage. Brain Res 953:45–52
36. Jung KH, Chu K, Jeong SW, Han SY, Lee ST et al (2004) HMG-CoA reductase inhibitor, atorvastatin, promotes sensorimotor recovery, suppressing acute inflammatory reaction after experimental intracerebral hemorrhage. Stroke 35:1744–1749
37. Dziedzic T, Bartus S, Klimkowicz A, Motyl M, Slowik A et al (2002) Intracerebral hemorrhage triggers interleukin-6 and interleukin-10 release in blood. Stroke 33:2334–2335

38. Rincon F, Mayer SA (2004) Novel therapies for intracerebral hemorrhage. Curr Opin Crit Care 10:94–100
39. Castillo J, Davalos A, Alvarez-Sabin J, Pumar JM, Leira R et al (2002) Molecular signatures of brain injury after intracerebral hemorrhage. Neurology 58:624–629
40. Mayne M, Ni W, Yan HJ, Xue M, Johnston JB et al (2001) Antisense oligodeoxynucleotide inhibition of tumor necrosis factor-alpha expression is neuroprotective after intracerebral hemorrhage. Stroke 32:240–248
41. Oda H, Kumar S, Howley PM (1999) Regulation of the Src family tyrosine kinase Blk through E6AP-mediated ubiquitination. Proc Natl Acad Sci U S A 96:9557–9562
42. Biscardi JS, Ishizawar RC, Silva CM, Parsons SJ (2000) Tyrosine kinase signalling in breast cancer: epidermal growth factor receptor and c-Src interactions in breast cancer. Breast Cancer Res 2:203–210
43. Boggon TJ, Eck MJ (2004) Structure and regulation of Src family kinases. Oncogene 23:7918–7927
44. Tatosyan AG, Mizenina OA (2000) Kinases of the Src family: structure and functions. Biochemistry (Mosc) 65:49–58
45. Groveman BR, Feng S, Fang XQ, Pflueger M, Lin SX et al (2012) The regulation of N-methyl-D-aspartate receptors by Src kinase. FEBS J 279:20–28
46. Yu XM, Askalan R, Keil GJ 2nd, Salter MW (1997) NMDA channel regulation by channel-associated protein tyrosine kinase Src. Science 275:674–678
47. Salter MW, Kalia LV (2004) Src kinases: a hub for NMDA receptor regulation. Nat Rev Neurosci 5:317–328
48. Trepanier CH, Jackson MF, MacDonald JF (2012) Regulation of NMDA receptors by the tyrosine kinase Fyn. FEBS J 279:12–19
49. Choi UB, Xiao S, Wollmuth LP, Bowen ME (2011) Effect of Src kinase phosphorylation on disordered C-terminal domain of N-methyl-D-aspartic acid (NMDA) receptor subunit GluN2B protein. J Biol Chem 286:29904–29912
50. Liu Y, Wong TP, Aarts M, Rooyakkers A, Liu L et al (2007) NMDA receptor subunits have differential roles in mediating excitotoxic neuronal death both in vitro and in vivo. J Neurosci 27:2846–2857
51. Liu DZ, Ander BP (2011) Cell cycle phase transitions: signposts for aberrant cell cycle reentry in dying mature neurons. J Cytol Histol 2:5
52. Liu DZ, Sharp FR (2011) The dual role of SRC kinases in intracerebral hemorrhage. Acta Neurochir Suppl 111:77–81
53. Ardizzone TD, Lu A, Wagner KR, Tang Y, Ran R et al (2004) Glutamate receptor blockade attenuates glucose hypermetabolism in perihematomal brain after experimental intracerebral hemorrhage in rat. Stroke 35:2587–2591
54. Copani A, Nicoletti F (2005) Cell-cycle mechanisms and neuronal cell death. Kluwer Academic/Plenum, New York
55. Liu DZ, Ander BP (2012) Cell cycle inhibition without disruption of neurogenesis is a strategy for treatment of aberrant cell cycle diseases: an update. ScientificWorldJournal 2012:491737
56. Liu DZ, Ander BP, Sharp FR (2010) Cell cycle inhibition without disruption of neurogenesis is a strategy for treatment of central nervous system diseases. Neurobiol Dis 37:549–557
57. Rodriguez PL, Sahay S, Olabisi OO, Whitehead IP (2007) ROCK I-mediated activation of NF-kappaB by RhoB. Cell Signal 19:2361–2369
58. Grimmler M, Wang Y, Mund T, Cilensek Z, Keidel EM et al (2007) Cdk-inhibitory activity and stability of p27Kip1 are directly regulated by oncogenic tyrosine kinases. Cell 128:269–280
59. Kasahara K, Nakayama Y, Nakazato Y, Ikeda K, Kuga T et al (2007) Src signaling regulates completion of abscission in cytokinesis through ERK/MAPK activation at the midbody. J Biol Chem 282:5327–5339
60. Liu Z, Falola J, Zhu X, Gu Y, Kim LT et al (2004) Antiproliferative effects of Src inhibition on medullary thyroid cancer. J Clin Endocrinol Metab 89:3503–3509
61. Mishra R, Wang Y, Simonson MS (2005) Cell cycle signaling by endothelin-1 requires Src nonreceptor protein tyrosine kinase. Mol Pharmacol 67:2049–2056
62. Taylor SJ, Shalloway D (1993) The cell cycle and c-Src. Curr Opin Genet Dev 3:26–34
63. Ardizzone TD, Zhan X, Ander BP, Sharp FR (2007) SRC kinase inhibition improves acute outcomes after experimental intracerebral hemorrhage. Stroke 38:1621–1625
64. Park Y, Luo T, Zhang F, Liu C, Bramlett HM et al (2013) Downregulation of Src-kinase and glutamate-receptor phosphorylation after traumatic brain injury. J Cereb Blood Flow Metab 33:1642–1649
65. Bai Y, Xu G, Xu M, Li Q, Qin X (2014) Inhibition of Src phosphorylation reduces damage to the blood-brain barrier following transient focal cerebral ischemia in rats. Int J Mol Med 34:1473–1482
66. Kusaka G, Ishikawa M, Nanda A, Granger DN, Zhang JH (2004) Signaling pathways for early brain injury after subarachnoid hemorrhage. J Cereb Blood Flow Metab 24:916–925
67. Morse WR, Whitesides JG 3rd, LaMantia AS, Maness PF (1998) p59fyn and pp60c-src modulate axonal guidance in the developing mouse olfactory pathway. J Neurobiol 36:53–63
68. Encinas M, Tansey MG, Tsui-Pierchala BA, Comella JX, Milbrandt J et al (2001) c-Src is required for glial cell line-derived neurotrophic factor (GDNF) family ligand-mediated neuronal survival via a phosphatidylinositol-3 kinase (PI-3K)-dependent pathway. J Neurosci 21:1464–1472
69. Sperber BR, Boyle-Walsh EA, Engleka MJ, Gadue P, Peterson AC et al (2001) A unique role for Fyn in CNS myelination. J Neurosci 21:2039–2047
70. Heidinger V, Manzerra P, Wang XQ, Strasser U, Yu SP et al (2002) Metabotropic glutamate receptor 1-induced upregulation of NMDA receptor current: mediation through the Pyk2/Src-family kinase pathway in cortical neurons. J Neurosci 22:5452–5461
71. Rouer E (2010) Neuronal isoforms of Src, Fyn and Lck tyrosine kinases: a specific role for p56lckN in neuron protection. C R Biol 333:1–10
72. Parsons SJ, Parsons JT (2004) Src family kinases, key regulators of signal transduction. Oncogene 23:7906–7909
73. Umemori H, Wanaka A, Kato H, Takeuchi M, Tohyama M et al (1992) Specific expressions of Fyn and Lyn, lymphocyte antigen receptor-associated tyrosine kinases, in the central nervous system. Brain Res Mol Brain Res 16:303–310
74. Ross CA, Wright GE, Resh MD, Pearson RC, Snyder SH (1988) Brain-specific src oncogene mRNA mapped in rat brain by in situ hybridization. Proc Natl Acad Sci U S A 85:9831–9835
75. Stein PL, Vogel H, Soriano P (1994) Combined deficiencies of Src, Fyn, and Yes tyrosine kinases in mutant mice. Genes Dev 8:1999–2007
76. Hunter T (1987) A tail of two src's: mutatis mutandis. Cell 49:1–4
77. Okutani D, Lodyga M, Han B, Liu M (2006) Src protein tyrosine kinase family and acute inflammatory responses. Am J Physiol Lung Cell Mol Physiol 291:L129–L141
78. Salmond RJ, Filby A, Qureshi I, Caserta S, Zamoyska R (2009) T-cell receptor proximal signaling via the Src-family kinases, Lck and Fyn, influences T-cell activation, differentiation, and tolerance. Immunol Rev 228:9–22
79. Palacios EH, Weiss A (2004) Function of the Src-family kinases, Lck and Fyn, in T-cell development and activation. Oncogene 23:7990–8000
80. Place AT, Chen Z, Bakhshi FR, Liu G, O'Bryan JP et al (2011) Cooperative role of caveolin-1 and C-terminal Src kinase binding

protein in C-terminal Src kinase-mediated negative regulation of c-Src. Mol Pharmacol 80:665–672
81. Kaimachnikov NP, Kholodenko BN (2009) Toggle switches, pulses and oscillations are intrinsic properties of the Src activation/deactivation cycle. FEBS J 276:4102–4118
82. Zhang S, Yu D (2012) Targeting Src family kinases in anti-cancer therapies: turning promise into triumph. Trends Pharmacol Sci 33:122–128
83. Huveldt D, Lewis-Tuffin LJ, Carlson BL, Schroeder MA, Rodriguez F et al (2013) Targeting Src family kinases inhibits bevacizumab-induced glioma cell invasion. PLoS One 8, e56505
84. Park SI, Zhang J, Phillips KA, Araujo JC, Najjar AM et al (2008) Targeting SRC family kinases inhibits growth and lymph node metastases of prostate cancer in an orthotopic nude mouse model. Cancer Res 68:3323–3333
85. Herold CI, Chadaram V, Peterson BL, Marcom PK, Hopkins J et al (2011) Phase II trial of dasatinib in patients with metastatic breast cancer using real-time pharmacodynamic tissue biomarkers of Src inhibition to escalate dosing. Clin Cancer Res 17:6061–6070
86. Gucalp A, Sparano JA, Caravelli J, Santamauro J, Patil S et al (2011) Phase II trial of saracatinib (AZD0530), an oral SRC-inhibitor for the treatment of patients with hormone receptor-negative metastatic breast cancer. Clin Breast Cancer 11(5):306–311
87. Anbalagan M, Carrier L, Glodowski S, Hangauer D, Shan B et al (2011) KX-01, a novel Src kinase inhibitor directed toward the peptide substrate site, synergizes with tamoxifen in estrogen receptor alpha positive breast cancer. Breast Cancer Res Treat 132(2):391–409
88. Fujisaka Y, Onozawa Y, Kurata T, Yasui H, Goto I et al (2013) First report of the safety, tolerability, and pharmacokinetics of the Src kinase inhibitor saracatinib (AZD0530) in Japanese patients with advanced solid tumours. Invest New Drugs 31:108–114
89. Jiang XB, Ohno K, Qian L, Tominaga B, Kuroiwa T et al (2000) Changes in local cerebral blood flow, glucose utilization, and mitochondrial function following traumatic brain injury in rats. Neurol Med Chir (Tokyo) 40:16–28; discussion 28–19
90. Simon R, Shiraishi K (1990) N-methyl-D-aspartate antagonist reduces stroke size and regional glucose metabolism. Ann Neurol 27:606–611
91. Ohab JJ, Fleming S, Blesch A, Carmichael ST (2006) A neurovascular niche for neurogenesis after stroke. J Neurosci 26: 13007–13016
92. Palmer TD, Willhoite AR, Gage FH (2000) Vascular niche for adult hippocampal neurogenesis. J Comp Neurol 425:479–494
93. Bernabeu R, Sharp FR (2000) NMDA and AMPA/kainate glutamate receptors modulate dentate neurogenesis and CA3 synapsin-I in normal and ischemic hippocampus. J Cereb Blood Flow Metab 20:1669–1680
94. Liu J, Solway K, Messing RO, Sharp FR (1998) Increased neurogenesis in the dentate gyrus after transient global ischemia in gerbils. J Neurosci 18:7768–7778
95. Higashida T, Kreipke CW, Rafols JA, Peng C, Schafer S et al (2011) The role of hypoxia-inducible factor-1alpha, aquaporin-4, and matrix metalloproteinase-9 in blood-brain barrier disruption and brain edema after traumatic brain injury. J Neurosurg 114:92–101
96. Karni R, Dor Y, Keshet E, Meyuhas O, Levitzki A (2002) Activated pp60c-Src leads to elevated hypoxia-inducible factor (HIF)-1alpha expression under normoxia. J Biol Chem 277: 42919–42925
97. Madri JA (2009) Modeling the neurovascular niche: implications for recovery from CNS injury. J Physiol Pharmacol 60(Suppl 4):95–104
98. Hannon GJ (2002) RNA interference. Nature 418:244–251
99. Reynolds A, Leake D, Boese Q, Scaringe S, Marshall WS et al (2004) Rational siRNA design for RNA interference. Nat Biotechnol 22:326–330
100. de Fougerolles A, Vornlocher HP, Maraganore J, Lieberman J (2007) Interfering with disease: a progress report on siRNA-based therapeutics. Nat Rev Drug Discov 6:443–453
101. Eifler AC, Thaxton CS (2011) Nanoparticle therapeutics: FDA approval, clinical trials, regulatory pathways, and case study. Methods Mol Biol 726:325–338
102. Davis ME (2009) The first targeted delivery of siRNA in humans via a self-assembling, cyclodextrin polymer-based nanoparticle: from concept to clinic. Mol Pharm 6:659–668
103. Davis ME, Zuckerman JE, Choi CH, Seligson D, Tolcher A et al (2010) Evidence of RNAi in humans from systemically administered siRNA via targeted nanoparticles. Nature 464:1067–1070

Fucoidan from *Fucus vesiculosus* Fails to Improve Outcomes Following Intracerebral Hemorrhage in Mice

Sherrefa R. Burchell, Loretta O. Iniaghe, John H. Zhang, and Jiping Tang

Introduction

Intracerebral hemorrhage (ICH), the second most common form of stroke, accounting for 15–20 % of all stroke subtypes [38, 44], results from the rupture of small blood vessels within the basal ganglia, thalamus, pons, or cerebellum. This leads to the development of a hematoma, which may expand over time following the initial ictus [18]. Intracerebral hemorrhaging can also lead to a sudden increase in intracranial pressure, resulting in headaches, nausea, vomiting, unconsciousness, and death [17]. These fatal outcomes make ICH the least treatable and most mortal subtype, being associated with a 40–50 % mortality rate at 30 days [14, 41, 49]. After the first year, more than 75 % of patients are deceased or severely injured [58]; and of those who survive, 80 % do not regain normal function [14].

The hematoma is the main source of primary brain injury following ICH, as it causes mechanical damage to the surrounding tissue, and expansion of the hematoma can be an independent determinant of functional outcome [16, 52]. Immediately after hematoma formation, inflammation begins, and this also plays a major role in the pathophysiology of ICH, contributing to secondary brain injury and resulting in significant neurological deficits [9]. Current therapies for ICH have not been very successful. Consequently, it is imperative that an effective therapy be established to protect against the devastating sequelae of ICH.

Fucoidans are sulfated polysaccharides extracted from different species of brown seaweed. They are known to exhibit various biological properties: anticoagulant, anti-inflammatory, antiviral, antitumoral, and antioxidant [3, 15, 32]. Fucoidan, from *Fucus vesiculosus*, was reported to be a novel agonist of the platelet C-type Lectin-like receptor 2 (CLEC-2) [37], which may play a role in limiting bleeding after injury; thus, we aimed to investigate whether fucoidan from *Fucus vesiculosus* could reduce hemorrhaging after ICH. Additionally, fucoidan is known to exhibit anti-inflammatory characteristics. Therefore, we also aimed to examine whether fucoidan is neuroprotective, attenuating neurological deficits by reducing injury from inflammation after experimental intracerebral hemorrhage in mice.

Methods

Animals

All procedures were conducted in accordance with the NIH *Guide for the Care and Use of Laboratory Animals* and were approved by the Institutional Animal Care and Use Committee of Loma Linda University. Male CD-1 mice weighing 30–40 g ($n=70$) (Charles River, Wilmington, MA, USA) were housed in a light- and temperature-controlled environment with access to food and water *ad libitum*.

S.R. Burchell, BSc
Department of Physiology and Pharmacology, Loma Linda University, Loma Linda, CA, USA

L.O. Iniaghe, MSc
Department of Physiology and Pharmacology, Loma Linda University, Loma Linda, CA, USA

Department of Pharmacology and Toxicology, University of Benin, Benin City, Nigeria

J.H. Zhang, MD, PhD
Department of Physiology and Pharmacology, Loma Linda University, Loma Linda, CA, USA

Department of Neurosurgery, Loma Linda University, Loma Linda, CA, USA

J. Tang, MD (✉)
Department of Physiology and Pharmacology, Loma Linda University School of Medicine, Loma Linda, CA 92350, USA
e-mail: jtang@llu.edu

R.L. Applegate et al. (eds.), *Brain Edema XVI: Translate Basic Science into Clinical Practice*, Acta Neurochirurgica Supplement, Vol. 121,
DOI 10.1007/978-3-319-18497-5_34, © Springer International Publishing Switzerland 2016

Intracerebral Hemorrhage Induction

Experimental ICH was induced in mice by intrastriatal infusion of bacterial collagenase, as previously reported [29, 36]. Briefly, animals were anesthetized by intraperitoneal (IP) co-injection of ketamine (100 mg/kg) and xylazine (10 mg/kg). The skull was exposed by a midline scalp incision, and the skin was retracted laterally. Mice were placed in a prone position and a 1 mm cranial burr hole was made at the following coordinates, relative to the bregma: 0.2 mm rostral and 2.2 mm lateral. A 27-Gauge needle (Hamilton Company, Reno, NV, USA) was inserted ventrally 3.5 mm below the dura. Using a Namonite Syringe Pump (Harvard Apparatus, Holliston, MA, USA), 0.075 U of bacterial collagenase (Type VII-S, Sigma-Aldrich, St. Louis, MO, USA), dissolved in 0.75 µl saline, was infused into the right basal ganglia at a rate of 0.25 µl/min. The needle was left in place for 5 min after the completion of infusion to prevent the backflow of bacterial collagenase along the needle tract, and then withdrawn slowly, at a rate of 1 mm/min. The burr hole was sealed with bone wax, the incision site was closed with uninterrupted sutures, and the animals were allowed to recover under observation. Sham operation was performed with needle insertion only.

Experimental Groups

Animals were randomly divided into the following groups: sham, ICH + vehicle, and ICH + fucoidan (25, 75, and 100 mg/kg [33]. Fucoidan (from *Fucus vesiculosus*) was purchased from Sigma Aldrich (St. Louis, MO, USA) and dissolved in 5 % dimethyl sulfoxide (DMSO). The drug was administered by IP injection at a dose of 25, 75, or 100 mg/kg. Vehicle animals received the same volume of 5 % DMSO. All treatments were given at 1 h after ICH.

Brain Water Content (BWC) Evaluation

Brain water content was measured as described previously [56]. Mice were decapitated under deep anesthesia and the brains quickly removed. A 4-mm section around the point of injection was sliced and divided into five parts: ipsilateral and contralateral basal ganglia, ipsilateral and contralateral cortex, and cerebellum. The cerebellum was used as an internal control. All brain samples were weighed using an analytical microbalance (APX-60 Denver Instrument, Bohemia, NY, USA) to obtain the wet weight (WW). Tissues were then dried at 100 °C for 24 h and the dry weight (DW) obtained. BWC was calculated as (WW-DW)/WW × 100.

Neurobehavioral Assessment

Sensorimotor deficits were evaluated at 24 h after induction of ICH. An observer blinded to the treatment groups conducted the behavior tests.

Modified Garcia Neuroscore

The modified Garcia neuroscore consists of seven (7) individual tests, which evaluate the animal's spontaneous activity, body sensation, vibrissae proprioception, fore and hind limb symmetry, lateral turning, forelimb outstretching, and climbing. Each sub-test was scored from 0 (worst performance) to 3 (best performance), for a composite total of 21 points for the Garcia neuroscore [20, 51].

Corner Turn Test

Mice were allowed to approach a 30° corner made out of two Plexiglas walls. To exit the corner, animals had to turn either to the right or left side. The choice of turning was recorded for 10 trials and the score calculated as number of left turns/all turns x 100 [24, 51].

Forelimb Placement Test

Mice were evaluated for their reflexive motor ability to vibrissae stimulation by forward movement of their paws [24, 51]. Animals were held by the trunk, ensuring the forelimbs were not restrained, then oriented parallel to a table top and slowly moved vertically until the vibrissae on one side touched the surface. The number of successful left (contralateral) paw placements out of 10 consecutive vibrissae stimulations was recorded.

Hemoglobin Assay

The hemoglobin assay was conducted as previously described [56], with modifications. Twenty-four hours after ICH, mice were deeply anesthetized and transcardially perfused with ice-cold phosphate-buffered saline (PBS) and the brains were removed, snap-frozen with liquid nitrogen, and stored at −80 °C until the time of evaluation. To each sample, 1000 µL of PBS was added, and they were homogenized for 30 s, followed by 1 min of sonication on ice with an ultrasonicator.

Samples were centrifuged for 30 min at 14,000 g, and the supernatant collected. Then, 800 μL of Drabkin's reagent (Sigma Aldrich, St. Louis, MO, USA) was added to a 200 μL aliquot of the sample. The solution was allowed to react for 15 min and then measured on a spectrophotomer (Thermo Fisher Scientific Inc., Waltham, MA, USA) at an absorbance wavelength of 540 nm to assess hemoglobin content.

Statistical Analysis

Data are expressed as mean ± standard error of the mean (SEM) and were analyzed using one-way analysis of variance (ANOVA) followed by Tukey post hoc multiple comparison test. A p-value < 0.05 was considered statistically significant. All statistical analyses were conducted using GraphPad Prism Software, Version 6.0 for Mac.

Results

Fucoidan Treatment Did Not Ameliorate the ICH-Induced Increase in BWC at 24 h

ICH induced a significant increase in brain water content in the ipsilateral basal ganglia, in comparison to sham animals ($p<0.05$). Fucoidan treatment did not attenuate this increase in BWC, with these mice also having significantly higher brain water content than sham ($p<0.05$) (Fig. 1).

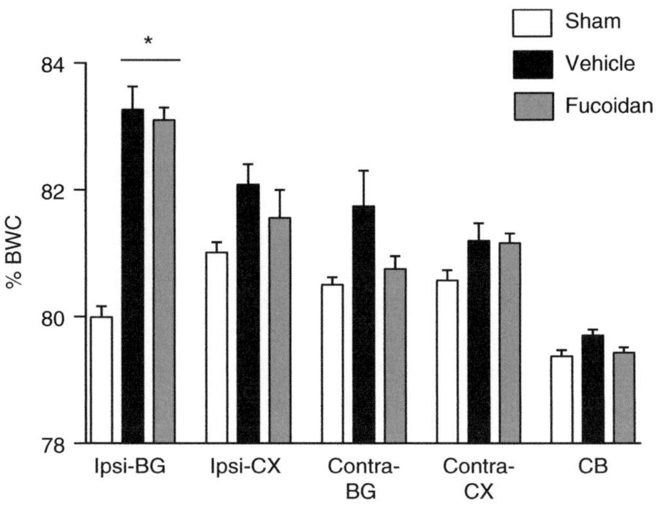

Fig. 1 Effect of fucoidan on brain water content (BWC) 24 h after ICH. There was a significant increase in brain water content in the ipsilateral basal ganglia after ICH. The fucoidan-treated group displayed a similar increase in BWC; treatment did not reverse the effects of ICH. Data are represented as mean ± SEM ($n=7$/group; $*=p<0.05$ vs. sham). *Ipsi-BG* ipsilateral basal ganglia, *Ipsi-CX* ipsilateral cortex, *Contra-BG* contralateral basal ganglia, *Contra-CX* contralateral cortex, *CB* cerebellum

Fucoidan Failed to Improve Neurological Outcomes at 24 h

Significant sensorimotor deficits were observed at 24 h after ICH in all behavior tests ($p<0.05$ vs. sham) (Fig. 2). Treatment with fucoidan at doses of 25, 75, and 100 mg/kg was not able to improve Garcia neuroscores ($p<0.05$ vs. sham) (Fig. 2a). Fucoidan was also not able to improve neurofunctional outcome in the corner turn and forelimb placement tests at 24 h with all three doses (Fig. 2b, c).

Treatment with Fucoidan Did Not Affect Hemoglobin Content 24 h after ICH

The hemoglobin content in the ipsilateral hemisphere of ICH mice was significantly increased compared with sham ($p<0.05$). Fucoidan at 100 mg/kg did not alter the hemoglobin content, in comparison to vehicle-treated animals ($p<0.05$ vs. sham) (Fig. 3).

Discussion

In the present study, we examined the effects of fucoidan, a polysaccharide isolated from the brown seaweed *Fucus vesiculosus*, on outcomes following experimental ICH in mice. We found that fucoidan failed to improve the worsened neurological outcomes induced by ICH and had no effect on brain water or hemoglobin contents.

Intracerebral hemorrhage most commonly affects the basal ganglia, as mimicked by our mouse model, and is well known to result in significant sensorimotor deficits, as well as a drastic deterioration in learning and memory capabilities [5, 53]. The collagenase infusion model of ICH employed in this study is clinically significant as it mimics the spontaneous vessel rupture and the re-bleeding that occurs post ictus [36]. ICH induces both primary and secondary brain injury: primary injury mainly from the mechanical disruption and mass effect of the hematoma [4], and secondary brain injury from the metabolic products of heme/erythrocyte breakdown [60]. Secondary brain injury involves edema formation and an infiltration of inflammatory cells around the hematoma [4, 29]. The cytotoxic products of inflammation after ICH all contribute to neuronal injury and death [22]. Moreover,

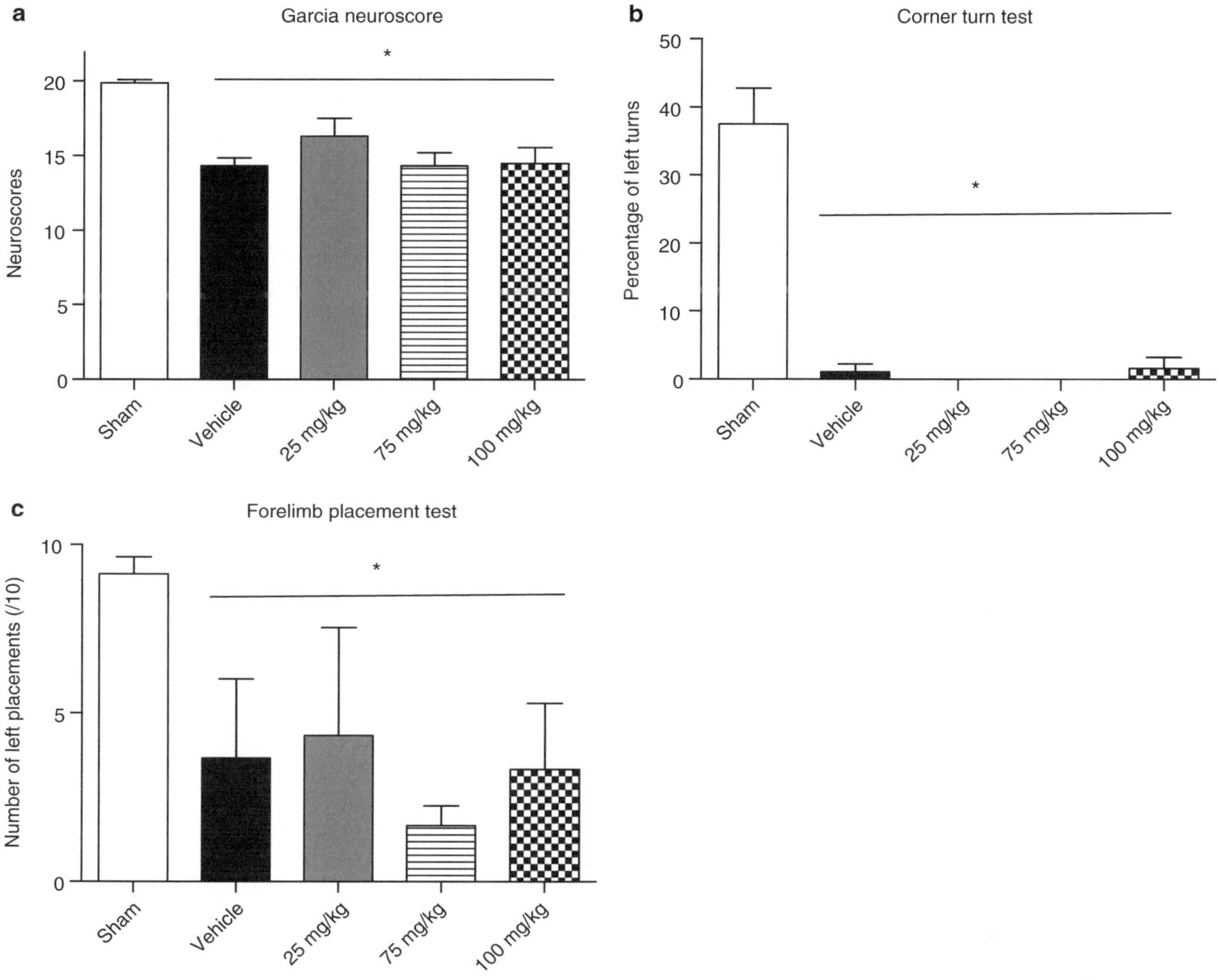

Fig. 2 Effect of treating with fucoidan on neurological function 24 h after ICH. ICH resulted in significant loss of neurological function, as assessed by Garcia neuroscore (**a**), corner turn test (**b**), and forelimb placement test (**c**). Mice were treated with 25, 75, or 100 mg/kg fucoidan, which failed to improve the sensorimotor deficits induced by ICH. Data are represented as mean ± SEM (n = 5–9/group; * = p < 0.05 vs. sham)

hematoma formation and the increased inflammation after ICH contribute to the occurrence of brain edema (increased brain water content) by reducing the integrity of the blood-brain barrier (BBB) [8, 64]. Thus, anti-inflammatory agents can alleviate BBB disruption and reverse the ICH-induced increase in BWC [9].

Fucoidan from *Fucus vesiculosus* has been shown to exhibit anti-inflammatory activities [15, 33, 35]; therefore, we hypothesized that treatment with this drug would provide neuroprotection after ICH by reducing inflammation. Additionally, Manne et al. [37] reported that fucoidan is a novel receptor for the platelet C-type Lectin-like receptor 2, which induces platelet aggregation upon activation. We proposed that this would result in a reduction in hematoma expansion after ICH, thus improving outcomes. We found that fucoidan treatment (at 25, 75, and 100 mg/kg) failed to attenuate neurological deficits after ICH, and had no effect on brain water content and hemorrhaging, thus making null our hypotheses.

Edible seaweeds are a rich source of dietary fiber and have been historically used in the diet and as traditional medicine, particularly in some Asian countries [7, 26, 65]. In brown seaweeds, the dietary fiber is composed of soluble polysaccharides such as alginates, fucans, and laminarans, along with insoluble fibers mainly made of cellulose. Fucans are cell wall polysaccharides that are classified into three families: fucoidans (homofucans), ascophyllans, and glycuronofuco-galactans sulfate. Fucoidans are fucose-containing sulfated polysaccharides (FCSPs), which consist mainly of a backbone of (1-3)- and (1-4)-linked α-L-fucopyranose residues that may be substituted with sulfate, single L-fucosyl residues, and/or short fucoside chains [3].

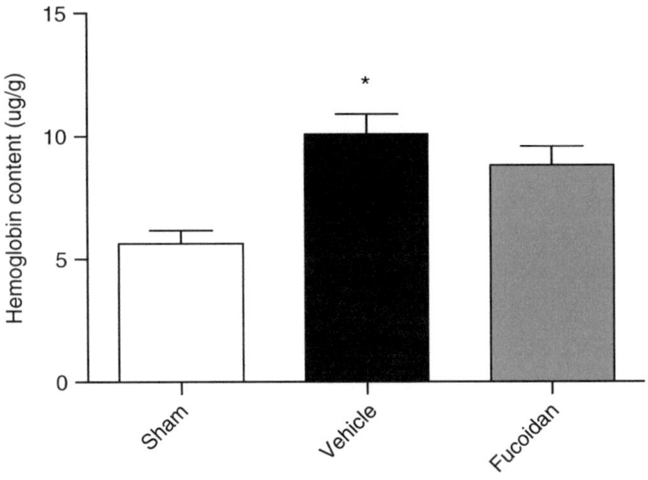

Fig. 3 Effect of fucoidan treatment on hemoglobin content 24 h after ICH. ICH significantly increased hemoglobin content in comparison with sham. Treatment with fucoidan was not able to attenuate this increase. Data are represented as mean ± SEM ($n = 5–9$/group; $* = p < 0.05$ vs. sham)

Research on fucoidan has increased greatly in the last decade, due to interest in its varied potentially beneficial biological activities [3]. Despite this, the mechanisms of fucoidan, and the particular structures or fractions that are responsible for different biological activities, are still unclear, owing to a lack of standardized extraction and purification protocols.

Li et al. [33] reported that fucoidan was protective in myocardial ischemia/reperfusion (I/R) injury through its anti-inflammatory properties; fucoidan treatment reduced the levels of tumor necrosis factor-α (TNF-α), interleukin-6 (IL-6), phospho-IκB-α, nuclear factor-κB (NF-κB), and the activity of myeloperoxidase (pro-inflammatory), while increasing the expression of IL-10 (an anti-inflammatory cytokine) following myocardial I/R. It has also been shown that treatment with fucoidan attenuated experimental autoimmune myocarditis by inhibiting macrophage and CD4-positive T-cell infiltration into the myocardium, thus exhibiting its anti-inflammatory actions [55]. Additionally, the anti-inflammatory effects of fucoidan were shown through its reduction of nitric oxide, prostaglandin E2, cyclooxygenase 2, and pro-inflammatory cytokines in lipopolysaccharide-induced BV2 microglia cells; the treatment also suppressed NF-κB activation and downregulation of ERK, JNK, p38 MAPK, and AKT pathways [46]. The regulation of the NF-κB signaling pathway by fucoidan was shown to be protective against diabetic nephropathy both in vivo and in vitro as well [59]. Furthermore, Raghavendran et al. [50] reported that pretreatment with fucoidan provided protection against aspirin-induced gastric mucosal damage in rats through its immunomodulatory actions on interleukins, TNF-α, and interferon-γ (IFN-γ). It was against this background of significant protection by fucoidan in various models that we speculated that fucoidan would exhibit its anti-inflammatory actions after ICH and be neuroprotective. However, our results revealed an opposite effect: fucoidan failed to ameliorate deficits after ICH.

We postulate that this may be for several reasons. Firstly, the bioactive properties of fucoidan depend on its purity, sugar composition, degree of sulfation, and molecular weight [63]. Controversies exist about the therapeutic benefits of high- versus low-molecular-weight fucoidans [11, 25, 47, 65]. Generally, however, low-molecular-weight fucoidan (<10 kDa) has been shown to have more therapeutic potential than high-molecular-weight fucoidan (>18 kDa) [7, 23, 28, 62]. In this study, we used the crude version of fucoidan from Sigma Aldrich, which has a high molecular weight of 20–200 kDa. Thus, the therapeutic potential was possibly decreased.

Additionally, fucoidan from *Fucus vesiculosus* is known to have powerful anticoagulant activity, comparable to heparin, a sulfated glycosaminoglycan, with which it shares a similar structure [13, 30, 31, 42], making it a part of the group of heparinoids. The anticoagulant activity of fucoidan is related to antithrombin and heparin cofactor II-mediated activity, and it has been investigated as a possible replacement therapy for heparin clinically [21, 39, 43]. Importantly, it was demonstrated that higher-molecular-weight FCSPs (28 kDa and 50 kDa) have higher anticoagulant activity than lower-molecular-weight FCSPs (10 kDa) [45]. In fact, cleavage of fucans by only a small amount greatly reduced their effect on thrombin inactivation mediated by heparin cofactor II [48]. These data suggest that the high-molecular-weight fucoidan may have been exerting its anticoagulant actions in our ICH model, and this accounts for our finding that there was no reduction in hemoglobin content with treatment. The hemoglobin assay we utilized measures the absorbance of hemoglobin as a quantification of ICH and can be used to evaluate the effectiveness of potential thrombolytic or anticoagulant therapies [12]. Because our initial hypothesis was that fucoidan might reduce hemorrhaging via its activity on the platelet receptor CLEC-2 [37], we conducted the hemoglobin assay to test this outcome. Based on our contrasting findings, we postulate that the anticoagulant effect of crude fucoidan may be stronger than its potential procoagulant ability, especially because of its larger size, and/or that fucoidan exhibits its effects through various other pathways. It has been established that platelet CLEC-2 activates spleen tyrosine kinase (Syk), lymphocyte cystolic protein 2 (SLP-76), and phospholipase C (PLC)-γ downstream [6, 40, 54], while fucoidan has been shown to activate other downstream signaling pathways, including inhibition of the PI3K-Akt-mTOR pathway [32, 46, 57] and caspase and ERK pathways [1, 34], indicating that it functions via another receptor(s). L-selectin and P-selectin are known to be receptors for fucoidan [19], but are not defined as the only receptors for the polysaccharide, as inhibition of L-selectin did not reverse the inhibitory effect of fucoidan on proliferation, suggesting this occurred via activation of another receptor [1]. Alternatively, Zhang and colleagues [63] conducted a study evaluating the structure-activity relationship of the pro- and anticoagulant activity of fucoidan from *Fucus vesiculosus* and found that the polysaccharide could be pro- or anticoagulant, depending on its charge density, molecular weight, and sugar composition. Hence, in our report, fucoidan's anticoagulant effects seem to outweigh its potential procoagulant activity. This, interestingly, coincides with a study by Cheng and colleagues [10], in which they found that the extravascular effects of thrombin, which is known to exacerbate ischemic injury and is a possible target for the prevention of hemorrhagic transformation (owing to its role in hemostasis), resulted in ICH, implying that this effect could outweigh the normal hemostatic effects of thrombin.

Another reason we propose that fucoidan treatment was not neuroprotective in our study is that it has been shown to have proapoptotic effects in various cancers [1, 2, 27, 61]. In colon cancer cells, fucoidan was reported to attenuate the levels of the X-linked inhibitor of apoptosis protein and survivin, which both play a role in cell survival [27]. Treatment with fucoidan also enhanced mitochondrial membrane permeability, and increased levels of Bak and truncated Bid, as well as tumor necrosis factor-related apoptosis-inducing ligand, in these cells, all of which are signals for cell death [27]. In human breast cancer cell lines, fucoidan treatment increased the expression of truncated Bid, and induced activation of caspases 7, 8, and 9, along with other cell death mechanisms [61]. Further, crude fucoidan was shown to reduce cell viability in lung carcinoma and melanoma cells, and to activate natural killer cell activity in mice *in vivo* [2]. These data suggest that fucoidan could have enhanced the apoptotic pathways occurring after ICH, increasing cell death. The heightened loss of neurons could then account for the significant neurological deficits (including the reduction in learning and memory capabilities) and the lack of amelioration with fucoidan treatment. Conversely, it has been reported that low-molecular-weight fucoidan (at 50 and 100 mg/kg/day for 3 months) alleviated cardiac dysfunction in diabetic cardiomyopathy in rats by reducing reactive oxygen species production and cardiomyocyte apoptosis [62]. Low-molecular-weight fucoidan also ameliorated injuries from renal I/R via inhibition of the MAPK signaling pathway, which resulted in reduced ratios of Bax/Bcl2 and cleaved caspase-3/caspase-3 [7]. Moreover, Li et al. [34] found that fucoidan protected ARPE-19 cells from glucose-induced oxidative stress and apoptosis through a Ca^{2+}-dependent ERK signaling pathway. This coincides with our previous discussion that our treatment was ineffective against ICH due largely to its higher molecular weight. However, these conflicting results on the effects of fucoidan treatment also highlight the fact that the mechanisms of its activity are still not completely understood, and more studies are needed on the molecular weights and particular fractions of fucoidan that may be most beneficial in the varying pathologies.

Our study has several limitations. Several groups have treated with fucoidan chronically (over several days) and found improvements in outcomes [7, 62]. It would therefore be prudent to examine whether chronic fucoidan treatment may be neuroprotective after ICH. Additionally, it may be beneficial to fractionate the crude fucoidan and examine the effects of the various fractions on outcomes after ICH. Finally, another approach to the study would be to investigate the effects of low-molecular-weight fucoidan on ICH-induced inflammation, edema, hematoma expansion, and neurological deficits.

Conclusion

We examined the effects of fucoidan from *Fucus vesiculosus* on brain water content, hemorrhaging, and neurological outcomes after ICH. Our findings revealed that fucoidan did not reduce brain water or hemoglobin contents after ICH, nor did it attenuate neurological deficits. Although there have been various studies highlighting the protective effects of fucoidan through its anti-inflammatory activities, we conclude that our findings were contradicting because of the use of crude fucoidan, which has a high molecular weight and may be proapoptotic and anticoagulant, essentially negating any anti-inflammatory effects. Low-molecular-weight fucoidan has shown greater therapeutic efficacy. Additionally, there are various fractions of fucoidan and multiple ways of fractionating, making it hard to differentiate the effects of this treatment and highlighting the need for more studies to determine which fraction of fucoidan shows the most therapeutic potential.

Conflicts of Interest The authors declare no conflicts of interest.

Funding This work was funded by National Institutes of Health grant NS082184 to JHZ and JT.

References

1. Aisa Y, Miyakawa Y, Nakazato T, Shibata H, Saito K, Ikeda Y, Kizaki M (2005) Fucoidan induces apoptosis of human HS-sultan cells accompanied by activation of caspase-3 and down-regulation of ERK pathways. Am J Hematol 78:7–14
2. Ale MT, Maruyama H, Tamauchi H, Mikkelsen JD, Meyer AS (2011) Fucoidan from *Sargassum* sp. and *Fucus vesiculosus* reduces cell viability of lung carcinoma and melanoma cells in vitro and activates natural killer cells in mice in vivo. Int J Biol Macromol 49:331–336

3. Ale MT, Mikkelsen JD, Meyer AS (2011) Important determinants for fucoidan bioactivity: a critical review of structure-function relations and extraction methods for fucose-containing sulfated polysaccharides from brown seaweeds. Mar Drugs 9:2106–2130
4. Aronowski J, Zhao X (2011) Molecular pathophysiology of cerebral hemorrhage: secondary brain injury. Stroke 42:1781–1786
5. Bhatia KP, Marsden CD (1994) The behavioural and motor consequences of focal lesions of the basal ganglia in man. Brain 117:859–876
6. Boulaftali Y, Hess PR, Getz TM, Cholka A, Stolla M, Mackman N, Owens AP 3rd, Ware J, Kahn ML, Bergmeier W (2013) Platelet ITAM signaling is critical for vascular integrity in inflammation. J Clin Invest 123:908–916
7. Chen J, Wang W, Zhang Q, Li F, Lei T, Luo D, Zhou H, Yang B (2013) Low molecular weight fucoidan against renal ischemia-reperfusion injury via inhibition of the MAPK signaling pathway. PLoS One 8, e56224
8. Chen Q, Zhang J, Guo J, Tang J, Tao Y, Li L, Feng H, Chen Z (2014) Chronic hydrocephalus and perihematomal tissue injury developed in a rat model of intracerebral hemorrhage with ventricular extension. Transl Stroke Res 6:125–32
9. Chen S, Yang Q, Chen G, Zhang JH (2015) An update on inflammation in the acute phase of intracerebral hemorrhage. Transl Stroke Res 6:4–8
10. Cheng Y, Xi G, Jin H, Keep RF, Feng J, Hua Y (2014) Thrombin-induced cerebral hemorrhage: role of protease-activated receptor-1. Transl Stroke Res 5:472–475
11. Cho ML, Lee BY, You SG (2010) Relationship between oversulfation and conformation of low and high molecular weight fucoidans and evaluation of their in vitro anticancer activity. Molecules 16:291–297
12. Choudhri TF, Hoh BL, Solomon RA, Connolly ES, Pinsky DJ (1997) Use of a spectrophotometric hemoglobin assay to objectively quantify intracerebral hemorrhage in mice. Stroke 28:2296–2302
13. Church FC, Meade JB, Treanor RE, Whinna HC (1989) Antithrombin activity of fucoidan. The interaction of fucoidan with heparin cofactor II, antithrombin III, and thrombin. J Biol Chem 264:3618–3623
14. Counsell C, Sandercock P (1995) Use of anticoagulants in patients with acute ischemic stroke. Stroke 26:522–523
15. Cumashi A, Ushakova NA, Preobrazhenskaya ME, D'Incecco A, Piccoli A, Totani L, Tinari N, Morozevich GE, Berman AE, Bilan MI, Usov AI, Ustyuzhanina NE, Grachev AA, Sanderson CJ, Kelly M, Rabinovich GA, Iacobelli S, Nifantiev NE, Consorzio Interuniversitario Nazionale per la Bio-Oncologia, Italy (2007) A comparative study of the anti-inflammatory, anticoagulant, antiangiogenic, and antiadhesive activities of nine different fucoidans from brown seaweeds. Glycobiology 17:541–552
16. Davis SM, Broderick J, Hennerici M, Brun NC, Diringer MN, Mayer SA, Begtrup K, Steiner T, Recombinant Activated Factor VIIIHTI (2006) Hematoma growth is a determinant of mortality and poor outcome after intracerebral hemorrhage. Neurology 66:1175–1181
17. Elijovich L, Patel PV, Hemphill JC 3rd (2008) Intracerebral hemorrhage. Semin Neurol 28:657–667
18. Emiru T, Bershad EM, Zantek ND, Datta YH, Rao GH, Hartley EW, Divani AA (2013) Intracerebral hemorrhage: a review of coagulation function. Clin Appl Thromb Hemost 19:652–662
19. Frenette PS, Weiss L (2000) Sulfated glycans induce rapid hematopoietic progenitor cell mobilization: evidence for selectin-dependent and independent mechanisms. Blood 96:2460–2468
20. Garcia JH, Wagner S, Liu KF, Xj H (1995) Neurological deficit and extent of neuronal necrosis attributable to middle cerebral artery occlusion in rats: statistical validation. Stroke 26:627–635
21. Grauffel V, Kloareg B, Mabeau S, Durand P, Jozefonvicz J (1989) New natural polysaccharides with potent antithrombic activity: fucans from brown algae. Biomaterials 10:363–368
22. Guo-Yuan Y, Betz AL, Thomas LC, James AB, Julian TH (1994) Experimental intracerebral hemorrhage: relationship between brain edema, blood flow, and blood-brain barrier permeability in rats. J Neurosurg 81:93–102
23. Hlawaty H, Suffee N, Sutton A, Oudar O, Haddad O, Ollivier V, Laguillier-Morizot C, Gattegno L, Letourneur D, Charnaux N (2011) Low molecular weight fucoidan prevents intimal hyperplasia in rat injured thoracic aorta through the modulation of matrix metalloproteinase-2 expression. Biochem Pharmacol 81:233–243
24. Hua Y, Schallert T, Keep RF, Wu J, Hoff JT, Xi G (2002) Behavioral tests after intracerebral hemorrhage in the rat. Stroke 33:2478–2484
25. Jang JY, Moon SY, Joo HG (2014) Differential effects of fucoidans with low and high molecular weight on the viability and function of spleen cells. Food Chem Toxicol 68:234–238
26. Jiao G, Yu G, Zhang J, Ewart HS (2011) Chemical structures and bioactivities of sulfated polysaccharides from marine algae. Mar Drugs 9:196–223
27. Kim EJ, Park SY, Lee JY, Park JH (2010) Fucoidan present in brown algae induces apoptosis of human colon cancer cells. BMC Gastroenterol 10:96
28. Kim KJ, Yoon KY, Lee BY (2012) Low molecular weight fucoidan from the sporophyll of *Undaria pinnatifida* suppresses inflammation by promoting the inhibition of mitogen-activated protein kinases and oxidative stress in RAW264.7 cells. Fitoterapia 83:1628–1635
29. Krafft PR, Rolland WB, Duris K, Lekic T, Campbell A, Tang J, Zhang JH (2012) Modeling intracerebral hemorrhage in mice: injection of autologous blood or bacterial collagenase. J Vis Exp 67:e4289(electronic)
30. Kusaykin M, Bakunina I, Sova V, Ermakova S, Kuznetsova T, Besednova N, Zaporozhets T, Zvyagintseva T (2008) Structure, biological activity, and enzymatic transformation of fucoidans from the brown seaweeds. Biotechnol J 3:904–915
31. Kwak KW, Cho KS, Hahn OJ, Lee KH, Lee BY, Ko JJ, Chung KH (2010) Biological effects of fucoidan isolated from *Fucus vesiculosus* on thrombosis and vascular cells. Korean J Hematol 45:51–57
32. Lee H, Kim JS, Kim E (2012) Fucoidan from seaweed *Fucus vesiculosus* inhibits migration and invasion of human lung cancer cell via PI3K-Akt-mTOR pathways. PLoS One 7, e50624
33. Li C, Gao Y, Xing Y, Zhu H, Shen J, Tian J (2011) Fucoidan, a sulfated polysaccharide from brown algae, against myocardial ischemia-reperfusion injury in rats via regulating the inflammation response. Food Chem Toxicol 49:2090–2095
34. Li X, Zhao H, Wang Q, Liang H, Jiang X (2015) Fucoidan protects ARPE-19 cells from oxidative stress via normalization of reactive oxygen species generation through the Ca2+-dependent ERK signaling pathway. Mol Med Rep 11:3746–3752
35. Lim JD, Lee SR, Kim T, Jang SA, Kang SC, Koo HJ, Sohn E, Bak JP, Namkoong S, Kim HK, Song IS, Kim N, Sohn EH, Han J (2015) Fucoidan from *Fucus vesiculosus* protects against alcohol-induced liver damage by modulating inflammatory mediators in mice and HepG2 cells. Mar Drugs 13:1051–1067
36. Ma Q, Manaenko A, Khatibi NH, Chen W, Zhang JH, Tang J (2011) Vascular adhesion protein-1 inhibition provides antiinflammatory protection after an intracerebral hemorrhagic stroke in mice. J Cereb Blood Flow Metab 31:881–893
37. Manne BK, Getz TM, Hughes CE, Alshehri O, Dangelmaier C, Naik UP, Watson SP, Kunapuli SP (2013) Fucoidan is a novel platelet agonist for the C-type lectin-like receptor 2 (CLEC-2). J Biol Chem 288:7717–7726
38. Martin M, Conlon LW (2013) Does platelet transfusion improve outcomes in patients with spontaneous or traumatic intracerebral hemorrhage? Ann Emerg Med 61:58–61
39. Mauray S, Sternberg C, Theveniaux J, Millet J, Sinquin C, Tapon-Bretaudiere J, Fischer AM (1995) Venous antithrombotic and anti-

coagulant activities of a fucoidan fraction. Thromb Haemost 74:1280–1285
40. May F, Hagedorn I, Pleines I, Bender M, Vogtle T, Eble J, Elvers M, Nieswandt B (2009) CLEC-2 is an essential platelet-activating receptor in hemostasis and thrombosis. Blood 114:3464–3472
41. Mayer SA, Brun NC, Begtrup K, Broderick J, Davis S, Diringer MN, Skolnick BE, Steiner T, Recombinant Activated Factor VIIHTI (2005) Recombinant activated factor VII for acute intracerebral hemorrhage. N Engl J Med 352:777–785
42. Mourao P (2004) Use of sulfated fucans as anticoagulant and antithrombotic agents: future perspectives. Curr Pharm Des 10: 967–981
43. Mourão P (1999) Searching for alternatives to heparin sulfated fucans from marine invertebrates. Trends Cardiovasc Med 9:225–232
44. Nieswandt B, Pleines I, Bender M (2011) Platelet adhesion and activation mechanisms in arterial thrombosis and ischaemic stroke. J Thromb Haemost 9(Suppl 1):92–104
45. Nishino T, Aizu Y, Nagumo T (1991) The influence of sulfate content and molecular weight of a fucan sulfate from the brown seaweed *Ecklonia kurome* on its antithrombin activity. Thromb Res 64:723–731
46. Park HY, Han MH, Park C, Jin CY, Kim GY, Choi IW, Kim ND, Nam TJ, Kwon TK, Choi YH (2011) Anti-inflammatory effects of fucoidan through inhibition of NF-kappaB, MAPK and Akt activation in lipopolysaccharide-induced BV2 microglia cells. Food Chem Toxicol 49:1745–1752
47. Park SB, Chun KR, Kim JK, Suk K, Jung YM, Lee WH (2010) The differential effect of high and low molecular weight fucoidans on the severity of collagen-induced arthritis in mice. Phytother Res 24:1384–1391
48. Pomin VH, Pereira MS, Valente AP, Tollefsen DM, Pavao MS, Mourao PA (2005) Selective cleavage and anticoagulant activity of a sulfated fucan: stereospecific removal of a 2-sulfate ester from the polysaccharide by mild acid hydrolysis, preparation of oligosaccharides, and heparin cofactor II-dependent anticoagulant activity. Glycobiology 15:369–381
49. Qureshi AI, Mohammad YM, Yahia AM, Suarez JI, Siddiqui AM, Kirmani JF, Suri MF, Kolb J, Zaidat OO (2005) A prospective multicenter study to evaluate the feasibility and safety of aggressive antihypertensive treatment in patients with acute intracerebral hemorrhage. J Intensive Care Med 20:34–42
50. Raghavendran HR, Srinivasan P, Rekha S (2011) Immunomodulatory activity of fucoidan against aspirin-induced gastric mucosal damage in rats. Int Immunopharmacol 11:157–163
51. Rolland WB, Lekic T, Krafft PR, Hasegawa Y, Altay O, Hartman R, Ostrowski R, Manaenko A, Tang J, Zhang JH (2013) Fingolimod reduces cerebral lymphocyte infiltration in experimental models of rodent intracerebral hemorrhage. Exp Neurol 241:45–55
52. Schlunk F, Schulz E, Lauer A, Yigitkanli K, Pfeilschifter W, Steinmetz H, Lo EH, Foerch C (2014) Warfarin pretreatment reduces cell death and MMP-9 activity in experimental intracerebral hemorrhage. Transl Stroke Res 6:133–9
53. Su CY, Chen HM, Kwan AL, Lin YH, Guo NW (2007) Neuropsychological impairment after hemorrhagic stroke in basal ganglia. Arch Clin Neuropsychol 22:465–474
54. Suzuki-Inoue K, Fuller GL, Garcia A, Eble JA, Pohlmann S, Inoue O, Gartner TK, Hughan SC, Pearce AC, Laing GD, Theakston RD, Schweighoffer E, Zitzmann N, Morita T, Tybulewicz VL, Ozaki Y, Watson SP (2006) A novel Syk-dependent mechanism of platelet activation by the C-type lectin receptor CLEC-2. Blood 107:542–549
55. Tanaka K, Ito M, Kodama M, Tomita M, Kimura S, Hoyano M, Mitsuma W, Hirono S, Hanawa H, Aizawa Y (2011) Sulfated polysaccharide fucoidan ameliorates experimental autoimmune myocarditis in rats. J Cardiovasc Pharmacol Ther 16:79–86
56. Tang J, Liu J, Zhou C, Alexander JS, Nanda A, Granger DN, Zhang JH (2004) Mmp-9 deficiency enhances collagenase-induced intracerebral hemorrhage and brain injury in mutant mice. J Cereb Blood Flow Metab 24:1133–1145
57. Teruya T, Tatemoto H, Konishi T, Tako M (2009) Structural characteristics and in vitro macrophage activation of acetyl fucoidan from *Cladosiphon okamuranus*. Glycoconj J 26:1019–1028
58. van Asch CJ, Oudendijk JF, Rinkel GJ, Klijn CJ (2010) Early intracerebral hematoma expansion after aneurysmal rupture. Stroke 41:2592–2595
59. Wang Y, Nie M, Lu Y, Wang R, Li J, Yang B, Xia M, Zhang H, Li X (2015) Fucoidan exerts protective effects against diabetic nephropathy related to spontaneous diabetes through the NF-kappaB signaling pathway in vivo and in vitro. Int J Mol Med 4(35):1067–1073
60. Xiong XY, Wang J, Qian ZM, Yang QW (2014) Iron and intracerebral hemorrhage: from mechanism to translation. Transl Stroke Res 5:429–441
61. Yamasaki-Miyamoto Y, Yamasaki M, Tachibana H, Yamada K (2009) Fucoidan induces apoptosis through activation of caspase-8 on human breast cancer MCF-7 cells. J Agric Food Chem 57:8677–8682
62. Yu X, Zhang Q, Cui W, Zeng Z, Yang W, Zhang C, Zhao H, Gao W, Wang X, Luo D (2014) Low molecular weight fucoidan alleviates cardiac dysfunction in diabetic Goto-Kakizaki rats by reducing oxidative stress and cardiomyocyte apoptosis. J Diabetes Res 2014:420929
63. Zhang Z, Till S, Jiang C, Knappe S, Reutterer S, Scheiflinger F, Szabo CM, Dockal M (2014) Structure-activity relationship of the pro- and anticoagulant effects of *Fucus vesiculosus* fucoidan. Thromb Haemost 111:429–437
64. Zhao X, Sun G, Zhang H, Ting SM, Song S, Gonzales N, Aronowski J (2014) Polymorphonuclear neutrophil in brain parenchyma after experimental intracerebral hemorrhage. Transl Stroke Res 5:554–561
65. Zhu Z, Zhang Q, Chen L, Ren S, Xu P, Tang Y, Luo D (2010) Higher specificity of the activity of low molecular weight fucoidan for thrombin-induced platelet aggregation. Thromb Res 125:419–426

Zinc Protoporphyrin Attenuates White Matter Injury after Intracerebral Hemorrhage

Yuxiang Gu, Ye Gong, Wen-quan Liu, Richard F. Keep, Guohua Xi, and Ya Hua

Introduction

About 60,000 people in the United States suffer an intracerebral hemorrhage (ICH) each year, and there is currently no proven therapy for ICH other than supportive care [11, 17]. White matter injury occurs in ICH, and iron has a role in ICH-induced white matter damage [18].

Heme oxygenase (HO) is the key enzyme in hemoglobin degradation, which metabolizes heme to biliverdin, iron, and carbon monoxide [9, 12]. Heme oxygenase-1 [12] is upregulated after ICH [15]. An inhibitor of heme oxygenase, zinc protoporphyrin (ZnPP), reduced ICH-induced brain injury in animal experiments [2, 4, 7].

In this study, we examined white matter injury at different time points after ICH and determined the effect of ZnPP on ICH-induced white matter injury.

Y. Gu • Y. Gong
Department of Neurosurgery, University of Michigan,
Ann Arbor, MI, USA

Department of Neurosurgery, Huashan Hospital, Fudan University,
Shanghai, China

W.-q. Liu • R.F. Keep • G. Xi
Department of Neurosurgery, University of Michigan,
Ann Arbor, MI, USA

Y. Hua, MD (✉)
Department of Neurosurgery, University of Michigan,
Ann Arbor, MI, USA

R5005, BSRB, University of Michigan,
Ann Arbor, MI 48109, USA
e-mail: yahua@umich.edu

Materials and Methods

Animal Preparation and Intracerebral Infusion

The protocols for these animal studies were approved by the University of Michigan Committee on the Use and Care of Animals. Adult male Sprague-Dawley rats (275–325 g, Charles River Laboratories, Portage, MI, USA) were anesthetized with pentobarbital (45 mg/kg, intraperitoneally (IP)). Body temperature was maintained at 37.5 °C using a feedback-controlled heating pad.

The rats were positioned in a stereotactic frame (Kopf Instrument, Tujunga, CA, USA). The scalp was incised along the sagittal midline using sterile technique. A cranial burr hole (1 mm) was drilled near the right coronal suture 4.0 mm lateral to the midline, and a 26-gauge needle was inserted stereotaxically into the right basal ganglia (coordinates: 0.2 mm anterior, 5.5 mm ventral, and 4.0 mm lateral to the bregma) [1]. Autologous blood (100 μl) was infused into the right caudate nucleus at a rate of 10 μl per minute using a microinfusion pump. The needle was removed and the skin incisions were closed with sutures after infusion. Animals were then allowed to recover.

Experimental Groups

This study was divided into two parts. In part 1, rats (four for each group) received either a sham operation (needle insertion) or a 100 μl autologous blood injection into the right basal ganglia. Animals were euthanized at 1 h, 1, 3, 7, 14, or 28 days after blood injection and the brains were used to determine the number of myelin basic protein (MBP)-labeled fiber bundles and their area. In part 2, all rats had intracerebral infusion of 100 μl autologous blood. An intraperitoneal osmotic minipump was implanted immediately after ICH to deliver vehicle

R.L. Applegate et al. (eds.), *Brain Edema XVI: Translate Basic Science into Clinical Practice*, Acta Neurochirurgica Supplement, Vol. 121,
DOI 10.1007/978-3-319-18497-5_35, © Springer International Publishing Switzerland 2016

or a heme oxygenase inhibitor, ZnPP (1 nmol/h), intraperitoneally for up to 14 days. Rats were euthanized at day 28 ($n=6$ for each group) and the brains used to determine the number and area of MBP-labeled fiber bundles.

Immunohistochemistry

Rats were reanesthetized with pentobarbital (60 mg/kg, IP) and perfused with 4 % paraformaldehyde in 0.1 M pH 7.4 phosphate-buffered saline (PBS). Removed brains were kept in 4 % paraformaldehyde for 6 h then immersed in 25 % sucrose for 3–4 days at 4 °C. The brains were embedded in OCT compound (Sakura Finetek USA Inc., Torrance, CA, USA) and sectioned on a cryostat (18 μm thick). Sections were incubated according to the avidin-biotin complex technique. Primary antibodies were myelin basic protein (MBP) antibody (1:400 dilution; Chemicon International, Inc., Temecula, CA, USA). Sections were then treated with secondary antibody (1:800). Immunoreactivity was visualized subsequently by the avidin-biotin complex method (Vectastatin; Vector Laboratories, Burlingame, CA, USA) [5].

Quantitation of Immunostaining Data

Images of the total caudate nucleus were digitized at ×10 magnification to quantify the number and area of MBP-positive bundles. NIH Object-Image software was used to calculate these parameters using the grayscale threshold setting, which includes all pixels above a specified grayscale value. This application permits isolating MBP from background staining. The MBP index was calculated as (sum of ipsilateral MBP area)/(sum of corresponding contralateral MBP area) and (sum of ipsilateral MBP bundles count)/(sum of corresponding contralateral MBP bundles count).

Statistical Analysis

All data in this study are presented as mean ± standard deviation. Data were analyzed with analysis of variance (ANOVA) or Student's t-test. Significance levels were set at $p<0.05$.

Results

The ipsilateral basal ganglia of sham-operated animals and the contralateral of the ICH animals did not show any obvious changes in the MBP fiber bundles. The number of MBP-positive bundles was significantly lower in the ipsilateral basal ganglia 4 weeks after ICH compared with sham-operated rats (Fig. 1a). The number of MBP-positive bundles and their area showed a progressive reduction from day 1 to day 28. There was an almost 50 % reduction at day 14, and a continued decline to day 28. The MBP positive area ($p<0.05$) and the number of MBP positive bundles ($p<0.01$) were significantly reduced in the ipsilateral basal ganglia at 2 weeks after blood injection vs. sham-operated animals (Fig. 1b).

Treatment with ZnPP, delivered by intraperitoneal osmotic mini-pump, significantly attenuated the reduction in MBP positive area (0.82 ± 0.03 vs. 0.44 ± 0.04 in the vehicle, $p<0.01$, Fig. 2a) and the number of bundles (0.87 ± 0.02 vs. 0.45 ± 0.02 in the vehicle, $p<0.01$, Fig. 2b) at 28 days following ICH.

Discussion

Intracerebral hemorrhage leads to secondary brain injury and severe neurological deficits. Such brain injury involves both gray and white matter [16]. However, most studies on experimental ICH-induced brain injury have focused on neuronal and gray matter alterations [6]. To date, few studies have quantified histological changes in white matter.

Oligodendrocytes are the major white matter cell type. MBP is produced by oligodendrocytes and it is the most abundant protein in the myelin sheath. Takahiro et al. [8] reported that myelin changes are the primary pathological event in cerebral white matter and the alteration in axons that occur with chronic hypoperfusion. In the present study, there was a time-dependent white matter injury after ICH. The decrease in both the number of MBP-labeled bundles in the ipsilateral caudate nucleus and their total area was almost 50 %. Degenerating myelin sheaths may be phagocytosed by macrophages.

The mechanisms of brain injury after ICH are complex. Hemoglobin and iron, its degradation product, are not only major factors responsible for acute brain edema formation and brain injury after ICH [4, 10, 16], but they also play a key role in persistent neurological deficits, even after the period when ICH-induced edema had resolved [3]. In the present study, we showed that ICH-induced white matter injury is progressive over the period of 1–28 days.

Heme oxygenases (HO) are key enzymes in heme degradation. There are three separate isozymes, HO-1, HO-2, and HO-3 [9]. HO-1 is markedly upregulated in the brain after ICH [4, 13, 15]. Our previous studies on HO inhibitors, including SnPP and ZnPP, showed that they can attenuate ICH- and hemoglobin-induced brain edema in rat ICH models [2, 4]. Similar results were found in a pig ICH model, with SnPP reducing both edema and clot volumes at 24 h after hematoma induction [14]. The present study shows that

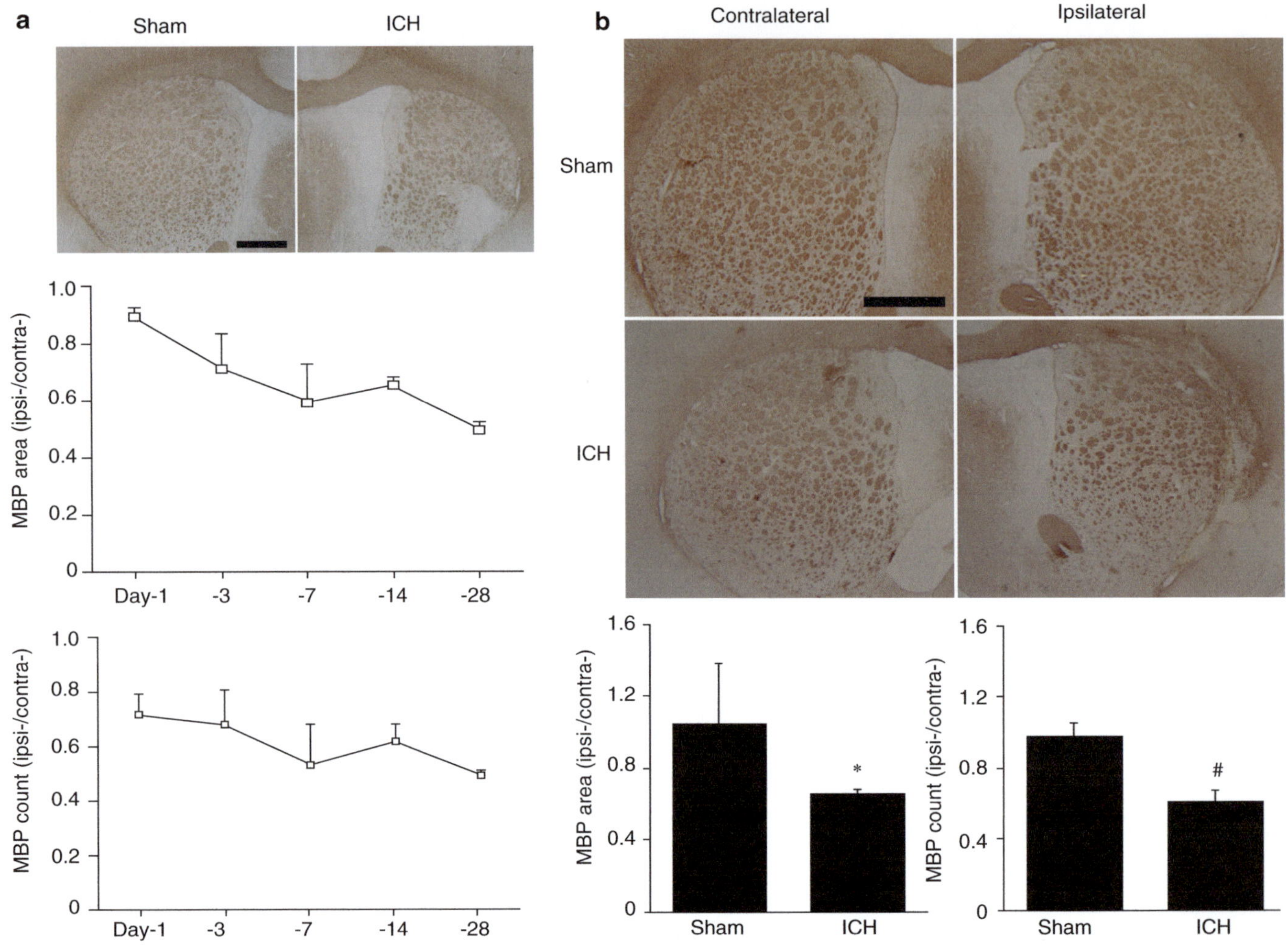

Fig. 1 (**a**) Myelin basic protein (*MBP*) immunoreactivity in the ipsilateral caudate after a sham operation or a 100 μl blood injection (*ICH*) into the right caudate at 4 weeks after surgery, along with the time course of changes in MBP total area and number of bundles expressed as ipsilateral/contralateral ratios. Scale bar=5 mm. (**b**) MBP immunoreactivity in the ipsi- and contralateral caudate in rats at 2 weeks after a sham operation or a 100 μl blood injection. Scale bar=5 mm. Bar graphs displaying MBP total area and number of bundles in the ipsilateral caudate 2 weeks after 100 μl blood injection or a needle insertion. Values are means ± SD, #$p<0.01$, *$p<0.05$ by Student's *t*-test

systemically administered ZnPP can markedly reduce myelin sheath injury after ICH and suggests that the brain protective effects of HO inhibitors are partly due to reductions in white matter injury.

In conclusion, progressive white matter injury occurs after ICH. ZnPP attenuated ICH-induced white matter injury, suggesting a role of heme degradation products in such damage.

Acknowledgment This study was supported by grants NS-073595, NS-079157 and NS-084049 from the National Institutes of Health (NIH) and 973 Program-2014CB541600.

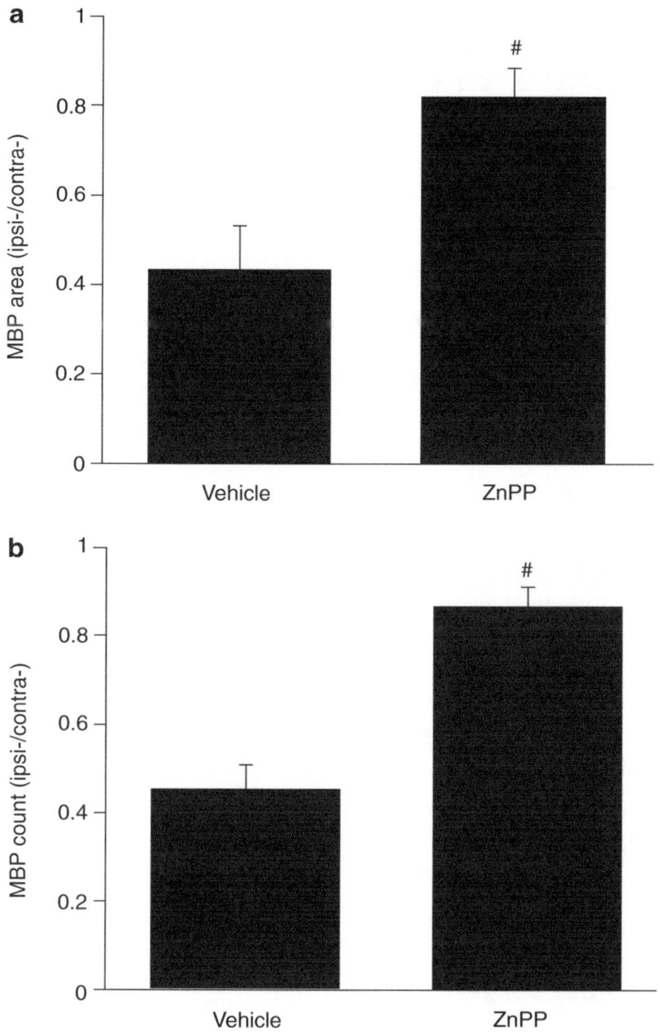

Fig. 2 Effects of ZnPP or vehicle treatment on (**a**) the myelin basic protein (*MBP*)-positive area and (**b**) the number of MBP-positive bundles in the ipsilateral caudate of rats 4 weeks after ICH. Values (± SD) are expressed as a ratio to the contralateral caudate. $\#p<0.01$ by Student's *t*-test

References

1. Cheng Y, Xi G, Jin H, Keep RF, Feng J, Hua Y (2014) Thrombin-induced cerebral hemorrhage: role of protease-activated receptor-1. Transl Stroke Res 5:472–475
2. Gong Y, Tian H, Xi G, Keep RF, Hoff JT, Hua Y (2006) Systemic zinc protoporphyrin administration reduces intracerebral hemorrhage-induced brain injury. Acta Neurochir Suppl 96:232–236
3. Hua Y, Nakamura T, Keep R, Wu J, Schallert T, Hoff J, Xi G (2006) Long-term effects of experimental intracerebral hemorrhage: the role of iron. J Neurosurg 104:305–312
4. Huang F, Xi G, Keep RF, Hua Y, Nemoianu A, Hoff JT (2002) Brain edema after experimental intracerebral hemorrhage: role of hemoglobin degradation products. J Neurosurg 96:287–293
5. Jin H, Xi G, Keep RF, Wu J, Hua Y (2013) DARPP-32 to quantify intracerebral hemorrhage-induced neuronal death in basal Ganglia. Transl Stroke Res 4:130–134
6. Keep RF, Hua Y, Xi G (2012) Intracerebral haemorrhage: mechanisms of injury and therapeutic targets. Lancet Neurol 11:720–731
7. Koeppen AH, Dickson AC, Smith J (2004) Heme oxygenase in experimental intracerebral hemorrhage: the benefit of tin-mesoporphyrin. J Neuropathol Exp Neurol 63:587–597
8. Kurumatani T, Kudo T, Ikura Y, Takeda M (1998) White matter changes in the gerbil brain under chronic cerebral hypoperfusion. Stroke 29:1058–1062
9. Maines MD (1997) The heme oxygenase system: a regulator of second messenger gases. Ann Rev Pharmacol Toxicol 37: 517–554
10. Nakamura T, Keep RF, Hua Y, Schallert T, Hoff JT, Xi G (2003) Deferoxamine-induced attenuation of brain edema and neurological deficits in a rat model of intracerebral hemorrhage. Neurosurg Focus 15:ECP4
11. Pandey AS, Xi G (2014) Intracerebral hemorrhage: a multimodality approach to improving outcome. Transl Stroke Res 5:313–315
12. Sharp FR, Zhan X, Liu DZ (2013) Heat shock proteins in the brain: role of Hsp70, Hsp 27, and HO-1 (Hsp32) and their therapeutic potential. Transl Stroke Res 4:685–692
13. Turner CP, Bergeron M, Matz P, Zegna A, Noble LJ, Panter SS, Sharp FR (1998) Heme oxygenase-1 is induced in glia throughout brain by subarachnoid hemoglobin. J Cerebral Blood Flow Metab 18:257–273
14. Wagner KR, Hua Y, de Courten-Myers GM, Broderick JP, Nishimura RN, Lu SY, Dwyer BE (2000) Tin-mesoporphyrin, a potent heme oxygenase inhibitor, for treatment of intracerebral hemorrhage: in vivo and in vitro studies. Cell Mol Biol 46:597–608
15. Wu J, Hua Y, Keep R, Schallert T, Hoff J, Xi G (2002) Oxidative brain injury from extravasated erythrocytes after intracerebral hemorrhage. Brain Res 953:45
16. Xi G, Keep RF, Hoff JT (2006) Mechanisms of brain injury after intracerebral haemorrhage. Lancet Neurol 5:53–63
17. Xi G, Strahle J, Hua Y, Keep RF (2014) Progress in translational research on intracerebral hemorrhage: is there an end in sight? Prog Neurobiol 115:45–63
18. Xie Q, Gu Y, Hua Y, Liu W, Keep RF, Xi G (2014) Deferoxamine attenuates white matter injury in a piglet intracerebral hemorrhage model. Stroke 45:290–292

Cyclooxygenase-2 Inhibition Provides Lasting Protection Following Germinal Matrix Hemorrhage in Premature Infant Rats

Tim Lekic, Paul R. Krafft, Damon Klebe, William B. Rolland, Jerry Flores, Jiping Tang, and John H. Zhang

Introduction

Germinal matrix hemorrhage (GMH) is the most common neurological disease of premature infants, partly because this germinal region is most vulnerable to spontaneous bleeding within the first 3 days of preterm life [1]. Intracerebroventricular expansion partly contributes to long-term brain injury through mechanical compression of surrounding tissues [2–4]. Devastating outcomes include hydrocephalus, mental retardation, and cerebral palsy [1, 5, 6]. Current treatment modalities are largely ineffective, and GMH has been thus far not preventable [7].

Importantly, the blood constituent thrombin is an established factor in hydrocephalus formation [8–10], which binds and trans-activates a subfamily of G protein-coupled receptors named proteinase-activated receptors (specifically PAR-1 and PAR-4) [11], theoretically leading to increased COX-2 expression [12]. Therefore, we hypothesized that modulation of brain injury through thrombin, PAR-1,-4, and COX-2 could be an eventual strategy to help improve outcomes after GMH.

T. Lekic • P.R. Krafft • D. Klebe • W.B. Rolland • J. Flores
J. Tang
Division of Physiology and Pharmacology, School of Medicine, Loma Linda, CA, USA

J.H. Zhang, MD, PhD (✉)
Division of Physiology and Pharmacology, School of Medicine, Loma Linda, CA, USA

Department of Neurosurgery, School of Medicine, Loma Linda, CA, USA

Department of Physiology and Pharmacology, Loma Linda University School of Medicine, 11041 Campus Street, Risley Hall Rm 219, Loma Linda, CA 92354, USA
e-mail: johnzhang3910@yahoo.com

Methods

All studies, protocols, and procedures were approved by the Institutional Animal Care and Use Committee at Loma Linda University. Postnatal day 7 (P7) neonatal rats were subjected to stereotactic ganglionic eminence collagenase infusion. Groups were as follows: animals were euthanized at either of two time points 72 h (short-term) or 4 weeks (long-term). Short-term COX-2 expression was evaluated in the context of PAR-1 (SCH-79797) and PAR-4 (P4pal10) inhibition; pups in the long-term group were administered the selective COX-2 inhibitor (NS-398) as routinely performed [13].

Animal Surgeries

P7 Sprague-Dawley rat pups (14–19 g) were randomly allocated to either GMH or sham operation. A stereotactically guided, 0.3 U bacterial collagenase infusion model was used to model preterm right-sided ganglionic eminence bleeds [14–16]. Timed pregnant rats were purchased from Harlan Laboratories (Indianapolis, IN, USA), and pups of equally both genders were subjected to collagenase infusion [15]. Briefly, general anesthesia was obtained by using isoflurane (3 % in 30/70 % oxygen/medical air). Anesthetized pups were positioned prone, with heads secured onto the neonatal stereotactic frame (Kopf Instruments, Tujunga, CA, USA). The scalp was then sterilized (using betadine solution), and a small midline incision made to expose the bregma. Using a standard dental drill, a 1-mm cranial burr hole was made (bregma coordinates: 1.8 mm anterior, 1.5 mm lateral, 2.8 mm deep), through which a 26-gauge needle was lowered, and at this position, clostridial collagenase VII-S (0.3 U: Sigma, St. Louis, MO, USA) was infused at 0.25 μl/min into the right basal ganglion. Needles were left in place for 10 min after infusion to prevent backflow. Thereafter, the needle was slowly withdrawn at rate of 1 mm/min; burr holes

R.L. Applegate et al. (eds.), *Brain Edema XVI: Translate Basic Science into Clinical Practice*, Acta Neurochirurgica Supplement, Vol. 121, DOI 10.1007/978-3-319-18497-5_36,

were sealed with bone wax; and the scalp was sutured closed. All animals were allowed to recover under observation on a 37 °C warm heating blanket before being returned to their dams. Shams received all the above without collagenase infusion, as routinely performed [13].

Animal Perfusion and Tissue Extraction

The animals were fatally anesthetized with isoflurane (≥5 %) followed by cardiovascular perfusion with ice-cold PBS for Western blot analyses. Forebrains were dissected and snap-frozen with liquid nitrogen and then stored in –80 °C freezer, awaiting quantification as routinely performed [13].

Western Blotting

For the protein immunoblot [13], the concentration was determined using the DC protein assay (Bio-Rad, Hercules, CA, USA). The samples were then subjected to SDS-PAGE on 4–20 % gels, and then transferred to nitrocellulose membrane X 100 min at 100 V (Bio-Rad). Blotting membranes were incubated for 1 h with 5 % nonfat milk in Tris-buffered saline containing 0.1 % Tween 20, and these were then incubated overnight with the primary antibody, anti-COX2 (1:200; Cayman Chemical, Ann Arbor, MI, USA). Membranes were then incubated using secondary antibodies (1:1,000; Santa Cruz Biotechnology, Santa Cruz, CA, USA) and processed with an ECL Plus kit (GE Healthcare and Life Science, Piscataway, NJ, USA). For an internal control, the same membrane was probed using an antibody against β-actin (1:1,000; Santa Cruz Biotechnology, Santa Cruz, CA, USA) after being stripped. Relative densities of resultant protein immunoblot images were semiquantitatively analyzed by Image J software (4.0, Media Cybernetics, Silver Spring, MD, USA) as described elsewhere [17].

Neurological Deficits

All neurobehavior assessments were conducted in a blinded manner by experienced investigators [13–16]. Animals were assessed using a series of tests. Neurological deficit was quantified using a series of six tests measuring functional deficits (100 = severe, 50 = moderate, 0 = none): (1) proprioceptive limb placing, (2) lateral limb placement, (3) forelimb placement, (4) postural reflex, (5) back pressure toward edge, and (6) lateral pressure toward edge. These are routinely performed in brain-injured juvenile rats [18]. A T-maze was used to assess short-term (working) memory ability [19]; for each trial, rat were placed into the stem (40 cm × 10 cm) of the T-maze and allowed to explore until either the left or right path was chosen. Following a sequence of 10 trials, the rate of spontaneous alternation (0 % = none and 100 % = complete; alternations/trial) was recorded [18, 20].

Histological Slides

Animals were terminally anesthetized with isoflurane (≥5 %), followed by cardiovascular perfusion with ice-cold PBS and 10 % paraformaldehyde. Brains were removed and separated from surrounding tissues and post-fixed in 10 % paraformaldehyde and then 30 % sucrose (weight/volume) for total of 3 days. Histopathological pictographs used 10-μm thick coronal sections, caudally cut every 600 μm on a cryostat (Leica Microsystems LM3050S), then mounted and stained on poly-L-lysine-coated slides.

Statistical Analysis

Significance was based on <0.05. Data were statistically analyzed using one-way ANOVA, followed by Tukey post hoc test for significant analyses. Statistical analyses were performed using SigmaPlot version 10.0 for Windows.

Results

Early combined PAR-1 and PAR-4 signal inhibition reduced COX-2 expression ($p<0.05$; Fig. 1) in a dose-responsive manner measured 72 h after collagenase infusion. Thereafter, in a separate cohort of animals, direct inhibition of COX-2 by NS-398 further reduced hydrocephalus (Fig. 2) and also improved long-term neurobehavioral outcome ($p<0.05$; Fig. 3).

Conclusion

Translational stroke studies, in particular those involving animal modeling, are greatly needed to safely integrate basic preclinical investigations ahead of eventual clinical applications [21–25]. This study therefore investigated the value of modulating thrombin–PAR-1 and PAR-4 with reversing COX-2 upregulation, as well as the effect of direct COX-2 inhibition on post-hemorrhagic hydrocephalus and on neurological deficits. In prior studies, others hypothesized that hydrocephalus mechanisms involved increased production of infiltrating extracellular matrix (ECM) proteins throughout the cerebroventricular system and that these would lead to the obstruction of CSF outflow [1, 2, 10, 14, 15, 26–30]. Our data suggest that thrombin-induced PAR-1, -4 stimulation could upregulate harmful signaling, exacerbating inflammatory signaling (i.e., COX-2 mediated) upstream of ECM dysregulation [1, 8, 12, 14, 15, 31–34]. Thus, we hypothesized that thrombin binding to PAR-1, -4 receptors could consequently upregulate COX-2 protein. Furthermore, we investigated inhibition of PAR-1, -4 using a combined treatment with SCH79797 (PAR-1 antagonist) and p4pal10 (PAR-4 antagonist), which also significantly improved COX-2 after 72 h. Next, we asked whether directly inhibiting COX-2 following GMH could circumvent long-term negative outcomes. Our findings demonstrated that vehicle-treated animals had significantly worsened outcomes compared with shams, and treatment with NS398 (COX-2 inhibitor) significantly improved not only neuropathology but also and neurological ability. Therefore, by decreasing the early inflammatory COX-2 signaling pathway, we improved long-term outcome in juvenile animals. In summary, this study is the first to show that normalization of thrombin–PAR-1, -4 signals positively affect early COX-2 expression levels and improve long-term outcomes following collagenase infusion-mediated GMH.

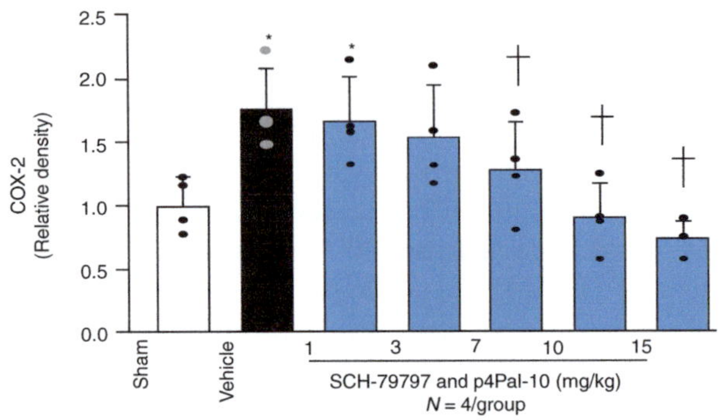

Brain COX-2 epression 3 days post GMH following SCH-79797 and p4Pal-10 co-administration.

Fig. 1 COX-2 expression post-GMH; dose response following PAR-1 and PAR-4 co- administration; 72 h after collagenase infusion; (*asterisk*) <0.05 compared with sham; (*cross*) <0.05 compared with GMH (vehicle); *SEM* standard error of the mean; *n*=4/group

Acknowledgment This study was partially supported by National Institutes of Health grant RO1 NS078755 (Dr. Zhang).

Disclosures None

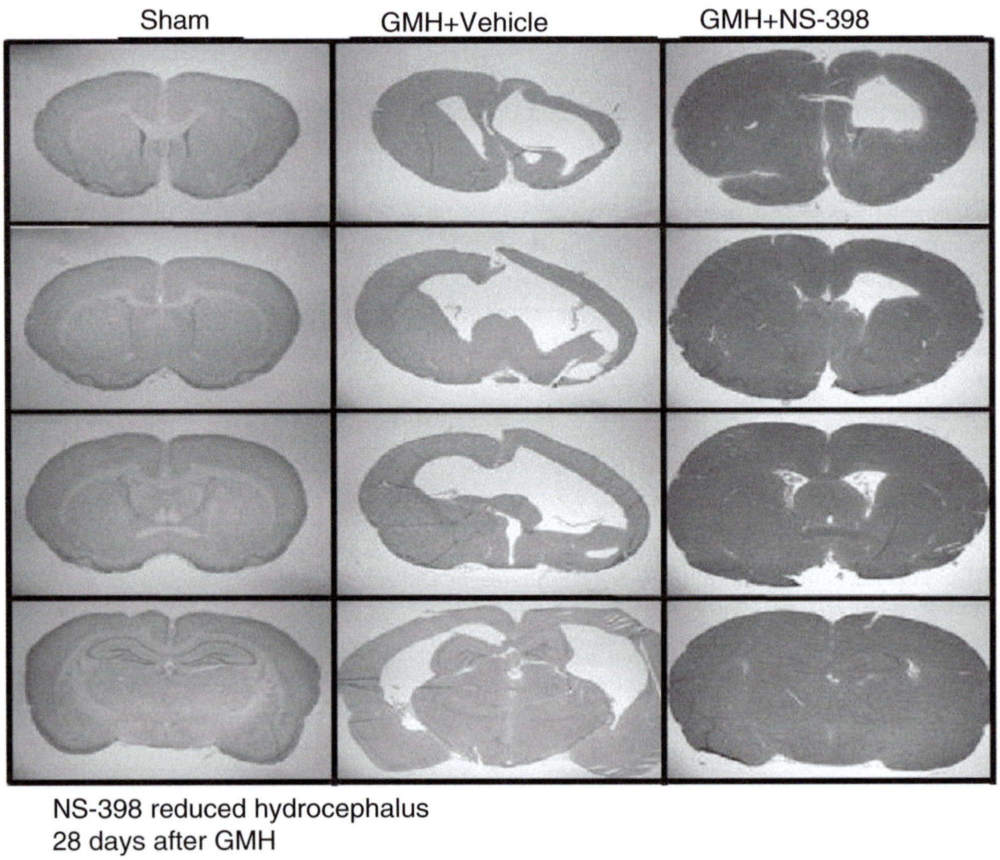

Fig. 2 Pictographs showing relative cortical thickness, ventricular and overall brain size between groups

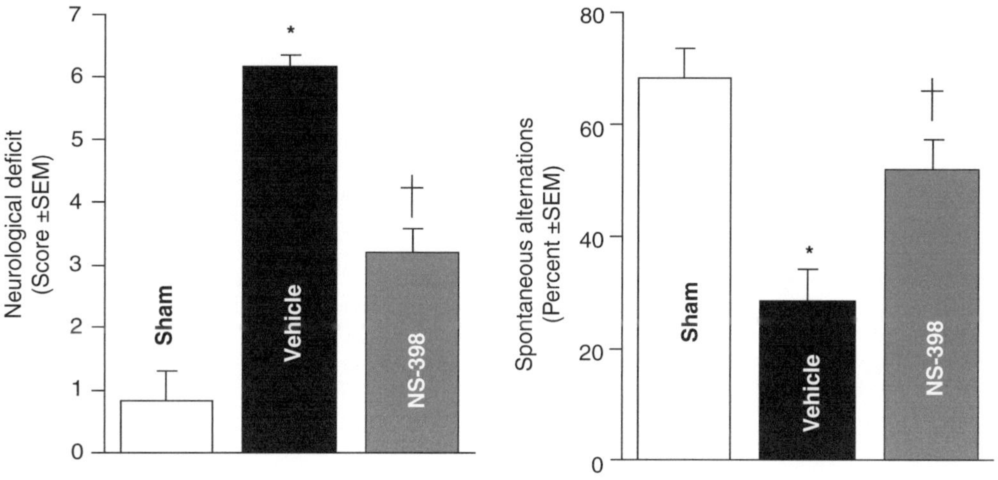

Fig. 3 *Left panel*, Neurological deficits (sensorimotor skill); *Right panel*, T-maze (spontaneous alterations) measured 1 month following collagenase infusion; (*asterisk*) <0.05 compared with sham; *SEM* standard error of the mean; $n = 4$/group

References

1. Ballabh P (2010) Intraventricular hemorrhage in premature infants: mechanism of disease. Pediatr Res 67:1–8
2. Aquilina K, Chakkarapani E, Love S, Thoresen M (2011) Neonatal rat model of intraventricular haemorrhage and post-haemorrhagic ventricular dilatation with long-term survival into adulthood. Neuropathol Appl Neurobiol 37:156–165
3. Chen Q, Zhang J, Guo J, Tang J, Tao Y, Li L, Feng H, Chen Z (2014) Chronic hydrocephalus and perihematomal tissue injury developed in a rat model of intracerebral hemorrhage with ventricular extension. Transl Stroke Res. doi:10.1007/s12975-014-0367-5
4. Zhao J, Chen Z, Xi G, Keep RF, Hua Y (2014) Deferoxamine attenuates acute hydrocephalus after traumatic brain injury in rats. Transl Stroke Res 5:586–594
5. Heron M, Sutton PD, Xu J, Ventura SJ, Strobino DM, Guyer B (2010) Annual summary of vital statistics: 2007. Pediatrics 125:4–15
6. Uria-Avellanal C, Robertson NJ (2014) Na(+)/H(+) exchangers and intracellular pH in perinatal brain injury. Transl Stroke Res 5:79–98
7. Whitelaw A (2001) Intraventricular haemorrhage and posthaemorrhagic hydrocephalus: pathogenesis, prevention and future interventions. Semin Neonatol 6:135–146
8. Gao F, Liu F, Chen Z, Hua Y, Keep RF, Xi G (2014) Hydrocephalus after intraventricular hemorrhage: the role of thrombin. J Cereb Blood Flow Metab 34:489–494
9. Cheng Y, Xi G, Jin H, Keep RF, Feng J, Hua Y (2014) Thrombin-induced cerebral hemorrhage: role of protease-activated receptor-1. Transl Stroke Res 5:472–475
10. Siler DA, Gonzalez JA, Wang RK, Cetas JS, Alkayed NJ (2014) Intracisternal administration of tissue plasminogen activator improves cerebrospinal fluid flow and cortical perfusion after subarachnoid hemorrhage in mice. Transl Stroke Res 5:227–237
11. Kataoka H, Hamilton JR, McKemy DD, Camerer E, Zheng YW, Cheng A, Griffin C, Coughlin SR (2003) Protease-activated receptors 1 and 4 mediate thrombin signaling in endothelial cells. Blood 102:3224–3231
12. Lo HM, Chen CL, Tsai YJ, Wu PH, Wu WB (2009) Thrombin induces cyclooxygenase-2 expression and prostaglandin E2 release via PAR1 activation and ERK1/2- and p38 MAPK-dependent pathway in murine macrophages. J Cell Biochem 108:1143–1152
13. Lekic T, Rolland W, Hartman R, Kamper J, Suzuki H, Tang J, Zhang JH (2011) Characterization of the brain injury, neurobehavioral profiles, and histopathology in a rat model of cerebellar hemorrhage. Exp Neurol 227:96–103
14. Manaenko A, Lekic T, Barnhart M, Hartman R, Zhang JH (2014) Inhibition of transforming growth factor-beta attenuates brain injury and neurological deficits in a rat model of germinal matrix hemorrhage. Stroke 45:828–834
15. Lekic T, Manaenko A, Rolland W, Krafft PR, Peters R, Hartman RE, Altay O, Tang J, Zhang JH (2012) Rodent neonatal germinal matrix hemorrhage mimics the human brain injury, neurological consequences, and post-hemorrhagic hydrocephalus. Exp Neurol 236:69–78
16. Leitzke AS, Rolland WB, Krafft PR, Lekic T, Klebe D, Flores JJ, Van Allen NR, Applegate RL 2nd, Zhang JH (2013) Isoflurane post-treatment ameliorates GMH- induced brain injury in neonatal rats. Stroke 44:3587–3590
17. Tang J, Liu J, Zhou C, Alexander JS, Nanda A, Granger DN, Zhang JH (2004) Mmp-9 deficiency enhances collagenase-induced intracerebral hemorrhage and brain injury in mutant mice. J Cereb Blood Flow Metab 24:1133–1145
18. Fathali N, Ostrowski RP, Lekic T, Jadhav V, Tong W, Tang J, Zhang JH (2010) Cyclooxygenase-2 inhibition provides lasting protection against neonatal hypoxic-ischemic brain injury. Crit Care Med 38:572–578
19. Hughes RN (2004) The value of spontaneous alternation behavior (SAB) as a test of retention in pharmacological investigations of memory. Neurosci Biobehav Rev 28:497–505
20. Zhou Y, Fathali N, Lekic T, Tang J, Zhang JH (2009) Glibenclamide improves neurological function in neonatal hypoxia-ischemia in rats. Brain Res 1270:131–139
21. Tso MK, Macdonald RL (2014) Subarachnoid hemorrhage: a review of experimental studies on the microcirculation and the neurovascular unit. Transl Stroke Res 5:174–189
22. Marbacher S, Nevzati E, Croci D, Erhardt S, Muroi C, Jakob SM, Fandino J (2014) The rabbit shunt model of subarachnoid haemorrhage. Transl Stroke Res 5:669–680
23. Pluta RM, Bacher J, Skopets B, Hoffmann V (2014) A non-human primate model of aneurismal subarachnoid hemorrhage (SAH). Transl Stroke Res 5:681–691
24. Zhang YP, Cai J, Shields LB, Liu N, Xu XM, Shields CB (2014) Traumatic brain injury using mouse models. Transl Stroke Res 5:454–471
25. Wada K, Makino H, Shimada K, Shikata F, Kuwabara A, Hashimoto T (2014) Translational research using a mouse model of intracranial aneurysm. Transl Stroke Res 5:248–251
26. Strahle J, Garton HL, Maher C, Muraszko K, Keep R, Xi G (2012) Mechanisms of hydrocephalus after neonatal and adult intraventricular hemorrhage. Transl Stroke Res 3:25–38

27. Crews L, Wyss-Coray T, Masliah E (2004) Insights into the pathogenesis of hydrocephalus from transgenic and experimental animal models. Brain Pathol 14:312–316
28. Sorensen SS, Nygaard AB, Nielsen MY, Jensen K, Christensen T (2014) miRNA expression profiles in cerebrospinal fluid and blood of patients with acute ischemic stroke. Transl Stroke Res 5:711–718
29. Yamauchi T, Saito H, Ito M, Shichinohe H, Houkin K, Kuroda S (2014) Platelet lysate and granulocyte-colony stimulating factor serve safe and accelerated expansion of human bone marrow stromal cells for stroke therapy. Transl Stroke Res 5:701–710
30. Khanna A, Kahle KT, Walcott BP, Gerzanich V, Simard JM (2014) Disruption of ion homeostasis in the neurogliovascular unit underlies the pathogenesis of ischemic cerebral edema. Transl Stroke Res 5:3–16
31. Jiang X, Zhu S, Panetti TS, Bromberg ME (2008) Formation of tissue factor- factor VIIa-factor Xa complex induces activation of the mTOR pathway which regulates migration of human breast cancer cells. Thromb Haemost 100:127–133
32. Gao C, Du H, Hua Y, Keep RF, Strahle J, Xi G (2014) Role of red blood cell lysis and iron in hydrocephalus after intraventricular hemorrhage. J Cereb Blood Flow Metab 34:1070–1075
33. Reuter B, Rodemer C, Grudzenski S, Meairs S, Bugert P, Hennerici MG, Fatar M (2014) Effect of simvastatin on MMPs and TIMPs in human brain endothelial cells and experimental stroke. Transl Stroke Res. doi:10.1007/s12975-014-0381-7
34. Badaut J, Bix GJ (2014) Vascular neural network phenotypic transformation after traumatic injury: potential role in long-term sequelae. Transl Stroke Res 5:394–406

Intranasal IGF-1 Reduced Rat Pup Germinal Matrix Hemorrhage

Tim Lekic, Jerry Flores, Damon Klebe, Desislava Doycheva, William B. Rolland, Jiping Tang, and John H. Zhang

Introduction

Germinal matrix hemorrhage (GMH) is the most common neurological disease of premature infants, partly because this germinal region is most vulnerable to spontaneous bleeding within the first 3 days of preterm life [1]. Intracerebroventricular expansion partly contributes to long-term brain injury through mechanical compression of surrounding tissues [2–4]. Devastating outcomes include hydrocephalus, mental retardation, and cerebral palsy [1, 5]. Current treatment modalities are largely ineffective, and GMH has thus far not been preventable [6]. Insulin-like growth factor 1 (IGF-1) is an endogenous protein shown to have multiple neuroprotective properties [7, 8]. We therefore hypothesize that IGF-1 could reduce brain injury after GMH.

Methods

All studies, protocols, and procedures were approved by the Institutional Animal Care and Use Committee at Loma Linda University. Postnatal day 7 (P7) neonatal rats were subjected to stereotactic ganglionic eminence collagenase infusion. The following groups were studied: (1) sham, (2) GMH + vehicle, (3) GMH + intranasal IGF-1. Three days later (i.e., 72 h) animals were evaluated using righting-reflex, blood-brain barrier (BBB) permeability by Evans blue dye leakage, and hemoglobin assay, as routinely performed [9].

Animal Surgeries

P7 Sprague-Dawley rat pups (14–19 g) were randomly allocated to either GMH or sham operation. A stereotactically guided, 0.3 U bacterial collagenase infusion model was used to model preterm right-sided ganglionic eminence bleeds [10–12]. Timed pregnant rats were purchased from Harlan Laboratories (Indianapolis, IN, USA) and pups of equally both genders were subjected to collagenase infusion [11]. Briefly, general anesthesia was obtained by using isoflurane (3 % in 30/70 % oxygen/medical air). Anesthetized pups were positioned prone, with heads secured onto the neonatal stereotactic frame (Kopf Instruments, Tujunga, CA, USA). The scalp was then sterilized (using betadine solution), and a small midline incision made to expose the bregma. A 1 mm cranial burr hole was made using a standard dental drill (bregma coordinates: 1.8 mm anterior, 1.5 mm lateral, 2.8 mm deep) through which a 26-gauge needle was lowered, and at this position, clostridial collagenase VII-S (0.3 U, Sigma; St. Louis, MO, USA) was infused at 0.25 μl/min into the right basal ganglion. The needle was left in place for 10 min following infusion to prevent backflow. Thereafter, the needle was slowly withdrawn at rate of 1 mm/min; burr holes were sealed with bone wax; and the scalp was sutured closed. All animals were allowed to recover under observation on a 37 °C warm heating blanket before being returned to their dams. Shams received all the above without collagenase infusion, as routinely performed [9].

T. Lekic • J. Flores • D. Klebe • D. Doycheva • W.B. Rolland
J. Tang
Division of Physiology and Pharmacology, School of Medicine, Loma Linda, CA, USA

J.H. Zhang, MD, PhD (✉)
Division of Physiology and Pharmacology, School of Medicine, Loma Linda, CA, USA

Department of Neurosurgery, School of Medicine, Loma Linda, CA, USA

Department of Physiology and Pharmacology, Loma Linda University School of Medicine, 11041 Campus Street, Risley Hall Rm 219, Loma Linda, CA 92354, USA
e-mail: johnzhang3910@yahoo.com

R.L. Applegate et al. (eds.), *Brain Edema XVI: Translate Basic Science into Clinical Practice*, Acta Neurochirurgica Supplement, Vol. 121, DOI 10.1007/978-3-319-18497-5_37, © Springer International Publishing Switzerland 2016

Assessment of Neurological Deficits

Acquisition of developmental milestones was assessed after collagenase infusion. For negative geotropism, the time needed for complete rotation (180°) after being placed head down on a slope (20° angle) was recorded [13]. All neurobehavior assessments were conducted in a blinded manner by experienced investigators [10–12]. The maximum allotted time was 60 s per trial (two trials/day) for these tests as routinely performed [9].

Animal Perfusion and Tissue Extraction

The animals were fatally anesthetized with isoflurane (≥5 %) followed by cardiovascular perfusion with ice-cold PBS for hemoglobin assay and Evans blue analyses. Forebrains were dissected and snap-frozen with liquid-nitrogen, and then stored in a –80 °C freezer awaiting spectrophotometric quantification as routinely performed [9].

Hemoglobin Assay

The spectrophotometric measurement of hemorrhage [14] was performed using established protocols [15, 16]. Extracted forebrain tissue was placed into test tubes with 3 mL PBS; homogenized for 60 s (Tissue Miser Homogenizer; Fisher Scientific, Pittsburgh, PA, USA); after ultrasonication for 1 min, lysed erythrocyte membranes products were then centrifuged for 30 min; and Drabkin's reagent was added (Sigma-Aldrich, St. Louis, MO, USA) into aliquots of supernatant, which reacted for 15 min. The measurement of absorbance, using a spectrophotometer (540 nm; Genesis 10uv; Thermo Fisher Scientific, Waltham, MA, USA) was plotted onto a graph as a conversion into blood volume (μL) on the basis of standard curves, as routinely performed [9].

Evans Blue

The spectrophotometric measurement of the dye of Evans blue [17, 18] was initiated through dye injected intraperitoneally (IP) after GMH to measure BBB permeability. Under anesthesia, Evans blue (Sigma-Aldrich) in normal saline (2 %, 4 ml/kg) was infused. For quantitative measurements, brain tissue was homogenized in 3 ml of N, N- dimethylformamide (Sigma-Aldrich), incubated for 18 h at 55 °C, then centrifuged. Supernatants were analyzed at 620 nm by spectrophotometer, as routine [9].

Statistical Analysis

Significance was based on $p<0.05$. Data were statistically analyzed using one-way analysis of variance (ANOVA), followed by Tukey post hoc test for significant analyses. Statistical analyses were performed using SigmaPlot version 10.0 for Windows.

Results

GMH significantly delayed development of negative geotropism reflex by 72 h after collagenase infusion compared with sham (Fig. 1) and was significantly improved using IGF-1 therapy. Figures 2 and 3 demonstrate the GMH animal model having significant amount of bleeding and BBB rupture, more so on the right hemisphere than the left, and these parameters tended to be improved in the IGF-1-treated animals.

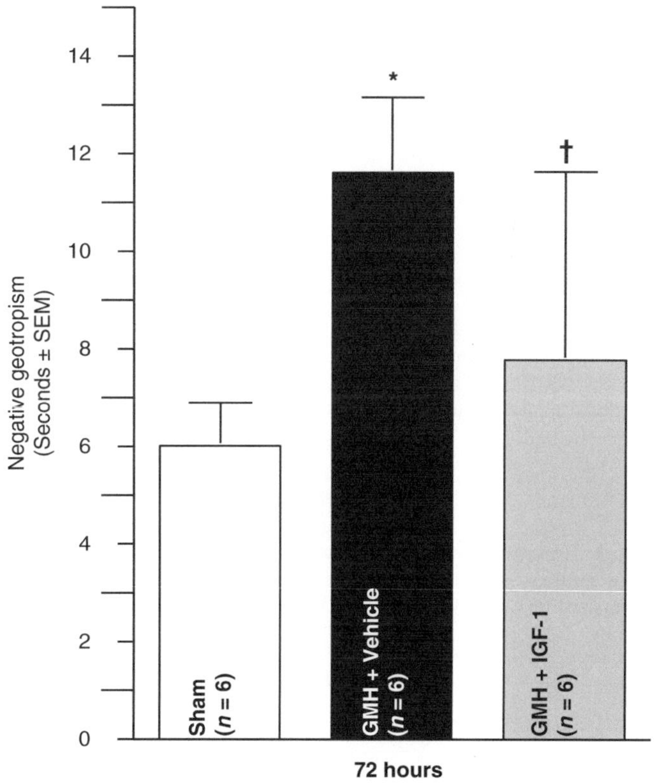

Fig. 1 Developmental milestone, measured by negative geotropism (*seconds*), 72 h after collagenase infusion; (*asterisk*) <0.05 compared with sham; (*cross*) <0.05 compared with GMH (*vehicle*); *SEM* standard error of the mean; $n=6$/group

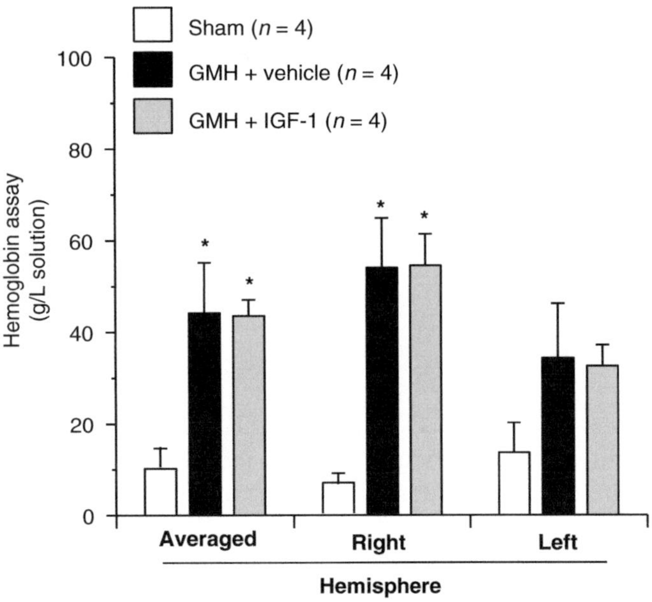

Fig. 2 Hemoglobin assay, measured by spectrophotometer, 72 h after collagenase infusion; (*asterisk*) <0.05 compared with sham; *SEM* standard error of the mean; $n = 4$/group

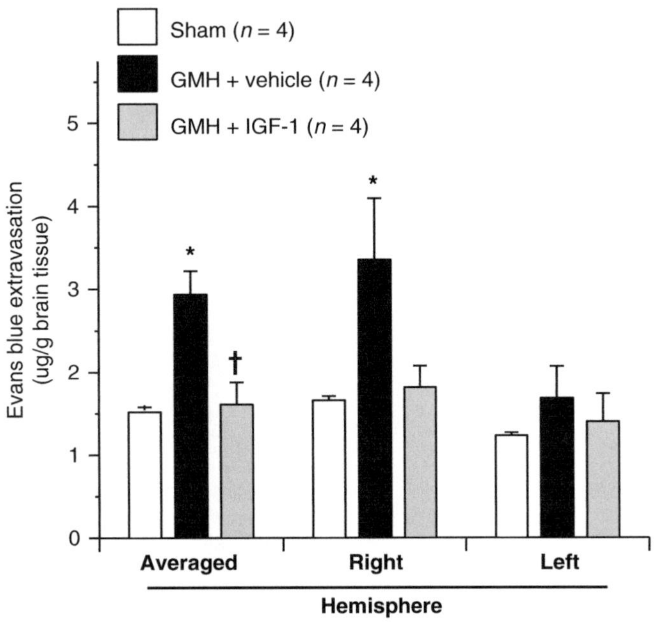

Fig. 3 Evans blue, measured by spectrophotometer, 72 h after collagenase infusion; (*asterisk*) <0.05 compared with sham; (*cross*) <0.05 compared with GMH (*vehicle*); *SEM* standard error of the mean; $n = 4$/group

Conclusion

Translational stroke studies, in particular those involving animal modeling, are greatly needed to safely integrate basic preclinical scientific principles ahead of further clinical applications [19–23]. This study showed that intranasal IGF-1 treated animals had improved neurological function and amelioration of BBB permeability, edema, and rebleeding. Therefore, IGF-1 may eventually be shown to play a part in protective brain signaling following GMH. Our observed protective effect may thus offer new promise for potential novel investigations of treatment targeting this vulnerable patient population.

Acknowledgment This study was partially supported by the National Institutes of Health grant RO1 NS078755 (Dr. Zhang).

Disclosures None

References

1. Ballabh P (2010) Intraventricular hemorrhage in premature infants: mechanism of disease. Pediatr Res 67:1–8
2. Zhao J, Chen Z, Xi G, Keep RF, Hua Y (2014) Deferoxamine attenuates acute hydrocephalus after traumatic brain injury in rats. Transl Stroke Res 5:586–594
3. Aquilina K, Chakkarapani E, Love S, Thoresen M (2011) Neonatal rat model of intraventricular haemorrhage and post-haemorrhagic ventricular dilatation with long-term survival into adulthood. Neuropathol Appl Neurobiol 37:156–165
4. Chen Q, Zhang J, Guo J, Tang J, Tao Y, Li L, Feng H, Chen Z (2014) Chronic hydrocephalus and perihematomal tissue injury developed in a rat model of intracerebral hemorrhage with ventricular extension. Transl Stroke Res. doi:10.1007/s12975-014-0367-5
5. Heron M, Sutton PD, Xu J, Ventura SJ, Strobino DM, Guyer B (2010) Annual summary of vital statistics: 2007. Pediatrics 125:4–15
6. Whitelaw A (2001) Intraventricular haemorrhage and posthaemorrhagic hydrocephalus: pathogenesis, prevention and future interventions. Semin Neonatol 6:135–146
7. Ploughman M, Austin MW, Glynn L, Corbett D (2015) The effects of poststroke aerobic exercise on neuroplasticity: a systematic review of animal and clinical studies. Transl Stroke Res 6:13–28
8. Fernandez AM, de la Vega AG, Torres-Aleman I (1998) Insulin-like growth factor I restores motor coordination in a rat model of cerebellar ataxia. Proc Natl Acad Sci U S A 95:1253–1258
9. Lekic T, Rolland W, Hartman R, Kamper J, Suzuki H, Tang J, Zhang JH (2011) Characterization of the brain injury, neurobehavioral profiles, and histopathology in a rat model of cerebellar hemorrhage. Exp Neurol 227:96–103
10. Manaenko A, Lekic T, Barnhart M, Hartman R, Zhang JH (2014) Inhibition of transforming growth factor-beta attenuates brain injury and neurological deficits in a rat model of germinal matrix hemorrhage. Stroke 45:828–834
11. Lekic T, Manaenko A, Rolland W, Krafft PR, Peters R, Hartman RE, Altay O, Tang J, Zhang JH (2012) Rodent neonatal germinal matrix hemorrhage mimics the human brain injury, neurological consequences, and post-hemorrhagic hydrocephalus. Exp Neurol 236:69–78
12. Leitzke AS, Rolland WB, Krafft PR, Lekic T, Klebe D, Flores JJ, Van Allen NR, Applegate RL 2nd, Zhang JH (2013) Isoflurane post-treatment ameliorates GMH-induced brain injury in neonatal rats. Stroke 44:3587–3590
13. Thullier F, Lalonde R, Cousin X, Lestienne F (1997) Neurobehavioral evaluation of lurcher mutant mice during ontogeny. Brain Res Dev Brain Res 100:22–28

14. Schlunk F, Schulz E, Lauer A, Yigitkanli K, Pfeilschifter W, Steinmetz H, Lo EH, Foerch C (2014) Warfarin pretreatment reduces cell death and MMP-9 activity in experimental intracerebral hemorrhage. Transl Stroke Res. doi:10.1007/s12975-014- 0377-3
15. Tang J, Liu J, Zhou C, Alexander JS, Nanda A, Granger DN, Zhang JH (2004) Mmp-9 deficiency enhances collagenase-induced intracerebral hemorrhage and brain injury in mutant mice. J Cereb Blood Flow Metab 24:1133–1145
16. Choudhri TF, Hoh BL, Solomon RA, Connolly ES Jr, Pinsky DJ (1997) Use of a spectrophotometric hemoglobin assay to objectively quantify intracerebral hemorrhage in mice. Stroke 28:2296–2302
17. Merali Z, Leung J, Mikulis D, Silver F, Kassner A (2015) Longitudinal assessment of imatinib's effect on the blood-brain barrier after ischemia/reperfusion injury with permeability MRI. Transl Stroke Res 6:39–49
18. Li H, Gao A, Feng D, Wang Y, Zhang L, Cui Y, Li B, Wang Z, Chen G (2014) Evaluation of the protective potential of brain microvascular endothelial cell autophagy on blood-brain barrier integrity during experimental cerebral ischemia-reperfusion injury. Transl Stroke Res 5:618–626
19. Tso MK, Macdonald RL (2014) Subarachnoid hemorrhage: a review of experimental studies on the microcirculation and the neurovascular unit. Transl Stroke Res 5:174–189
20. Marbacher S, Nevzati E, Croci D, Erhardt S, Muroi C, Jakob SM, Fandino J (2014) The rabbit shunt model of subarachnoid haemorrhage. Transl Stroke Res 5:669–680
21. Pluta RM, Bacher J, Skopets B, Hoffmann V (2014) A non-human primate model of aneurismal subarachnoid hemorrhage (SAH). Transl Stroke Res 5:681–691
22. Zhang YP, Cai J, Shields LB, Liu N, Xu XM, Shields CB (2014) Traumatic brain injury using mouse models. Transl Stroke Res 5:454–471
23. Wada K, Makino H, Shimada K, Shikata F, Kuwabara A, Hashimoto T (2014) Translational research using a mouse model of intracranial aneurysm. Transl Stroke Res 5:248–251

PAR-1, -4, and the mTOR Pathway Following Germinal Matrix Hemorrhage

Tim Lekic, Paul R. Krafft, Damon Klebe, Jerry Flores, William B. Rolland, Jiping Tang, and John H. Zhang

Introduction

Germinal matrix hemorrhage (GMH) is the most common neurological disease of premature infants, partly because this germinal region is most vulnerable to spontaneous bleeding within the first 3 days of preterm life [1]. Intracerebroventricular expansion partly contributes to long-term brain injury through mechanical compression of surrounding tissues [2–4]. Devastating outcomes include hydrocephalus, mental retardation, and cerebral palsy [1, 5, 6]. Current treatment modalities are largely ineffective, and GMH has been thus far not preventable [7]. Importantly, the blood constituent thrombin is an established factor in hydrocephalus formation [8, 9] that binds and trans-activates a subfamily of G protein-coupled receptors named proteinase-activated-receptors (specifically PAR-1 and PAR-4) [10], theoretically leading to phosphorylation and activation of the mammalian target of rapamycin (mTOR) [11, 12]. Therefore, we hypothesized that modulation of brain injury using the thrombin–PAR-1, -4–mTOR pathway could be an eventual strategy to help improve outcomes after GMH.

T. Lekic • P.R. Krafft • D. Klebe • J. Flores • W.B. Rolland
J. Tang
Division of Physiology and Pharmacology, School of Medicine, Loma Linda, CA, USA

J.H. Zhang, MD, PhD (✉)
Division of Physiology and Pharmacology, School of Medicine, Loma Linda, CA, USA

Department of Neurosurgery, School of Medicine, Loma Linda, CA, USA

Department of Physiology and Pharmacology, Loma Linda University School of Medicine, 11041 Campus Street, Risley Hall Rm 219, Loma Linda, CA 92354, USA
e-mail: johnzhang3910@yahoo.com

Methods

All studies, protocols, and procedures were approved by the Institutional Animal Care and Use Committee at Loma Linda University. Postnatal day 7 (P7) neonatal rats were subjected to stereotactic ganglionic eminence collagenase infusion. Rodents were euthanized at 72 h (short-term) or 4 weeks (long-term). Short-term mTOR expression was evaluated by Western blot in the context of PAR-1 (SCH-79797) and PAR-4 (P4pal10) inhibition. Pups in the long-term group were administered the selective mTOR inhibitor (rapamycin), and neurobehavioral examinations were performed at 4 weeks [13].

Animal Surgeries

P7 Sprague-Dawley rat pups (14–19 g) were randomly allocated to either GMH or sham operation. A stereotactically guided, 0.3 U bacterial collagenase infusion model was used to model preterm right-sided ganglionic eminence bleeds [14–16]. Timed pregnant rats were purchased from Harlan Laboratories (Indianapolis, IN, USA) and pups of equally both genders were subjected to collagenase infusion [15]. Briefly, general anesthesia was obtained by using isoflurane (3 % in 30/70 % oxygen/medical air). Anesthetized pups were positioned prone, with heads secured onto the neonatal stereotactic frame (Kopf Instruments, Tujunga, CA, USA). The scalp was then sterilized (using betadine solution), followed by a small midline incision to expose the bregma. A 1-mm cranial burr hole was made using a standard dental drill (bregma coordinates: 1.8 mm anterior, 1.5 mm lateral, 2.8 mm deep) through which a 26-gauge needle was lowered, and at this position, clostridial collagenase VII-S (0.3 U; Sigma, St. Louis, MO, USA) was infused at 0.25 μl/min into the right basal ganglion. The needle was left in place for 10 min following infusion to prevent backflow. Thereafter,

R.L. Applegate et al. (eds.), *Brain Edema XVI: Translate Basic Science into Clinical Practice*, Acta Neurochirurgica Supplement, Vol. 121, DOI 10.1007/978-3-319-18497-5_38,

the needle was slowly withdrawn at rate of 1 mm/min, the burr hole was sealed with bone wax, and the scalp was sutured closed. All animals were allowed to recover under observation on a 37 °C warm heating blanket before being returned to their dams. Shams received all of the above without collagenase infusion, as routinely performed [13].

Animal Perfusion and Tissue Extraction

The animals were fatally anesthetized with isoflurane (≥5 %) followed by cardiovascular perfusion with ice-cold phosphate-buffered saline (PBS) for thrombin and Western blot analyses. Forebrains were dissected and snap-frozen with liquid-nitrogen, and then stored in a −80 °C freezer awaiting quantification per routine [13].

Thrombin Assay

Animals were sacrificed at 6 h, 1 day, 5 days, 7 days, 10 days, and 21 days following GMH in accordance with standard protocols [14–16]. Brain samples were homogenized and thrombin amidolytic activity measured by thrombin-specific chromogenic substrate, S2238 (Anaspec, Fremont, CA, USA) [17]. Final concentrations of S2238 solution were in 20 mM in phosphate-buffered saline, and thrombin standards were made using rat thrombin (Sigma Aldrich, St. Louis, MO, USA) at concentrations of 0, 1.5625, 3.125, 6.25, 12.5, 25, and 50 mU/ml. Further reaction mixtures consisted of 10 μl of brain sample supernatant and 1.5 μl of s2238 chromogenic mixture, which were admixed to the 90 μl of PBS. These reaction mixtures were then allowed to incubate for 1 h at room temperature, after which sample absorbance was spectrophotometrically determined using 405 nm.

Western Blotting

For the protein immunoblot [13], the concentration was determined using the DC protein assay (Bio-Rad, Hercules, CA, USA). The samples were then subjected to SDS-PAGE on 4–20 % gels, and then transferred to nitrocellulose membrane X 100 min at 100 V (Bio-Rad). Blotting membranes were incubated for 1 h with 5 % nonfat milk in Tris-buffered saline containing 0.1 % Tween 20, and these were then incubated overnight with the primary antibody, anti-phospho-mTOR (1:1,000; Cell Signaling Technology, Danvers, MA, USA). Membranes were then incubated using secondary antibodies (1:1,000; Santa Cruz Biotechnology, Santa Cruz, CA, USA) and processed with an ECL Plus kit (GE Healthcare and Life Science, Piscataway, NJ, USA). For an internal control, the same membrane was probed using an antibody against β-actin (1:1,000; Santa Cruz Biotechnology, Santa Cruz, CA, USA) after being stripped. Relative densities of resultant protein immunoblot images were semiquantitatively analyzed by Image J software (4.0, Media Cybernetics, Silver Spring, MD, USA) as described elsewhere [18].

Neurological Deficit

Assessments were conducted in a blinded manner by experienced investigators [13–16]. The T-maze assessed short-term (working) memory ability [19]. For each trial, rats were placed into the stem (40 cm × 10 cm) of a T-maze and allowed to explore until either the left or right path was chosen. Following a sequence of 10 trials, the rate of spontaneous alternation (0 % = none and 100 % = complete; alternations/trial) was recorded [20, 21].

Statistical Analysis

Significance was based on $p<0.05$. Data were statistically analyzed using one-way analysis of variance (ANOVA), followed by Tukey post hoc test for significant analyses. Statistical analyses were performed using SigmaPlot version 10.0 for Windows.

Results

Thrombin increased early after collagenase infusion in a time-dependant manner (Fig. 1). Corresponding combined PAR-1 and PAR-4 signal inhibition normalized increased mTOR activation ($p<0.05$; Fig. 2) in a dose responsive manner measured 72 h after collagenase infusion. Thereafter, in a separate cohort of animals, direct inhibition of mTOR by rapamycin improved long-term neurobehavior ($p<0.05$; Fig. 3).

Conclusion

Translational stroke studies, in particular those involving animal modeling, are greatly needed to safely integrate basic preclinical investigations ahead of eventual clinical applications

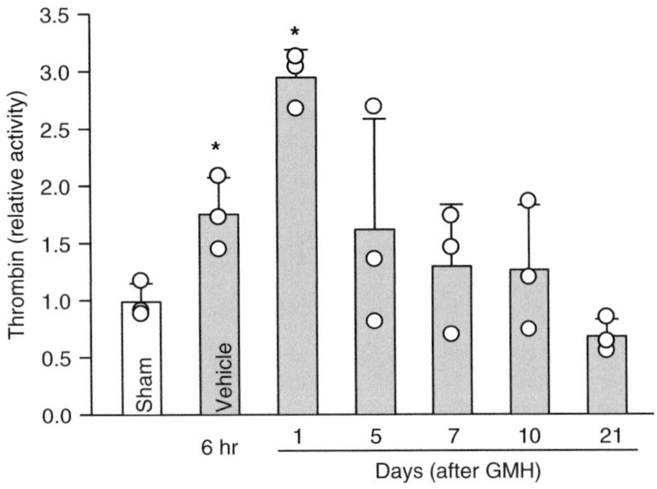

Fig. 1 Thrombin activity following GMH, timed levels using standard assay

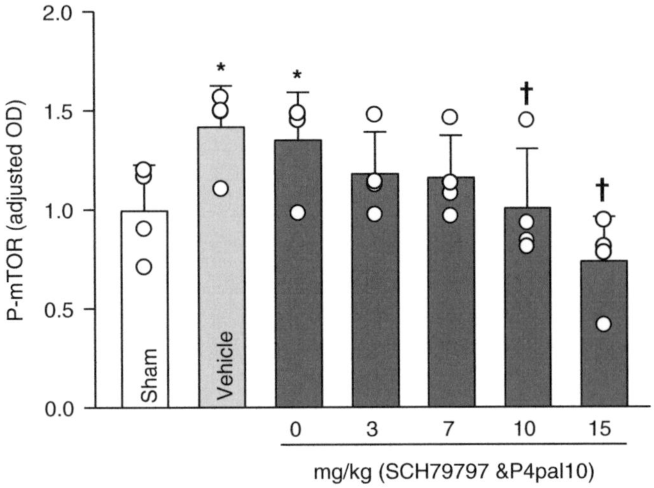

Fig. 2 mTOR activity post-GMH; dose-response following PAR-1 and PAR-4 co- administration; 72 h after collagenase infusion; (*asterisk*) <0.05 compared with sham; (*cross*) <0.05 compared with GMH (*vehicle*); *SEM* standard error of the mean; $n=4$/group

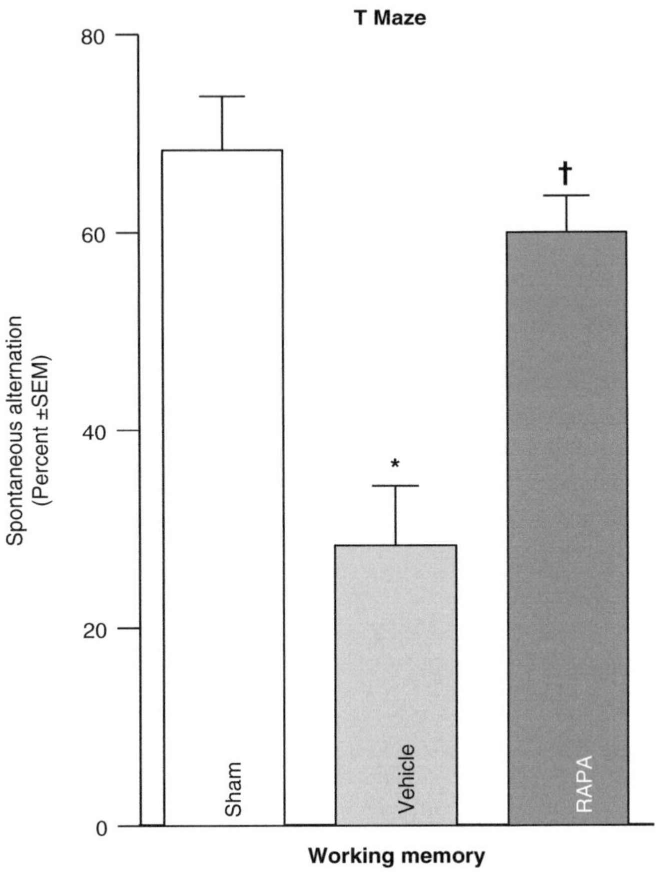

Fig. 3 T-maze (spontaneous alterations) measured 1 month after collagenase infusion; (*asterisk*) <0.05 compared with sham; *SEM* standard error of the mean; and the $n=4$/group

[22–26]. This study therefore investigated the modulation of thrombin–PAR-1 and PAR-4 in reversing p-mTOR upregulation, as well as the effect of direct p-mTOR inhibition on neurological deficits. Prior studies hypothesized mechanisms of hydrocephalus involving increased production of infiltrating extracellular matrix (ECM) proteins of the cerebroventricular system, thus leading to the disruption of cerebrospinal fluid (CSF) outflow [1, 2, 14, 15, 27–32]. Our results suggested that thrombin-induced PAR-1,-4 stimulation could upregulate detrimental proliferative responses (i.e., p-mTOR mediated), possibly upstream of ECM dysregulation [1, 8, 11, 14, 15, 33–35]. To address the question of molecular mediators, we demonstrated that intraparenchymal infusion of collagenase generated thrombin with greatest activity in the acute phase between 6 and 24 h post-GMH, and then hypothesized that thrombin binds to PAR-1, -4 receptors, consequently upregulating p-mTOR. Because thrombin is most active in the early time frame, we examined levels at 72 h after GMH and found that p-mTOR was significantly greater in vehicle animals compared with shams. Then, inhibiting PAR-1, -4 through combined therapy using SCH-79797 (PAR-1 antagonist) and p4pal10 (PAR-4 antagonist) significantly ameliorated p-mTOR by day 3 after GMH. We then asked whether direct inhibition of p-mTOR could improve long-term outcome. Our findings showed that vehicle-treated animals significantly worsened outcome compared with shams, and treating with rapamycin (mTOR inhibitor) could significantly improve neurological ability. Thus, by decreasing early proliferative (i.e., p-mTOR) signaling, we improved long-term juvenile outcome. In sum, this study showed that thrombin-PAR-1, -4 signal inhibitions normalized early p-mTOR expression, and may improve long-term GMH outcome.

Acknowledgment This study was partially supported by the National Institutes of Health grant RO1 NS078755 (Dr. Zhang).

Disclosures None

References

1. Ballabh P (2010) Intraventricular hemorrhage in premature infants: mechanism of disease. Pediatr Res 67:1–8
2. Aquilina K, Chakkarapani E, Love S, Thoresen M (2011) Neonatal rat model of intraventricular haemorrhage and post-haemorrhagic ventricular dilatation with long-term survival into adulthood. Neuropathol Appl Neurobiol 37:156–165
3. Chen Q, Zhang J, Guo J, Tang J, Tao Y, Li L, Feng H, Chen Z (2014) Chronic hydrocephalus and perihematomal tissue injury developed in a rat model of intracerebral hemorrhage with ventricular extension. Transl Stroke Res. doi:10.1007/s12975-014-0367-5
4. Zhao J, Chen Z, Xi G, Keep RF, Hua Y (2014) Deferoxamine attenuates acute hydrocephalus after traumatic brain injury in rats. Transl Stroke Res 5:586–594
5. Heron M, Sutton PD, Xu J, Ventura SJ, Strobino DM, Guyer B (2010) Annual summary of vital statistics: 2007. Pediatrics 125:4–15
6. Uria-Avellanal C, Robertson NJ (2014) Na(+)/H(+) exchangers and intracellular pH in perinatal brain injury. Transl Stroke Res 5:79–98
7. Whitelaw A (2001) Intraventricular haemorrhage and posthaemorrhagic hydrocephalus: pathogenesis, prevention and future interventions. Semin Neonatol 6:135–146
8. Gao F, Liu F, Chen Z, Hua Y, Keep RF, Xi G (2014) Hydrocephalus after intraventricular hemorrhage: the role of thrombin. J Cereb Blood Flow Metab 34:489–494
9. Cheng Y, Xi G, Jin H, Keep RF, Feng J, Hua Y (2014) Thrombin-induced cerebral hemorrhage: role of protease-activated receptor-1. Transl Stroke Res 5:472–475
10. Kataoka H, Hamilton JR, McKemy DD, Camerer E, Zheng YW, Cheng A, Griffin C, Coughlin SR (2003) Protease-activated receptors 1 and 4 mediate thrombin signaling in endothelial cells. Blood 102:3224–3231
11. Jiang X, Zhu S, Panetti TS, Bromberg ME (2008) Formation of tissue factor- factor VIIa-factor Xa complex induces activation of the mTOR pathway which regulates migration of human breast cancer cells. Thromb Haemost 100:127–133
12. Li H, Gao A, Feng D, Wang Y, Zhang L, Cui Y, Li B, Wang Z, Chen G (2014) Evaluation of the protective potential of brain microvascular endothelial cell autophagy on blood-brain barrier integrity during experimental cerebral ischemia-reperfusion injury. Transl Stroke Res 5:618–626
13. Lekic T, Rolland W, Hartman R, Kamper J, Suzuki H, Tang J, Zhang JH (2011) Characterization of the brain injury, neurobehavioral profiles, and histopathology in a rat model of cerebellar hemorrhage. Exp Neurol 227:96–103
14. Manaenko A, Lekic T, Barnhart M, Hartman R, Zhang JH (2014) Inhibition of transforming growth factor-beta attenuates brain injury and neurological deficits in a rat model of germinal matrix hemorrhage. Stroke 45:828–834
15. Lekic T, Manaenko A, Rolland W, Krafft PR, Peters R, Hartman RE, Altay O, Tang J, Zhang JH (2012) Rodent neonatal germinal matrix hemorrhage mimics the human brain injury, neurological consequences, and post-hemorrhagic hydrocephalus. Exp Neurol 236:69–78
16. Leitzke AS, Rolland WB, Krafft PR, Lekic T, Klebe D, Flores JJ, Van Allen NR, Applegate RL 2nd, Zhang JH (2013) Isoflurane post-treatment ameliorates GMH-induced brain injury in neonatal rats. Stroke 44:3587–3590
17. Gong Y, Xi G, Hu H, Gu Y, Huang F, Keep RF, Hua Y (2008) Increase in brain thrombin activity after experimental intracerebral hemorrhage. Acta Neurochir Suppl 105:47–50
18. Tang J, Liu J, Zhou C, Alexander JS, Nanda A, Granger DN, Zhang JH (2004) Mmp-9 deficiency enhances collagenase-induced intracerebral hemorrhage and brain injury in mutant mice. J Cereb Blood Flow Metab 24:1133–1145
19. Hughes RN (2004) The value of spontaneous alternation behavior (SAB) as a test of retention in pharmacological investigations of memory. Neurosci Biobehav Rev 28:497–505
20. Fathali N, Ostrowski RP, Lekic T, Jadhav V, Tong W, Tang J, Zhang JH (2010) Cyclooxygenase-2 inhibition provides lasting protection against neonatal hypoxic-ischemic brain injury. Crit Care Med 38:572–578
21. Zhou Y, Fathali N, Lekic T, Tang J, Zhang JH (2009) Glibenclamide improves neurological function in neonatal hypoxia-ischemia in rats. Brain Res 1270:131–139
22. Tso MK, Macdonald RL (2014) Subarachnoid hemorrhage: a review of experimental studies on the microcirculation and the neurovascular unit. Transl Stroke Res 5:174–189
23. Marbacher S, Nevzati E, Croci D, Erhardt S, Muroi C, Jakob SM, Fandino J (2014) The rabbit shunt model of subarachnoid haemorrhage. Transl Stroke Res 5:669–680
24. Pluta RM, Bacher J, Skopets B, Hoffmann V (2014) A non-human primate model of aneurismal subarachnoid hemorrhage (SAH). Transl Stroke Res 5:681–691
25. Zhang YP, Cai J, Shields LB, Liu N, Xu XM, Shields CB (2014) Traumatic brain injury using mouse models. Transl Stroke Res 5:454–471
26. Wada K, Makino H, Shimada K, Shikata F, Kuwabara A, Hashimoto T (2014) Translational research using a mouse model of intracranial aneurysm. Transl Stroke Res 5:248–251
27. Strahle J, Garton HL, Maher C, Muraszko K, Keep R, Xi G (2012) Mechanisms of hydrocephalus after neonatal and adult intraventricular hemorrhage. Transl Stroke Res 3:25–38
28. Crews L, Wyss-Coray T, Masliah E (2004) Insights into the pathogenesis of hydrocephalus from transgenic and experimental animal models. Brain Pathol 14:312–316
29. Siler DA, Gonzalez JA, Wang RK, Cetas JS, Alkayed NJ (2014) Intracisternal administration of tissue plasminogen activator improves cerebrospinal fluid flow and cortical perfusion after subarachnoid hemorrhage in mice. Transl Stroke Res 5:227–237
30. Khanna A, Kahle KT, Walcott BP, Gerzanich V, Simard JM (2014) Disruption of ion homeostasis in the neurogliovascular unit underlies the pathogenesis of ischemic cerebral edema. Transl Stroke Res 5:3–16
31. Yamauchi T, Saito H, Ito M, Shichinohe H, Houkin K, Kuroda S (2014) Platelet lysate and granulocyte-colony stimulating factor serve safe and accelerated expansion of human bone marrow stromal cells for stroke therapy. Transl Stroke Res 5:701–710
32. Sorensen SS, Nygaard AB, Nielsen MY, Jensen K, Christensen T (2014) miRNA expression profiles in cerebrospinal fluid and blood of patients with acute ischemic stroke. Transl Stroke Res 5:711–718
33. Lo HM, Chen CL, Tsai YJ, Wu PH, Wu WB (2009) Thrombin induces cyclooxygenase-2 expression and prostaglandin E2 release via PAR1 activation and ERK1/2- and p38 MAPK-dependent pathway in murine macrophages. J Cell Biochem 108:1143–1152
34. Gao C, Du H, Hua Y, Keep RF, Strahle J, Xi G (2014) Role of red blood cell lysis and iron in hydrocephalus after intraventricular hemorrhage. J Cereb Blood Flow Metab 34:1070–1075
35. Badaut J, Bix GJ (2014) Vascular neural network phenotypic transformation after traumatic injury: potential role in long-term sequelae. Transl Stroke Res 5:394–406

Intranasal Osteopontin for Rodent Germinal Matrix Hemorrhage

Jay Malaguit, Darlene Casel, Brandon Dixon, Desislava Doycheva, Jiping Tang, John H. Zhang, and Tim Lekic

Introduction

Germinal matrix hemorrhage (GMH) is the most common neurological disease of premature infants, partly because this germinal region is most vulnerable to spontaneous bleeding within the first 3 days of preterm life [1]. Intracerebroventricular expansion partly contributes to long-term brain injury through mechanical compression of surrounding tissues [2–4]. Devastating outcomes include hydrocephalus, mental retardation, and cerebral palsy [1, 5, 6]. Current treatment modalities are largely ineffective, and GMH has been thus far not preventable [7].

Osteopontin (OPN) is an endogenous neuroprotective protein that has been shown to be neuroprotective in multiple animal models of stroke [8–13]. Therefore, we hypothesized that modulation of brain injury using OPN treatment could be a promising strategy to improve outcomes after GMH.

J. Malaguit • B. Dixon • D. Doycheva • J. Tang
Division of Physiology and Pharmacology, School of Medicine, Loma Linda, CA, USA

D. Casel
Departments of Neonatology, School of Medicine, Loma Linda, CA, USA

J.H. Zhang
Division of Physiology and Pharmacology, School of Medicine, Loma Linda, CA, USA

Neurosurgery, School of Medicine, Loma Linda, CA, USA

T. Lekic, MD, PhD (✉)
Division of Physiology and Pharmacology, School of Medicine, Loma Linda, CA, USA

Department of Physiology, Loma Linda University School of Medicine, 11041 Campus Street, Risley Hall Rm 129, Loma Linda, CA 92354, USA
e-mail: tlekic@llu.edu

Methods

All studies, protocols, and procedures were approved by the Institutional Animal Care and Use Committee at Loma Linda University. Postnatal day 7 (P7) neonatal rats were subjected to stereotactic ganglionic eminence collagenase infusion. Groups were as follows: (1) sham, (2) GMH + vehicle, (3) GMH + intranasal OPN. Seventy-two hours later, the animals were evaluated using righting reflex, blood-brain barrier (BBB) permeability by Evans blue dye leakage, and hemoglobin assay, as routinely performed [14].

Animal Surgeries

P7 Sprague-Dawley rat pups (14–19 g) were randomly allocated to either GMH or sham operation. A stereotactically guided, 0.3 U bacterial collagenase infusion model was used to model preterm right-sided ganglionic eminence bleeds [15–17]. Timed pregnant rats were purchased from Harlan Laboratories (Indianapolis, IN, USA) and pups of equally both genders were subjected to collagenase infusion [16]. Briefly, general anesthesia was obtained by using isoflurane (3 % in 30/70 % oxygen/medical air). Anesthetized pups were positioned prone, with heads secured onto the neonatal stereotactic frame (Kopf Instruments, Tujunga, CA, USA). The scalp was then sterilized (using betadine solution), followed by a small midline incision to expose the bregma. A 1-mm cranial burr hole was made using a standard dental drill (bregma coordinates: 1.8 mm anterior, 1.5 mm lateral, 2.8 mm deep) through which a 26-gauge needle was lowered, and at this position, clostridial collagenase VII-S (0.3 U, Sigma; St. Louis, MO, USA) was infused at 0.25 μl/min into the right basal ganglion. The needle was left in place for 10 min following infusion to prevent backflow. Thereafter, the needle was slowly withdrawn at rate of 1 mm/min, the burr hole sealed with bone wax, and the scalp was sutured

R.L. Applegate et al. (eds.), *Brain Edema XVI: Translate Basic Science into Clinical Practice*, Acta Neurochirurgica Supplement, Vol. 121,
DOI 10.1007/978-3-319-18497-5_39,

closed. All animals were allowed to recover under observation on a 37 °C warm heating blanket before being returned to their dams. Shams received all of the above without collagenase infusion, as routinely performed [14].

Assessment of Neurological Deficits

Acquisition of developmental milestone was assessed following collagenase infusion. For negative geotropism, the time needed for complete rotation (180°) after being placed head down on a slope (20° angle) was recorded [18]. All neurobehavior assessments were conducted in a blinded manner by experienced investigators [15–17]. The maximum allotted time was 60 s per trial (two trials/day) for these tests as routinely performed [14].

Animal Perfusion and Tissue Extraction

The animals were fatally anesthetized with isoflurane (≥5 %) followed by cardiovascular perfusion with ice-cold phosphate-buffered saline (PBS) for hemoglobin assay, and Evans blue analyses. Forebrains were dissected and snap-frozen with liquid-nitrogen, and then stored in a −80 °C freezer awaiting spectrophotometric quantification as routinely performed [14].

Hemoglobin Assay

Spectrophotometric measurement of hemorrhage [19] was performed using established protocols [20, 21]. Extracted forebrain tissue was placed into test tubes with 3 mL PBS, homogenized for 60 s (Tissue Miser Homogenizer; Fisher Scientific, Pittsburgh, PA, USA), and, after ultrasonication for 1 min, lysed erythrocyte membrane products were then centrifuged for 30 min and Drabkin's reagent was added (Sigma-Aldrich) into aliquots of supernatant, which reacted for 15 min. The measurement of absorbance, using a spectrophotometer (540 nm; Genesis 10 uv; Thermo Fisher Scientific, Waltham, MA, USA) was plotted onto a graph as a conversion into blood volume (μL) on the basis of standard curves, as routinely performed [14].

Evans Blue

The spectrophotometric measurement of the dye of Evans blue [22, 23] was initiated through dye injected intraperitoneally (IP) after GMH to measure BBB permeability. Under anesthesia, Evans blue (Sigma-Aldrich) in normal saline (2 %, 4 ml/kg) was infused. For quantitative measurements, brain tissue was homogenized in 3 ml of N, N- dimethylformamide (Sigma-Aldrich), incubated for 18 h at 55 °C, then centrifuged. Supernatants were analyzed at 620 nm by spectrophotometer, as routine [14].

Statistical Analysis

Significance was based on $p<0.05$. Data were statistically analyzed using one-way analysis of variance (ANOVA), followed by Tukey post hoc test for significant analyses. Statistical analyses were performed using SigmaPlot version 10.0 for Windows.

Results

GMH significantly delayed development of the negative geotropism reflex by 72 h after collagenase infusion compared with sham (see Fig. 1) and was significantly improved using OPN therapy. Figures 2 and 3 demonstrate the GMH animal model having a significant amount of bleeding and BBB rupture, more so on the right hemisphere than the left, and these parameters tended to be improved in the OPN-treated animals.

Conclusion

OPN may play an important role in enhancing neuroprotective brain signaling following GMH. Translational stroke studies, including animal modeling, are greatly needed to safely integrate basic preclinical scientific principles ahead of clinical application [24–28]. Intranasal OPN improved outcomes after GMH by attenuation of brain swelling, BBB function, re-bleeding, and neurological outcomes. These observed effects may offer novel possibilities for eventual therapy in this patient population. Further study is needed to evaluate the mechanisms of this neuroprotection.

Acknowledgment This study was partially supported by the National Institutes of Health grant RO1 NS078755 (Dr. Zhang) and American Heart Association CRP 17380009 (Dr. Lekic).

Disclosures None

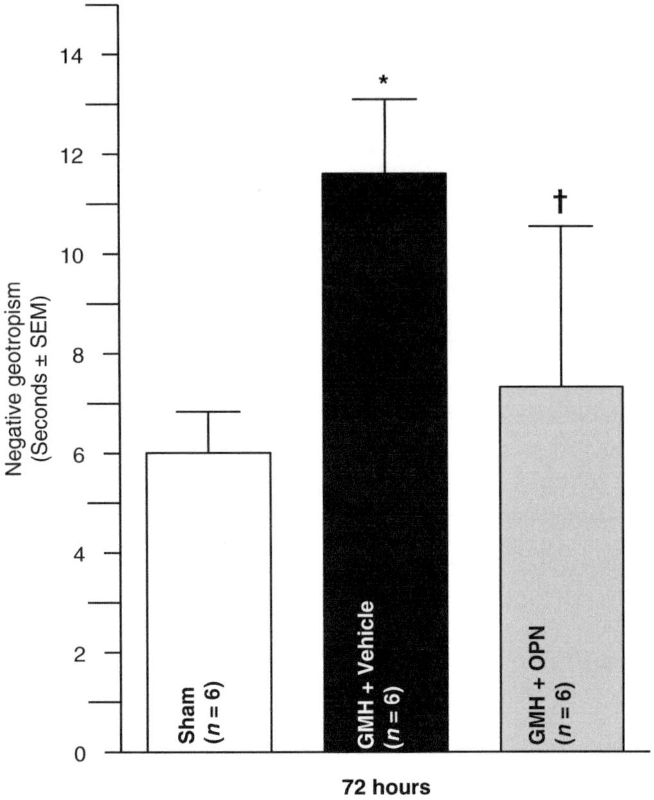

Fig. 1 Developmental milestone, measured by negative geotropism (*seconds*), 72 h after collagenase infusion; (*asterisk*) <0.05 compared with sham; (*cross*) <0.05 compared with GMH (*vehicle*); *SEM* standard error of the mean; *n* = 6/group

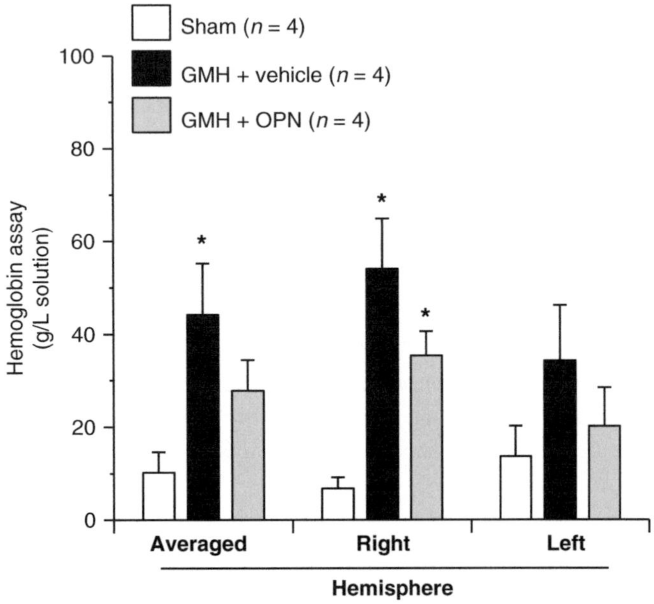

Fig. 2 Hemoglobin assay, measured by spectrophotometer, 72 h after collagenase infusion; (*asterisk*) <0.05 compared with sham; *SEM* standard error of the mean; *n* = 4/group

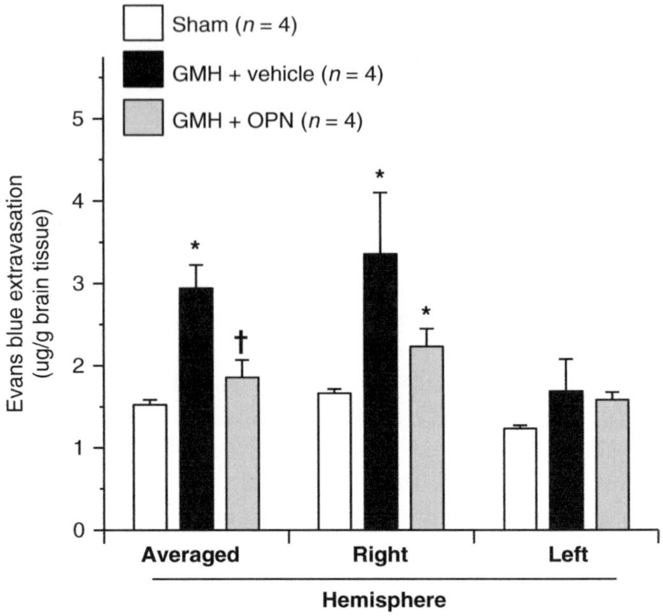

Fig. 3 Evans blue, measured by spectrophotometer, 72 h after collagenase infusion; (*asterisk*) <0.05 compared with sham; (*cross*) <0.05 compared with GMH (*vehicle*); *SEM* standard error of the mean; *n* = 4/group

References

1. Ballabh P (2010) Intraventricular hemorrhage in premature infants: mechanism of disease. Pediatr Res 67:1–8
2. Aquilina K, Chakkarapani E, Love S, Thoresen M (2011) Neonatal rat model of intraventricular haemorrhage and post-haemorrhagic ventricular dilatation with long-term survival into adulthood. Neuropathol Appl Neurobiol 37:156–165
3. Chen Q, Zhang J, Guo J, Tang J, Tao Y, Li L, Feng H, Chen Z (2014) Chronic hydrocephalus and perihematomal tissue injury developed in a rat model of intracerebral hemorrhage with ventricular extension. Transl Stroke Res. doi:10.1007/s12975-014-0367-5
4. Zhao J, Chen Z, Xi G, Keep RF, Hua Y (2014) Deferoxamine attenuates acute hydrocephalus after traumatic brain injury in rats. Transl Stroke Res 5:586–594
5. Heron M, Sutton PD, Xu J, Ventura SJ, Strobino DM, Guyer B (2010) Annual summary of vital statistics: 2007. Pediatrics 125:4–15
6. Uria-Avellanal C, Robertson NJ (2014) Na(+)/H(+) exchangers and intracellular pH in perinatal brain injury. Transl Stroke Res 5:79–98
7. Whitelaw A (2001) Intraventricular haemorrhage and posthaemorrhagic hydrocephalus: pathogenesis, prevention and future interventions. Semin Neonatol 6:135–146
8. Topkoru BC, Altay O, Duris K, Krafft PR, Yan J, Zhang JH (2013) Nasal administration of recombinant osteopontin attenuates early brain injury after subarachnoid hemorrhage. Stroke 44:3189–3194
9. Chen W, Ma Q, Suzuki H, Hartman R, Tang J, Zhang JH (2011) Osteopontin reduced hypoxia-ischemia neonatal brain injury by suppression of apoptosis in a rat pup model. Stroke 42:764–769
10. van Velthoven CT, Heijnen CJ, van Bel F, Kavelaars A (2011) Osteopontin enhances endogenous repair after neonatal hypoxic-ischemic brain injury. Stroke 42:2294

11. Suzuki H, Hasegawa Y, Chen W, Kanamaru K, Zhang JH (2010) Recombinant osteopontin in cerebral vasospasm after subarachnoid hemorrhage. Ann Neurol 68:650–660
12. Suzuki H, Hasegawa Y, Kanamaru K, Zhang JH (2010) Mechanisms of osteopontin-induced stabilization of blood-brain barrier disruption after subarachnoid hemorrhage in rats. Stroke 41:1783–1790
13. Suzuki H, Ayer R, Sugawara T, Chen W, Sozen T, Hasegawa Y, Kanamaru K, Zhang JH (2010) Protective effects of recombinant osteopontin on early brain injury after subarachnoid hemorrhage in rats. Crit Care Med 38:612–618
14. Lekic T, Rolland W, Hartman R, Kamper J, Suzuki H, Tang J, Zhang JH (2011) Characterization of the brain injury, neurobehavioral profiles, and histopathology in a rat model of cerebellar hemorrhage. Exp Neurol 227:96–103
15. Manaenko A, Lekic T, Barnhart M, Hartman R, Zhang JH (2014) Inhibition of transforming growth factor-beta attenuates brain injury and neurological deficits in a rat model of germinal matrix hemorrhage. Stroke 45:828–834
16. Lekic T, Manaenko A, Rolland W, Krafft PR, Peters R, Hartman RE, Altay O, Tang J, Zhang JH (2012) Rodent neonatal germinal matrix hemorrhage mimics the human brain injury, neurological consequences, and post-hemorrhagic hydrocephalus. Exp Neurol 236:69–78
17. Leitzke AS, Rolland WB, Krafft PR, Lekic T, Klebe D, Flores JJ, Van Allen NR, Applegate RL 2nd, Zhang JH (2013) Isoflurane post-treatment ameliorates GMH-induced brain injury in neonatal rats. Stroke 44:3587–3590
18. Thullier F, Lalonde R, Cousin X, Lestienne F (1997) Neurobehavioral evaluation of lurcher mutant mice during ontogeny. Brain Res Dev Brain Res 100:22–28
19. Schlunk F, Schulz E, Lauer A, Yigitkanli K, Pfeilschifter W, Steinmetz H, Lo EH, Foerch C (2014) Warfarin pretreatment reduces cell death and MMP-9 activity in experimental intracerebral hemorrhage. Transl Stroke Res. doi:10.1007/s12975-014- 0377-3
20. Tang J, Liu J, Zhou C, Alexander JS, Nanda A, Granger DN, Zhang JH (2004) Mmp-9 deficiency enhances collagenase-induced intracerebral hemorrhage and brain injury in mutant mice. J Cereb Blood Flow Metab 24:1133–1145
21. Choudhri TF, Hoh BL, Solomon RA, Connolly ES Jr, Pinsky DJ (1997) Use of a spectrophotometric hemoglobin assay to objectively quantify intracerebral hemorrhage in mice. Stroke 28:2296–2302
22. Merali Z, Leung J, Mikulis D, Silver F, Kassner A (2014) Longitudinal assessment of imatinib's effect on the blood-brain barrier after ischemia/reperfusion injury with permeability MRI. Transl Stroke Res 6:39–49
23. Li H, Gao A, Feng D, Wang Y, Zhang L, Cui Y, Li B, Wang Z, Chen G (2014) Evaluation of the protective potential of brain microvascular endothelial cell autophagy on blood-brain barrier integrity during experimental cerebral ischemia-reperfusion injury. Transl Stroke Res 5:618–626
24. Tso MK, Macdonald RL (2014) Subarachnoid hemorrhage: a review of experimental studies on the microcirculation and the neurovascular unit. Transl Stroke Res 5:174–189
25. Marbacher S, Nevzati E, Croci D, Erhardt S, Muroi C, Jakob SM, Fandino J (2014) The rabbit shunt model of subarachnoid haemorrhage. Transl Stroke Res 5:669–680
26. Pluta RM, Bacher J, Skopets B, Hoffmann V (2014) A non-human primate model of aneurismal subarachnoid hemorrhage (SAH). Transl Stroke Res 5:681–691
27. Zhang YP, Cai J, Shields LB, Liu N, Xu XM, Shields CB (2014) Traumatic brain injury using mouse models. Transl Stroke Res 5:454–471
28. Wada K, Makino H, Shimada K, Shikata F, Kuwabara A, Hashimoto T (2014) Translational research using a mouse model of intracranial aneurysm. Transl Stroke Res 5:248–251

Brain Ischemia Section

Novel Imaging Markers of Ischemic Cerebral Edema and Its Association with Neurological Outcome

W. Taylor Kimberly, Thomas W.K. Battey, Ona Wu, Aneesh B. Singhal, Bruce C.V. Campbell, Stephen M. Davis, Geoffrey A. Donnan, and Kevin N. Sheth

Introduction

Stroke is the fourth leading cause of death and a leading cause of disability in the United States. With nearly 700,000 ischemic stroke victims annually, the burden of illness is substantial [1]. Although successful efforts in acute therapy to date have focused on reperfusion [2–5], only a minority of stroke patients is eligible for this type of treatment.

Ischemic cerebral edema (ICE) is a well-known complication after stroke, yet remarkably little is known about the scope of its impact. Fulminant edema is a widely recognized component of the malignant infarction syndrome, leading to rapid decline, poor functional outcome, and death in up to 75 % of patients [6–8]. Decompressive craniectomy can reduce the risk of death from malignant edema and, in some instances, leads to better outcomes [9, 10]. These data unequivocally confirm that cerebral edema directly contributes to poor outcome after stroke.

We hypothesized that malignant cerebral edema after large infarction is only the most visible example of a more prevalent problem. While smaller volume strokes may not be associated with fulminant deterioration, edema may nevertheless hinder recovery. Because the time course of developing ICE spans hours to days, ICE also represents an attractive translational target for intervention [8]. We sought to fill a critical gap in the study of ICE by developing validated intermediate endpoints and a detailed characterization of its impact on neurological outcome.

Existing Strategies to Quantify Edema

Few methods are currently available that are capable of precisely quantifying edema. The existing method for measuring brain edema after stroke is an "indirect" approach that measures the change in hemisphere volume between baseline and follow-up scans. We have previously shown that this approach quantitatively assesses ICE in large hemispheric strokes [11]. Accordingly, a greater increase in hemispheric volumes was associated with early neurological deterioration [11]. However, this method also has several limitations. First, there is substantial variance in the hemispheric volume measurements, reducing the ability to detect differences in the magnitude of ICE. Second, it is insensitive to smaller volume strokes that occupy <20 % of the hemisphere volume. Third, the indirect method does not distinguish between ICE, infarct growth into new anatomic territory, or hemorrhagic transformation (HT). Thus, in the absence of a more discriminating measure of swelling, only the most severe stroke patients can be evaluated using this method.

W.T. Kimberly, MD, PhD (✉)
Department of Neurology, Massachusetts General Hospital, Lunder 644, 55 Fruit Street, Boston, MA 02114, USA
e-mail: wtkimberly@mgh.harvard.edu

T.W.K. Battey • A.B. Singhal
Department of Neurology, Massachusetts General Hospital, 55 Fruit Street, Boston, MA, USA

O. Wu
Department of Radiology, Massachusetts General Hospital, 55 Fruit Street, Boston, MA, USA

B.C.V. Campbell • S.M. Davis
Department of Medicine and Neurology, Melbourne Brain Centre, Royal Melbourne Hospital, University of Melbourne, Parkville, Victoria, Australia

G.A. Donnan
Florey Institute of Neuroscience and Mental Health, University of Melbourne, Parkville, Victoria, Australia

K.N. Sheth
Department of Neurology, Yale New Haven Hospital, New Haven, CT, USA

R.L. Applegate et al. (eds.), *Brain Edema XVI: Translate Basic Science into Clinical Practice*, Acta Neurochirurgica Supplement, Vol. 121,
DOI 10.1007/978-3-319-18497-5_40,

Novel Strategies to Measure Edema

In an effort to develop new tools to measure edema, we first assessed for the presence of swelling and/or infarct growth in a categorical manner. We reasoned that this approach could be used to separately evaluate the potential effects of lesion expansion due to infarct growth into new anatomic territory and space-occupying brain edema. We defined swelling as the presence of mass effect in affected gyri, new distortion of adjacent tissue, midline shift, or effacement of sulci. Infarct growth was defined as lesion involvement into new anatomical territory, as classified by the Alberta Stroke Program Early CT Score (ASPECTS) system [12], a validated and reproducible method of quantifying the neuroanatomic territories involved in a stroke. Using these assignments, we found evidence of ICE in 67 % of stroke patients, infarct growth in 43 %, and parenchymal hemorrhage in 12 % [13].

The change in stroke lesion volume between baseline and follow-up magnetic resonance imaging (MRI) (delta diffusion weighted imaging (DWI)) is a quantitative measure that is often used as an imaging surrogate in patients [14]. Delta DWI is consistently shown to predict outcome in a variety of settings, both with and without thrombolysis [13–16]. However, it represents a composite measure encompassing infarct growth, HT, and ICE. As a result, its specificity for reflecting the true impact of ICE is limited because of the confounding contributions of infarct growth and HT.

We therefore developed an alternative method to directly and specifically quantify ICE in a broad array of stroke volume and severity. We generated a "direct" method that assesses baseline and follow-up images, using triplanar co-registration of the stroke lesion. By comparing merged baseline and follow-up images, this has the added advantage of differentiating between ICE, infarct growth, and HT with a volume assignment for each process. Figure 1 demonstrates a representative example of the technique in a patient with distinct regions of infarct growth and ICE.

Brain Edema Portends Worse Outcome

First, using the categorical designations we found that patients with ICE had a greater likelihood of poor outcome (defined as modified Rankin Scale (mRS) 3-6; univariate $p<0.002$; Fig. 2). In this cohort, infarct growth did not have an impact on outcome until a change in ASPECTS of >1 was used. Volumetric analysis of ICE showed that patients with poor outcome had higher ICE volume than those who did not (Fig. 3). Multivariate adjustment confirmed that swelling volume was an independent predictor of poor outcome ($p=0.02$) [13]. Receiver operating characteristic (ROC) curve analysis showed that 11 mL of swelling volume had the highest sensitivity and specificity for distinguishing good versus poor outcome [13]. Together, these data suggest that ICE not only predicts worse outcome, but that an edema volume of >11 mL is sufficient to impair recovery.

Predictors of Brain Edema

To understand the underlying mechanisms that contribute to ICE, our group has also studied the lesional properties of the stroke and assessed the association with subsequent

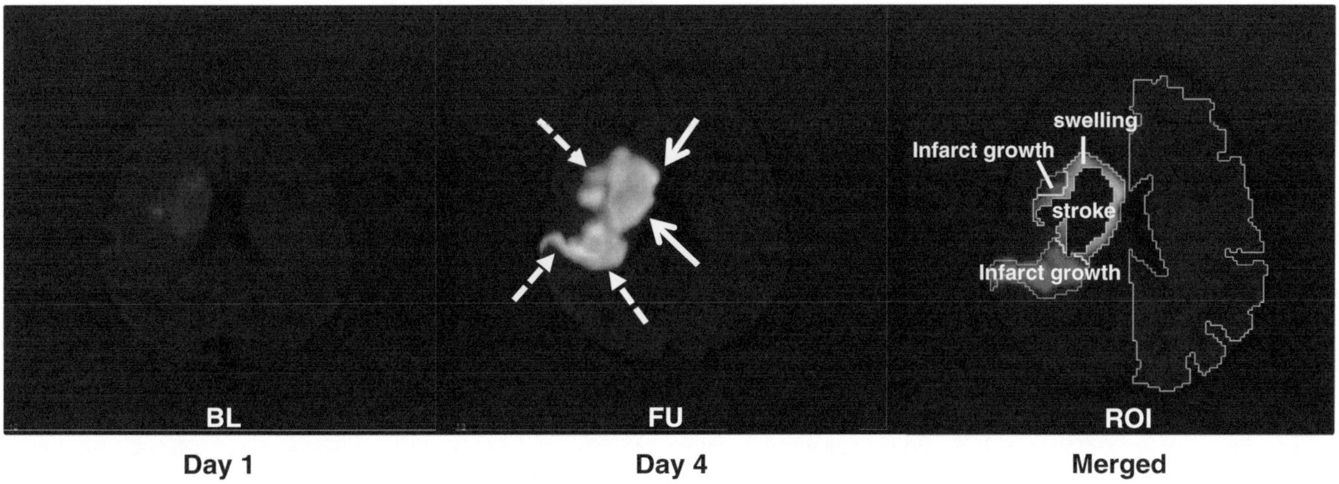

Fig. 1 Example of swelling and infarct growth in a stroke patient. Baseline DWI (*left panel*) was compared with the co-registered follow-up DWI (*middle panel*) to assess the presence of swelling or infarct growth. Region of interest (ROI) defining the stroke at baseline and the stroke at follow-up were co-registered and merged to assign volumes for edema, infarct growth, and, as appropriate, hemorrhage (*right panel*) (From Battey et al. [13])

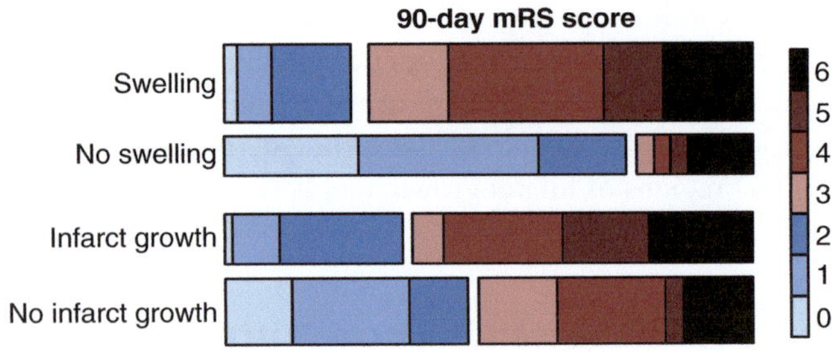

Fig. 2 The distribution of 90-day modified Rankin Scale (mRS) scores for subjects with and without swelling or infarct growth. The distribution for swelling and infarct growth are shown, with the right-hand color key representing each category of mRS as labeled. The height of each bar graph is representative of the percentage of the cohort with each characteristic (From Battey et al. [13])

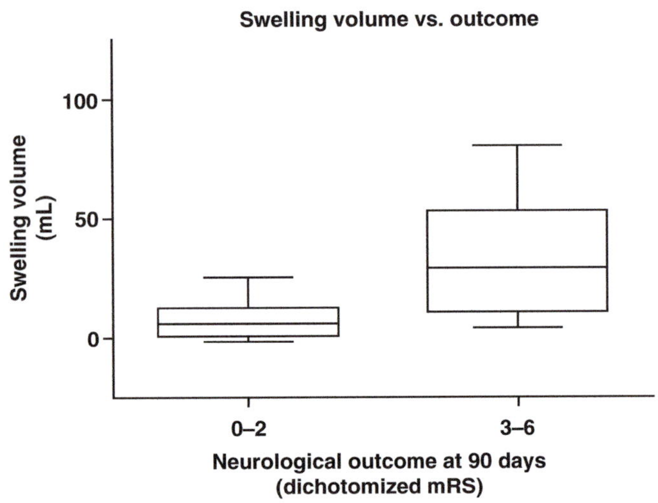

Fig. 3 Increased swelling volume is associated with poor neurological outcome at 90 days. The volume of swelling in subjects with mRS of 3–6 was significantly higher than those with mRS of 0–2 ($p<0.001$) (From Battey et al. [13])

ICE. Little is known about the biological factors underlying ICE that lead to poor outcome in stroke patients. Prior studies have demonstrated that high admission National Institutes of Health Stroke Scale (NIHSS) score and the initial stroke volume are key factors that determine the development of ICE [17, 18]. Indeed, our own studies confirm that stroke volume predicts ICE across a broader range of stroke volumes [13].

In addition, the severity of the initial cytotoxic injury can influence subsequent brain swelling [19–21], which is dependent on blood flow [22, 23]. Previously published data from our group provides further support that the severity of cytotoxic injury is predictive of ICE and is measurable using clinically available apparent diffusion coefficient (ADC) imaging [13]. Taken together, these data suggest that the degree of the cytotoxic injury plays a central role in determining the severity of ICE.

Significance for Clinical Trial Design

The development of imaging biomarkers of ICE has relevance for prognosis after stroke and also for clinical trial design and interpretation. As stroke size and cytotoxic injury (measured on apparent diffusion coefficient (ADC)) both predict ICE severity, these factors can be used to identify stroke patients at elevated risk for developing clinically significant edema. These patients may warrant closer observation for secondary neurological decline and also avoidance of factors that may worsen edema such as hypotonic solutions.

Our imaging biomarkers can also be used for selection of patients for inclusion in clinical trials targeting novel anti-edema therapies or as treatment response biomarkers. Accordingly, our ongoing evaluation of intravenous glyburide for the prevention of malignant edema see chap. 3 represents the ideal setting to test and validate these intermediate surrogate endpoints in the clinical development of anti-edema therapies.

Conclusions

Brain edema after stroke is a significant clinical problem with few current treatment options. The development and validation of neuroimaging biomarkers represents an important step in the further study of ICE. These surrogate endpoints can be used to assess prognosis and for treatment response in ongoing clinical trials.

References

1. Go AS, Mozaffarian D, Roger VL et al (2014) Heart disease and stroke statistics–2014 update: a report from the American Heart Association. Circulation 129(3):e28–e292
2. Emberson J, Lees KR, Lyden P et al (2014) Effect of treatment delay, age, and stroke severity on the effects of intravenous thrombolysis with alteplase for acute ischaemic stroke: a meta-analysis of individual patient data from randomised trials. Lancet 384(9958):1929–1935
3. Berkhemer OA, Fransen PS, Beumer D et al (2015) A randomized trial of intraarterial treatment for acute ischemic stroke. N Engl J Med 372(1):11–20
4. Hacke W, Kaste M, Bluhmki E et al (2008) Thrombolysis with alteplase 3 to 4.5 hours after acute ischemic stroke. N Engl J Med 359(13):1317–1329
5. Tissue plasminogen activator for acute ischemic stroke. The National Institute of Neurological Disorders and Stroke rt-PA Stroke Study Group (1995) N Engl J Med 333(24): 1581–1587
6. Hacke W, Schwab S, Horn M, Spranger M, De Georgia M, von Kummer R (1996) 'Malignant' middle cerebral artery territory

infarction: clinical course and prognostic signs. Arch Neurol 53(4):309–315
7. Kimberly WT, Sheth KN (2011) Approach to severe hemispheric stroke. Neurology 76(7 Suppl 2):S50–S56
8. Wijdicks EF, Sheth KN, Carter BS et al (2014) Recommendations for the management of cerebral and cerebellar infarction with swelling: a statement for healthcare professionals from the American Heart Association/American Stroke Association. Stroke J Cereb Circ 45(4):1222–1238
9. Vahedi K (2009) Decompressive hemicraniectomy for malignant hemispheric infarction. Curr Treat Options Neurol 11(2):113–119
10. Juttler E, Unterberg A, Woitzik J et al (2014) Hemicraniectomy in older patients with extensive middle-cerebral-artery stroke. N Engl J Med 370(12):1091–1100
11. Yoo AJ, Sheth KN, Kimberly WT et al (2013) Validating imaging biomarkers of cerebral edema in patients with severe ischemic stroke. J Stroke Cerebrovasc Dis 22(6):742–749
12. Barber PA, Demchuk AM, Zhang J, Buchan AM (2000) Validity and reliability of a quantitative computed tomography score in predicting outcome of hyperacute stroke before thrombolytic therapy. ASPECTS Study Group Alberta Stroke Programme Early CT Score. Lancet 355(9216):1670–1674
13. Battey TW, Karki M, Singhal AB et al (2014) Brain edema predicts outcome after nonlacunar ischemic stroke. Stroke 45(12): 3643–3648
14. Barrett KM, Ding YH, Wagner DP, Kallmes DF, Johnston KC, Investigators A (2009) Change in diffusion-weighted imaging infarct volume predicts neurologic outcome at 90 days: results of the Acute Stroke Accurate Prediction (ASAP) trial serial imaging substudy. Stroke 40(7):2422–2427
15. Baird AE, Benfield A, Schlaug G et al (1997) Enlargement of human cerebral ischemic lesion volumes measured by diffusion-weighted magnetic resonance imaging. Ann Neurol 41(5):581–589
16. Beaulieu C, de Crespigny A, Tong DC, Moseley ME, Albers GW, Marks MP (1999) Longitudinal magnetic resonance imaging study of perfusion and diffusion in stroke: evolution of lesion volume and correlation with clinical outcome. Ann Neurol 46(4):568–578
17. Thomalla GJ, Kucinski T, Schoder V et al (2003) Prediction of malignant middle cerebral artery infarction by early perfusion- and diffusion-weighted magnetic resonance imaging. Stroke 34(8): 1892–1899
18. Thomalla G, Hartmann F, Juettler E et al (2010) Prediction of malignant middle cerebral artery infarction by magnetic resonance imaging within 6 hours of symptom onset: a prospective multicenter observational study. Ann Neurol 68(4):435–445
19. Todd NV, Picozzi P, Crockard A, Russell RW (1986) Duration of ischemia influences the development and resolution of ischemic brain edema. Stroke 17(3):466–471
20. Bell BA, Symon L, Branston NM (1985) CBF and time thresholds for the formation of ischemic cerebral edema, and effect of reperfusion in baboons. J Neurosurg 62(1):31–41
21. Crockard A, Iannotti F, Hunstock AT, Smith RD, Harris RJ, Symon L (1980) Cerebral blood flow and edema following carotid occlusion in the gerbil. Stroke 11(5):494–498
22. Ayata C, Ropper AH (2002) Ischaemic brain oedema. J Clin Neurosci 9(2):113–124
23. Klatzo I (1967) Presidental address. Neuropathological aspects of brain edema. J Neuropathol Exp Neurol 26(1):1–14

Methylene Blue Ameliorates Ischemia/Reperfusion-Induced Cerebral Edema: An MRI and Transmission Electron Microscope Study

Qing Fang, Xu Yan, Shaowu Li, Yilin Sun, Lixin Xu, Zhongfang Shi, Min Wu, Yi Lu, Liping Dong, Ran Liu, Fang Yuan, and Shao-Hua Yang

Q. Fang • X. Yan • S. Li • Y. Sun • L. Xu • Z. Shi • M. Wu • Y. Lu
L. Dong
Beijing Key Laboratory of Central Nervous System Injury, Beijing Neurosurgical Institute, Beijing Tiantan Hospital, Capital Medical University, Beijing 100050, China

Beijing Key Laboratory of Translational Medicine for Cerebrovascular Disease, Beijing Tiantan Hospital, Capital Medical University, Beijing 100050, China

China National Clinical Research Center for Neurological Diseases, Beijing Tiantan Hospital, Capital Medical University, Beijing 100050, China

R. Liu
Department of Pharmacology and Neuroscience, University of North Texas Health Science Center, 3500 Camp Bowie Boulevard, Fort Worth, TX 76107, USA

F. Yuan, MD, PhD (✉)
Department of Pathophysiology, Beijing Neurosurgical Institute, Capital Medical University,
Tiantanxili 6, Dongcheng District, Beijing 100050, China

Beijing Key Laboratory of Central Nervous System Injury, Beijing Neurosurgical Institute, Beijing Tiantan Hospital, Capital Medical University, Beijing 100050, China

Beijing Key Laboratory of Translational Medicine for Cerebrovascular Disease, Beijing Tiantan Hospital, Capital Medical University, Beijing 100050, China

China National Clinical Research Center for Neurological Diseases, Beijing Tiantan Hospital, Capital Medical University, Beijing 100050, China
e-mail: florayuan@vip.sina.com

S.-H. Yang, MD, PhD (✉)
Beijing Key Laboratory of Central Nervous System Injury, Beijing Neurosurgical Institute, Beijing Tiantan Hospital, Capital Medical University, Beijing 100050, China

Beijing Key Laboratory of Translational Medicine for Cerebrovascular Disease, Beijing Tiantan Hospital, Capital Medical University, Beijing 100050, China

China National Clinical Research Center for Neurological Diseases, Beijing Tiantan Hospital, Capital Medical University, Beijing 100050, China

Department of Pharmacology and Neuroscience, University of North Texas Health Science Center, 3500 Camp Bowie Boulevard, Fort Worth, TX 76107, USA
e-mail: shaohua.yang@unthsc.edu

Abbreviation

ADC	Apparent diffusion coefficient
AP	Astrocytic foot process
BBB	Blood–brain barrier
E	Endothelial cell
L	Lumen
MB	Methylene blue
MRI	Magnetic resonance imaging
REP	Reperfusion
rtPA	Recombinant tissue plasminogen activator
T2WI	T2-weighted Imaging
tMCAO	Transient middle cerebral artery occlusion
TTC	2,3,5-triphenyltetrazolium chloride

Introduction

Stroke ranks as the second leading cause of death in the world [9]. Until 1995, treatment of stroke consisted exclusively of efforts to prevent recurrence. Since that time, the introduction of recombinant tissue plasminogen activator (rtPA) treatment has significantly improved morbidity and mortality of ischemic stroke [1]. Almost two decades after its clinical application, rtPA remains the only choice for acute treatment in ischemic stroke patient. However, its overall impact in ischemic stroke is limited given the short therapeutic window. In addition, there is increasing evidence indicating that, in addition to the unquestionable beneficial effect, rtPA has deleterious effects on the ischemic brain, including increasing blood-brain barrier (BBB) permeability and cytotoxicity, which can further enhance postischemic brain edema and hemorrhagic transformation [22, 31, 38]. Neuroprotective interventions alone and in combination with rtPA have been extensively explored for the treatment of ischemic stroke. However, despite decades of research, none of the current neuroprotective approaches has been found to be effective against ischemic stroke in clinical settings [14].

R.L. Applegate et al. (eds.), *Brain Edema XVI: Translate Basic Science into Clinical Practice*, Acta Neurochirurgica Supplement, Vol. 121, DOI 10.1007/978-3-319-18497-5_41, © Springer International Publishing Switzerland 2016

Brain edema, the accumulation of fluid in the intracellular and extracellular space, is a life-threatening complication of ischemic stroke. Postischemic brain edema is a complex pathophysiological process that causes brain swelling, intracranial hypertension, and may ultimately lead to brain herniation and death [13]. Several therapeutic strategies have been proposed to control brain edema and reduce intracranial pressure, including osmotherapeutics, hyperventilation, hypothermia, steroids, and barbiturates [3]. However, none of these interventions has been proved to be beneficial in clinical trials, even when combined with rtPA thrombolysis [3, 33]. Thus, no evidence-based recommendation on the use of any of these conventional strategies for postischemic brain edema has been made [3, 37]. Encouragingly, decompressive surgery with hemicraniectomy has been found to be beneficial for malignant middle cerebral artery (MCA) infarction in selected patients [37]. Nonetheless, the mechanistic basis of postischemic brain edema remains to be clarified and advanced novel therapeutics are urgently needed.

Methylene blue (MB) was first synthesized in 1876 and has been used as treatment for malaria, methemoglobinemia, and cyanide poisoning [29]. MB has been demonstrated to be neuroprotective in models of ischemic stroke and Parkinson's disease because of its capability as an alternative mitochondria electron carrier [28, 36]. However, it is unclear whether MB has effects on postischemic brain edema. The goal of the current research was to evaluate the therapeutic efficacy of MB for postischemic brain edema in a rat ischemic stroke model using magnetic resonance imaging (MRI) and transmission electron microscopy (TEM).

Material and methods

Animal

All animal procedures were conducted in accordance with the Guidelines for Care and Use of Laboratory Animals and were approved by the Animal Care and Use Committee at Beijing Neurosurgical Institute. Male Sprague-Dawley rats (280–320 g, $n=54$), purchased from Vital River Laboratories (Beijing, China) were housed in polypropylene cages, maintained under controlled laboratory conditions with a 12 h dark–light cycle, and allowed free access to food and water.

Transient Focal Cerebral Ischemia

Transient middle cerebral artery occlusion (tMCAO) was induced as described previously [36]. Briefly, Rats were anesthetized with chloral hydrate dissolved in normal saline (350 mg/kg intraperitoneally (IP)). Core temperature (rectal) was maintained at 37 °C throughout the surgical procedure using a heating blanket and thermo-controlled operating table. A midline incision was made, and the left common carotid artery, external carotid artery, and internal carotid artery were exposed under an operating microscope. A 0.38-mm diameter silicon-coated filament was advanced from the lumen of the external carotid artery into the internal carotid artery until resistance was felt, which ensured the occlusion of the origin of the middle cerebral artery. The filament was allowed to remain in place for 1 h, after which it was gently retracted to allow reperfusion of the ischemic territory. Sham-operated animals were subjected to the same surgical procedure without the filament insertion.

Experimental Design

Animals were randomly assigned to three groups: (1) stroke with MB treatment group ($n=21$), (2) stroke with vehicle treatment ($n=21$), and (3) sham surgery group ($n=6$). For MB treatment, MB (Sigma Aldrich, St. Louis, MO) was infused intravenously through a tail vein (3 mg/kg,over 30 min), started immediately after reperfusion and again at 3 h post-occlusion (1.5 mg/kg, over 15 min). The same volume of normal saline was infused intravenously for vehicle-treated rats. The experimental design is summarized in Fig. 1. Six rats prematurely died of subarachnoid hemorrhage and were excluded from further analysis.

MR Imaging

Sequential MRI was performed in 15 rats (MRI: $n=7$ for MB-treated rats, $n=8$ for vehicle-treated rats) at 0.5, 2.5, and 48 h post-occlusion on a 7.0 T scanner (BioSpec, Bruker, Billerica, Germany) with a four-channel phased-array rat-head coil. Diffusion-weighted images (DWI) were acquired using a spin-echo echo-planar-imaging sequence with the following parameters: field of view (FOV)=4×4 cm, matrix=128×108, slice thickness (THK)=1 mm, repetition time (TR)=4500 ms, echo time (TE)=35 ms, number of averages (NA)=1, b values=1000 s/mm^2. Quantitative maps of the apparent diffusion coefficient (ADC) were calculated based on two different b-values (0, 1,000 s/mm^2). T2-weighted turbo-spin echo images (T2WI) were acquired using a fast spin echo sequence (FOV=4×4 cm, matrix=320×240, THK=1 mm, NS=20, NA=1, TR=3140 ms, TE=37 ms). Image analysis was performed using OsiriX software (http://www.osirix-viewer.com). For the lesion size quantification on T2WI and ADC maps, the lesion and brain areas in the

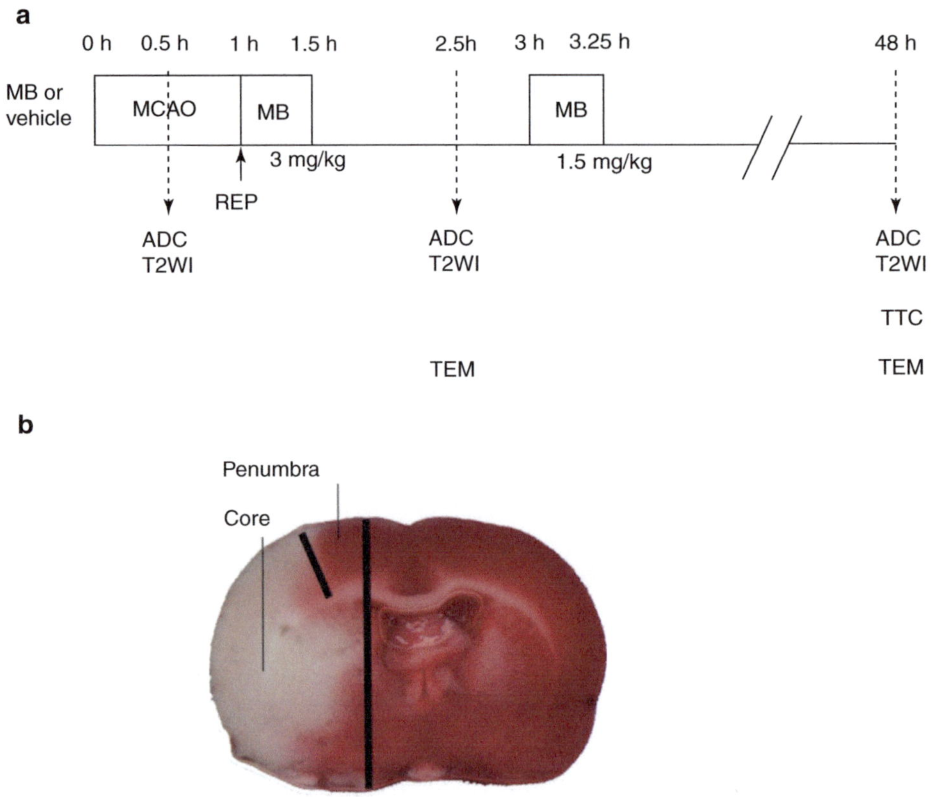

Fig. 1 (**a**) Schematic drawings of experimental design. (**b**) Schematic drawing of samples dissection and collection at the ischemic penumbra for TEM assays. *MB* methylene blue; *REP* reperfusion; *MCAO* middle cerebral artery occlusion; *TEM* transmission electron microscope; *ADC* apparent diffusion coefficient; *T2WI* T2-weighted Imaging; *TTC* 2,3,5-triphenyltetrazolium chloride

same slice were delineated by two people by consensus using an operator-defined region of interest (ROI) on each of the lesion-containing slices, and the volume of the lesion and brain regions were then summed for each animal. The contralateral brain area was also measured using the same methods. The area of the different structures involved in the ischemic process was delineated on the images according to rescaled drawings from the Paxinos and Watson atlas [25]. The hyperintense pixels in T2WI and hypointense pixels in ADC in the ipsilateral cortex were then selected as those with a significantly higher or lower signal ($p<0.05$) than in the contralateral hemisphere. The lesion volume on T2WI (Vu) and ADC were determined as the sum of the hyper- or hypointense area in each slice multiplied by the slice thickness. To compensate for the effects of brain swelling, a corrected lesion volume (Ve %) and brain swelling (Swelling %), expressed as the volume increase of the affected hemisphere, were calculated using following equation as previously described [10]:

$$\mathrm{Ve} = \mathrm{Vc} + \mathrm{Vi} - (\mathrm{Vc} + \mathrm{Vi} - \mathrm{Vu})\frac{\mathrm{Vc} + \mathrm{Vi}}{2\mathrm{Vc}}$$

$$\mathrm{Ve}\,\% = \frac{2\mathrm{Ve}}{\mathrm{Vc} + \mathrm{Vi}} \cdot 100$$

$$\mathrm{Swelling}\,\% = \frac{2(\mathrm{Ve} - \mathrm{Vu})}{\mathrm{Vc} + \mathrm{Vi}} \cdot 100$$

where Ve and Vu indicate corrected and uncorrected lesion volume, respectively, and Vi and Vc indicate volume of the ischemic and contralateral hemisphere, respectively.

2,3,5-Triphenyltetrazolium Chloride (TTC) Staining

TTC staining was performed in separate groups of rats at 48 h after stroke for final lesion volume analysis ($n=8$ for MB-treated rats, $n=7$ for vehicle-treated rats). The rats were deeply re-anesthetized with chloral hydrate at a dose of 800 mg/kg. The rats were sacrificed by decapitation and brains were harvested and cut into 2-mm-thick coronal sections. The sections were incubated in 2 % solution of TTC (Sigma Chemical, St. Louis, MO) for 15 min and then fixed in 4 % buffered formaldehyde solution for 24 h. Images of the stained sections were captured using a scanner (N-TEK NuScan 900, San Jose CA. USA) and analyzed for infarct volume using Image-J (NIH, Bethesda, Maryland). Percentage of infarct volume (Infarct %) was calculated using the following equation as previous described [34]:

$$\text{Infarct}\,\% = \frac{\text{Vc} - \text{Vl}}{\text{Vc}} \cdot 100$$

where Vc is the volume of contralateral hemisphere and Vl is the volume of nonischemic tissue in the lesion hemisphere. Brain swelling (Swelling %) was calculated as previously described [10]:

$$\text{Swelling}\,\% = \frac{\text{Vi} - \text{Vc}}{\text{Vc}} \cdot 100$$

where Vi is volume of ischemic hemisphere.

Transmission Electron Microscopy

For the TEM study, three rats from each group were sacrificed at 2.5 or 48 h after tMCAO or sham surgery ($n=3$ each). Rats were anesthetized and perfused with 4 % paraformaldehyde and 2.5 % glutaraldehyde buffer (pH 7.4). The brains were harvested and the ischemic penumbra was dissected as described previously [2]. Briefly, a 2-mm section was cut at 5 mm from the anterior tip of the frontal lobe. A longitudinal cut was made from top to bottom approximately 2 mm from the midline through the ischemic hemisphere of this section. Then, a transverse diagonal cut was made at approximately the "one o'clock" position to separate the core (i.e., striatum and overlying cortex) from the penumbra. Brain blocks ($1 \times 1 \times 1$ mm^3) were separated from the penumbra region (Fig. 1B). The samples were then fixed in 1 % osmium tetroxide, dehydrated in graded ethyl alcohol, and embedded in epoxy resin. The epoxy-embedded blocks were sectioned with an ultramicrotome (Leica, UC6, Wetzlar, Germany), placed on 200-mesh copper grids, and then stained in saturated uranyl acetate and lead citrate. Sections (40-nm thick) were analyzed using H-7650 transmission electron microscope (Hitachi, Chiyoda, Tokyo).

Statistical Analysis

The data are presented as mean ± standard error of the mean (SEM). Independent *t*-test and the Mann-Whitney *U*-test were performed to compare the differences between the MB-treated and vehicle-treated group. A two-tailed value of $p<0.05$ was taken to be statistically significant.

Results

Acute Treatment of MB Reduced ADC and T2WI Lesion Volume Induced by Transient Focal Cerebral Ischemia

We determined the effect of acute MB treatment on the progression of ADC and T2WI lesion induced by transient focal cerebral ischemia. At 0.5 h after tMCAO, ADC detected ischemic lesion within the MCA territory, including basal ganglia and the frontoparietal cortex, in both vehicle and MB treated rats. No significant difference was found in ADC lesion between vehicle- and MB-treated groups, which were 266.5 ± 15.13 and 284.31 ± 18.73 mm^3, respectively ($p>0.05$, Fig. 2a, b). The ADC-defined ischemic lesion was partially recovered at 1.5 h after reperfusion (2.5 h after stroke) in both vehicle- and MB-treated rats, which were 70.19 ± 20.37 and 53.99 ± 13.29 mm^3, respectively ($p>0.05$). At 48 h after stroke, the ADC lesion increased, accompanied by T2WI lesion. The final ADC lesion volume at 48 h after MCAO was 346.76 ± 15.01 and 219.6 ± 16.58 mm^3 in vehicle-treated and MB-treated groups, respectively ($p<0.001$, Fig. 2a, b).

T2WI failed to detect lesions in both groups at 0.5 and 2.5 h after tMCAO (Fig. 2a). At 48 h after stroke, T2WI lesion volume was 372.45 ± 21.15 and 254.56 ± 14.30 mm^3 in vehicle and MB groups, respectively ($p<0.001$, Fig. 2a, c). MB treatment significantly decreased ischemic brain swelling as compared with vehicle treatment, which was 20.03 ± 0.93 and 14.95 ± 1.43 % in vehicle and MB group, respectively ($p<0.01$, Fig. 2e). The corrected T2WI lesion volume was 31.42 ± 2.46 and 22.51 ± 1.16 % in vehicle and MB group, respectively ($p<0.01$, Fig. 2d).

Consistently, neuropathological analysis demonstrated that MB decreased the final infarct lesion volume induced by transient focal cerebral ischemia. At 48 h after tMCAO, the TTC-staining defined infarct lesion volume was 36.90 ± 1.49 and 30.52 ± 2.06 % in vehicle and MB groups, respectively (Fig. 3a, b, $p<0.05$). In addition, MB treatment significantly ameliorated ischemic brain swelling, which was 14.39 ± 1.50 and 9.54 ± 1.38 % in the vehicle and MB groups, respectively ($p<0.05$) (Fig. 3c).

Acute Treatment of MB Attenuated Edema of Neurovascular Unit Component

We determined the effect of MB on edema in neurovascular components induced by transient focal cerebral ischemia using TEM. The cortical capillary of sham-operated rats

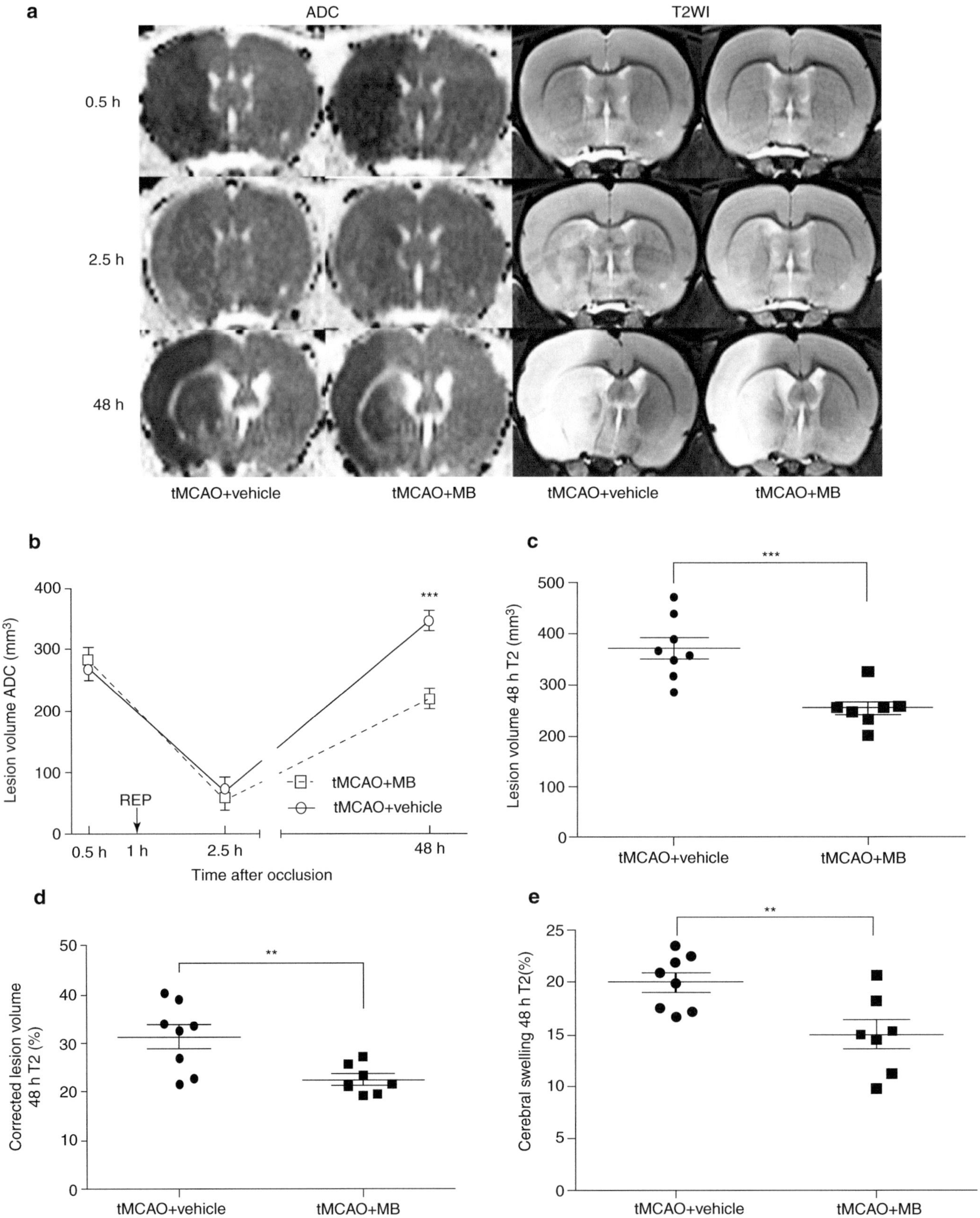

Fig. 2 (**a**) Representative ADC, T2WI images at 0.5, 2.5 and 48 h after tMCAO from vehicle-treated and MB-treated rats. (**b**) Temporal evolution of apparent diffusion coefficient (ADC)-defined ischemic lesion volumes in vehicle (*circles*) and MB groups. *Arrow* indicates reperfusion (REP). (**c**) Quantitative analysis of T2WI-defined lesion volume in vehicle and MB-treated groups at 48 h after stroke. (**d**) Quantitative analysis of corrected T2WI lesion volume in vehicle and MB-treated groups at 48 h after stroke. (**e**) Quantitative analysis of cerebral swelling estimated in T2WI at 48 h after stroke. Values are the mean ± SEM., $^{**}p<0.01$ vs. vehicle; $^{***}p<0.001$ vs. vehicle

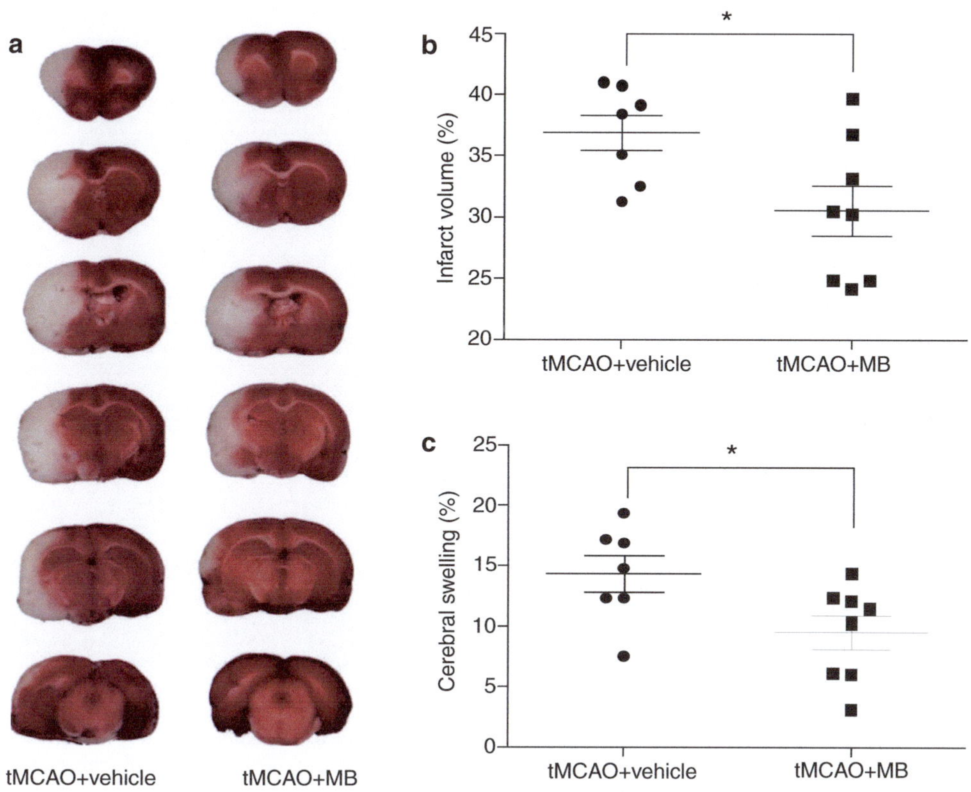

Fig. 3 (**a**) Representative TTC staining of brain sections in vehicle- and MB-treated rats at 48 h following the tMCAO. (**b**) Quantitative analysis of TTC-defined lesion volume in vehicle and MB groups. (**c**) Quantitative analysis of brain swelling in vehicle and MB groups. Values are the mean ± SEM. $*p<0.05$ vs. vehicle

have normal endothelial cells, basal lamina, and astrocyte foot processes (Fig. 4a, b). In the vehicle-treated stroke rat brains, swollen astrocyte foot processes were observed in the penumbra regions at 2.5 h after stroke (Fig. 4c). The enlargement of astrocyte foot process was even more severe at 48 h after stroke, accompanied by detachment of astrocyte foot processes, plasma membrane from the basal lamina and endothelial cell swelling were observed (Fig. 4d). In the MB-treated rats, very mild edema was found at the astrocyte foot processes at 2.5 h after stroke (Fig. 4e). At 48 h after stroke, less edema was observed at the astrocyte foot process in MB-treated rats compared with vehicle-treated animals (Fig. 4f).

In the cortex of sham-operated rats, neurons have well-defined nuclei with prominent nucleoli (Fig. 5a, b). In the vehicle-treated stroke rats, TEM at 2.5 h after stroke demonstrated that most neurons at the penumbra were shrunken, accompanied with a lack of perikaryal cytoplasm and triangular nuclei, surrounded by swollen vacuoles and astrocytic processes (Fig. 5c). At 48 h after stroke, necrotic neurons show cytoplasmic and nuclear disintegration with marked chromatin clumping and discontinuous cellular membranes (Fig. 5d). In the MB-treated rats, the neuron damage was remarkably alleviated with only mild nuclei deformation observed at the penumbra region at 48 h after stroke (Fig. 5e, f).

In the sham-operated rats, cortical astrocytes had defined nuclei and scanty cytoplasm dispersed with intact mitochondria (Fig. 6a, b). In the vehicle-treated stroke rats, TEM revealed a significant astrocyte edema at 2.5 h after stroke evidenced by the vacuolated cytoplasm with swollen mitochondria (Fig. 6c). At 48 h after stroke, the perikaryal space was even wider, extremely lucent, and virtually devoid of organelles (Fig. 6d). On the other hand, TEM revealed that MB treatment rats had relatively normal astrocytes at the penumbra area with only mild nuclei deformation at 2.5 h after stroke (Fig. 6e). At 48 h after stroke, astrocytic swelling at the penumbra area was substantially attenuated in MB-treated rats (Fig. 6f).

Discussion

In recent years, increasing numbers of studies have focused on the energy-enhancing and antioxidant properties effects of MB [18, 28, 30]. In addition, acute treatment has been demonstrated to attenuate infarct volume in experimental ischemic stroke model [28, 30, 36]. In the present study, we applied serial ADC and T2 MRI and TEM to test the hypothesis that acute MB treatment attenuates postischemic brain

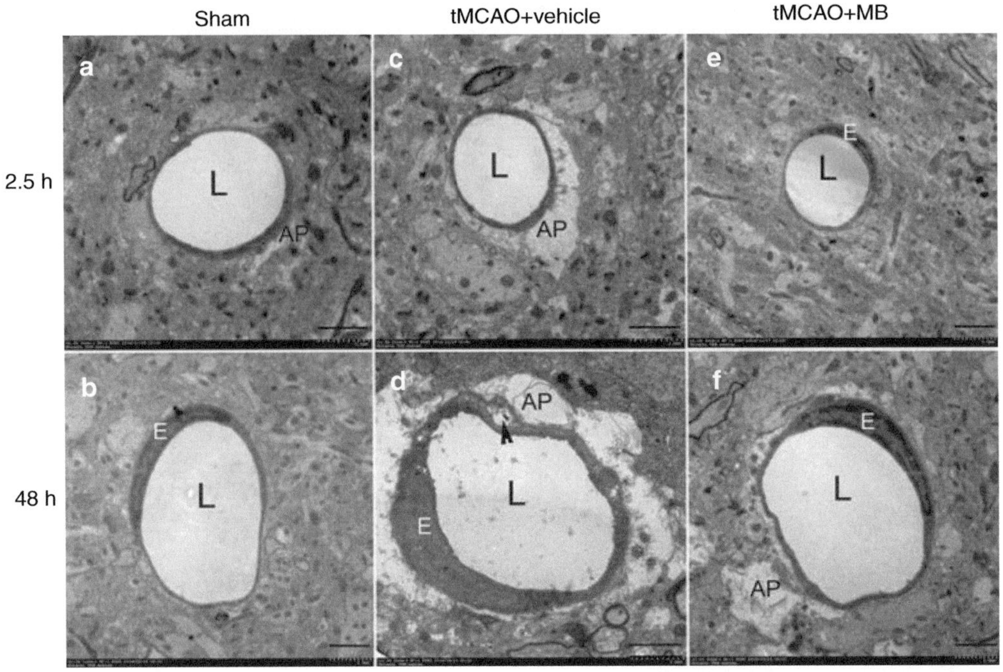

Fig. 4 Representative electron microscopy images of cortical vessels in the ischemic penumbra at 2.5 or 48 h after tMCAO. (**a**, **b**) cortical capillary in a sham-operated rat. The lumen (*L*) is circular, the endothelial cells nucleus is crescent shaped, and the cytoplasmic rim is thin and compact. Perivascular astrocytic foot processes (*AP*) are relatively flat and difficult to delineate. (**c**) Cortical capillary with highly swollen perivascular astrocytic foot processes in a vehicle-treated rat at 2.5 h after stroke. (**d**) In the penumbra of a vehicle-treated rat at 48 h after stroke, cortical capillary lumen became irregular, and astrocyte foot processes were seriously enlarged. The cytoplasm of the endothelial cell is expanded. Detachment of the foot process plasma membrane from the basal lamina was observed (*arrowhead*). (**e**) In the penumbra of a MB-treated rat at 2.5 h after stroke, cortical capillary with normal endothelial cells, basal lamina, and astrocyte foot processes. (**f**) In the penumbra of a MB-treated rat at 48 h after stroke, cortical capillary with mild enlargement of perivascular spaces. *L* lumen, *AP* astrocytic foot process, *E* endothelial cell. Bar = 2 μm

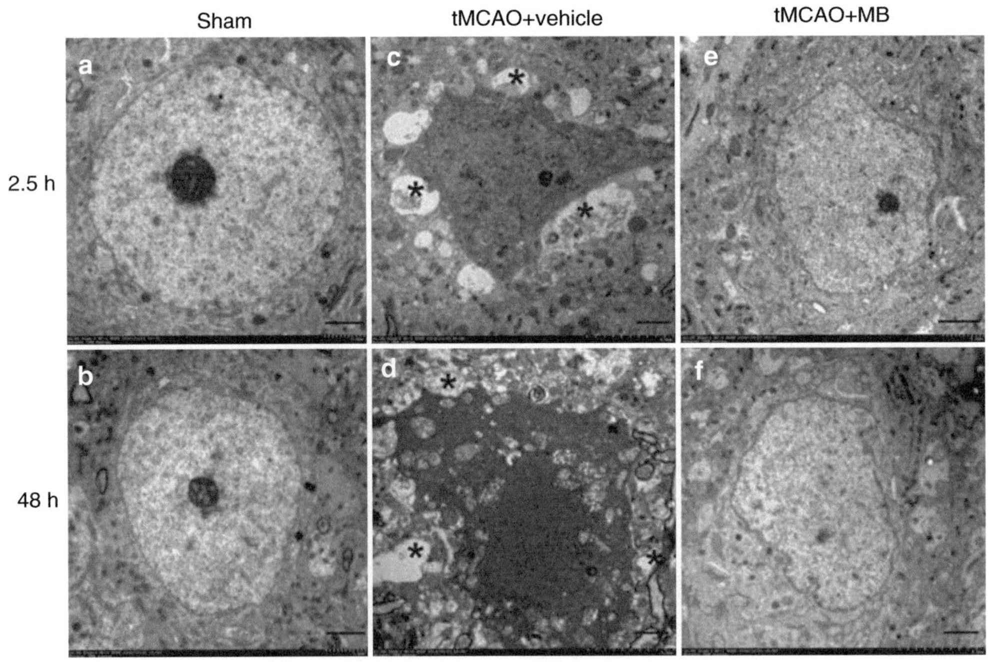

Fig. 5 Representative electron microscopy images of neurons in the ischemic penumbra at 2.5 or 48 h after the ischemic stroke. (**a**, **b**) Normal neuron with a large circular nucleus containing a dark nucleolus and a 1–2-μm-thick rim of perikaryal cytoplasm. (**c**) In a vehicle-treated rat at 2.5 h after stroke, shrunken neurons with condensed nuclei and cytoplasm are surrounded by a ring of swollen astrocytic processes (marked by *asterisks*). (**d**) In a vehicle-treated rat at 2.5 h after stroke, necrotic neurons show cytoplasmic and nuclear disintegration with marked chromatin clumping and discontinuous cellular membranes. (**e**, **f**) In MB-treated rats at 2.5 or 48 h after stroke, neuron with mild nuclei deformation. Bar = 2 μm

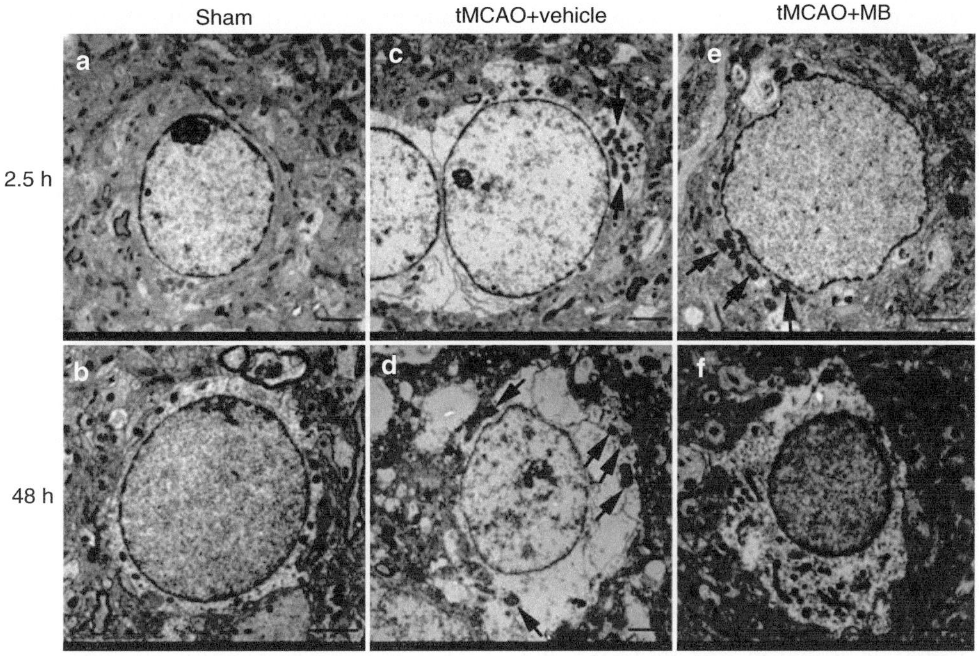

Fig. 6 Representative electron microscopy images of astrocytes in ischemic penumbra at 2.5 or 48 h after the ischemic insult. (**a**, **b**) Cortical astrocyte from sham-operated rats at 2.5 or 48 h after surgery show oval nucleus and scant cytoplasm. (**c**) In a vehicle-treated rat at 2.5 h after stroke, severely swollen astrocyte with extensive and vacuolated cytoplasm, and a few contracted mitochondria (*arrowhead*). (**d**) In a vehicle-treated rat at 48 h after stroke, an irreversibly astrocyte with watery cytoplasm, and severely swollen mitochondria (*arrowhead*). (**e**) In a MB-treated rat at 2.5 h after stroke, astrocyte with nuclei deformation and a few contracted mitochondria (*arrowhead*). (**f**) In a MB-treated rat at 48 h after stroke, swollen astrocyte with clumps of heterochromatin around the edge of its nucleus and an abnormally wide rim of watery perikaryal cytoplasm. Bar = 2 μm m

edema. Our study demonstrated that acute MB treatment (i) decreased infarct lesion volume induced by tMCAO, (ii) attenuated postischemic brain edema, and (iii) ameliorated damage of neurovascular unit component after ischemic stroke.

Postischemic brain edema is a critical condition that warrants immediate intervention. Two types of edema are present after ischemic stroke, cytotoxic and vasogenic edema. Cytotoxic edema is the initial type of brain edema after ischemic stroke, primarily caused by energy metabolism failure and dissipation of transmembrane ion gradients in the ischemic territory. Vasogenic edema is the second phase of ischemic brain edema and is caused by the breakdown of the BBB [12]. MRI is considered the most promising noninvasive approach for examining brain edema formation in real time [6, 11]. Cerebral ischemic-induced ADC reduction has been found to occur within minutes after cerebral ischemia, which is closely related to cytotoxic edema [4, 5, 2, 35]. T2WI has been used for evaluation of vasogenic edema and infarct lesion after ischemic stroke [23]. In the current study, we observed similar ADC-defined lesions within 30 min after ischemia in both vehicle- and MB-treated animals, suggesting that tMCAO induced same degree of ischemic insult in both vehicle and MB treatment group animals before treatment. Interestingly, temporal recovery of the initial ADC lesion was found almost equally in both vehicle- and MB-treated rats at 1.5 h after reperfusion. At 2 days after stroke, the ADC-defined lesion increased accompanied with T2WI lesion in both vehicle and MB treated groups. MB treatment significantly decreased both ADC and T2WI-defined lesions as compared with vehicle treatment. In addition, cerebral swelling was significantly attenuated upon MB treatment. Consistently, our histological study demonstrated that acute MB treatment reduced ischemic lesion volume and cerebral swelling at 2 days after stroke. Temporal and permanent recovery of the initial ADC and DWI lesion upon on reperfusion has been found previously [15, 17, 21]. Furthermore, studies have indicated that even permanent reversibility of initial ADC and DWI lesion was not associated with histological recovery [16]. Our MRI result is in line with those previous studies, and our ultrastructural analysis demonstrated that MB treatment could protect neurovascular unit components and attenuate postischemic brain edema.

Astrocyte swelling has been indicated to be the primary event contributing to the cytotoxic brain edema, given that it is the most abundant cell type in CNS and its highly selective function is implicated in ion and water fluxes [11, 24]. Consistently, our TEM study demonstrated that cytotoxic edema was mainly observed in astrocytes. On the other hand, neuron shrinkage was observed after cerebral ischemia [19]. Similarly, our ultrastructural study demonstrated cytotoxic edema in astrocytes and capillary endothelial cells concurrent with neuronal shrinkage at the ischemic penumbra at 2.5 h after ischemia. Thus, the transient recovery of ADC in cortex at 2.5 h may be caused by the combined effects of neuronal shrinkage and astrocyte swelling. Although similar ADC-defined lesion was observed in both vehicle and MB treatment groups at 2.5 h after stroke, our TEM study indicated that MB attenuated astrocyte edema and neuron shrinkage. Furthermore, the action of MB was unlikely simply a delay of lesion progression, as even more profound protection was observed at 48 h after stroke.

Our previous study demonstrated the neuroprotective function of MB as an alternative electron carrier bypassing complex I/III blockage, which accepts electrons from NADH and transfers them to cytochrome *c* [36]. This mechanism was further supported by findings that MB enhances brain metabolism [18]. We speculated that the alternative mitochondrial electron transfer action of MB preserves mitochondrial function and ATP production after ischemic stroke, maintains Na/K ATPase and transmembrane potential, thus, attenuates sodium influx and cytotoxic edema after ischemic stroke. In our ultrastructual study, we found that MB protected the BBB components, including endothelium and astrocyte foot processes, from ischemia-induced cytotoxic edema at 1.5 after reperfusion when T2WI lesion was still undetectable, indicating that the primary effect of MB is likely the amelioration of cytotoxic edema due to its mitochondrial election transfer action.

The second phase postischemic brain edema represents vasogenic edema and occurs in the setting of BBB disruption, causing intravascular fluid to move to brain parenchyma [8, 32]. Furthermore, the increase of water in brain parenchyma could further compromise cerebral blood flow and, hence, augment cytotoxic edema. Indeed, we observed even more severe astrocyte swelling and concurrent neuron necrosis at 48 h after stroke. One study has indicated that MB ameliorated the BBB disruption induced by cardiac arrest and resuscitation [20]. T2WI is frequently used to study vasogenic edema and final lesion volume induced by ischemia/reperfusion [27]. The present study demonstrated that MB reduced final T2WI lesion, which was further verified by a histological study. In addition, postischemic brain swelling was significantly reduced by MB treatment. Our TEM demonstrated that MB treatment protected BBB structures, evidenced by the attenuation of swelling of astrocyte, astrocyte foot processes, and endothelial cells at 48 h after stroke. The protective effects of MB against vasogenic edema could be interpreted by its primary action on cytotoxic edema due to its alternative mitochondrial electron transfer. Nonetheless, the alternative electron transfer function of MB could also provide protective action against reperfusion-induced superoxide overproduction. Complex I and III blockage are the major causes of superoxide and free radical production [7]. The action of MB to bypass complex I and III could attenuate free radical overproduction during reperfusion [26, 36].

In conclusion, the present study provides additional experimental evidence that MB, a century-old drug, exerts a protective effect against transient ischemic stroke. Using both MRI and TEM ultrastructural analysis, our study indicated that MB, as an alternative mitochondrial electron transfer carrier, attenuates postischemic brain edema induced by transient ischemic stroke. Given that MB has already been used in different clinical conditions and has well-established pharmacokinetics in humans, our study, together with previous studies [36, 28, 30], shows that further clinical investigation of MB for the treatment of ischemic stroke is warrented.

Acknowledgments This work was supported by National Institutes of Health grants NS054651, NS088596, and NS087209, and National Natural Science Foundation of China Grants 81228009 and 81271286.

References

1. (1995) Tissue plasminogen activator for acute ischemic stroke. The National Institute of Neurological Disorders and Stroke rt-PA Stroke Study Group. N Engl J Med 333:1581–1587
2. Ashwal S, Tone B, Tian HR, Cole DJ, Pearce WJ (1998) Core and penumbral nitric oxide synthase activity during cerebral ischemia and reperfusion. Stroke 29:1037–1046; discussion 1047
3. Bardutzky J, Schwab S (2007) Antiedema therapy in ischemic stroke. Stroke 38:3084–3094
4. Benveniste H, Hedlund LW, Johnson GA (1992) Mechanism of detection of acute cerebral ischemia in rats by diffusion-weighted magnetic resonance microscopy. Stroke 23:746–754
5. Busza AL, Allen KL, King MD, van Bruggen N, Williams SR, Gadian DG (1992) Diffusion-weighted imaging studies of cerebral ischemia in gerbils. Potential relevance to energy failure. Stroke 23:1602–1612
6. Chalouhi N, Jabbour P, Magnotta V, Hasan D (2014) Molecular imaging of cerebrovascular lesions. Transl Stroke Res 5:260–268
7. Cocheme HM, Murphy MP (2008) Complex I is the major site of mitochondrial superoxide production by paraquat. J Biol Chem 283:1786–1798
8. Donkin JJ, Vink R (2010) Mechanisms of cerebral edema in traumatic brain injury: therapeutic developments. Curr Opin Neurol 23:293–299
9. Feigin VL, Forouzanfar MH, Krishnamurthi R, Mensah GA, Connor M, Bennett DA, Moran AE, Sacco RL, Anderson L, Truelsen T, O'Donnell M, Venketasubramanian N, Barker-Collo S, Lawes CM, Wang W, Shinohara Y, Witt E, Ezzati M, Naghavi M, Murray C (2014) Global and regional burden of stroke during 1990–2010: findings from the Global Burden of Disease Study 2010. Lancet 383:245–254
10. Gerriets T, Stolz E, Walberer M, Müller C, Kluge A, Bachmann A, Fisher M, Kaps M, Bachmann G (2004) Noninvasive quantification of brain edema and the space-occupying effect in rat stroke models using magnetic resonance imaging. Stroke 35:566–571
11. Jayakumar AR, Valdes V, Tong XY, Shamaladevi N, Gonzalez W, Norenberg MD (2014) Sulfonylurea receptor 1 contributes to the astrocyte swelling and brain edema in acute liver failure. Transl Stroke Res 5:28–37

12. Kahle KT, Simard JM, Staley KJ, Nahed BV, Jones PS, Sun D (2009) Molecular mechanisms of ischemic cerebral edema: role of electroneutral ion transport. Physiology (Bethesda) 24:257–265
13. Khanna A, Kahle KT, Walcott BP, Gerzanich V, Simard JM (2014) Disruption of ion homeostasis in the neurogliovascular unit underlies the pathogenesis of ischemic cerebral edema. Transl Stroke Res 5:3–16
14. Lai TW, Zhang S, Wang YT (2014) Excitotoxicity and stroke: identifying novel targets for neuroprotection. Prog Neurobiol 115:157–188
15. Li F, Han SS, Tatlisumak T, Liu KF, Garcia JH, Sotak CH, Fisher M (1999) Reversal of acute apparent diffusion coefficient abnormalities and delayed neuronal death following transient focal cerebral ischemia in rats. Ann Neurol 46:333–342
16. Li F, Liu KF, Silva MD, Omae T, Sotak CH, Fenstermacher JD, Fisher M, Hsu CY, Lin W (2000) Transient and permanent resolution of ischemic lesions on diffusion-weighted imaging after brief periods of focal ischemia in rats: correlation with histopathology. Stroke 31:946–954
17. Li F, Silva MD, Liu KF, Helmer KG, Omae T, Fenstermacher JD, Sotak CH, Fisher M (2000) Secondary decline in apparent diffusion coefficient and neurological outcomes after a short period of focal brain ischemia in rats. Ann Neurol 48:236–244
18. Lin A-L, Poteet E, Du F, Gourav RC, Liu R, Wen Y, Bresnen A, Huang S, Fox PT, Yang S-H (2012) Methylene blue as a cerebral metabolic and hemodynamic enhancer. PLoS One 7, e46585
19. Liu KF, Li F, Tatlisumak T, Garcia JH, Sotak CH, Fisher M, Fenstermacher JD (2001) Regional variations in the apparent diffusion coefficient and the intracellular distribution of water in rat brain during acute focal ischemia. Stroke 32:1897–1905
20. Miclescu A, Sharma HS, Martijn C, Wiklund L (2010) Methylene blue protects the cortical blood–brain barrier against ischemia/reperfusion-induced disruptions*. Crit Care Med 38:2199–2206
21. Minematsu K, Li L, Sotak CH, Davis MA, Fisher M (1992) Reversible focal ischemic injury demonstrated by diffusion-weighted magnetic resonance imaging in rats. Stroke 23:1304–1310; discussion 1310–1311
22. Ning M, Sarracino DA, Buonanno FS, Krastins B, Chou S, McMullin D, Wang X, Lopez M, Lo EH (2010) Proteomic protease substrate profiling of tPA treatment in acute ischemic stroke patients: a step toward individualizing thrombolytic therapy at the bedside. Transl Stroke Res 1:268–275
23. Obenaus A, Ashwal S (2012) Neuroimaging of stroke and ischemia in animal models. Transl Stroke Res 3:4–7
24. Pasantes-Morales H, Vazquez-Juarez E (2012) Transporters and channels in cytotoxic astrocyte swelling. Neurochem Res 37:2379–2387
25. Paxinos G, Watson C (2006) The rat brain in stereotaxic coordinates: hard cover edition. Academic Press, Waltham, Massachusetts
26. Poteet E, Winters A, Yan LJ, Shufelt K, Green KN, Simpkins JW, Wen Y, Yang SH (2012) Neuroprotective actions of methylene blue and its derivatives. PLoS One 7, e48279
27. Rivers CS, Wardlaw JM, Armitage PA, Bastin ME, Carpenter TK, Cvoro V, Hand PJ, Dennis MS (2006) Do acute diffusion- and perfusion-weighted MRI lesions identify final infarct volume in ischemic stroke? Stroke 37:98–104
28. Rodriguez P, Jiang Z, Huang S, Shen Q, Duong TQ (2014) Methylene blue treatment delays progression of perfusion-diffusion mismatch to infarct in permanent ischemic stroke. Brain Res 1588:144–149
29. Scheindlin S (2008) Something old… something blue. Mol Interv 8:268–273
30. Shen Q, Du F, Huang S, Rodriguez P, Watts LT, Duong TQ (2013) Neuroprotective efficacy of methylene blue in ischemic stroke: an MRI study. PLoS One 8, e79833
31. Siler DA, Gonzalez JA, Wang RK, Cetas JS, Alkayed NJ (2014) Intracisternal administration of tissue plasminogen activator improves cerebrospinal fluid flow and cortical perfusion after subarachnoid hemorrhage in mice. Transl Stroke Res 5:227–237
32. Spatz M (2010) Past and recent BBB studies with particular emphasis on changes in ischemic brain edema. In: Brain edema XIV. Springer, Wien, New York City, New York, pp 21–27
33. Strbian D, Meretoja A, Putaala J, Kaste M, Tatlisumak T (2013) Cerebral edema in acute ischemic stroke patients treated with intravenous thrombolysis. Int J Stroke 8:529–534
34. Swanson RA, Morton MT, Tsao-Wu G, Savalos RA, Davidson C, Sharp FR (1990) A semiautomated method for measuring brain infarct volume. J Cereb Blood Flow Metab 10:290–293
35. Wang Y, Hu W, Perez-Trepichio AD, Ng TC, Furlan AJ, Majors AW, Jones SC (2000) Brain tissue sodium is a ticking clock telling time after arterial occlusion in rat focal cerebral ischemia. Stroke 31:1386–1392
36. Wen Y, Li W, Poteet EC, Xie L, Tan C, Yan L-J, Ju X, Liu R, Qian H, Marvin MA (2011) Alternative mitochondrial electron transfer as a novel strategy for neuroprotection. J Biol Chem 286:16504–16515
37. Wijdicks EF, Sheth KN, Carter BS, Greer DM, Kasner SE, Kimberly WT, Schwab S, Smith EE, Tamargo RJ, Wintermark M (2014) Recommendations for the management of cerebral and cerebellar infarction with swelling: a statement for healthcare professionals from the American Heart Association/American Stroke Association. Stroke 45:1222–1238
38. Yepes M, Roussel BD, Ali C, Vivien D (2009) Tissue-type plasminogen activator in the ischemic brain: more than a thrombolytic. Trends Neurosci 32:48–55

Acute Hyperglycemia Is Associated with Immediate Brain Swelling and Hemorrhagic Transformation After Middle Cerebral Artery Occlusion in Rats

Devin W. McBride, Julia Legrand, Paul R. Krafft, Jerry Flores, Damon Klebe, Jiping Tang, and John H. Zhang

Introduction

Stroke is a devastating disease that disproportionally affects diabetic patients and hyperglycemic patients, accounting for up to 40 % of stroke cases [10], with increased morbidity, mortality, and poorer outcome, associated with larger infarct volume, cerebral edema, and hemorrhagic transformation [4, 14, 16]. Hemorrhagic transformation of ischemic stroke, with a 48 % occurrence rate [2, 8], is a large contributor to post-ictus debilitation of patients, and clinically arises 2–3 days after the initial stroke [24]. Several risk factors have been identified in hemorrhagic transformation, including hypertension and hyperglycemia [1, 27].

Experimental models of hemorrhagic transformation have been developed to better understand its mechanisms and to develop treatments targeted at prevention and reduction of the bleeding. In diabetic and hyperglycemic models of transient middle cerebral artery occlusion (MCAO), the rate of hemorrhagic transformation is as high as 100 % [5, 7]. Numerous studies have focused on understanding the mechanism or development of therapies for hemorrhagic transformation models, yet none have examined the progression of brain swelling and hemorrhagic transformation after reperfusion. In this study, we measure the development of the infarction, brain swelling, and hemorrhagic transformation following transient MCAO in hyperglycemic rats.

D.W. McBride • J. Legrand • P.R. Krafft • J. Flores
D. Klebe • J. Tang
Department of Physiology and Pharmacology, Loma Linda University School of Medicine, Loma Linda, CA 92350, USA

J.H. Zhang, MD, PhD (✉)
Department of Physiology and Pharmacology, Loma Linda University School of Medicine, Loma Linda, CA 92350, USA

Department of Neurosurgery, Loma Linda University School of Medicine, Loma Linda, CA, USA
e-mail: jhzhang@llu.edu

Materials and Methods

All experiments were approved by the Institutional Animal Care and Use Committee at Loma Linda University. Adult male Sprague-Dawley rats (260–290 g) were used in all experiments. Animal groups were sham ($n=5$), MCAO sacrificed 15 min after MCAO ($n=5$), MCAO sacrificed 1 h after MCAO ($n=5$), MCAO sacrificed 3 h after MCAO ($n=5$), and MCAO sacrificed 24 h after MCAO ($n=5$).

Middle Cerebral Artery Occlusion Model

Male rats were either subjected to 90 min of middle cerebral artery occlusion (MCAO) or sham surgery as previously described [12]. Animals were anesthetized with an intraperitoneal (IP) injection mixture of ketamine (80 mg/kg) and xylazine (20 mg/kg), then given a dose of atropine (0.1 mg/kg, subcutaneously (SC)). After reaching an adequate plane of anesthesia, determined by loss of paw pinch reflex, 50 % dextrose (6 ml/kg, IP) was injected 15 min before surgery.

Animals were placed supine and surgery began. Briefly, the right common, internal, and external carotid arteries were surgically exposed. The external carotid artery was isolated and ligated, leaving a 3–4 mm stump. Then the internal carotid artery was isolated and the pterygopalatine artery was ligated close to its origin with the internal carotid artery. A vascular clip was used to clamp the internal carotid artery closed, and another was used to close the common carotid artery. The stump of the external carotid artery was then opened and a 4.0 monofilament nylon suture with a rounded tip was advanced up through the internal carotid artery until resistance was felt. The suture remained in place for 90 min, after which the suture was removed from the internal carotid artery through the external carotid artery stump, beginning reperfusion. The stump of the external carotid artery was then ligated shut, and the skin was sutured. Animals were

R.L. Applegate et al. (eds.), *Brain Edema XVI: Translate Basic Science into Clinical Practice*, Acta Neurochirurgica Supplement, Vol. 121, DOI 10.1007/978-3-319-18497-5_42,

then given buprenorphine (0.02 mg/kg, SC) and yohimbine (1 mg/kg, IP). Animals were placed in a recovery chamber until fully awake.

Blood glucose was measured before dextrose injection (15 min before MCAO), 1 min before beginning MCAO surgery, 5 min after starting reperfusion, and 24 h after MCAO. Animals were sacrificed 15 min, 1 h, 3 h, or 24 h after MCAO for histological analysis of infarct volume, brain swelling, and hemoglobin volume.

Infarct Volume, Brain Swelling, and Hemoglobin Assay

Animals, sacrificed at 15 min, 1 h, 3 h, or 24 h ($n=5$/group) were used for quantification of infarct volume, brain swelling, and hemoglobin volume. Animals were deeply anesthetized with 5 % isoflurane in O_2, then transcardially perfused with 1 M phosphate-buffered saline (PBS) until the right atrium outflow was colorless. The brains were then quickly removed, sliced into 2-mm-thick coronal sections, then stained with 2 % 2,3,5-triphenyltetrazolium (TTC) for 30 min at room temperature [25]. TTC stained slices were then imaged and ImageJ (National Institutes of Health) used for tracing the areas of the contralateral hemispheres, C_i, and noninfarcted hemispheric tissue (unstained), N_i. Infarct volume was calculated using

$$\text{Infarct volume}(\%) = \left(\frac{\sum_i (C_i - N_i)}{2\left(\sum_i C_i\right)} \right) 100.$$

Swelling of the ipsilateral hemisphere was computed using the area of the contralateral and ipsilateral, I_i, slices with

$$\text{Swelling volume}(\%) = \left(\frac{\sum_i (I_i - C_i)}{\left(\sum_i C_i\right)} \right) 100.$$

After taking an image of the TTC-stained tissue, the slices were cut into left and right hemispheres. The right hemisphere pieces were combined, flash frozen, and stored at −80 °C. Hemorrhagic transformation was quantified using the hemoglobin assay, as previously described [3, 6]. Hemispheric brain tissue, added to 3 ml PBS, was homogenized for 30 s, followed by sonication on ice for 1 min, and centrifugation at 13,000 rpm and 4 °C for 30 min. After this, 0.2 ml of supernatant was added to 0.8 ml of Drabkin's reagent (Bio-Rad, Hercules, CA, USA), and allowed to stand in the dark for 15 min at room temperature. Optical density at 540 nm was measured with a spectrophotometer (Genesys 10S, Thermoscientific, Waltham, MA, USA). A standard curve was used to obtain the hemoglobin volume of each sample; error was propagated through all calculations. The standard curve was created by adding known amounts of blood to naïve hemispheric brain tissue, measuring absorbance following the above protocol, and then performing linear regression analysis of the absorbance versus hemoglobin volume.

All measures are presented as the mean ± SEM. Data were analyzed using one-way analysis of variance (ANOVA) with Tukey post hoc tests for the infarct volume, swelling volume, and hemoglobin volume. Blood glucose data were analyzed using one-way repeated measures ANOVA with Tukey post hoc test. A $p < 0.05$ was considered statistically significant.

Results

Blood glucose of sham and MCAO animals at the beginning of MCAO surgery (1 min pre-MCAO, sham: 242.3±46.4 mg/dl, MCAO: 194.0±22.5 mg/dl) and immediately after reperfusion (5 min post-MCAO, sham: 285.0±46.9 mg/dl, MCAO: 209.3±17.9 mg/dl) were significantly higher than that of sham and MCAO animals 15 min pre-MCAO (15 min pre-MCAO, sham: 75.8±4.3 mg/dl, MCAO: 81.8±2.2 mg/dl) and 24 h post-MCAO (24 h post-MCAO, sham: 75.5±3.3 mg/dl, MCAO: 67.5±3.3 mg/dl) (sham: $p<0.05$ vs 15 min pre-MCAO and $p<0.05$ vs 24 h post-MCAO for the both the 1 min pre-MCAO and 5 min post-MCAO groups; MCAO: $p<0.05$ vs 15 min pre-MCAO and $p<0.05$ vs 24 h post-MCAO for the both the 1 min pre-MCAO and 5 min post-MCAO groups) (Table 1).

Progression of Infarct Volume

Within 15 min post-MCAO, the infarct volume (15 min post-reperfusion, 14.9 ± 2.59 %) was significantly higher than sham animals (0.3 ± 0.30 %; $p < 0.05$), and reached its maximum. No difference in infarct volume was observed between any of the groups after 15 min ($p > 0.05$ for all group comparisons between 15 min, 1, 3, and 24 h post-reperfusion) and all were significantly higher than sham animals ($p < 0.05$ vs sham for all groups). The infarct volumes were 10.75 ± 0.79 %, 11.8 ± 3.53 %, and 13.1 ± 1.81 % for the 1, 3, and 24 h post-reperfusion, respectively (Fig. 1).

Progression of Ipsilateral Hemisphere Swelling

Swelling of the ipsilateral hemisphere was elevated at 15 min (4.3 ± 1.34 %) and 1 h post-reperfusion (6.2 ± 1.50 %) but not significantly different from sham (−0.7 ± 0.66 %) ($p > 0.05$ vs sham for the 15 min and 1 h post-reperfusion groups). By 3 h after reperfusion, ipsilateral hemisphere swelling reached statistically significant values (9.7 ± 1.91 %; $p > 0.05$) and continued to increase to the 24 h time point (14.5 ± 2.69 %; $p < 0.05$ vs sham for 3 and 24 h post-reperfusion groups). At 24 h, the ipsilateral swelling was also significantly higher than the 15 min and 1 h post-reperfusion time points ($p < 0.05$ vs 15 min and 1 h post-reperfusion) (Fig. 2a).

Table 1 Blood glucose measurements

	Sham	MCAO
15 min pre-MCAO	75.8 ± 4.3	81.8 ± 2.2
1 min pre-MCAO	242.3 ± 46.4*	194.0 ± 22.5*
5 min post-MCAO	285.0 ± 46.9*	209.3 ± 17.9*
24 h post-MCAO	75.5 ± 3.3	67.5 ± 3.3

Blood glucose (mg/dL) was measured before dextrose injection (15 min pre-MCAO), at the beginning of surgery (1 min pre-MCAO), at the beginning of reperfusion (5 min post-MCAO, and 24 h after MCAO (24 h post-MCAO) ($n = 5$/group))
*$p < 0.05$ vs 15 min pre-MCAO baseline and 24 h post-MCAO

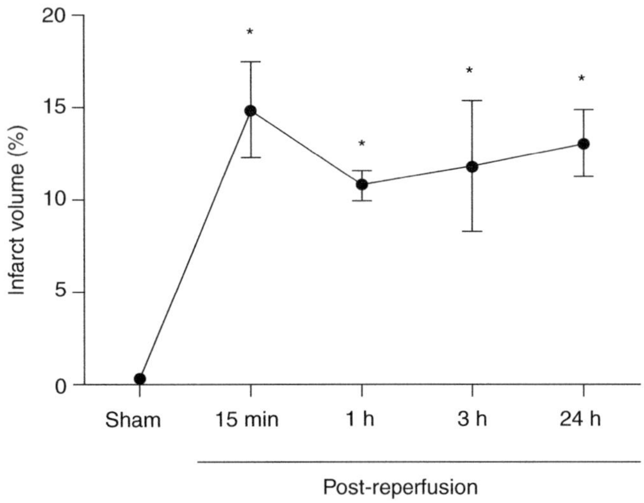

Fig. 1 Development of infarct volume after MCAO. Infarct volume (%) time course after MCAO. * $p < 0.05$ vs sham. $n = 5$/group

Development of Hemorrhagic Transformation

The amount of hemoglobin in the brain tissue was not significantly elevated 15 min after reperfusion (15 min post-reperfusion, 2.0 ± 1.33 μl) compared with sham (0.4 ± 1.03 μl) ($p > 0.05$). However, 1 h post-reperfusion, the hemoglobin volume (1 h post-reperfusion, 7.7 ± 1.31 μl) was significantly higher than sham and continued to rise to the 3 (9.0 ± 1.90 μl) and 24 h (12.3 ± 2.15 μl) time points ($p < 0.05$ vs sham for the 1, 3, and 24 h post-reperfusion groups). Additionally, the hemoglobin volume at 3 and 24 h after reperfusion was significantly higher than the 15 min time point ($p < 0.05$ vs 15 min post-reperfusion for the 3 h, and 24 h post-reperfusion groups) (Fig. 2b).

Discussion

Hemorrhagic transformation occurs in a large number of ischemic stroke patients and contributes to the morbidity and mortality after stroke [11]. Several risk factors have been identified for causing hemorrhagic transformation, including tPA [19], hyperglycemia [9], and hypertension [9]. Clinically,

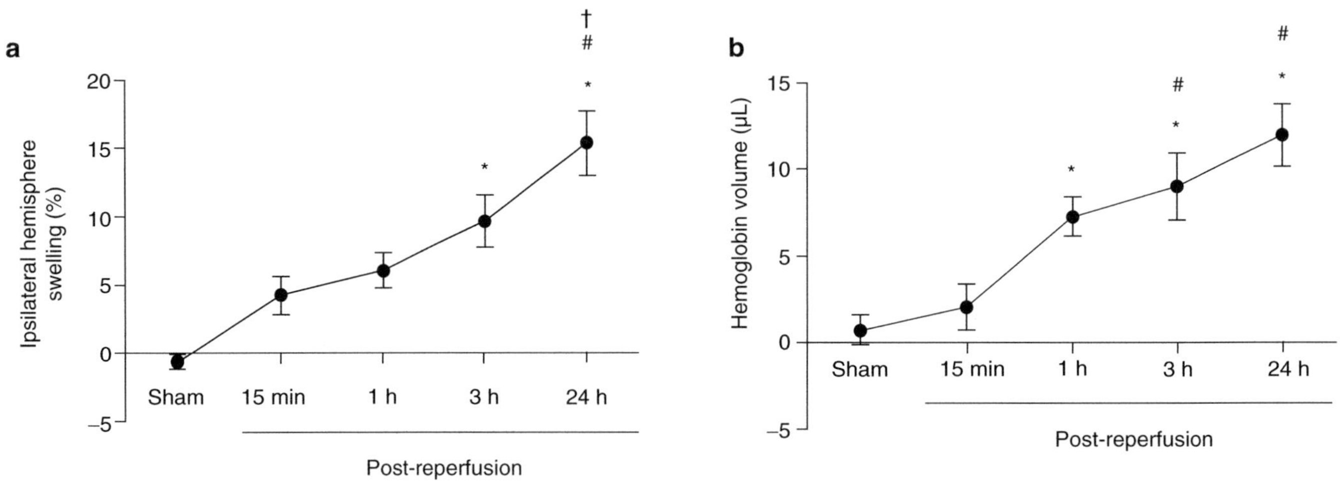

Fig. 2 Development of brain swelling and hemorrhagic transformation after MCAO. (**a**) Ipsilateral hemispheric swelling (%) time course after MCAO. *$p < 0.05$ vs sham. #$p < 0.05$ vs 15 min. †$p < 0.05$ vs 1 h. $n = 5$/group. (**b**) Hemoglobin volume (μL) describes hemorrhagic transformation after MCAO. *$p < 0.05$ vs sham. #$p < 0.05$ vs 15 min. $n = 5$/group, † $p < 0.05$ vs 1 h. $n = 5$/group

treatment of hemorrhagic transformation relies primarily on surgical interventions, which may be ineffective [18]. Furthermore, pharmacologic interventions of hemorrhagic transformation are almost non-existent [1, 15, 18]. Thus it is critically important to develop novel therapeutics which can prevent the occurrence of, as well as treat, hemorrhagic transformation.

In order to study and ultimately achieve promising therapies for prevention and treatment of hemorrhagic transformation, experimental models in which hemorrhagic transformation of ischemic injury occurs are utilized. The most widely used rodents models of hemorrhagic transformation are the hyperglycemic MCAO model [20, 26], diabetic MCAO model [7], and tissue plasminogen activator (tPA) embolic model [17, 22, 23]. Understanding the progression of bleeding following ischemic injury is essential for discerning the mechanisms of and the effects a treatment has on hemorrhagic transformation.

To provide more insight into hemorrhagic transformation, the objective of the current study was to determine the initiation and progression of hemorrhage after MCAO in hyperglycemic rats. Our results show that the infarct develops within 15 min after beginning reperfusion, but swelling of the ipsilateral hemisphere continues to increase over 24 h after MCAO [13, 21].

This study indicates that this model is not an ideal candidate for investigation of the novel therapeutics aimed at preventing or reducing hemorrhagic transformation; the administration of treatments to target post-reperfusion bleeding should work on a timescale faster than that of hemorrhagic transformation. Therefore, the most appropriate animal model should be utilized. The model described herein, pre-hyperglycemia with transient MCAO, has a therapeutic window of less than 1 h, which would put a severe time constraint on tested treatments. We expect a similar time course of hemorrhagic transformation for the long-term MCAO model, but this remains to be studied. We suggest using an alternative model, such as inducing hyperglycemia 2–3 h after starting reperfusion in the MCAO rat model.

Acknowledgments This work was supported by National Institutes of Health grant R01 NS043338 (JHZ).

Disclosure The authors have no conflicts of interest to report.

References

1. Alvarez-Sabin J, Maisterra O, Santamarina E, Kase CS (2013) Factors influencing haemorrhagic transformation in ischaemic stroke. Lancet Neurol 12:689–705
2. Arnould MC, Grandin CB, Peeters A, Cosnard G, Duprez TP (2004) Comparison of CT and three MR sequences for detecting and categorizing early (48 hours) hemorrhagic transformation in hyperacute ischemic stroke. Am J Neuroradiol 25:939–944
3. Asahi M, Asahi K, Wang X, Lo EH (2000) Reduction of tissue plasminogen activator-induced hemorrhage and brain injury by free radical spin trapping after embolic focal cerebral ischemia in rats. J Cereb Blood Flow Metab 20:452–457
4. Bruno A, Biller J, Adams HP, Clarke WR, Woolson RF, Williams LS, Hansen MD, Investigators T (1999) Acute blood glucose level and outcome from ischemic stroke. Neurology 52:280–284
5. Chen C, Ostrowski RP, Zhou C, Tang J, Zhang JH (2010) Suppression of hypoxia-inducible factor-1 alpha and its downstream genes reduces acute hyperglycemia-enhanced hemorrhagic transformation in a rat model of cerebral ischemia. J Neurosci Res 88:2046–2055
6. Choudhri TF, Hoh BL, Solomon RA, Connolly ES Jr, Pinsky DJ (1997) Use of a spectrophotometric hemoglobin assay to objectively quantify intracerebral hemorrhage in mice. Stroke 28:2296–2302
7. Ergul A, Elgebaly MM, Middlemore M-L, Li W, Elewa H, Switzer JA, Hall C, Kozak A, Fagan SC (2007) Increased hemorrhagic transformation and altered infarct size and localization after experimental stroke in a rat model type 2 diabetes. BMC Neurol 7:33
8. Fagan SC, Lapchak PA, Liebeskind DS, Ishrat T, Ergul A (2013) Recommendations for preclinical research in hemorrhagic transformation. Transl Stroke Res 4:322–327
9. Go AS, Mozaffarian D, Roger VL, Benjamin EJ, Berry JD, Borden WB, Bravata DM, Dai S, Ford ES, Fox CS, Franco S, Fullerton HJ, Gillespie C, Hailpern SM, Heit JA, Howard VJ, Huffman MD, Kissela BM, Kittner SJ, Lackland DT, Lichtman JH, Lisabeth LD, Magid D, Marcus GM, Marelli A, Matchar DB, McGuire DK, Mohler ER, Moy CS, Mussolino ME, Nichol G, Paynter NP, Schreiner PJ, Sorlie PD, Stein J, Turan TN, Virani SS, Wong ND, Woo D, Turner MB (2013) Heart disease and stroke statistics–2013 update: a report from the American Heart Association. Circulation 127:e6–e245
10. Hafez S, Coucha M, Bruno A, Fagan SC, Ergul A (2014) Hyperglycemia, acute ischemic stroke, and thrombolytic therapy. Transl Stroke Res 5:442–453
11. Hornig CR, Dorndorf W, Agnoli AL (1986) Hemorrhagic cerebral infarction–a prospective study. Stroke 17:179–185
12. Kawamura S, Yasui N, Shirasawa M, Fukasawa H (1991) Rat middle cerebral artery occlusion using an intraluminal thread technique. Acta Neurochir 109:126–132
13. Khanna A, Kahle KT, Walcott BP, Gerzanich V, Simard JM (2014) Disruption of ion homeostasis in the neurogliovascular unit underlies the pathogenesis of ischemic cerebral edema. Transl Stroke Res 5:3–16
14. Kissela BM, Ewing I, Khoury J, Moomaw CJ, Kleindorfer D, Szaflarski JP, Woo D, Gebel J, Schneider A, Shukla R, Alwell K, Broderick JP, Miller R (2005) Epidemiology of ischemic stroke in patients with diabetes – the greater Cincinnati/Northern Kentucky Stroke Study. Diabetes Care 28:355–359
15. Lapchak PA (2002) Hemorrhagic transformation following ischemic stroke: significance, causes, and relationship to therapy and treatment. Curr Neurol Neurosci Rep 2:38–43
16. Mandava P, Martini SR, Munoz M, Dalmeida W, Sarma AK, Anderson JA, Fabian RH, Kent TA (2014) Hyperglycemia worsens outcome after rt-PA primarily in the large-vessel occlusive stroke subtype. Transl Stroke Res 5:519–525
17. Marinescu M, Bouley J, Chueh J, Fisher M, Henninger N (2014) Clot injection technique affects thrombolytic efficacy in a rat embolic stroke model: implications for translaboratory collaborations. J Cereb Blood Flow Metab 34:677–682
18. Morgenstern LB, Frankowski RF, Shedden P, Pasteur W, Grotta JC (1998) Surgical treatment for intracerebral hemorrhage (STICH) – a single-center, randomized clinical trial. Neurology 51:1359–1363
19. Orso F, Baldasseroni S, Maggioni AP (2008) The role of thrombolysis in acute ischemic stroke. Herz 33:498–506

20. Pulsinelli WA, Waldman S, Rawlinson D, Plum F (1982) Moderate hyperglycemia augments ischemic brain damage: a neuropathologic study in the rat. Neurology 32:1239–1246
21. Song M, Yu SP (2014) Ionic regulation of cell volume changes and cell death after ischemic stroke. Transl Stroke Res 5:17–27
22. Sumii T, Lo EH (2002) Involvement of matrix metalloproteinase in thrombolysis-associated hemorrhagic transformation after embolic focal ischemia in rats. Stroke 33:831–836
23. Tejima E, Katayama Y, Suzuki Y, Kano T, Lo EH (2001) Hemorrhagic transformation after fibrinolysis with tissue plasminogen activator: evaluation of role of hypertension with rat thromboembolic stroke model. Stroke 32:1336–1340
24. Thanvi B, Treadwell S, Robinson T (2008) Early neurological deterioration in acute ischaemic stroke: predictors, mechanisms and management. Postgrad Med J 84:412–417
25. Yin D, Zhou C, Kusaka I, Calvert JW, Parent AD, Nanda A, Zhang JH (2003) Inhibition of apoptosis by hyperbaric oxygen in a rat focal cerebral ischemic model. J Cereb Blood Flow Metab 23:855–864
26. Yip PK, He YY, Hsu CY, Garg N, Marangos P, Hogan EL (1991) Effect of plasma glucose on infarct size in focal cerebral ischemia-reperfusion. Neurology 41:899–905
27. Zhang Z, Yan J, Shi H (2013) Hyperglycemia as a risk factor of ischemic stroke. J Drug Metab Toxicol 4:1000153

The Effects of Clinically Relevant Hypertonic Saline and Conivaptan Administration on Ischemic Stroke

David Decker, Lisa Collier, Tsz Lau, Raul Olivera, Glenn Roma, Christopher Leonardo, Hilary Seifert, Derrick Rowe, and Keith R. Pennypacker

Introduction

Cerebral edema is characterized by pathologic increase in brain water content, one of the most important mechanisms of secondary injury and early mortality after ischemic stroke [29]. Despite the prevalence of this disorder, therapeutic options remain limited. In the case of ischemic stroke, cytotoxic edema is regarded by many to be the predominant injury mechanism in the early phase after stroke [13]. As injured brain tissue swells within the fixed volume of the skull and displaces healthy tissue, intracranial pressure (ICP) rises and cerebral perfusion is further decreased. These events promote additional ischemic events and herniation syndromes. In the clinical setting, the major goal of therapy is to preserve viable tissue by reducing ICP and maintaining cerebral blood flow.

Osmotherapy is the mainstay of treatment for cerebral edema [6]. Hypertonic saline (HS) has many of the properties of an ideal osmotherapeutic agent in that it is nontoxic [7], only slowly permeates or disrupts the blood-brain barrier (BBB) [8], and promotes the maintenance of intravascular volume [15]. Despite increasing use of HS, there is currently no optimized, validated clinical protocol for the treatment of cerebral edema. In current clinical practice, a target serum osmolality of 310–320 mOsm/L is commonly used. However, this target is largely arbitrary and insufficient for full therapeutic effect [6]. A number of recent animal studies examining different dosing strategies have determined that achieving higher serum osmolality levels (≥350 mOsm/l) with infusion of 7.5 % saline results in a robust attenuation of cerebral edema, and is well tolerated [7, 8, 31].

Although HS effectively reduces ICP and cerebral edema [27, 31], the mechanism of action is not fully understood and little is known regarding the net effect on neurodegenerative tissue damage. The benefits of HS are thought to arise from establishment of an osmotic gradient along which water travels from brain tissue into the intravascular compartment [8]. Astrocytic expression of the water channel aquaporin 4 (AQP4) has been shown to be involved in the rate-limiting effect on the bulk flow of water across membranes [36], suggesting that alterations in AQP4 expression and/or function may be linked to the therapeutic benefits of osmotherapy, including HS.

Interestingly, reduction of cerebral edema may not be the sole mechanism by which osmotherapy could promote tissue survival. Clinical data also suggest that HS may attenuate inflammation after brain injury [25]. Microgliosis is one of the most important components of post-stroke neuroinflammation [21], characterized by microglial activation that triggers intracellular signaling pathways. The net effect of these processes is production of cytotoxic and inflammatory mediators that facilitate tissue injury. Inflammation has also been linked to increased BBB permeability at both early and delayed time points after stroke [9], thereby promoting vasogenic edema [33], peripheral immune cell extravasation into brain parenchyma [18], and cytokine/chemokine production/release [14].

Targeting arginine vasopressin (AVP) signaling has been reported to be an effective osmotherapeutic therapy to reduce stroke-induced edema and infarct [7, 10, 17]. Evidence suggests that AVP has pro-inflammatory effects in traumatic brain injury and oxidative stress in the brain following dehydration [12, 30]. Conivaptan is a US Food and Drug Administration (FDA)-approved pan-AVP receptor antagonist and its osmotherapeutic and anti-inflammatory properties suggest a potential treatment for stroke. The present study was conducted to examine the effect of multiple HS

D. Decker • T. Lau • R. Olivera
Department of Neurology, Morsani College of Medicine, University of South Florida, 12901 Bruce B. Downs Blvd., Tampa, FL 33612, USA

L. Collier • G. Roma • C. Leonardo • H. Seifert • D. Rowe
K.R. Pennypacker (✉)
Department of Molecular Pharmacology and Physiology, Morsani College of Medicine, University of South Florida, 12901 Bruce B. Downs Blvd., Tampa, FL 33612, USA
e-mail: kpennypa@health.usf.edu

R.L. Applegate et al. (eds.), *Brain Edema XVI: Translate Basic Science into Clinical Practice*, Acta Neurochirurgica Supplement, Vol. 121,
DOI 10.1007/978-3-319-18497-5_43, © Springer International Publishing Switzerland 2016

and conivaptan administration strategies on brain edema, infarct volume, and neuroinflammation after ischemic stroke.

Methods

Animal Care

All animal procedures were conducted in accordance with the National Institutes of Health Guide for the Care and Use of Laboratory Animals with a protocol approved by the Institutional Animal Care and Use Committee at the University of South Florida. Male Sprague-Dawley rats (300–350 g), purchased from Harlan Labs (Indianapolis, IN, USA), were used for the experiments.

Laser Doppler Blood Flow Measurement, Permanent Focal Ischemia, and Jugular Catheter Placement

Blood perfusion in the brain was detected using the Moor Instruments Ltd. Laser Doppler (Devon, England) with MoorLAB proprietary Windows-based software on a standard laptop as previously described [1]. Rats that did not show ≥60 % reduction in perfusion during MCAO were excluded from the study [1].

MCAO surgery was performed using the intraluminal method originally described by Longa et al. [22] and previously reported [1]. An i-STAT handheld clinical analyzer was used to measure physiological blood parameters including hemoglobin, hematocrit, ionized calcium, glucose, sodium, potassium, pH, pCO_2, HCO_3, TCO_2, base excess, pO_2, and O_2. No differences in these were found between groups of rats used in the treatment studies.

Following MCAO, the right jugular vein was exposed. Using forceps, two pieces of equal length of suture were passed under the jugular vein. The more distal suture was tied tightly to occlude blood flow from the head region. A small cut was made into the jugular vein between the two ligatures. A catheter filled with saline was inserted into the vein and threaded 0.5 cm toward the heart. The ligature closest to the heart was tightened around the vein and catheter to prevent dislodgement. The ends of the distal ligature were tied between the cuffs on the catheter for additional anchorage. After confirming patency, the catheter was tunneled subcutaneously and exteriorized at the nape of the neck. This incision was closed with a staple. The catheter was filled with lock solution (saline:glycerol 50:50 ratio). The neck was sutured closed and the rat was allowed to wake in a fresh cage. Following recovery, animals were randomly assigned into treatment groups.

Treatment Regimens

A series of injections were given intravenous (IV; jugular catheter) at 6 and 9 h post-MCAO, then every 4 h starting at 8:00 AM until 8:00 PM on the first day postoperatively, and a single 8:00 AM injection the second day postoperatively for a total of seven injections for every rat. Two treatment paradigms were used with treatment starting at either 6 h (Early) or 24 h (Late) post-stroke. The five treatment groups were normal saline (0.9 %, NS, control), 5 % saline infusion +5 % saline maintenance (HS), conivaptan only (Con), conivaptan +5 % saline maintenance (Con + HS), and conivaptan +5 % saline bolus +5 % saline maintenance (Con + HSb). The experimental dosages were chosen based on a weight-based extrapolation of typical human dosages. The initial dose of conivaptan was 0.35 mg/kg (0.5 ml of a 0.2 mg/ml stock) with follow-up doses of 0.7 mg/kg (0.1 ml). Treatment schedules for each group are summarized (Table 1).

Tissue Preparation and Fluoro-Jade Histochemistry

Animals were euthanized at 48 h post-MCAO and perfused with 0.9 % saline followed by 4 % paraformaldehyde in phosphate buffer (pH 7.4). The brains were harvested and processed as previously described [1]. Sections were collected from six bregma points, ranging from 1.7 to −2.3 mm. For determination of infarct volume, Fluoro-Jade (Histochem, Jefferson, AR, USA) staining was performed to label degenerating neurons. This method was adapted from that originally developed by Schmued et al. [26] and has been subsequently detailed [11].

Immunohistochemistry

Immunohistochemistry was performed to detect activated microglia [12]. Sections were incubated overnight at 4 °C with mouse anti-rat CD11b antibody (Ox-42; 1:3,000; Serotec, Raleigh, NC, USA) in PBS with 2 % goat serum, 0.3 % Triton X-100. The following day, slides were washed with PBS and incubated 1 h at room temperature with horse anti-mouse secondary antibody (1:300; Vector Laboratories Inc., Burlingame, CA, USA) in antibody solution (2 % serum, 0.3 % Triton X-100 in PBS). Slides were then washed

Table 1 Treatment groups and timeline of experimental intervention

Treatments'	Surgery day		Post-op day 1		Post-op day 2	
6 h post-op "Early" start	*6 h post-op*	*9 h post-op*	*Every 4 h: 8 AM until 8 PM*		*8 AM*	*12 PM*
NS	1.4 ml NS	1.4 ml NS	1.4 ml NS		1.4 ml NS	E
HS	Bolus 2.4 ml HS	1.4 ml HS	1.4 ml HS		1.4 ml HS	E
Con	Bolus 0.5 ml Con	0.1 ml Con	0.1 ml Con		1.4 ml NS	E
Con+HS	Bolus 0.5 ml Con	0.1 ml Con+1.4 ml HS	0.1 ml Con+1.4 ml HS		1.4 ml HS	E
Con+HSb	Bolus 0.5 ml Con+2.4 ml HS	0.1 ml Con+1.4 ml HS	0.1 ml Con+1.4 ml HS		1.4 ml HS	E
24 h post-op "Late" start	*6 h post-op*	*9 h post-op*	*8 AM*	*Every 4 h: 12 pm until 8 PM*	*8 AM*	*12 PM*
NS	1.4 ml NS	1.4 ml NS	1.4 ml NS	1.4 ml NS	1.4 ml NS	E
HS	1.4 ml NS	1.4 ml NS	Bolus 2.4 ml HS	1.4 ml HS	1.4 ml HS	E
Con	1.4 ml NS	1.4 ml NS	Bolus 0.5 ml Con	0.1 ml Con	0.1 ml Con	E
Con+HS	1.4 ml NS	1.4 ml NS	Bolus 0.5 ml Con	0.1 ml Con+1.4 ml HS	0.1 ml Con+1.4 ml HS	E
Con+HSb	1.4 ml NS	1.4 ml NS	Bolus 0.5 ml Con+2.4 ml HS	0.1 ml Con+1.4 ml HS	0.1 ml Con+1.4 ml HS	E

The five treatment groups were: Normal Saline (0.9 %, control) [NS], Hypertonic (5 %) Saline [HS], Conivaptan only [Con], Conivaptan+HS maintenance [Con+HS], and Conivaptan/HS Bolus+Conivaptan/HS maintenance [Con+HSb]
E euthanized

with PBS and incubated in Avidin-Biotin Complex (ABC; Vector Laboratories Inc.) mixture for 1 h. Next the slides were washed and then visualized using a DAB/peroxide solution (Vector Laboratories Inc.).

Image Analyses

Images of the brain sections were taken with a 1× objective (for Fluoro-Jade and brain edema) on a Zeiss Axioskop2 microscope (Carl Zeiss Inc., Thornwood, NY, USA) using Open Lab software (Improvision Ltd., Lexington, MA, USA). Hemispheric areas were measured using Image J software (National Institutes of Health). Photomicrographs were processed using Jasc Paint Shop Pro to sharpen and enhance contrast to the same specifications for all slides.

Fluoro-Jade stained slides were used to calculate infarct volume. Total area of positive staining was measured in the ipsilateral and contralateral hemispheres for each section. The area values for six representative bregma points throughout the infarct were totaled for each animal, and infarct volumes were calculated as the percent of the contralateral hemisphere.

For edema, thaw-mounted slides were air-dried overnight before imaging. The area of each hemisphere was measured and the ventricular areas were subtracted from the hemispheric area. The total adjusted area for each hemisphere was determined across all six bregma points, and edema for each animal was calculated as a percentage of the contralateral hemisphere.

For CD11b immunohistochemistry, images were taken with a 10× objective. Three regions of the striatum were imaged (upper right, middle left, and lower center) for the first four bregma points collected (1.7 to −1.3). The area fraction of CD11b-positive staining was calculated for each image, and data are expressed as the average area fraction for each group.

Statistical Analyses

Data from all experiments were quantified and analyzed using GraphPad Prism 6.0 (GraphPad, La Jolla, CA, USA) software. For all statistical tests, the threshold for significant differences between groups was set at $p<0.05$. For behavioral tests, significant effects of treatment were determined using unpaired, two-tailed t-tests with Welch's correction. For all other data, main effects were determined using one-way or two-way analysis of variance (ANOVA) followed by Fisher's least squares difference test for pairwise comparisons between treatment groups.

Results

Infarct Volume

Infarct volume was measured with Fluoro-Jade staining to determine the efficacy of HS and conivaptan, both alone and in combination, when administered either 6 h or 24 h following MCAO. Total area occupied by staining was calculated for each animal and was expressed as a percentage of Fluoro-Jade positive area in the ischemic hemisphere relative to the contralateral hemisphere.

Both HS and conivaptan elicited protection when administered 6 h after MCAO (Fig. 1). NS controls showed large expanses of Fluoro-Jade throughout the striatum and adjacent cerebral cortex (Fig. 1a), whereas staining appeared markedly reduced in sections from animals treated with HS or Con (Fig. 1b, c). Quantification of total infarct volume (Fig. 1d) showed significant reductions in the 6 h HS ($p = 0.0411$, $t = 1.825$) and Con ($p = 0.050$, $t = 1.678$) relative to NS controls, whereas there were no significant differences in the combined Con + HS ($p = 0.0922$, $t = 1.370$) or Con + HSb groups ($p = 0.3296$, $t = 0.4489$) compared to NS controls.

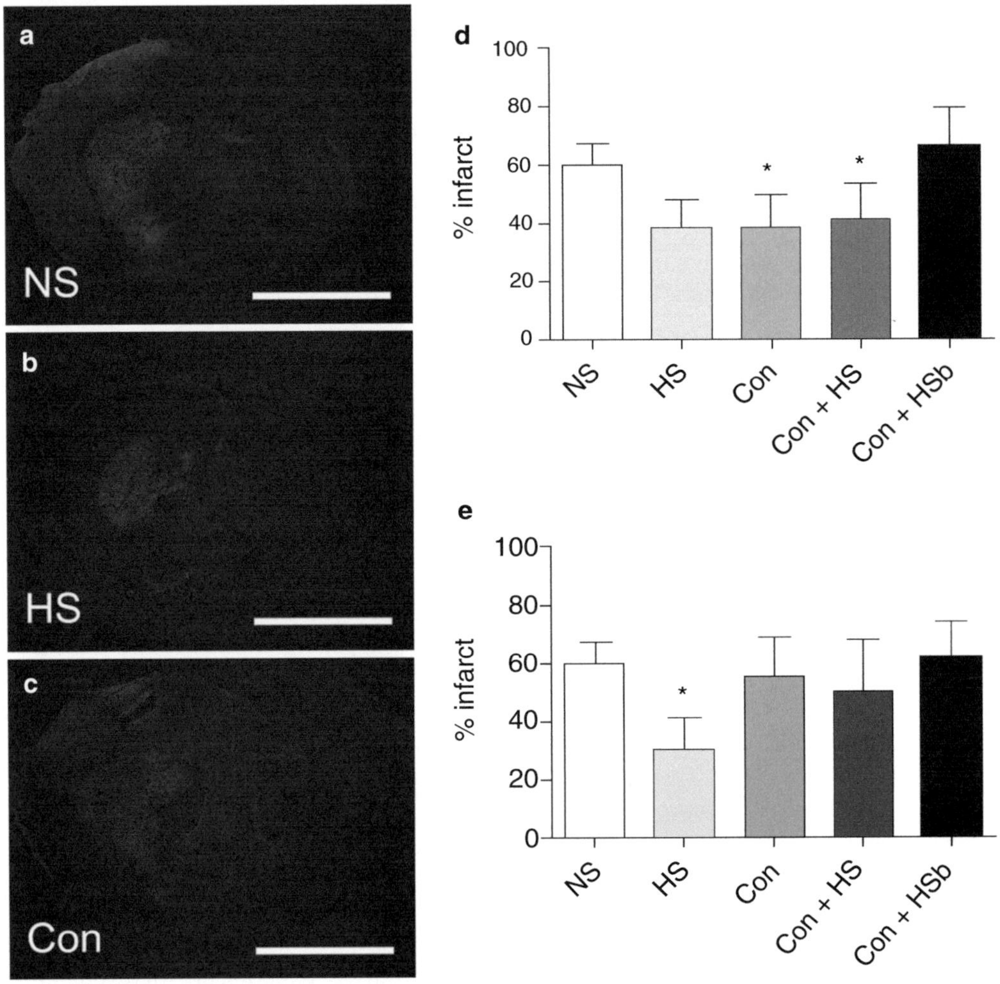

Fig. 1 (**a–c**) Representative micrographs of Fluoro-Jade stained sections from rats treated with NS, HS, or Con 6 h after MCAO. Fluoro-Jade staining was abundant throughout the striatum and cerebral cortex after treatment with NS (**a**), whereas staining was markedly reduced in sections from rats treated with HS (**b**) and Con (**c**). Quantification of infarct volume (**d**) showed significant reductions in rats treated with HS or Con ($p<0.05$), whereas there was no significant difference between NS controls and rats that received Con + HS or Con + HSb. *$p<0.05$, $n=4$–6 per group. Scale bars = 2 mm. NS, normal (0.9 %) saline. HS, hypertonic (5 %) saline. Con, conivaptan. Con + HS, conivaptan + hypertonic (5 %) saline maintenance. Con + HSb, conivaptan/hypertonic (5 %) saline bolus + hypertonic (5 %) saline maintenance. Quantification of infarct volume in rats treated with NS, Con, Con + HS, or Con + HSb 24 h after MCAO (**e**). Data show a significant reduction in infarct volume following treatment with HS relative to NS controls ($p<0.05$), whereas there were no significant differences after treatment with Con. Combined treatments produced no protective effect, as the Con + HS and Con + HSb groups showed no significant differences relative to NS controls. *$p<0.05$, $n=4$–6 per group. NS, normal (0.9 %) saline. HS, hypertonic (5 %) saline. Con, conivaptan. Con + HS, conivaptan + hypertonic (5 %) saline maintenance. Con + HSb, conivaptan/hypertonic (5 %) saline bolus + conivaptan/hypertonic (5 %) saline maintenance

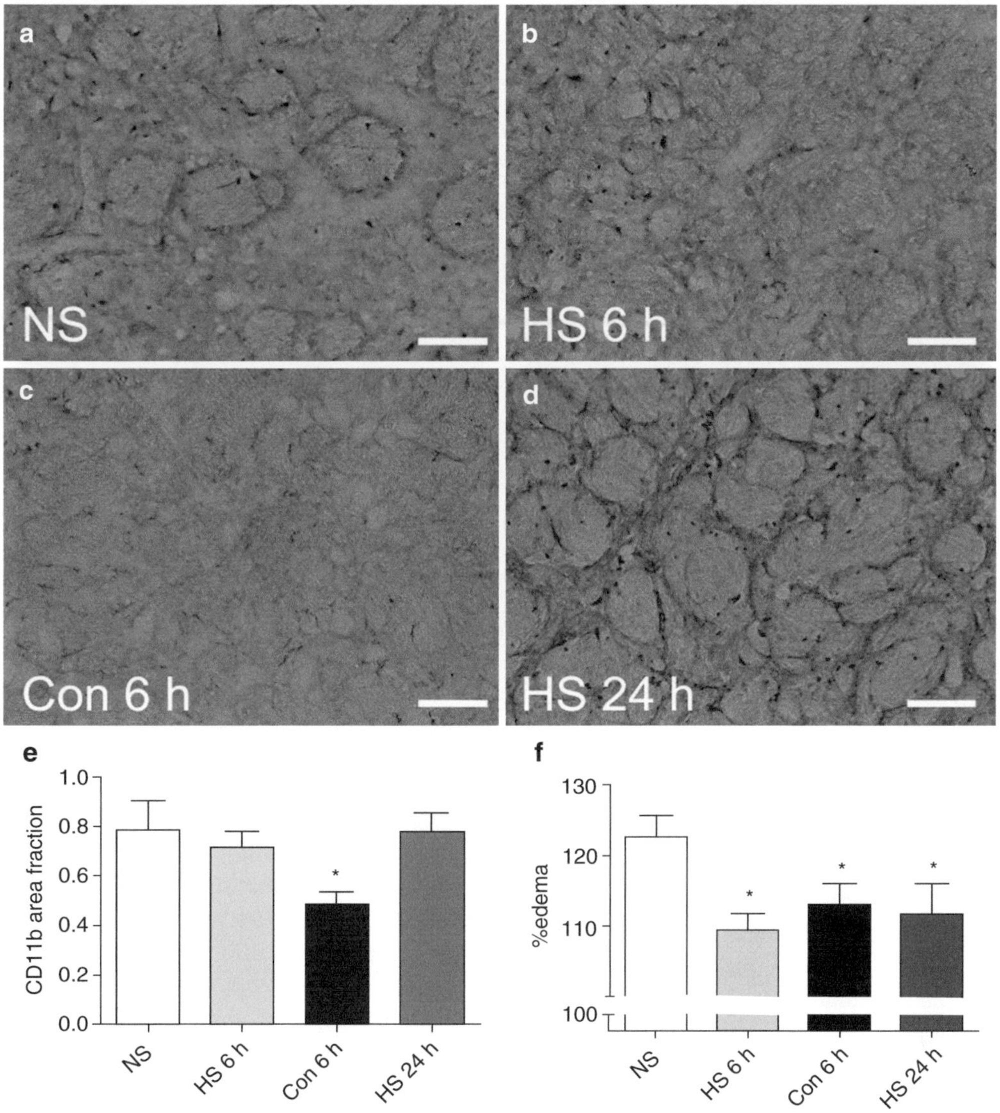

Fig. 2 (**a–d**) Representative micrographs of CD11b immunohistochemistry in sections from rats treated with HS or Con 6 h after MCAO, or HS 24 h after MCAO. Immunohistochemical staining shows a profile of ubiquitous CD11b-positive cells within the striatum of an NS control (**a**) that resembles sections from rats treated with HS (**b**, **d**). Treatment with Con 6 h after MCAO resulted in reduced numbers of CD11b-positive cells (**c**). Quantification revealed a significant reduction in the area occupied by CD11b staining in the 6 h Con group ($p<0.05$) relative to NS controls and HS groups. $*p<0.05$, $n=4$–6 per group (**e**). Quantification of brain swelling in rats treated with HS or Con 6 h after MCAO, or HS 24 h after MCAO (**f**). Brain swelling was calculated in groups that showed efficacy in reducing Fluoro-Jade staining to assess whether edema might account for the observed effects. Data show significantly reduced brain edema in 6 h HS, 6 h Con and 24 h HS rats relative to NS controls ($p<0.05$), thus establishing a relationship between neurodegenerative injury and brain swelling. $*p<0.05$, $n=4$–6 per group. NS, normal (0.9 %) saline. HS 6 h, hypertonic (5 %) saline administered 6 h after MCAO. Con 6 h, conivaptan administered 6 h after MCAO. HS 24 h, hypertonic (5 %) saline administered 24 h after MCAO. Scale bars = 50 μm. NS, normal (0.9 %) saline. HS 6 h, hypertonic (5 %) saline administered 6 h after MCAO. Con 6 h, conivaptan administered 6 h after MCAO. HS 24 h, hypertonic (5 %) saline administered 24 h after MCAO

Interestingly, the results from the 24 h post-treatment groups were not entirely consistent with those obtained from the 6 h groups (Fig. 2). Similar to the 6 h treatments, animals that received HS 24 h after MCAO showed significant reductions in infarct volume ($p=0.0207$, $t=2.217$) relative to NS controls, while there were no significant differences from controls in the combined Con + HS ($p=0.2722$, $t=0.6204$) or Con + HSb ($p=0.4399$, $t=0.1532$) groups. However, unlike the 6 h treatment, animals that received Con 24 h after MCAO showed no significant difference in infarct volume ($p=0.3753$, $t=0.3235$) compared with NS controls.

Microglia/Macrophage Activation

Adjacent sections were immunostained for the microglia/macrophage cell surface marker CD11b to gain insight into the anti-inflammatory effects of HS and Con (Fig. 2). Cells labeled with CD11b were abundant in sections from NS controls, particularly throughout the striatum (Fig. 2a) but also within the cortical tissue. Sections from animals treated with HS also displayed ubiquitous staining for CD11b (Fig. 2b, d) that resembled those of NS controls. However, sections from animals treated with Con 6 h after MCAO showed far fewer numbers of CD11b – positive cells, particularly within the striatum (Fig. 2c). Quantification (Fig. 2e) showed a significant reduction in the area occupied by CD11b staining for the 6 h Con group relative to NS ($p=0.0455$, $t=1.786$), 6 h HS ($p=0.0091$, $t=2.651$) and 24 h HS ($p=0.0031$, $t=3.450$). There were no significant differences between the NS controls and 6 h HS ($p=0.3231$, $t=0.4659$) or 24 h HS ($p=0.4872$, $t=0.03247$) groups.

Brain Swelling

Based on initial results, brain swelling was calculated for the treatment groups that showed reduced infarct volume to determine whether the protective doses of HS and Con also reduced brain edema (Fig. 2f). Brain edema in the ipsilateral hemisphere was measured by image analysis and expressed as a percentage of the contralateral hemisphere. Consistent with the Fluoro-Jade staining, animals that were protected from neurodegenerative injury also showed less brain edema. HS significantly attenuated brain swelling when administered either 6 h ($p=0.0015$, $t=3.434$) or 24 h ($p=0.0278$, $t=2.102$) after MCAO compared with NS controls, and Con significantly reduced brain swelling when administered 6 h following MCAO ($p=0.0221$, $t=2.197$).

Discussion

The present study evaluated the potential of two therapeutic strategies, both alone and in combination, to improve histological and functional outcomes when administered at clinically relevant time points after stroke onset. Although osmotherapy has been shown to be effective in reducing ICP and brain edema [6], studies that assess the relationship between these outcomes and neurodegenerative injury provide varied results [5, 24]. The 6 h HS and conivaptan groups showed significant reductions in both infarct volume and brain edema relative to controls, linking the effects of limiting edema to reduced cellular injury. Furthermore, HS significantly reduced edema even when administered 24 h after stroke onset. These data highlight the importance of controlling edema throughout the period of delayed infarct expansion [13] and establish a connection between brain swelling, neurodegenerative injury, and survival.

The mechanism of action of HS is not fully understood, but HS is believed to work primarily by establishment of an osmotic gradient along which water travels from brain tissue into the intravascular compartment through an intact BBB [8]. While cellular membranes are freely permeable to water, diffusion through membranes is relatively slow. For water in the capillary lumen to enter the astrocytic compartment in the brain, it must pass through three plasma membranes (luminal endothelial, abluminal endothelial, and luminal perivascular). Aquaporin channels allow cells to modulate the rapid bulk flow of water across cell membranes. AQP4 is the most abundant water channel in the brain. This channel has been implicated in the pathogenesis of cerebral edema, and also been shown to be a rate-limiter for water influx during edema formation [2, 34] and water efflux in the setting of an osmotic gradient created by hypertonic saline [37]. Expression levels of AQP4 also correlate with brain water content in untreated animals after ischemic stroke [35]. In ischemic stroke studies using transgenic mice, the deletion of AQP4 was shown to impair water uptake by ischemic cells and led to increased survival with improved neurologic outcomes [23]. This is consistent with other studies demonstrating the neuroprotective effects of limiting edema [8].

In addition to the effect of osmolar gradients on the development of cerebral edema, several lines of evidence suggest that AVP plays an important and complementary role. Elevated AVP levels have been demonstrated after ischemic stroke and other forms of brain injury [3, 7, 17]. Intracerebroventricular injections of AVP exacerbated acute ischemic brain edema, whereas injection of AVP antiserum significantly decreased cerebral edema [16]. Cerebral edema after ischemic stroke was also attenuated in vasopressin-deficient rats [10], while pharmacological AVP receptor inhibitors attenuated postischemic cerebral edema [4, 17, 19, 20, 28]. Indeed, a study by Chang et al. [4] demonstrated that treatment with HS led to a reduction in plasma AVP levels following experimental stroke in rats, which supports the idea that HS might have limited edema and infarction here through modulation of AVP.

It has been demonstrated that receptor antagonism of V1a, but not V2, reduced infarct volume and brain water content while increasing AQP4 expression following experimental stroke [28]. Conivaptan is a V1 and V2 receptor antagonist [32] that is currently FDA-approved for the treatment of hyponatremia. Based on this mechanism of action, conivaptan would be expected to increase serum sodium and osmolality, but may also reduce cerebral edema by accentuating AQP4 expression. This potential effect has not yet been investigated. However, the fact that conivaptan was ineffective in reducing infarct volume or edema when administered 24 h after MCAO suggests that its mechanism of action is likely distinct, at least in part, from that of HS. Notably, the 6 h conivaptan treatment also decreased microglial activation, which is implicated in delayed expansion of the infarct, while initiation of conivaptan treatment at 24 h did not alter microglial activation/recruitment. Vasopressin has been shown to exert pro-inflammatory effects in a model of traumatic brain injury [30], suggesting that conivaptan is blunting the stroke-induced neuroinflammatory response through vasopressin receptor antagonism. This finding suggests a potential additional mechanism to explain the beneficial effects of conivaptan on survival, tissue injury, and functional recovery that is independent of its role in fluid homeostasis.

Our results showed a positive result from HS or conivaptan alone but did not show a synergistic effect between HS and conivaptan. This suggests that conivaptan should be explored as a potentially useful alternative osmotherapeutic agent. The pharmacologic properties of conivaptan, that is, increasing serum sodium while reducing blood volume, may be particularly useful for treating patients who cannot tolerate the additional volume load associated with HS, such as those with congestive heart failure. In addition, the novel finding of reduced microglial activation offers a new potential mechanism to be exploited as means of improving outcomes after ischemic stroke.

Acknowledgments This work was supported by the University of South Florida Neuroscience Collaborative.

References

1. Ajmo CT Jr, Vernon DO, Collier L, Hall AA, Garbuzova-Davis S, Willing A, Pennypacker KR (2008) The spleen contributes to stroke-induced neurodegeneration. J Neurosci Res 86:2227–2234
2. Amiry-Moghaddam M, Ottersen OP (2003) The molecular basis of water transport in the brain. Nat Rev Neurosci 4:991–1001
3. Barreca T, Gandolfo C, Corsini G, Del Sette M, Cataldi A, Rolandi E, Franceschini R (2001) Evaluation of the secretory pattern of plasma arginine vasopressin in stroke patients. Cerebrovasc Dis 11:113–118
4. Bemana I, Nagao S (1999) Treatment of brain edema with a nonpeptide arginine vasopressin V1 receptor antagonist OPC-21268 in rats. Neurosurgery 44:148–154, discussion 154–145
5. Bhardwaj A, Harukuni I, Murphy SJ, Alkayed NJ, Crain BJ, Koehler RC, Hurn PD, Traystman RJ (2000) Hypertonic saline worsens infarct volume after transient focal ischemia in rats. Stroke 31:1694–1701
6. Bhardwaj A, Ulatowski JA (2004) Hypertonic saline solutions in brain injury. Curr Opin Crit Care 10:126–131
7. Chang Y, Chen TY, Chen CH, Crain BJ, Toung TJ, Bhardwaj A (2006) Plasma arginine-vasopressin following experimental stroke: effect of osmotherapy. J Appl Physiol 100:1445–1451
8. Chen CH, Toung TJ, Sapirstein A, Bhardwaj A (2006) Effect of duration of osmotherapy on blood–brain barrier disruption and regional cerebral edema after experimental stroke. J Cereb Blood Flow Metab 26:951–958
9. Danton GH, Dietrich WD (2003) Inflammatory mechanisms after ischemia and stroke. J Neuropathol Exp Neurol 62:127–136
10. Dickinson LD, Betz AL (1992) Attenuated development of ischemic brain edema in vasopressin-deficient rats. J Cereb Blood Flow Metab 12:681–690
11. Duckworth EA, Butler TL, De Mesquita D, Collier SN, Collier L, Pennypacker KR (2005) Temporary focal ischemia in the mouse: technical aspects and patterns of Fluoro-Jade evident neurodegeneration. Brain Res 1042:29–36
12. Faraco G, Wijasa TS, Park L, Moore J, Anrather J, Iadecola C (2014) Water deprivation induces neurovascular and cognitive dysfunction through vasopressin-induced oxidative stress. J Cereb Blood Flow Metab 34(5):852–860
13. Forsyth LL, Liu-DeRyke X, Parker D Jr, Rhoney DH (2008) Role of hypertonic saline for the management of intracranial hypertension after stroke and traumatic brain injury. Pharmacotherapy 28:469–484
14. Hanisch UK, Kettenmann H (2007) Microglia: active sensor and versatile effector cells in the normal and pathologic brain. Nat Neurosci 10:1387–1394
15. Harukuni I, Kirsch JR, Bhardwaj A (2002) Cerebral resuscitation: role of osmotherapy. J Anesth 16:229–237
16. Hertz L, Chen Y, Spatz M (2000) Involvement of non-neuronal brain cells in AVP-mediated regulation of water space at the cellular, organ, and whole-body level. J Neurosci Res 62:480–490
17. Ikeda Y, Toda S, Kawamoto T, Teramoto A (1997) Arginine vasopressin release inhibitor RU51599 attenuates brain oedema following transient forebrain ischaemia in rats. Acta Neurochir (Wien) 139:1166–1171, discussion 1171–1162
18. Jander S, Kraemer M, Schroeter M, Witte OW, Stoll G (1995) Lymphocytic infiltration and expression of intercellular adhesion molecule-1 in photochemically induced ischemia of the rat cortex. J Cereb Blood Flow Metab 15:42–51
19. Kagawa M, Nagao S, Bemana I (1996) Arginine vasopressin receptor antagonists for treatment of vasogenic brain edema: an experimental study. J Neurotrauma 13:273–279
20. Laszlo FA, Varga C, Nakamura S (1999) Vasopressin receptor antagonist OPC-31260 prevents cerebral oedema after subarachnoid haemorrhage. Eur J Pharmacol 364:115–122
21. Leonardo CC, Hall AA, Collier LA, Ajmo CTJ, Willing AE, Pennypacker KR (2010) Human umbilical cord blood cell therapy blocks the morphological change and recruitment of CD-11b-expressing isolectin-binding proinflammatory cells after middle cerebral artery occlusion. J Neurosci Res 88:1213–1222
22. Longa E, Weinstein P, Carlson S, Cummins R (1989) Reversible middle cerebral artery occlusion without craniectomy in rats. Stroke 20:84–91
23. Manley GT, Fujimura M, Ma T, Noshita N, Filiz F, Bollen AW, Chan P, Verkman AS (2000) Aquaporin-4 deletion in mice reduces brain edema after acute water intoxication and ischemic stroke. Nat Med 6:159–163
24. Papangelou A, Toung TJ, Gottschalk A, Mirski MA, Koehler RC (2013) Infarct volume after hyperacute infusion of hypertonic saline in a rat model of acute embolic stroke. Neurocrit Care 18:106–114
25. Rhind SG, Crnko NT, Baker AJ, Morrison LJ, Shek PN, Scarpelini S, Rizoli SB (2010) Prehospital resuscitation with hypertonic saline-dextran modulates inflammatory, coagulation and endothelial activation marker profiles in severe traumatic brain injured patients. J Neuroinflammation 7:5
26. Schmued LC, Albertson C, Slikker W Jr (1997) Fluoro-Jade: a novel fluorochrome for the sensitive and reliable histochemical localization of neuronal degeneration. Brain Res 751:37–46

27. Schwarz S, Georgiadis D, Aschoff A, Schwab S (2002) Effects of hypertonic (10%) saline in patients with raised intracranial pressure after stroke. Stroke 33:136–140
28. Shuaib A, Xu Wang C, Yang T, Noor R (2002) Effects of nonpeptide V(1) vasopressin receptor antagonist SR-49059 on infarction volume and recovery of function in a focal embolic stroke model. Stroke 33:3033–3037
29. Silver FL, Norris JW, Lewis AJ, Hachinski VC (1984) Early mortality following stroke: a prospective review. Stroke 15:492–496
30. Szmydynger-Chodobska J, Fox LM, Lynch KM, Zink BJ, Chodobski A (2010) Vasopressin amplifies the production of proinflammatory mediators in traumatic brain injury. J Neurotrauma 27:1449–1461
31. Toung TJ, Chang Y, Lin J, Bhardwaj A (2005) Increases in lung and brain water following experimental stroke: effect of mannitol and hypertonic saline. Crit Care Med 33:203–208, discussion 259–260
32. Udelson JE, Smith WB, Hendrix GH, Painchaud CA, Ghazzi M, Thomas I, Ghali JK, Selaru P, Chanoine F, Pressler ML, Konstam MA (2001) Acute hemodynamic effects of conivaptan, a dual V(1A) and V(2) vasopressin receptor antagonist, in patients with advanced heart failure. Circulation 104:2417–2423
33. Uenohara H, Imaizumi S, Yoshimoto T, Suzuki J (1988) Correlation among lipid peroxidation, brain energy metabolism and brain oedema in cerebral ischaemia. Neurol Res 10:194–199
34. Vajda Z, Pedersen M, Fuchtbauer EM, Wertz K, Stodkilde-Jorgensen H, Sulyok E, Doczi T, Neely JD, Agre P, Frokiaer J, Nielsen S (2002) Delayed onset of brain edema and mislocalization of aquaporin-4 in dystrophin-null transgenic mice. Proc Natl Acad Sci U S A 99:13131–13136
35. Yang M, Gao F, Liu H, Yu WH, Sun SQ (2009) Temporal changes in expression of aquaporin-3, -4, -5 and -8 in rat brains after permanent focal cerebral ischemia. Brain Res 1290:121–132
36. Zeynalov E, Chen CH, Froehner SC, Adams ME, Ottersen OP, Amiry-Moghaddam M, Bhardwaj A (2008) The perivascular pool of aquaporin-4 mediates the effect of osmotherapy in postischemic cerebral edema. Crit Care Med 36:2634–2640
37. Ziai WC, Toung TJ, Bhardwaj A (2007) Hypertonic saline: first-line therapy for cerebral edema? J Neurol Sci 261:157–166

Acute Hyperglycemia Does Not Affect Brain Swelling or Infarction Volume After Middle Cerebral Artery Occlusion in Rats

Devin W. McBride, Nathanael Matei, Justin R. Câmara, Jean-Sébastien Louis, Guillaume Oudin, Corentin Walker, Loic Adam, Xiping Liang, Qin Hu, Jiping Tang, and John H. Zhang

Introduction

Stroke disproportionally affects diabetic and hyperglycemic patients, with increased incidence, higher morbidity and mortality, and worse outcome, and is associated with larger infarct volume and more cerebral edema [2–4, 6, 12]. After the initial insult, secondary injury follows, consisting of delayed neuronal apoptosis, cerebral edema, and inflammation [3, 7, 9, 11, 15, 16]. A major contributor to the outcome of stroke patients is brain edema; thus, gaining a better understanding of its mechanisms and potential therapeutics is of the utmost importance.

A number of experimental models have been developed to examine the effects of blood glucose and diabetes on stroke pathophysiology, and to identify and test novel therapeutics for stroke in these patient populations [3, 11]. The most widely used experimental model of hyperglycemic stroke is the intraluminal suture middle cerebral artery occlusion (MCAO) model conducted on acutely hyperglycemic rats [3, 7]. While these rats present with high brain water content and brain swelling [11], to date, no study has examined whether these outcomes are significantly elevated compared with normo-glycemic animals subjected to MCAO. Thus, the objective of this study is to evaluate the amount of brain swelling in the injured hemisphere and the infarct volume after MCAO in hyperglycemic rats, and to compare these outcomes with those of normo-glycemic rats. Our primary hypothesis is that acute hyperglycemia will be associated with increased brain swelling of the injured hemisphere compared with normo-glycemic animals after MCAO. Our secondary hypothesis is that after MCAO, acutely hyperglycemic rats will have infarct volumes that are indistinguishable from those of normo-glycemic rats.

D.W. McBride • N. Matei • J.R. Câmara • J.-S. Louis
G. Oudin • C. Walker • L. Adam • X. Liang • Q. Hu • J. Tang
Department of Physiology and Pharmacology, Loma Linda University School of Medicine, Loma Linda, CA, USA

J.H. Zhang, M.D., Ph.D. (✉)
Department of Physiology and Pharmacology, Loma Linda University School of Medicine, Loma Linda, CA, USA

Department of Neurosurgery, Loma Linda University School of Medicine, Loma Linda, CA, USA
e-mail: jhzhang@llu.edu

Materials and Methods

All experiments were approved by the Institutional Animal Care and Use Committee at Loma Linda University. Fifty-four adult male Sprague-Dawley rats (270–290 g) were used in all experiments. Animal groups were normo-glycemic sham ($n=9$), hyperglycemic sham ($n=10$), normo-glycemic MCAO ($n=21$), and hyperglycemic MCAO ($n=14$).

Middle Cerebral Artery Occlusion Model

MCAO for 90 min or sham surgery was performed on adult rats, as previously described [8]. Briefly, animals were anesthetized with a mixture of ketamine (80 mg/kg) and xylazine (20 mg/kg) given intraperitoneally (IP), followed by a dose of atropine (0.1 mg/kg, subcutaneously (SC)). Upon reaching an adequate plane of anesthesia, assessed by loss of paw pinch reflex, 50 % dextrose (6 mL/kg) was injected IP 15 min before surgery (for the animals allotted to the hyperglycemic sham and hyperglycemic MCAO groups). Blood glucose measurements took place before dextrose injection (15 min before MCAO), 1 min before beginning surgery, 5 min after beginning reperfusion, and 24 h after reperfusion.

Briefly, the right common, internal, and external carotid arteries were surgically exposed, and the external carotid artery ligated, leaving a 3–4 mm stump. The internal

R.L. Applegate et al. (eds.), *Brain Edema XVI: Translate Basic Science into Clinical Practice*, Acta Neurochirurgica Supplement, Vol. 121,
DOI 10.1007/978-3-319-18497-5_44, © Springer International Publishing Switzerland 2016

carotid artery was then isolated and the pterygopalatine artery was ligated. A vascular clip was placed on the internal carotid artery, and another was placed on the common carotid artery. A 4.0 monofilament nylon suture with a rounded tip was advanced through the stump of the external carotid artery and up the internal carotid artery until resistance was felt. The suture was left in place for 90 min, after which the suture was removed, beginning reperfusion. The external carotid artery was the ligated, and the skin was sutured. Animals were given buprenorphine (0.02 mg/kg, SC) and yohibime (1 mg/kg, IP) and allowed to recover.

Histological Analysis

Animals were sacrificed 24 h after MCAO for histological analysis of hemispheric brain swelling and infarct volume. Twenty-four hours after reperfusion, animals were sacrificed, their brains removed, the brains sectioned into 2-mm-thick slices, and slices stained using 2 % TTC for 30 min at room temperature. Brain slices were then photographed. ImageJ (ImageJ, National Institutes of Health) was used to determine the areas of the contralateral hemisphere (C_i), ipsilateral hemisphere (I_i), and the nonischemic ipsilateral hemisphere (N_i). Hemispheric brain swelling was calculated using Eq. 1 [5, 10, 13] and infarct volume was calculated using Eq. 2 [17].

$$\text{Ipsilateral hemispheric swelling } (\%) = \left(\frac{\sum_i (I_i - C_i)}{\left(\sum_i C_i\right)} \right) 100 \quad (1)$$

$$\text{Infarct volume } (\%) = \left(\frac{\sum_i (C_i - N_i)}{2\left(\sum_i C_i\right)} \right) 100 \quad (2)$$

Data Analysis

Data are presented as the mean ± standard error of the mean (SEM). Data was analyzed using one-way analysis of variance (ANOVA) with Tukey post hoc tests for the effects of blood glucose on brain swelling and infarct volume. Blood glucose data was analyzed using one-way repeated measures ANOVA with Tukey post hoc test (Table 1). A $p<0.05$ was considered statistically significant.

Table 1 Blood glucose for animals given dextrose

	Sham	MCAO
15 min pre-MCAO	73.3 ± 3.8	81.1 ± 2.1
1 min pre-MCAO	239.3 ± 43.9[a]	198.5 ± 20.1[a]
5 min post-MCAO	278.1 ± 44.2[a]	213.1 ± 19.7[a]
24 h post-MCAO	71.2 ± 5.9	67.4 ± 4.5

Blood glucose (mg/dl) was measured before dextrose injection (15 min pre-MCAO), at the beginning of surgery (1 min pre-MCAO), at the beginning of reperfusion (5 min post-MCAO), and 24 h after MCAO (24 h post-MCAO)

[a]$p<0.05$ vs 15 min pre-MCAO baseline and 24 h post-MCAO

Results

Baseline blood glucose levels for animals in the hyperglycemic groups were 73.3 ± 3.8 mg/dL and 81.1 ± 2.1 mg/dL for the hyperglycemic sham and hyperglycemic MCAO groups, respectively. Acute hyperglycemia was achieved before surgery began (1 min pre-MCAO, Sham: 239.3 ± 43.9 mg/dL, MCAO: 198.5 ± 20.1 mg/dL) and remained elevated at the beginning of reperfusion (5 min post-MCAO, Sham: 278.1 ± 44.2 mg/dL, MCAO: 213.1 ± 19.7 mg/dL) ($p<0.05$ for 1 min pre-MCAO vs 15 min pre-MCAO for both sham and MCAO groups, $p<0.05$ for 5 min post-MCAO vs 15 min pre-MCAO for both sham and MCAO groups, and $p>0.05$ for 1 min pre-MCAO vs 5 min post-MCAO for both sham and MCAO groups). At the time of sacrifice, the blood glucose had returned to baseline levels (24 h post-MCAO, Sham: 71.2 ± 5.9 mg/dL, MCAO: 67.4 ± 4.5 mg/dL) ($p<0.05$ for both sham and MCAO groups vs 1 min pre-MCAO and 5 min-post MCAO, and $p>0.05$ for both sham and MCAO groups vs 15 min pre-MCAO) (Table 1).

Hemispheric Brain Swelling

The sham groups, normo-glycemic and hyperglycemic, did not have any hemispheric brain swelling (Normo-glycemic Sham: 0.6 ± 1.74 %, $n=9$; Hyperglycemic Sham: −2.6 ± 1.24 %, $n=10$). However, both normo-glycemic and hyperglycemic animals subjected to MCAO presented with hemispheric brain swelling (Normo-glycemic MCAO: 7.2 ± 1.60 %, $n=21$; Hyperglycemic MCAO: 12.4 ± 1.54 %, $n=14$) (Fig. 1).

Regardless of blood glucose, the hemispheric swelling for sham animals was not statistically different from each other

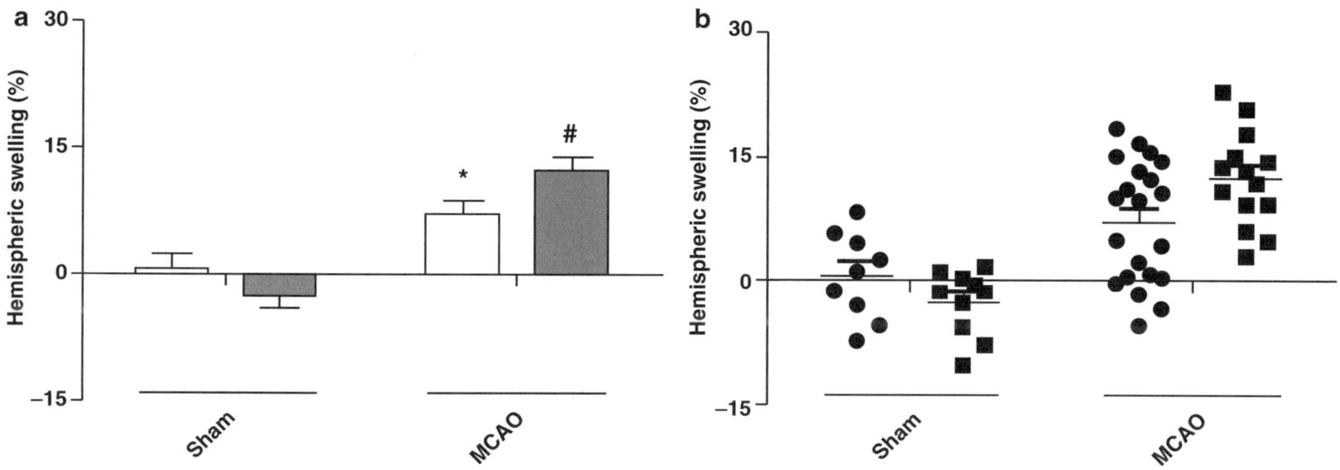

Fig. 1 Hemispheric brain swelling 24 h after MCAO. Hemispheric brain swelling (%) for normo-glycemic (*white bars, circles*) and hyperglycemic (*gray bars, squares*) animals. Swelling of the ipsilateral hemisphere is significantly higher in both normo-glycemic and hyperglycemic animals after MCAO compared with their respective shams ($p<0.001$). *$p<0.001$ vs Normo-glycemic Sham, #$p<0.001$ vs Hyperglycemic Sham. $n=9$–21/group. (**a**) Bar Graphs. (**b**) Scatter Plots

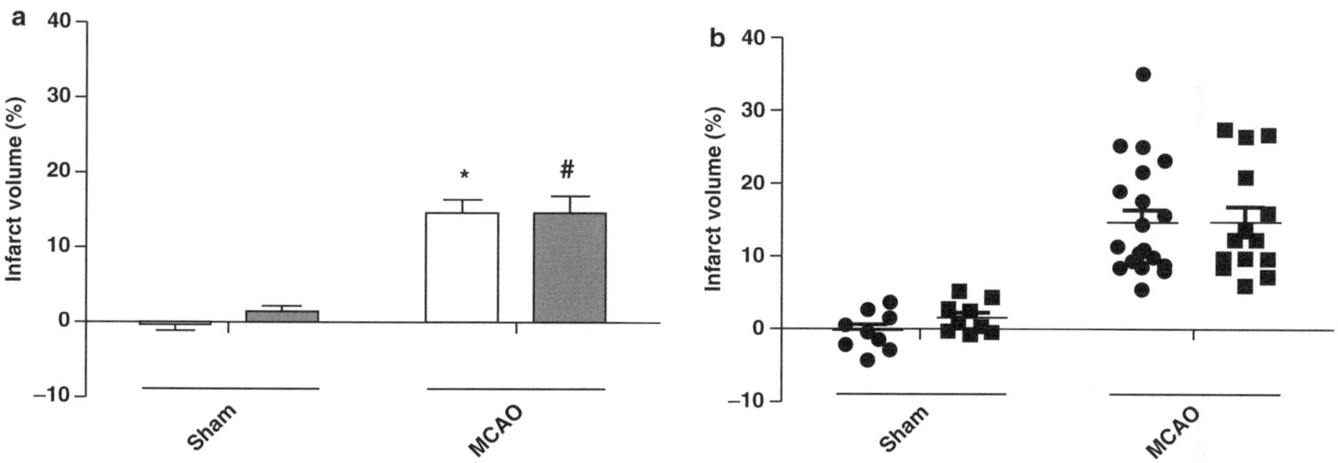

Fig. 2 Infarct volume 24 h after MCAO. Infarct volume (%) for normo-glycemic (*white bars, circles*) and hyperglycemic (*gray bars, squares*) animals. Infarct volume is significantly higher in both normo-glycemic and hyperglycemic animals after MCAO compared with their respective shams. *$p<0.001$ vs Normo-glycemic Sham, #$p<0.001$ vs Hyperglycemic Sham. $n=9$–21/group. (**a**) Bar Graphs. (**b**) Scatter Plots

($p>0.05$ for Normo-glycemic Sham vs Hyperglycemic Sham). Interestingly, animals subjected to MCAO had indistinguishable hemispheric swelling for normo-glycemic and hyperglycemic animals ($p>0.05$ for Normo-glycemic MCAO vs Hyperglycemic MCAO) (Fig. 1).

Although no significance was observed for the hemispheric swelling with respect to blood glucose levels for either injury group, the hemispheric swelling between animals subjected to MCAO and sham surgery is significantly different for both the normo-glycemic ($p<0.001$ for Normo-glycemic MCAO vs Normo-glycemic MCAO) and hyperglycemic animals ($p<0.001$ for Hyperglycemic MCAO vs Hyperglycemic Sham) (Fig. 1).

Infarct Volume

Normo-glycemic and hyperglycemic sham animals had essentially no infarcts (Normo-glycemic Sham: −0.4 ± 0.89 %, $n=9$; Hyperglycemic Sham: 1.5 ± 0.65 %, $n=10$). MCAO caused normo-glycemic and hyperglycemic animals to have large infarcts (Normo-glycemic MCAO: 14.6 ± 1.66 %, $n=21$; Hyperglycemic MCAO: 14.7 ± 2.03 %, $n=14$) (Fig. 2).

The infarct volumes for normo-glycemic and hyperglycemic sham animals were not significantly different from each other ($p>0.05$ for Normo-glycemic Sham vs Hyperglycemic Sham). Similarly, the infarct volumes of MCAO animals were not statistically different for either the normo-glycemic or hyperglycemic cases ($p > 0.05$ for Normo-glycemic MCAO vs Hyperglycemic MCAO) (Fig. 2).

The infarct volumes between the sham and MCAO animals were significantly different for both the normoglycemic ($p < 0.001$ for Normo-glycemic MCAO vs Normo-glycemic MCAO) and hyperglycemic cases ($p < 0.001$ for Hyperglycemic MCAO vs Hyperglycemic Sham) (Fig. 2).

Discussion

Herein, we investigated the effect of blood glucose on brain swelling and infarction volume after MCAO. To this end, the intraluminal suture MCAO model was performed on 54 SD rats that either had normal blood glucose levels (normo-glycemia, $n = 30$) or high blood glucose levels (hyperglycemia, $n = 24$).

Effect of Blood Glucose on Hemispheric Brain Swelling after MCAO

Our primary hypothesis that acute hyperglycemia would cause significantly more swelling of the ipsilateral, injured hemisphere after MCAO (compared with normo-glycemic controls) was wrong. Interestingly, hyperglycemia created by bolus injection of 50 % dextrose, did not induce more hemispheric swelling than normo-glycemic animals subjected to identical MCAO procedures. However, because normo-glycemic and hyperglycemic animals subjected to MCAO had more brain swelling than their respective controls, this study suggests that blood glucose is not a significant factor contributing to hemispheric swelling after MCAO.

A review of the literature confirms that animals after MCAO have more ipsilateral hemispheric swelling than sham animals for normo-glycemic and hyperglycemic cases [1, 7, 14, 19]; however, no study has compared brain swelling between normo-glycemic and hyperglycemic MCAO animals. Thus, this is the first time that the effect blood glucose has on ipsilateral hemispheric swelling has been examined.

The findings of this study do not disagree with the literature that blood glucose is a significant factor in the functional outcome of animals after MCAO. It is well documented that hyperglycemic MCAO animals perform worse on neurobehavior tests compared with normo-glycemic MCAO animals [3]. Because we identified no difference in the swelling of hyperglycemic animals subjected to MCAO compared with normo-glycemic animals subjected to MCAO, the likely cause of increased neurological deficits in hyperglycemic MCAO animals compared with normo-glycemic MCAO animals is likely the hemorrhagic transformation [3, 11, 14].

Effect of Blood Glucose on Infarction Volume after MCAO

Our secondary hypothesis that acute hyperglycemia would have no effect on infarct volume (compared with normo-glycemic controls) was supported by the results. Although no significance was observed for the infarct volume between any of the blood glucose pairings for the same injury type, the animals subjected to MCAO had significantly higher infarct volumes than their respective shams. Thus, blood glucose does not have any significantly effect on infarct volume after MCAO.

The role of blood glucose on infarct volume has been previously examined and mixed results have been observed in the MCAO model. In some cases, hyperglycemia increases infarct volume compared with normo-glycemia, whereas in others, hyperglycemia does not change the infarct volume compared with normo-glycemia [3, 18]. The findings herein found no effect of blood glucose on infarct volume. The reason(s) for the disagreement in blood glucose's role in infarct volume is unknown but may be caused by subtle procedural differences.

Conclusion

There is a tendency for the hemispheric brain swelling to be higher in the hyperglycemic MCAO group compared with the normo-glycemic MCAO group, however, it was not statistically significant with the animal numbers used herein. Inclusion of additional animals may make the hemispheric swelling in these two groups become statistically different. Based on the findings of this study, blood glucose has no effect on either the amount of hemispheric brain swelling or the infarction volume after MCAO in rats.

Acknowledgments This work was supported by National Institutes of Health grant R01 NS043338 (JHZ).

Disclosure The authors have no conflicts of interest to report.

References

1. Amiry-Moghaddam M, Otsuka T, Hurn PD, Traystman RJ, Haug FM, Froehner SC, Adams ME, Neely JD, Agre P, Ottersen OP, Bhardwaj A (2003) An alpha-syntrophin-dependent pool of AQP4 in astroglial end-feet confers bidirectional water flow between blood and brain. Proc Natl Acad Sci U S A 100:2106–2111
2. Bruno A, Biller J, Adams HP, Clarke WR, Woolson RF, Williams LS, Hansen MD, Investigators T (1999) Acute blood glucose level and outcome from ischemic stroke. Neurology 52:280–284

3. Chen C, Ostrowski RP, Zhou C, Tang J, Zhang JH (2010) Suppression of hypoxia-inducible factor-1 alpha and its downstream genes reduces acute hyperglycemia-enhanced hemorrhagic transformation in a rat model of cerebral ischemia. J Neurosci Res 88:2046–2055
4. Fagan SC, Lapchak PA, Liebeskind DS, Ishrat T, Ergul A (2013) Recommendations for preclinical research in hemorrhagic transformation. Transl Stroke Res 4:322–327
5. Gartshore G, Patterson J, Macrae IM (1997) Influence of ischemia and reperfusion on the course of brain tissue swelling and blood–brain barrier permeability in a rodent model of transient focal cerebral ischemia. Exp Neurol 147:353–360
6. Hafez S, Coucha M, Bruno A, Fagan SC, Ergul A (2014) Hyperglycemia, acute ischemic stroke, and thrombolytic therapy. Transl Stroke Res 5:442–453
7. Hu Q, Ma Q, Zhan Y, He Z, Tang J, Zhou C, Zhang J (2011) Isoflurane enhanced hemorrhagic transformation by impairing antioxidant enzymes in hyperglycemic rats with middle cerebral artery occlusion. Stroke 42:1750–1756
8. Kawamura S, Yasui N, Shirasawa M, Fukasawa H (1991) Rat middle cerebral artery occlusion using an intraluminal thread technique. Acta Neurochir 109:126–132
9. Khanna A, Kahle KT, Walcott BP, Gerzanich V, Simard JM (2014) Disruption of ion homeostasis in the neurogliovascular unit underlies the pathogenesis of ischemic cerebral edema. Transl Stroke Res 5:3–16
10. Kondo T, Reaume AG, Huang TT, Carlson E, Murakami K, Chen SF, Hoffman EK, Scott RW, Epstein CJ, Chan PH (1997) Reduction of CuZn-superoxide dismutase activity exacerbates neuronal cell injury and edema formation after transient focal cerebral ischemia. J Neurosci 17:4180–4189
11. Kusaka I, Kusaka G, Zhou C, Ishikawa M, Nanda A, Granger DN, Zhang JH, Tang J (2004) Role of AT1 receptors and NAD(P)H oxidase in diabetes-aggravated ischemic brain injury. Am J Physiol Heart Circ Physiol 286:H2442–H2451
12. Mandava P, Martini SR, Munoz M, Dalmeida W, Sarma AK, Anderson JA, Fabian RH, Kent TA (2014) Hyperglycemia worsens outcome after rt-PA primarily in the large-vessel occlusive stroke subtype. Transl Stroke Res 5:519–525
13. Osborne KA, Shigeno T, Balarsky AM, Ford I, McCulloch J, Teasdale GM, Graham DI (1987) Quantitative assessment of early brain damage in a rat model of focal cerebral ischaemia. J Neurol Neurosurg Psychiatry 50:402–410
14. Soejima Y, Ostrowski RP, Manaenko A, Fujii M, Tang J, Zhang JH (2012) Hyperbaric oxygen preconditioning attenuates hyperglycemia enhanced hemorrhagic transformation after transient MCAO in rats. Med Gas Res 2:9
15. Song M, Yu SP (2014) Ionic regulation of cell volume changes and cell death after ischemic stroke. Transl Stroke Res 5:17–27
16. Srinivasan K, Sharma SS (2011) Augmentation of endoplasmic reticulum stress in cerebral ischemia/reperfusion injury associated with comorbid type 2 diabetes. Neurol Res 33:858–865
17. Swanson RA, Morton MT, Tsao-Wu G, Savalos RA, Davidson C, Sharp FR (1990) A semiautomated method for measuring brain infarct volume. J Cereb Blood Flow Metab 10:290–293
18. Toung TK, Hurn PD, Traystman RJ, Sieber FE (2000) Estrogen decreases infarct size after temporary focal ischemia in a genetic model of type 1 diabetes mellitus. Stroke 31:2701–2706
19. Xing Y, Hua Y, Keep RF, Xi G (2009) Effects of deferoxamine on brain injury after transient focal cerebral ischemia in rats with hyperglycemia. Brain Res 1291:113–121

ZNT-1 Expression Reduction Enhances Free Zinc Accumulation in Astrocytes After Ischemic Stroke

Rong Pan and Ke Jian Liu

Introduction

The brain is highly rich in zinc, which is crucial for cellular development and survival [1, 2]. Some cytoarchitectonic regions of the brain contain 200–600 μM of rapidly exchangeable zinc. Stroke is a leading cause of disability and death [3–6]. It causes neuron, glia, astrocyte, and endothelial cell damage [7, 8]. When ischemic stroke occurs, zinc is released from a subset of glutamatergic terminals in the brain [9]. Kaspar Vogt et al. [10] reported synaptically released zinc could bring zinc concentration to more than 100 μM in the extracellular space. Our previous results showed that adding 100 μM extracellular zinc dramatically increased intracellular free zinc level in hypoxic astrocytes but not in normoxic astrocytes [11]. Other researchers' in vivo and in vitro experimental results also show that intracellular zinc increases after ischemic stroke [12–14]. However, the mechanism that leads to free zinc accumulation only in hypoxic astrocytes was unknown.

Two major protein groups are involved in transporting zinc into or out of the cells. The first is ZnTs (zinc transporter proteins), which mediate zinc efflux from cytoplasm. The second group is the ZIP (Zrt/IRT-like protein) family. The ZIP family is known to promote zinc influx to cytoplasm [15]. Although the effect of the ZnTs and ZIPs on zinc transportation was well investigated, there is no report on the change of ZnTs or ZIPs in hypoxic cells. In the present study, we tested the hypothesis that hypoxia-induced change in ZnTs and/or ZIPs is the cause of free zinc accumulation.

R. Pan
Department of Pharmaceutical Sciences,
College of Pharmacy, Albuquerque, NM 87131, USA

K.J. Liu (✉)
Department of Pharmaceutical Sciences,
College of Pharmacy, Albuquerque, NM 87131, USA

Department of Neurology, University of New Mexico
Health Sciences Center, Albuquerque, NM 87131, USA
e-mail: kliu@salud.unm.edu

Methods

Primary Culture of Rat Cortical Astrocytes

Primary astrocytes were isolated from the cortices of day 1 Sprague-Dawley rats as previously described [16–18]. Briefly, after decapitation, the brains of postnatal day 1 rats were immediately excised. Meninges and blood vessels were removed, and the forebrains were placed in Dulbecco's Modified Eagle medium (DMEM; Life Technologies, Carlsbad, CA, USA). The tissue was minced and placed in 0.05 % trypsin (Life Technologies) at 37 °C for 30 min. Trypsinization was completed by adding 10 % (v/v) FBS (Life Technologies) in DMEM. After dissociating tissue and passing through a 40 μM strainer, the cells were seeded in the flasks at a density of 1.5×10^5 cells/cm^2 in growth medium (90 % DMEM containing 4.5 g/l glucose, and 10 % fetal bovine serum (FBS)) and placed in the cell culture incubator at 37 °C with 95 % air/5 % CO_2.

Hypoxic Cellular Model

For hypoxic treatment, the cell culture medium was replaced with serum-free DMEM media, which had previously been bubbled with nitrogen for 15 min. The cells were then incubated in a polymer hypoxic glove chamber (Coy Laboratory Products Inc., Grass Lake, MI, USA) with 1 % O_2/95 % (5 % CO_2/95 % N_2) at 37 °C for 3 h. After hypoxia, reoxygenation was performed by removing the cells from the hypoxic chamber and adding FBS (final concentration 10 %). The

R.L. Applegate et al. (eds.), *Brain Edema XVI: Translate Basic Science into Clinical Practice*, Acta Neurochirurgica Supplement, Vol. 121,
DOI 10.1007/978-3-319-18497-5_45,

cells were then incubated in 5 % CO_2/95 % air at 37 °C for another 12 h.

Intracellular Zinc Detection by FluoZin-3 AM

Intracellular free zinc was measured by using FluoZin-3 AM (Life Technologies). FluoZin-3 AM is a selective fluorescent cell permeable probe to label the free zinc in cells. Astrocytes were plated onto glass cover slips. After hypoxia/reoxygenation treatment, cells were washed with DMEM to remove extracellular zinc before incubating with DMEM containing 2.5 μM FluoZin-3 for 45 min at room temperature. After washing with DMEM, the cover slips were mounted on a glass slide. Images were acquired using an inverted microscope (Olympus OX71, Tokyo, Japan) with a GFP dichroic mirror to visualize FluoZin-3 AM fluorescence.

Extracellular Zinc Detection by FluoZin-3 Cell Impermeant

Extracellular zinc level was measured by using the cell impermeable zinc probe FluoZin-3 Cell Impermeant (Life Technologies). FluoZin-3 Cell Impermeant only stains extracellular zinc in the media and will not be disturbed by intracellular zinc. Astrocytes (1.5×10^6 cells/well) were cultured in 6-well plates in 1 ml media. At the end of the 3-h hypoxia/12-h reoxygenation, 100 μl media in each well were transferred to a 96-well plate. 500 nM FluoZin-3 Cell Impermeant was added into the wells and incubated for 30 min at room temperature. The fluorescence of FluoZin-3 was excited at 494 nm and emission was measured at 516 nm by the SpectraMax M2 Multi-Mode Microplate Readers (Molecular Devices, Sunnyvale, CA, USA).

Western Blot Analysis for ZIP-1 and ZnT-1

At the end of the indicated treatments, cells were collected and lysed in RIPA buffer (Sigma, St. Louis, MO, USA). Total protein concentrations were determined using protein assay reagents (Bio-Rad, Hercules, CA, USA). Forty micrograms of protein lysate were separated on AnykD gels (Bio-Rad), and analyzed by Western immunoblot using Goat anti-ZIP-1 antibody (diluted 1:1000, Santa Cruz Biotechnology, Dallas, Texas, USA) or Goat anti-ZnT-1 antibody (diluted 1:1000, Santa Cruz Biotechnology) and IRDye 680LT Donkey anti-Goat IgG (diluted 1:10,000, LI-COR, Lincoln, NE, USA). Immunoblots were photographed using the Odyssey® Infrared Imaging System (LI-COR) with Molecular Imaging Software V4.0.

Results

Hypoxia Increased Intracellular Free Zinc

Evidence indicates that the increase of intracellular free zinc contributes to cell death in acute brain injury [19]. Ischemic injury can be categorized into two main phases: one is the hypoxic-ischemic phase and the other is the reperfusion phase [20]. To simulate these two phases, astrocytes were placed in 1 % O_2 for 3 h and then in 95 % air for 12 h. We used a cell-permeable Zn-specific sensor FluoZin-3 AM to visualize intracellular free zinc after hypoxia/reoxygenation. We found that at normoxia, little free zinc was detectable in astrocytes (Fig. 1), and adding 100 μM extracellular zinc barely increased intracellular free zinc. However, after the astrocytes were exposed to 3-h hypoxia and 12-h reoxygenation, the intracellular free zinc increased remarkably. Notably, with the treatment of the combination of 100 μM zinc and 3-h hypoxia/12-h reoxygenation, the FluoZin-3 fluorescence intensity was significant greater than that with zinc or 3-h hypoxia/12-h reoxygenation treatment alone. These results demonstrate that without exogenous zinc, hypoxia increased endogenous free zinc. Meanwhile, in the presence of exogenous zinc, the intracellular free zinc level dramatically increased only in hypoxia/reoxygenation astrocytes but not in normoxic astrocytes.

Hypoxia Decreased Extracellular Zinc

Obviously, hypoxia/reoxygenation increased endogenous free zinc level even when no zinc was added. However, what about that with zinc treatment? Is the increase of intracellular free zinc completely from endogenous zinc or is it also from exogenous zinc? We reasoned that if exogenous zinc uptake is a cause for the increase of intracellular free zinc, then extracellular zinc must decrease after hypoxia/reoxygenation treatment. Thus, following 100 μM zinc and the hypoxia/reoxygenation treatment, extracellular zinc was detected using a cell-impermeable zinc probe FluoZin-3 Cell Impermeant, which only stains zinc in the media. As shown in Fig. 2, just as we had predicted, the extracellular zinc decreased only after hypoxia/reoxygenation treatment, but not at normoxia, demonstrating that extracellular zinc uptake is, or at least is one of, the reasons for the increase in intracellular free zinc.

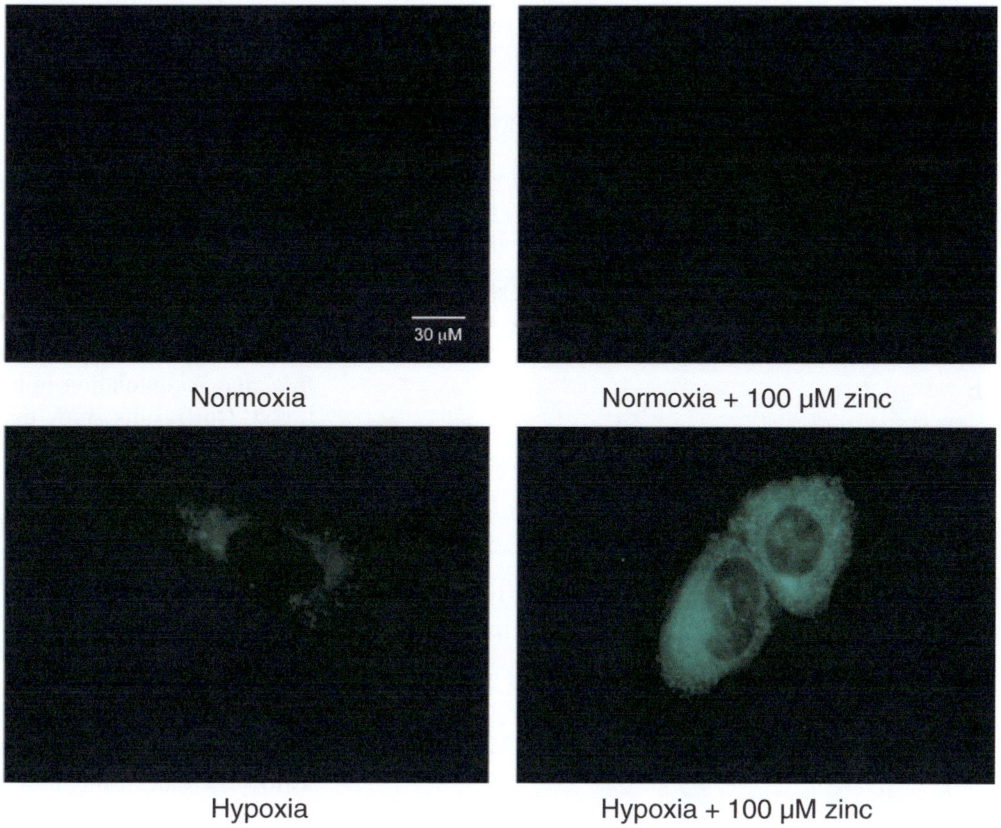

Fig. 1 Intracellular free zinc level in primary astrocytes. Primary astrocytes were treated with 0 or 100 μM zinc under 3 h hypoxia/12 h reoxygenation or 15 h normoxia condition. The intracellular free zinc was visualized using FluoZin-3 AM fluorescence probe

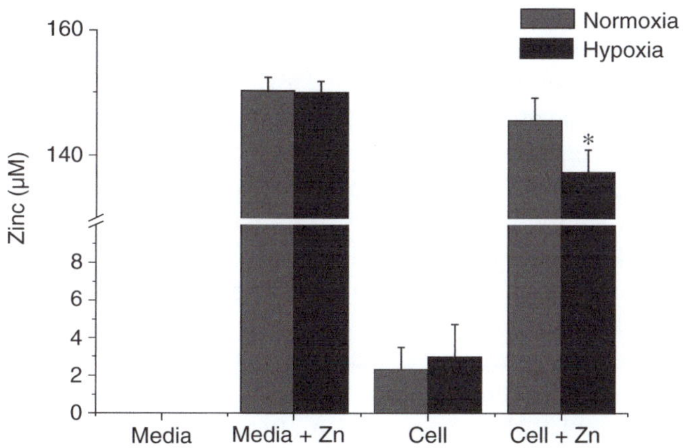

Fig. 2 Extracellular zinc level in the media. 100 μM zinc was added into the astrocytes culture media. After 3 h hypoxia/12 h reoxygenation or 15 h normoxia, zinc level in the media was measured by using FluoZin-3 Cell Impermeant probe. The experiments were repeated three times. Data were presented as mean ± standard error (SE). *$p < 0.05$ compared with the normoxia and zinc-treated group

Znt-1 Expression Reduced after Hypoxia/ Reoxygenation Treatment

The regulation of cellular zinc homeostasis is controlled tightly through zinc transporters ZIP family and ZnTs [15]. By measuring the ZIP-1 expression, we found that hypoxia/reoxygenation hardly changes the ZIP-1 level in astrocytes. However, for the ZnT-1 protein, hypoxia/reoxygenation dramatically decreased ZnT-1 expression, which is difficult to reverse by zinc, although zinc significantly increased its expression in normoxic conditions. Remarkably, these results gave us an interesting suggestion: Compared with normoxic conditions, in the hypoxia/reoxygenation condition, zinc influx remained at a same level while the efflux of zinc was severely hampered. This may be one of the reasons why intracellular free zinc increases with extracellular zinc addition only in hypoxia/reoxygenation but not in normoxia.

Discussion

Evidence shows that intracellular zinc increases after ischemic stroke [12]. Excess intracellular free zinc has a well-documented role in contributing to cell injury [21–23]. Understanding the mechanism of intracellular free zinc accumulation is critically important for ischemic stroke research. The present study demonstrates a zinc efflux blocking function of hypoxia/reoxygenation. Under hypoxia/reoxygenation conditions, the zinc efflux mediator protein ZnT-1

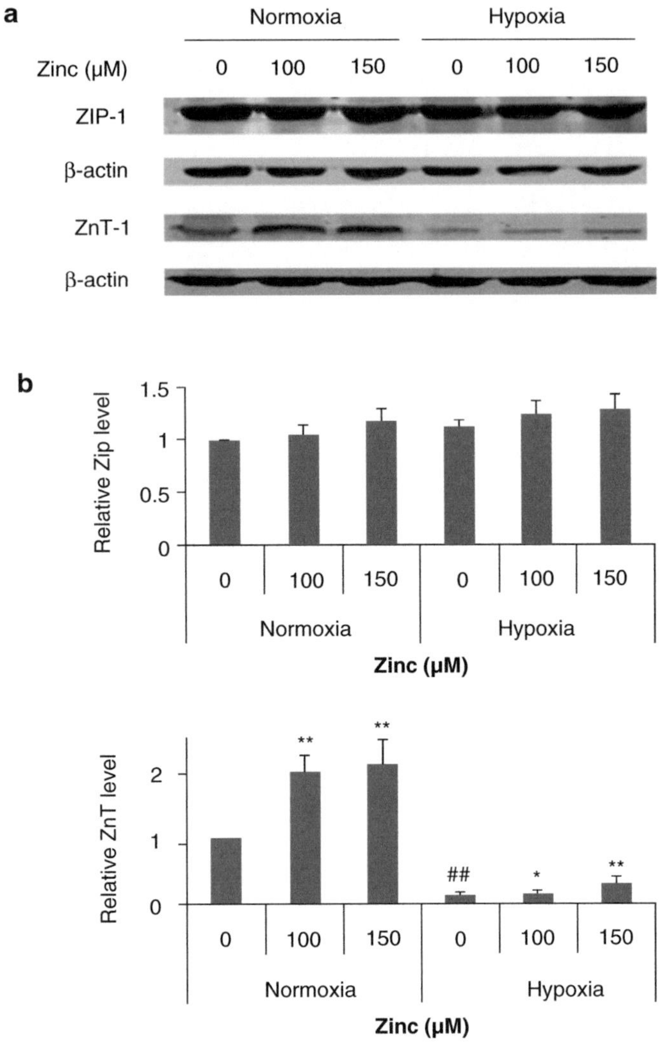

Fig. 3 The effect of zinc and hypoxia/reoxygenation on ZnT-1 and ZIP protein level. Astrocytes were treated with the indicated concentration of zinc under hypoxia/reoxygenation or normoxia. Representative immunoblots showing zinc transporter protein levels (**a**). Relative protein levels (**b**) were quantitated after normalization to β-actin. The experiments were repeated three times. Data were presented as mean ± SE. $^{*}p<0.05$, $^{**}p<0.01$ compared with the group without zinc treatment on each condition; $^{\#\#}p<0.01$ compared with normoxic astrocytes group

level declined to less than half the level of that under normoxia conditions (Fig. 3). Moreover, although zinc caused a substantial jump in ZnT-1 level at normoxia, it was unable to reverse the loss of ZnT-1 caused by hypoxia/reoxygenation. However, in this situation, hypoxia did not change the zinc influx mediate protein ZIP-1 level. In addition, the loss of extracellular zinc (Fig. 2) provided more direct evidence for zinc influx greater than zinc efflux in hypoxic astrocytes. Our results demonstrate that hypoxia/reoxygenation decreased ZnT-1 protein level, preventing zinc efflux from cell, leading to increase of intercellular free zinc. It is the first time hypoxia/reoxygenation interrupting zinc homeostasis in astrocytes has been shown.

Zinc homeostasis in cells is considered to be tightly regulated by 10 members of ZnT (zinc transporter protein) and 14 members of ZIP (Zrt/IRT-like protein) families [24]. Among them, ZnT-1 mediates zinc efflux from cytoplasm to the extracellular space. Evidences show that ZnT-1 protein mediates zinc efflux, at the same time the expression of the ZnT-1 gene is also regulated by zinc. The reaction of ZnT-1 and zinc regulates intercellular zinc level [25]. Qin et al. [13] found that zinc was locked in cultured cortical neurons after ZnT-1 silence. Although, ZnT-1 mediation of zinc efflux is well documented, whether ZnT-1 contributes to intercellular free zinc accumulation in hypoxic cells had not been illustrated. Our results show that ZnT-1 was downregulated by hypoxia/reoxgenation, leading to zinc trapping in cell. Regarding zinc influx, the ZIP family is known to promote zinc influx to cytoplasm [15], however, there is no report on the relationship of ZIPs and intercellular free zinc accumulation in hypoxic astrocytes. ZIP-1, -2, and -4 transport zinc from extracellular space to cytoplasm [26]. Franklin et al. [27] reported that ZIP-1 is the major zinc uptake transporter for the accumulation of zinc. Thus, we only measured ZIP-1 level after zinc and hypoxia treatment. We found that the expression of ZIP-1 was similar in normoxic and hypoxic astrocytes. Our results indicate that in normoxic conditions, zinc influx and efflux were regulated by ZnT-1 and ZIP-1, keeping intracellular zinc at a normal and nontoxic concentration. Notably, in the hypoxia/reoxygenation condition, zinc influx remained at a normal level, whereas the loss of ZnT-1 disabled the zinc efflux. Thus, zinc was trapped in the cells, accumulating to a high and toxic concentration, which may be one of the reasons why ischemic stroke-induced zinc release causes brain injury. However, how hypoxia/reoxygenation affect the ZnT-1 protein needs further study.

In addition to exogenous zinc, endogenous zinc may also be a cause of intercellular zinc increase after ischemic stroke. The metallothioneins (MTs) protein family, functioning in absorption and temporary storage of zinc, is known to be involved in managing zinc cellular level [15, 28]. The bond between zinc and MT is tightly regulated by redox [29, 30], suggesting that after ischemic stroke, the intercellular free zinc increase may be from endogenous MT-bound zinc release. Moreover, the increase of intracellular free zinc without adding exogenous zinc also indicated that endogenous zinc is a reason for zinc accumulation in hypoxic astrocytes. To investigate whether exogenous zinc contributed to free zinc accumulation in addition to endogenous zinc, we added zinc to the cell culture media, and measured the remaining zinc in the media after hypoxia/reoxygenation or nomorxia treatment. We found that extracellular zinc only decreased in hypoxic astrocytes but not in normoxic astrocytes, indicating that the uptake of exogenous zinc is at least one of the reasons for intercellular free zinc increase.

In conclusion, our results demonstrate that hypoxia/reoxygenation significantly decreased ZnT-1 protein level, whereas it did not change ZIP-1 protein level, leading to intercellular free zinc accumulation. We found that hypoxia/reoxygenation decreased ZnT-1 level, while ZIP remained at a similar level as in normoxia. Our results demonstrate that hypoxia/reoxygenation blocked zinc efflux, whereas it had no effect on zinc influx, and that hypoxia/reoxygenation interrupted zinc homeostasis in astrocytes by limiting zinc return to extracellular space, providing a novel way for intracellular free zinc accumulation after ischemic stroke. These findings provide a novel mechanism accounting for intercellular free zinc accumulation after ischemic stroke.

Acknowledgments This work was supported in part by grants from the National Institutes of Health (P20RR15636, P30GM103400, and R01AG031725).

References

1. MacDonald RS (2000) The role of zinc in growth and cell proliferation. J Nutr 130:1500S–1508S
2. Prasad AS (1988) Zinc in growth and development and spectrum of human zinc deficiency. J Am Coll Nutr 7:377–384
3. Qi Z, Liu W, Luo Y, Ji X, Liu KJ (2013) Normobaric hyperoxia-based neuroprotective therapies in ischemic stroke. Med Gas Res 3:2
4. Hafez S, Coucha M, Bruno A, Fagan SC, Ergul A (2014) Hyperglycemia, acute ischemic stroke, and thrombolytic therapy. Transl Stroke Res 5:442–453
5. Eckermann JM, Krafft PR, Shoemaker L, Lieberson RE, Chang SD et al (2012) Potential application of hydrogen in traumatic and surgical brain injury, stroke and neonatal hypoxia-ischemia. Med Gas Res 2:11
6. Chen X, Zhai X, Kang Z, Sun X (2012) Lactulose: an effective preventive and therapeutic option for ischemic stroke by production of hydrogen. Med Gas Res 2:3
7. Song M, Yu SP (2014) Ionic regulation of cell volume changes and cell death after ischemic stroke. Transl Stroke Res 5:17–27
8. Ouyang YB, Voloboueva LA, Xu LJ, Giffard RG (2007) Selective dysfunction of hippocampal CA1 astrocytes contributes to delayed neuronal damage after transient forebrain ischemia. J Neurosci 27:4253–4260
9. Galasso SL, Dyck RH (2007) The role of zinc in cerebral ischemia. Mol Med 13:380–387
10. Vogt K, Mellor J, Tong G, Nicoll R (2000) The actions of synaptically released zinc at hippocampal mossy fiber synapses. Neuron 26:187–196
11. Pan R, Chen C, Liu WL, Liu KJ (2013) Zinc promotes the death of hypoxic astrocytes by upregulating hypoxia-induced hypoxia-inducible factor-1alpha expression via poly(ADP-ribose) polymerase-1. CNS Neurosci Ther 19:511–520
12. Medvedeva YV, Lin B, Shuttleworth CW, Weiss JH (2009) Intracellular Zn2+ accumulation contributes to synaptic failure, mitochondrial depolarization, and cell death in an acute slice oxygen-glucose deprivation model of ischemia. J Neurosci 29:1105–1114
13. Qin Y, Thomas D, Fontaine CP, Colvin RA (2009) Silencing of ZnT1 reduces Zn2+ efflux in cultured cortical neurons. Neurosci Lett 450:206–210
14. Hattink J, De Boeck G, Blust R (2006) Toxicity, accumulation, and retention of zinc by carp under normoxic and hypoxic conditions. Environ Toxicol Chem 25:87–96
15. Szewczyk B (2013) Zinc homeostasis and neurodegenerative disorders. Front Aging Neurosci 5:33
16. Tabernero A, Bolanos JP, Medina JM (1993) Lipogenesis from lactate in rat neurons and astrocytes in primary culture. Biochem J 294(Pt 3):635–638
17. Kim EJ, Raval AP, Hirsch N, Perez-Pinzon MA (2010) Ischemic preconditioning mediates cyclooxygenase-2 expression via nuclear factor-kappa B activation in mixed cortical neuronal cultures. Transl Stroke Res 1:40–47
18. He Y, Hua Y, Lee JY, Liu W, Keep RF et al (2010) Brain alpha- and beta-globin expression after intracerebral hemorrhage. Transl Stroke Res 1:48–56
19. Lee SJ, Koh JY (2010) Roles of zinc and metallothionein-3 in oxidative stress-induced lysosomal dysfunction, cell death, and autophagy in neurons and astrocytes. Mol Brain 3:30
20. Cheng MY, Lee IP, Jin M, Sun G, Zhao H et al (2011) An insult-inducible vector system activated by hypoxia and oxidative stress for neuronal gene therapy. Transl Stroke Res 2:92–100
21. Cho E, Hwang JJ, Han SH, Chung SJ, Koh JY et al (2010) Endogenous zinc mediates apoptotic programmed cell death in the developing brain. Neurotox Res 17:156–166
22. Hamatake M, Iguchi K, Hirano K, Ishida R (2000) Zinc induces mixed types of cell death, necrosis, and apoptosis, in molt-4 cells. J Biochem 128:933–939
23. Seve M, Chimienti F, Favier A (2002) Role of intracellular zinc in programmed cell death. Pathol Biol (Paris) 50:212–221
24. Lichten LA, Cousins RJ (2009) Mammalian zinc transporters: nutritional and physiologic regulation. Annu Rev Nutr 29:153–176
25. Liuzzi JP, Blanchard RK, Cousins RJ (2001) Differential regulation of zinc transporter 1, 2, and 4 mRNA expression by dietary zinc in rats. J Nutr 131:46–52
26. John E, Laskow TC, Buchser WJ, Pitt BR, Basse PH et al (2010) Zinc in innate and adaptive tumor immunity. J Transl Med 8:118
27. Franklin RB, Ma J, Zou J, Guan Z, Kukoyi BI et al (2003) Human ZIP1 is a major zinc uptake transporter for the accumulation of zinc in prostate cells. J Inorg Biochem 96:435–442
28. Cherian MG (1977) Studies on the synthesis and metabolism of zinc-thionein in rats. J Nutr 107:965–972
29. Maret W (2000) The function of zinc metallothionein: a link between cellular zinc and redox state. J Nutr 130:1455S–1458S
30. Malaiyandi LM, Dineley KE, Reynolds IJ (2004) Divergent consequences arise from metallothionein overexpression in astrocytes: zinc buffering and oxidant-induced zinc release. Glia 45:346–353

Osteopontin-Rac1 on Blood-Brain Barrier Stability Following Rodent Neonatal Hypoxia-Ischemia

Brandon Dixon, Jay Malaguit, Darlene Casel, Desislava Doycheva, Jiping Tang, John H. Zhang, and Tim Lekic

Introduction

Neonatal hypoxic-ischemic (HI) brain injury remains a leading cause of mortality and morbidity, affecting 2–4 of 1,000 full-term and nearly 60 % of premature infants [1, 2]. Among survivors, 20–40 % develop significant neurological impairments, associated with life-long medical, social, and emotional difficulties [3]. Recent studies have demonstrated neuroprotective effects of intracerebroventricular (ICV) administration of recombinant osteopontin (rOPN) [4]. Previously, rOPN was shown to have reduced cell death, stabilized the blood-brain barrier (BBB), and improved neurological impairments in rodents subjected to brain injury [5].

In sum, osteopontin (OPN) is a neuroprotective molecule that is upregulated following rodent neonatal hypoxic-ischemic (nHI) brain injury [5, 6]. OPN, an extracellular matrix protein, stimulates cell surface integrin receptors, which induce the phosphorylation of focal adhesion kinase (FAK) [4, 7, 8], which induces Rac-1, a downstream target of FAK that has been shown to stabilize the BBB after HI insult [9]. Because Rac1 is a regulator of BBB stability [10–13], we hypothesized a role for this in OPN signaling.

Methods

Neonatal hypoxia-ischemia (nHI) was induced by unilateral ligation of the right carotid artery followed by hypoxia (8 % oxygen for 2 h) in P10 Sprague-Dawley rat pups. Intranasal (iN) OPN was administered at 1 h post-nHI. Groups consisted of: (1) Sham, (2) Vehicle, (3) OPN, and (4) OPN+Rac1 inhibitor (NSC23766). Evans blue dye extravasation (BBB permeability) was quantified 24 h post-nHI, brain edema at 48 h.

Animal Surgery

After induction of anesthesia, the neck of the rats was prepared and draped using standard sterile techniques. Skin preparation consisted of alcohol swabbing of the neck. Next, a small midline neck incision on the anterior neck was made with a No. 11 blade surgical knife. This incision was approximately 3–5 mm in length. Using gentle blunt dissection, the right carotid artery was isolated and gently separated from surrounding structures, including the vagus nerve, trachea, and esophagus. The carotid artery was then ligated with 5–0 surgical suture. All bleeding was controlled with gentle pressure and electocautery as needed. After the carotid artery was ligated, the surgical field was irrigated with several drops of saline, dried, and the skin closed with sutures. The entire surgical procedure took approximately 10 min. After the surgical procedure was completed, the rats were allowed

B. Dixon • J. Malaguit • D. Doycheva • J. Tang
Division of Physiology and Pharmacology, School of Medicine, 11041 Campus Street, Risley Hall Rm 129, Loma Linda, CA 92354, USA

D. Casel
Department of Neonatology, School of Medicine, Loma Linda, CA 92354, USA

J.H. Zhang
Division of Physiology and Pharmacology, School of Medicine, 11041 Campus Street, Risley Hall Rm 129, Loma Linda, CA 92354, USA

Department of Neurosurgery, School of Medicine, Loma Linda, CA 92354, USA

T. Lekic, MD, PhD (✉)
Division of Physiology and Pharmacology, School of Medicine, 11041 Campus Street, Risley Hall Rm 129, Loma Linda, CA 92354, USA

Department of Physiology, Loma Linda University School of Medicine, 11041 Campus Street, Risley Hall Rm 129, Loma Linda, CA 92354, USA
e-mail: tlekic@llu.edu

R.L. Applegate et al. (eds.), *Brain Edema XVI: Translate Basic Science into Clinical Practice*, Acta Neurochirurgica Supplement, Vol. 121,
DOI 10.1007/978-3-319-18497-5_46,

to wake and recover for 1 h. This recovery occurred in a temperature-controlled incubator. Throughout the surgical and postoperative period, temperature was controlled with heating blankets and incubators. After the rats recovered, they were returned to the care of their mother. After the 1-h recovery period, rats were exposed to hypoxia using the standard published protocols of the Rice-Vannucci model, done previously [14]. Exposure to hypoxia involved placing the animals in a temperature-controlled chamber and then exposing them to 8 % oxygen in balanced nitrogen gas for 2.5 h. This hypoxic treatment was rendered in a specially designed treatment chamber to prevent escape of the hypoxic gas mixture. Gas composition in the chamber was monitored continuously with a monitor that measures oxygen and carbon dioxide content. After hypoxic treatment all animals were monitored closely for any signs of distress, failure to thrive, infection, or serious disability. Immediately after hypoxia, animals were returned to the care of their mother.

ICV Injection

Animals were anesthetized with isoflurane. A scalp incision was made on the skull surface and the bregma exposed. Infusion of Rac1 inhibitor (NSC23766) was performed using a 10-μl syringe (Hamilton Co., Reno, NV, USA) at the location 1.5 mm posterior and 1.5 mm lateral to the bregma, and 1.7 mm deep to the skull surface at the contralateral hemisphere 24 h before HI. Control rats were injected with 2 % DMSO (2 μl/pup, diluted in saline; Sigma). The injection was completed in 5 min and the needle maintained in the injection position for an additional 2 min. Then the needle was removed slowly out of the brain and the wound sutured. After recovery from anesthesia, the pups were returned to their dams.

Evans Blue

The spectrophotometric measurement of Evans blue dye [15, 16] was initiated through intraperitoneal (IP) injection after nHI to measure BBB permeability. Under anesthesia, Evans blue (Sigma-Aldrich) in normal saline (2 %, 4 ml/kg) was infused. For quantitative measurements, the brain hemispheres (hemorrhage) were homogenized in 3 ml of N, N-dimethylformamide (Sigma-Aldrich), incubated for 18 h at 55 °C, and then centrifuged. Supernatants were analyzed at 620 nm by spectrophotometry, as routinely performed [17].

Brain Edema

Brain water content [15, 18–21] was measured using the wet-weight/dry-weight method [17]. Following sacrifice, the brains were removed and divided. Tissue weights were measured before and after drying for 24 h in a 100 °C oven. Weights were measured using an analytical microbalance (model AE 100; Mettler Instrument Co., Columbus, OH, USA) capable of precision within 1.0 μg. Brain edema was tabulated as percentage: (wet weight − dry weight)/wet weight × 100.

Statistical Analysis

Significance was based on $p < 0.05$. Data were statistically analyzed using one-way analysis of variance (ANOVA), followed by Tukey post hoc test for significant analyses. Statistical analyses were performed using SigmaPlot version 10.0 for Windows.

Results

A schematic of the proposed mechanism used as the basis of this preliminary work is outlined (Fig. 1). Experimental data show significantly increased BBB permeability (Fig. 2) and brain edema (Fig. 3) following nHI. These brain injuries were significantly improved in the OPN treatment group. However, the rat pups receiving OPN cotreatment with the Rac1 inhibitor experienced no improvement compared with vehicle (please see Fig. 2), mechanistically reversing neuroprotection.

Conclusion

Translational stroke studies, including animal modeling, are greatly needed to safely integrate basic preclinical scientific principles ahead of clinical application [22–26]. Numerous attempts to reduce HI-induced consequences have failed in the clinical setting. Therefore, it is imperative to create translatable studies that incorporate unique characteristics of the immature brain, such as its anatomical structure, physiological function, cellular composition, and its response to injury [14, 25, 27–36].

The specific objective of this study was to determine a mechanism by which rOPN affected BBB permeability and brain edema in a well-established animal model of neonatal HI. Our data demonstrate that administration of rOPN

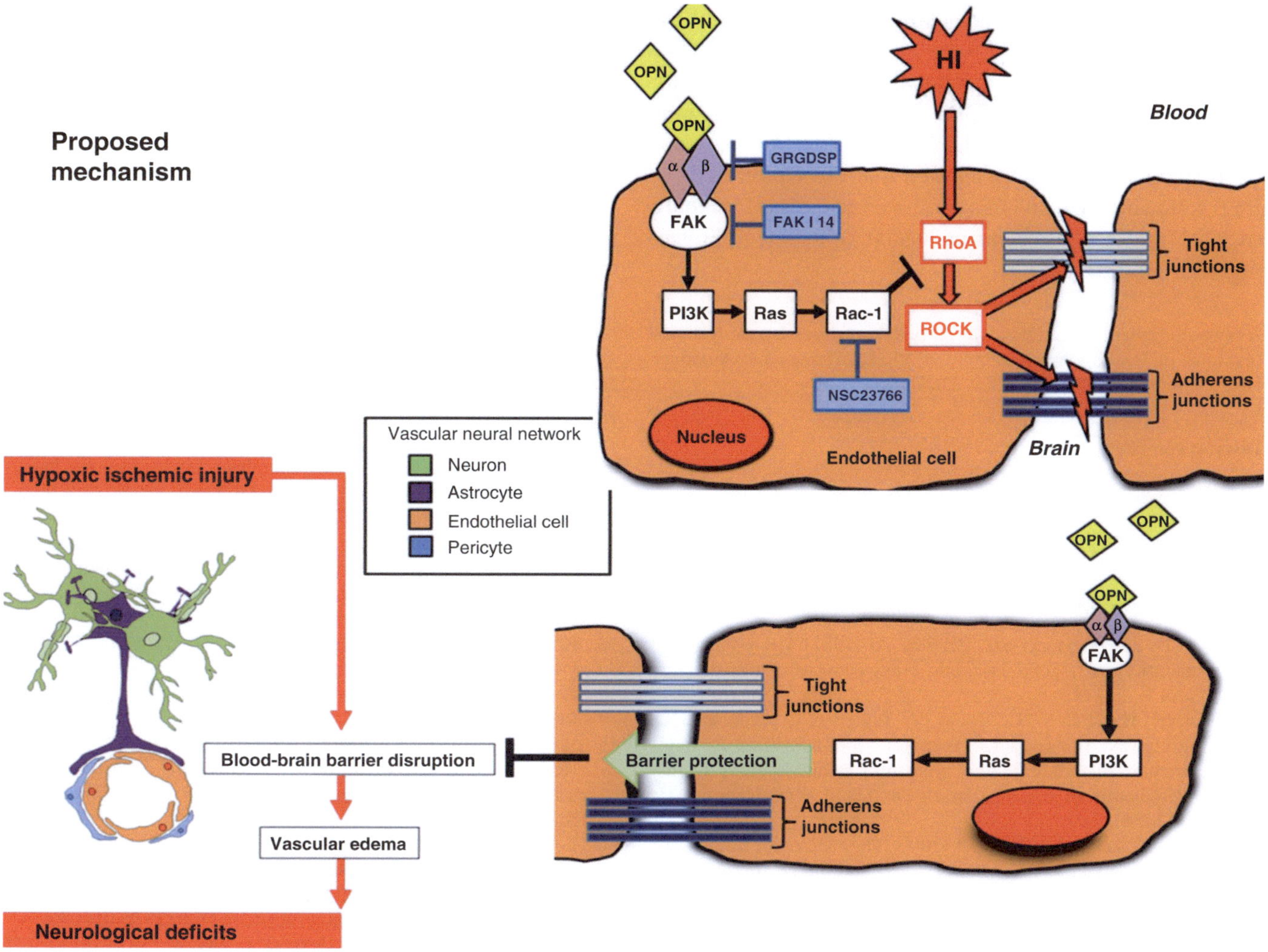

Fig. 1 Schematic, showing proposed mechanisms involving this preliminary investigation, directives of further study

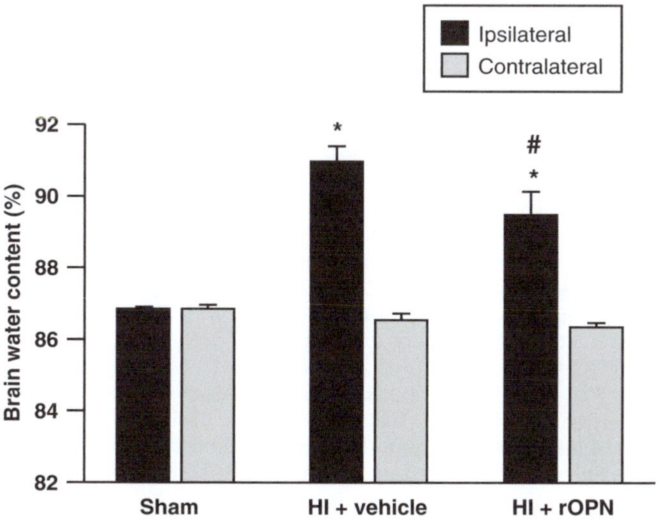

Fig. 2 OPN reduced brain edema. To determine the effects of OPN on BBB permeability, brain water content, which is a measure of brain edema, was evaluated. Brain edema was significantly increased in the ipsilateral hemisphere following HI induction. OPN significantly reduced brain edema compared with vehicle group. The contralateral hemisphere showed no increase in edema (*$p<0.05$ vs. sham; #$p<0.05$ vs. vehicle; $N=4$/group)

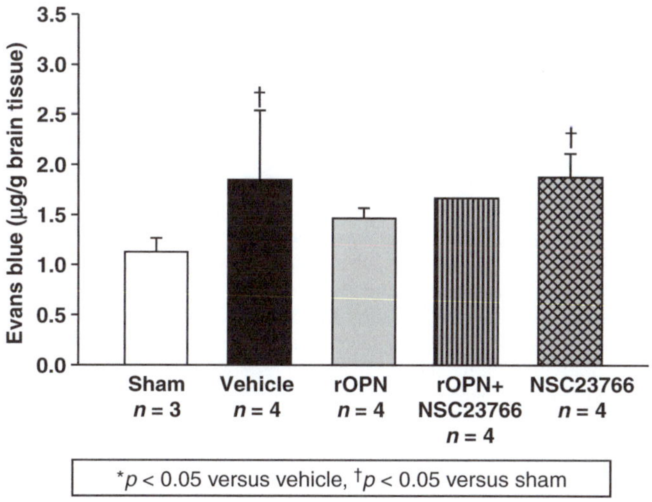

Fig. 3 OPN reduced BBB permeability. To determine the effect of OPN on BBB permeability, Evans blue dye extravasation as a measure of BBB permeability was evaluated. OPN (5 μg) was administered following HI induction, and HI significantly increased Evans blue dye extravasation, as seen in the ipsilateral hemisphere, which was significantly attenuated by OPN treatment

improves recovery after neonatal HI by stabilization of the BBB, possibly via integrin receptor signaling pathway. The long-term goal of this study is to provide a further basis for the clinical translation of rOPN as an effective therapeutic option with long-term benefits.

In summary, this study showed that OPN protected the BBB following nHI, and this was reversed by Rac1 inhibitor (NSC23766). The mechanisms mediating this neuroprotection warrant further study.

Acknowledgment This study was partially supported by the National Institutes of Health grant RO1 NS078755 (Dr. Zhang) and American Heart Association CRP 17380009 (Dr. Lekic).

Disclosures None

References

1. Rice JE 3rd, Vannucci RC, Brierley JB (1981) The influence of immaturity on hypoxic-ischemic brain damage in the rat. Ann Neurol 9:131–141
2. Murphy BP, Inder TE, Rooks V, Taylor GA, Anderson NJ, Mogridge N, Horwood LJ, Volpe JJ (2002) Posthaemorrhagic ventricular dilatation in the premature infant: natural history and predictors of outcome. Arch Dis Child Fetal Neonatal Ed 87:F37–F41
3. Kadri H, Mawla AA, Kazah J (2006) The incidence, timing, and predisposing factors of germinal matrix and intraventricular hemorrhage (GMH/IVH) in preterm neonates. Childs Nerv Syst 22:1086–1090
4. Suzuki H, Ayer R, Sugawara T, Chen W, Sozen T, Hasegawa Y, Kanamaru K, Zhang JH (2010) Protective effects of recombinant osteopontin on early brain injury after subarachnoid hemorrhage in rats. Crit Care Med 38:612–618
5. Chen W, Ma Q, Suzuki H, Hartman R, Tang J, Zhang JH (2011) Osteopontin reduced hypoxia-ischemia neonatal brain injury by suppression of apoptosis in a rat pup model. Stroke 42:764–769
6. van Velthoven CT, Heijnen CJ, van Bel F, Kavelaars A (2011) Osteopontin enhances endogenous repair after neonatal hypoxic-ischemic brain injury. Stroke 42:2294–2301
7. Suzuki H, Hasegawa Y, Chen W, Kanamaru K, Zhang JH (2010) Recombinant osteopontin in cerebral vasospasm after subarachnoid hemorrhage. Ann Neurol 68:650–660
8. Suzuki H, Hasegawa Y, Kanamaru K, Zhang JH (2010) Mechanisms of osteopontin-induced stabilization of blood-brain barrier disruption after subarachnoid hemorrhage in rats. Stroke 41:1783–1790
9. Topkoru BC, Altay O, Duris K, Krafft PR, Yan J, Zhang JH (2013) Nasal administration of recombinant osteopontin attenuates early brain injury after subarachnoid hemorrhage. Stroke 44:3189–3194
10. Quinn M, McMillin M, Galindo C, Frampton G, Pae HY, DeMorrow S (2014) Bile acids permeabilize the blood brain barrier after bile duct ligation in rats via Rac1- dependent mechanisms. Dig Liver Dis 46:527–534
11. Woollard SM, Li H, Singh S, Yu F, Kanmogne GD (2014) HIV-1 induces cytoskeletal alterations and Rac1 activation during monocyte-blood-brain barrier interactions: modulatory role of CCR5. Retrovirology 11:20
12. Huang B, Krafft PR, Ma Q, Rolland WB, Caner B, Lekic T, Manaenko A, Le M, Tang J, Zhang JH (2012) Fibroblast growth factors preserve blood-brain barrier integrity through RhoA inhibition after intracerebral hemorrhage in mice. Neurobiol Dis 46:204–214
13. Maruvada R, Zhu L, Pearce D, Zheng Y, Perfect J, Kwon-Chung KJ, Kim KS (2012) Cryptococcus neoformans phospholipase B1 activates host cell Rac1 for traversal across the blood-brain barrier. Cell Microbiol 14:1544–1553
14. Fathali N, Ostrowski RP, Hasegawa Y, Lekic T, Tang J, Zhang JH (2013) Splenic immune cells in experimental neonatal hypoxia-ischemia. Transl Stroke Res 4:208–219
15. Merali Z, Leung J, Mikulis D, Silver F, Kassner A (2014) Longitudinal assessment of imatinib's effect on the blood-brain barrier after ischemia/reperfusion injury with permeability MRI. Transl Stroke Res. doi:10.1007/s12975-014-0358-6
16. Li H, Gao A, Feng D, Wang Y, Zhang L, Cui Y, Li B, Wang Z, Chen G (2014) Evaluation of the protective potential of brain microvascular endothelial cell autophagy on blood-brain barrier integrity during experimental cerebral ischemia-reperfusion injury. Transl Stroke Res 5:618–626. doi:10.1007/s12975-014-0354-x
17. Lekic T, Rolland W, Hartman R, Kamper J, Suzuki H, Tang J, Zhang JH (2011) Characterization of the brain injury, neurobehavioral profiles, and histopathology in a rat model of cerebellar hemorrhage. Exp Neurol 227:96–103
18. Khanna A, Kahle KT, Walcott BP, Gerzanich V, Simard JM (2014) Disruption of ion homeostasis in the neurogliovascular unit underlies the pathogenesis of ischemic cerebral edema. Transl Stroke Res 5:3–16
19. Jayakumar AR, Valdes V, Tong XY, Shamaladevi N, Gonzalez W, Norenberg MD (2014) Sulfonylurea receptor 1 contributes to the astrocyte swelling and brain edema in acute liver failure. Transl Stroke Res 5:28–37
20. Schlunk F, Schulz E, Lauer A, Yigitkanli K, Pfeilschifter W, Steinmetz H, Lo EH, Foerch C (2014) Warfarin pretreatment reduces cell death and MMP-9 activity in experimental intracerebral hemorrhage. Transl Stroke Res. doi:10.1007/s12975-014- 0377-3
21. Hasegawa Y, Nakagawa T, Uekawa K, Ma M, Lin B, Kusaka H, Katayama T, Sueta D, Toyama K, Koibuchi N, Kim-Mitsuyama S (2014) Therapy with the combination of amlodipine and irbesartan has persistent preventative effects on stroke onset associated with BDNF preservation on cerebral vessels in hypertensive rats. Transl Stroke Res. doi:10.1007/s12975-014-0383-5
22. Tso MK, Macdonald RL (2014) Subarachnoid hemorrhage: a review of experimental studies on the microcirculation and the neurovascular unit. Transl Stroke Res 5:174–189. doi:10.1007/s12975-014-0323-4
23. Marbacher S, Nevzati E, Croci D, Erhardt S, Muroi C, Jakob SM, Fandino J (2014) The rabbit shunt model of subarachnoid haemorrhage. Transl Stroke Res 5:669–680
24. Pluta RM, Bacher J, Skopets B, Hoffmann V (2014) A non-human primate model of aneurismal subarachnoid hemorrhage (SAH). Transl Stroke Res 5:681–691
25. Zhang YP, Cai J, Shields LB, Liu N, Xu XM, Shields CB (2014) Traumatic brain injury using mouse models. Transl Stroke Res 5:454–471
26. Wada K, Makino H, Shimada K, Shikata F, Kuwabara A, Hashimoto T (2014) Translational research using a mouse model of intracranial aneurysm. Transl Stroke Res 5:248–251
27. Fathali N, Lekic T, Zhang JH, Tang J (2010) Long-term evaluation of granulocyte-colony stimulating factor on hypoxic-ischemic brain damage in infant rats. Intensive Care Med 36:1602–1608
28. Zhou Y, Fathali N, Lekic T, Tang J, Zhang JH (2009) Glibenclamide improves neurological function in neonatal hypoxia-ischemia in rats. Brain Res 1270:131–139

29. Souvenir R, Fathali N, Tong W, Lekic T, Chee P, Zhang J (2009) Janus kinase 2 and tissue inhibitor of matrix metalloproteinase-1 mediate the protective effects of erythropoietin in in-vitro model of hypoxia ischemia. FASEB J 23:614–620
30. Fathali N, Ostrowski RP, Lekic T, Jadhav V, Tong W, Tang J, Zhang JH (2010) Cyclooxygenase-2 inhibition provides lasting protection against neonatal hypoxic- ischemic brain injury. Crit Care Med 38:572–578
31. Zhou Y, Lekic T, Fathali N, Ostrowski RP, Martin RD, Tang J, Zhang JH (2010) Isoflurane posttreatment reduces neonatal hypoxic-ischemic brain injury in rats by the sphingosine-1-phosphate/phosphatidylinositol-3-kinase/Akt pathway. Stroke 41:1521–1527
32. Zhou Y, Fathali N, Lekic T, Ostrowski RP, Chen C, Martin RD, Tang J, Zhang JH (2011) Remote limb ischemic postconditioning protects against neonatal hypoxic-ischemic brain injury in rat pups by the opioid receptor/Akt pathway. Stroke 42:439–444
33. Souvenir R, Fathali N, Ostrowski RP, Lekic T, Zhang JH, Tang J (2011) Tissue inhibitor of matrix metalloproteinase-1 mediates erythropoietin-induced neuroprotection in hypoxia ischemia. Neurobiol Dis 44:28–37
34. Seifert HA, Pennypacker KR (2014) Molecular and cellular immune responses to ischemic brain injury. Transl Stroke Res 5:543–553
35. Chen D, Yu SP, Wei L (2014) Ion channels in regulation of neuronal regenerative activities. Transl Stroke Res 5:156–162
36. Brathwaite S, Macdonald RL (2014) Current management of delayed cerebral ischemia: update from results of recent clinical trials. Transl Stroke Res 5:207–226

Early Use of Statin in Patients Treated with Alteplase for Acute Ischemic Stroke

Jieli Geng, Yeping Song, Zhihao Mu, Qun Xu, Guowen Shi, Yameng Sun, Ying Chen, Yan Lin, Yuanmei Pan, Lin Yu, Guo-Yuan Yang, and Yansheng Li

Introduction

Following the SPARCL (Stroke Prevention with Aggressive Reductions in Cholesterol Levels) study, hydroxymethylglutaryl-CoA reductase inhibitors (statins) became the fundamental therapy for secondary stroke prevention that was recommended by guidelines [1]. A great number of studies have shown that pretreatment or early administration of statins can reduce infarct volumes and improve functional outcomes in animal stroke models [2, 3]. Furthermore, statin treatment before or after the onset of ischemic stroke improved clinical outcomes by its possible neuroprotective effect, independent of its cholesterol-lowering effects [4–6].

It is a widely accepted concept that secondary stroke prevention treatment should begin earlier. Thus, to examine the safety of statin treatment at the early stage of a stroke is fundamental to determine the time of initiation in a patient who receives thrombolytic treatment. Several studies have focused on the impacts of pretreatment with statins in patients who received thrombolytic therapy [7–14] and very few have studied the impact of statin usage in the early stage of ischemic stroke after thrombolysis [15, 16]. A meta-analysis of 27 studies revealed that statin treatment at stroke onset improved functional outcome at 90 days, but this favorable effect was not seen in patients who received thrombolysis [17]. Scheitz [18] found a statistically significant dose response relationship between previous statin use and symptomatic intracerebral hemorrhage (sICH). However, another study found that the discontinuation of statin after hemorrhagic stroke was still associated with an increased risk of death and other disadvantageous or harmful outcomes [19].

The aim of this study was to investigate the risk of intracerebral hemorrhage (ICH) and clinical functional outcomes of statin treatment within 24 h of stroke onset in patients treated with intravenous (IV) alteplase.

Material and Methods

Design and Patient Selection

We again studied the data of 119 consecutive patients with acute ischemic stroke who received IV alteplase at Shanghai Renji Hospital from April 2008 to December 2012. The inclusion and exclusion criteria as well as the thrombolytic protocol were strictly followed according to the European Cooperative Acute Stroke Study (ECASS) II criteria [20]. ECASS III criteria were used to treat patients with the onset time between 3 and 4.5 h [21]. All patients with a clinical diagnosis of ischemic stroke and a National Institutes of

J. Geng
Department of Neurology, Ruijin Hospital,
Shanghai Jiao Tong University, School of Medicine,
Shanghai 200025, China

Department of Neurology,
Renji Hospital, Shanghai Jiao Tong University,
School of Medicine, 1630 Dongfang Road,
Shanghai 200127, China

Y. Song • Q. Xu • G. Shi • Y. Sun • Y. Chen • Y. Lin • Y. Pan
L. Yu • Y. Li (✉)
Department of Neurology, Renji Hospital,
Shanghai Jiao Tong University, School of Medicine,
1630 Dongfang Road, Shanghai 200127, China
e-mail: lliyans@hotmail.com

Z. Mu
Department of Neurology, Ruijin Hospital,
Shanghai Jiao Tong University, School of Medicine,
Shanghai 200025, China

G.-Y. Yang (✉)
Department of Neurology, Ruijin Hospital,
Shanghai Jiao Tong University, School of Medicine,
Shanghai 200025, China

Neuroscience and Neuroengineering Research Center,
Med-X Research Institute and School of Biomedical Engineering,
Shanghai Jiao Tong University, 1954 Huashan Road,
Shanghai 200030, China
e-mail: gyyang0626@gmail.com

R.L. Applegate et al. (eds.), *Brain Edema XVI: Translate Basic Science into Clinical Practice*, Acta Neurochirurgica Supplement, Vol. 121, 269
DOI 10.1007/978-3-319-18497-5_47,

Health Stroke Scale (NIHSS) [22] score of less than 24 received IV alteplase (0.9 mg/kg) within 4.5 h of stroke onset after obtaining informed consent.

The time of initiation of the statin therapy and its dosages was decided by the physician treating the stroke. In this study, early statin use is defined as starting the treatment within 24 h of stroke onset. Patients who used statin before or within 24 h of stroke onset but stopped during the acute phase (within 1 week following stroke onset) were excluded, as were those using statin after 24 h of stroke onset. Patients diagnosed with cardioembolic or other rare causes of stroke were also excluded.

Within 24 h of onset, patients in the statin-treated group received 20–40 mg atorvastatin (Pfizer, New York, NY). After 2 weeks, all patients were treated with atorvastatin (20 mg daily) as a standard dose for secondary stroke prevention. Other early management and secondary stroke prevention treatment such as antiplatelet and antihypertensive treatment were prescribed strictly according to the Chinese and American Heart Association (AHA)/American Stroke Association (ASA) guidelines for the management of acute ischemic stroke [23].

Data Collection and Definition

We collected the following information: (1) demographic characteristics; (2) vascular risk factors such as hypertension, diabetes mellitus, atrial fibrillation, hyperlipidemia (total cholesterol greater than 5.6 mmol/l and/or total triglyceride greater than 1.7 mmol/l and/or low-density lipoprotein cholesterol greater than 3.4 mmol/l and/or high-density lipoprotein cholesterol less than 0.9 mmol/l), previous stroke or transient ischemic attack (TIA), and current cigarette smoker for more than 3 months [24]; (3) baseline neurologic deficit assessed by the NIHSS; (4) arterial blood pressure before thrombolytic treatment; (5) times from symptom onset to initiation of rtPA; (6) initiation time and dosage of statin; (7) laboratory findings including plasma glucose level before thrombolytic treatment and fasting lipid levels within 24 h of stroke onset; (8) imaging information including a computed tomography (CT) scan after 24 h after thrombolytic treatment and a magnetic resonance imaging (MRI) scan within 1 week after stroke onset; (9) classification of stroke subtype according to the TOAST criteria [25]; and (10) 90-day functional outcomes assessed by the modified Rankin Scale (mRS) [26].

Outcomes

The outcomes assessed include the risk of ICH, functional outcome, and all-cause mortality at 90 days. ICHs were detected by CT/MRI and classified according to the criteria of the ECASS II into hemorrhagic infarction 1 (HI1), hemorrhagic infarction 2 (HI2), parenchymal hemorrhage (PH1), and parenchymal hemorrhage (PH2) [20]. sICH was defined as clinical neurologic deterioration (an increment of the NIHSS of scores of 4 or greater) in addition to any hemorrhage on the CT/MRI scan [20]. ICHs were further divided into early ICHs (within 36 h after thrombolytic treatment) or later ICHs (from 36 h to 7 days). The functional outcomes were assessed at 90 days by mRS and good functional outcomes were defined as mRS 0-1 [10]. The neurological deficit at baseline was categorized by NIHSS scores as mild ($\leq$5), moderate (6–13), or severe ($\geq$14). The cutoff points were made according to previous studies of stroke severity related to stroke outcomes, as well as in a recent clinical trial of a neuroprotective agent [27, 28].

Statistical Analysis

All statistical analyses were done using the SPSS 16.0 statistical package. Continuous variables were expressed as a median or mean, while categorical variables were expressed as numbers and percentages. Differences among groups were further assessed by the *t*-test, chi-square test, or Wilcoxon signed-rank test as appropriate. Significance was established at the two-tailed α level of 0.05. 2×2 Cross-tables were used to calculate odds ratios. The logistic regression model with a forward stepwise method was performed to assess whether statin treatment was an independent factor of different outcomes. Considered a predictor of ICH related to statin therapy, all variables were added to the regression model, including age, gender, risk factors, systolic and diastolic blood pressure, glucose and lipid levels, baseline NIHSS level, TOAST classification, and times from symptom onset to initiation of alteplase. Results were given as an odds ratio (OR) with an estimated relative risk within 95 % CI and an OR >1.0 that would indicate a greater likelihood of ICH, sICH, good outcomes, and mortality at 90 days after stroke.

Results

Baseline Characteristics

Among the 119 patients treated by IV alteplase, 71 patients received atorvastatin within 24 h of stroke onset as a statin group and 48 patients did not as a control group. There were no significant differences in demographics or vascular risk factors between the statin and control group ($p>0.05$). Furthermore, there were no significant differences between the two groups at baseline in blood pressure, blood glucose level, lipids, time from onset to thrombolytic treatment, NIHSS level, and stroke subtypes ($p>0.05$, Table 1).

Table 1 Baseline demographic and clinical characteristics between patients with or without statin treatment

Variable	Non-statin $N=48$	Statin $N=71$	Total $N=119$	*p*-value
Age, years, mean (SD)	64.5 ± 10.4	60.6 ± 10.9	62.2 ± 10.8	0.056[a]
Male, %	33 (68.8 %)	51 (71.8 %)	84 (70.6 %)	0.717[b]
Risk factors, %				
Hypertension	26 (54.2 %)	43 (60.6 %)	69 (58.0 %)	0.488[b]
Diabetes	8 (16.7 %)	18 (25.4 %)	26 (21.8 %)	0.261[b]
Hyperlipidemia	25 (52.1 %)	31 (43.7 %)	56 (47.1)	0.367[b]
Previous stroke or TIA	9 (18.8 %)	5 (7.0 %)	14 (11.8 %)	0.052[b]
Smoking	23 (45.8)	31 (43.7 %)	53 (44.5 %)	0.815[b]
Clinical measures				
SBP before thrombolysis, mmHg, median (IQR)	147 (130–160)	149 (130–161)	149 (130–160)	0.741[a]
DBP, before thrombolysis, mmHg, median (IQR)	87 (76–95)	85 (80–95)	86 (80–95)	0.728[a]
Blood glucose level, before thrombolysis, mmol/L, median (IQR)	6.6 (5.4–7.3)	7.0 (5.9–8.7)	6.7 (5.7–7.8)	0.066[c]
LDL, mmol/L, median (IQR)	2.9 (2.4–3.4)	2.9 (2.4–3.5)	2.9 (2.4–3.4)	0.993[a]
TC, mmol/L, median (IQR)	4.6 (4.0–5.4)	4.1 (4.7–5.5)	4.6 (4.1–5.5)	0.800[a]
Stroke severity				
NIHSS, *n* (%)				0.989[b]
≤5	9 (18.8 %)	13 (18.3 %)	22 (18.5 %)	
6–13	23 (47.9 %)	35 (49.3 %)	58 (48.7 %)	
≥14	16 (33.3 %)	23 (32.4 %)	39 (32.8 %)	
TOAST ischemic stroke subtype				0.410[b]
Large artery	29 (60.4 %)	36 (50.7 %)	65 (54.6 %)	
Small vessel	8 (16.7 %)	19 (26.8 %)	27 (22.7 %)	
Unknown etiology	11 (22.9 %)	16 (22.5 %)	27 (22.7 %)	
Time from onset to thrombolysis, min, median (IQR)	168 (136–210)	170 (150–211)	170 (144–210)	0.533[a]

Abbreviations: *DBP* diastolic blood pressure, *SBP* systolic blood pressure, *LDL* low density lipoprotein, *TC* total cholesterol, *NIHSS* National Institutes of Health Stroke Scale, *TOAST* Trial of Org 10172 in Acute Stroke Treatment, *IQR* interquartile range

[a]*t*-test

[b]Chi-square test

[c]Wilcoxon signed-rank test

Effect of Statin Treatment on ICH

A total of 24 (20.2 %) patients had ICH: 12 (16.9 %) in the statin group and 12 (25.0 %) in the non-statin group. Of these 24 patients, 11 developed ICH within 36 h after thrombolytic treatment (6 [8.5 %] in the statin group and 5 [10.4 %] in the non-statin group); and 13 developed ICH between 36 h and 7 days (6 [8.5 %] and 7 [14.6 %], respectively). Six (5.0 %) patients had sICH: 3 (4.2 %) in statin group and 3 (6.2 %) in the non-statin group. Statin treatment was not associated with an increased likelihood of ICH (OR 0.610, 95 % CI 0.248–1.502, $p=0.280$) or sICH (OR 0.662, 95 % CI 0.128–3.425, $p=0.684$, Table 2). After multivariate logistic regression analysis, there was still no significant association between the use of statin and occurrence of ICH or sICH (Table 3).

As shown in Table 4, among statin-treated groups, 15 patients received 40 mg of atorvastatin daily and others received 20 mg of atorvastatin daily. Although there were no statistically significant differences in ICH types between the two statin subgroups and the control group, there was a trend toward a lower rate of ICH among those taking a higher

Table 2 Univariate analyses regarding the intracerebral hemorrhage and functional outcome

	Non-statin	Statin	Total	OR (95 % CI)	
Outcome	*N*=48	*N*=71	*N*=119		*p*-value
ICH, *n* (%)	12 (25.0 %)	12 (16.9 %)	24 (20.2 %)	0.610 (0.248–1.502)	0.280
Early ICH[a]	5 (10.4 %)	6 (8.5 %)	11 (9.2 %)	0.794 (0.228–2.765)	0.755
Later ICH[b]	7 (14.6 %)	6 (8.5 %)	13 (10.9 %)	0.541 (0.170–1.722)	0.293
sICH *n* (%)[c]	3 (6.2 %)	3 (4.2 %)	6 (5.0 %)	0.662 (0.128–3.425)	0.684
Good functional outcome *n* (%)[d]	21 (43.8 %)	36 (50.7 %)	57 (47.9 %)	1.322 (0.634–2.761)	0.456
All-cause death	3 (6.0 %)	1 (1.4 %)	4 (3.3 %)	0.214 (0.022–2.124)	0.302

[a]Early ICHs (early intracerebral hemorrhage) defined as intracerebral hemorrhage within 36 h after thrombolytic treatment
[b]Later ICHs (later intracerebral hemorrhage) defined as intracerebral hemorrhage that occurred from 36 h to 7 days
[c]sICH (Symptomatic intracerebral hemorrhage) defined as clinical neurologic deterioration (an increase of 4 or more points in the NIHSS score) in addition to any hemorrhage on the follow-up CT/MRI scan
[d]Good outcome defined as 90-day mRS score of 0-1

Table 3 Adjusted ORs for the different outcome parameters

	Statin	
	OR	*p*-value
Any ICH	0.525 (0.184–1.504)	0.230
sICH	0.915 (0.060–13.941)	0.949
Good functional outcome	1.278 (0.515–3.176)	0.597
All-cause deaths	0.259 (0.022–3.100)	0.286

statin dose. Moreover, none of the patients on the 40 mg statin treatment had later or severe ICH. All patients with ICH in this subgroup were of HI1 type within 36 h of stroke onset.

Effect of Statin Treatment on Functional Outcomes

Among 119 patients, 57 (47.9 %) patients had good functional outcomes at 90 days (36 [50.7 %] in the statin group and 21 [43.8 %] in the non-statin group) and 4 (3.3 %) patients died (1 [1.4 %] in the statin group and 3 [6.0 %] in the non-statin group, respectively). Statin treatment showed a trend toward good functional outcomes (OR 1.322, 95 % CI 0.634–2.761, p=0. 456) and a lower rate of all-cause mortality (OR 0.214, 95 % CI 0.022–2.124, p=0.302, Table 2). However, after multivariate logistic regression analysis, statin treatment had no significant effect on the probability of a good functional outcomes or mortality (Table 3). As shown in Table 4, there were no significant differences in good functional outcomes (43.8, 50.0, 53.3 % in non-, 20 mg-, and 40 mg statin users, respectively, p=0.738) or all-cause mortality (6.2, 1.8 %, 0 in non-, 20 mg, and 40 mg statin users, respectively, p=0. 474) with higher statin doses.

Discussion

The 71 patients treated with alteplase showed that an early statin treatment was associated with similar good functional outcome at 90 days, risk of late ICH, sICH, and all-cause deaths to those who did not receive statins. Although statin therapy has become an essential part of secondary stroke prevention therapy with strong clinical evidence, it can potentially cause ICH, especially in patients receiving thrombolytic treatment and, therefore, still needs to be explored. Experimental studies have found that statins inhibit expression of matrix metalloproteinases (MMPs), ameliorate elevation in alteplase-induced MMP-9 [29, 30], inhibit coagulation [31], and decrease expression of plasminogen activator inhibitor-1 (PAI-1) [32]. Conversely, clinical studies on the relationship between statins and ICHs are lacking and, of these, most have studied the effects of statin treatment before stroke onset [7–14]. The Thrombolysis and Statins (TURaST) study reported that the risk of sICH was not affected by statin treatment [15]. An Italian study reported increased risk of sICH in patients treated with alteplase who used statin therapy before stroke and continued during the acute phase, but not within 24 h of stroke onset [16]. Although the authors suggested that ICHs were related to the excessive enhancement of the fibrinolytic effect of statin on rtPA, the correlation remains inconclusive.

Many factors, such as selection bias and confounding factors, can impact the outcome of any clinical study. The consistent and appropriate definition of ICH is undoubtedly important in conducting any studies related to ICHs. The timing of conducting an imaging study and the methods used are two important aspects in detecting ICH. In the classical thrombolytic trials, the timing of defining ICH was a CT scan of a brain within 10 days after the onset of stroke in the National Institute of Neurological Disorders and Stroke (NINDS) t-PA study [33]; within 7 days after the alteplase

Table 4 Hemorrhagic transformation and neurological functional outcome among different statin groups

Variable	Non-statin $N=48$	Statin (20 mg) $N=56$	Statin (40 mg) $N=15$	Total $N=119$	p-value
Hemorrhagic transformation					
Any ICH, n (%)	12 (25.0 %)	10 (17.9 %)	2 (13.3 %)	24 (20.2 %)	0.589
ICH					0.556
HI1, n (%)	2 (4.2 %)	4 (7.1 %)	2 (13.3 %)	8 (6.7 %)	
HI2, n (%)	7 (14.6 %)	4 (7.1 %)	0	11 (9.2 %)	
PH1, n (%)	1 (2.1 %)	0	0	1 (0.8 %)	
PH2, n (%)	2 (4.2 %)	2 (3.6 %)	0	4 (3.4 %)	
ICH time					0.547
Early ICH	5 (10.4 %)	4 (7.1 %)	2 (13.3 %)	11 (9.2 %)	
Later ICH	7 (14.6 %)	6 (10.7 %)	0	13 (10.9 %)	
sICH n (%)	3 (6.2 %)	3 (5.4 %)	0	6 (5.0 %)	1.000
Neurological function outcome					
Good functional outcome (mRS $\leq$ 1), n (%)	21 (43.8 %)	28 (50.0 %)	8 (53.3 %)	57 (47.9 %)	0.738
All-cause deaths	3 (6.2 %)	1 (1.8 %)	0	4 (3.4 %)	0.474

Abbreviations: *HI1* hemorrhagic infarction 1, *HI2* hemorrhagic infarction 2, *PH1* parenchymal hemorrhage, *PH2* parenchymal hemorrhage

treatment in ECASS II study [20]; and a CT or MRI scan within 36 h after alteplase treatment in ECASS III study [21]. The reported rate of ICH varied greatly: 10.5 %, 46.7 %, and 27 %, respectively. In this study, a total of 24 (20.2 %) patients had ICH, 11 of which were detected by CT and 13 detected by MRI. Because MRI is superior to CT in detecting chronic hemorrhage and micro-bleeding, both the time of imaging study and methods employed would have different impact on the sensitivity of finding ICH [34]. In a TURaST study [15], sICH was assessed within 36 h after IV thrombolysis, while statin treatment was limited to 72 h after IV thrombolysis; the possible effect of statin on hemorrhage may be underestimated. To avoid such ambiguity, 7 days was selected as the cutoff point of ICH in our study.

The present study also suggests that of the very few patients who developed ICH in the high-dose statin therapy, ICH is mild and the patients are in the early stage of stroke. Only two patients in the 40 mg atorvastatin group had HI1 type hemorrhage within 36 h after alteplase therapy. Because the sample size is so small, it should be interpreted with caution. The dose effect of statin at the early stage of stroke in patients receiving alteplase was not evaluated. The only related report was from a European intravenous thrombolysis study, which found that the higher the statin dose used before stroke attack, the higher the occurrence of sICH (2 %, 6 %, and 13 % in low-, medium-, and high-dose statin users, respectively, $p<0.01$) [18]. We believe that the different results may be due to the different bleeding time point we measured. Another possibility may be due to the type of statin given; we used atorvastatin whereas Scheitz used simvastatin, atorvastatin, pravastatin, fluvastatin, and rosuvastatin. Compared with statin treatment after thrombolysis, statin use before stroke significantly increased the fibrinolytic effect and disrupted homeostasis between coagulation and fibrinolysis [16]. Further work is needed to clarify the dose effect of statin in thrombolytic treatment and the development of ICH.

In our study, there is an insignificant trend toward a better functional outcome and lower mortality at day 90 of stroke onset in patients receiving higher doses of atorvastatin. Such benefit may be caused by the potential neuroprotective properties of statins, which would offset their hemorrhagic tendency.

Our study has limitations. First, the sample size was relatively small. Secondly, although neither total cholesterol nor LDL were associated with ICH, the baseline triglyceride (TG) level was not available. Uyttenboogaart et al. [12] reported that a high admission TG level was an independent risk factor for developing sICH after thrombolytic treatment for acute stroke. However, other studies have not shown the relationship between lipid profiles and sICH or functional outcome [11]. Therefore, further research is required. Third, information on leukoaraiosis, lacunes, and cerebral microbleeding by MRI were not available. Studies also suggest that moderate to severe leukoaraiosis of the deep white matter related to small vessel diseases is independently associated with sICH in patients receiving thrombolytic treatment [35]. Lastly, more patients had sICH compared with patients in the ECASS III (5.0 % vs 2.4 %), which may be related to the difference in cutoff points, in terms of timing, of sICH.

Conclusions

This study suggests that statin treatment in the early stage of ischemic stroke is safe and is associated with decreased risks of later development of sICH or death after IV treatment. Future randomized controlled trials with large sample sizes are needed to confirm these findings.

Acknowledgments The authors thank Yanping Song for assistance with statistical analysis. We also thank Xiaoyan Chen for her editorial assistance with the manuscript.

Conflict of Interest The authors declare that they have no conflicts of interest.

References

1. Amarenco P, Bogousslavsky J, Callahan A 3rd, Goldstein LB, Hennerici M, Rudolph AE, Sillesen H, Simunovic L, Szarek M, Welch KM, Zivin JA, Stroke Prevention by Aggressive Reduction in Cholesterol Levels (SPARCL) Investigators (2006) High-dose atorvastatin after stroke or transient ischemic attack. N Engl J Med 355(6):549–559
2. Chen J, Zhang ZG, Li Y, Wang Y, Wang L, Jiang H, Zhang C, Lu M, Katakowski M, Feldkamp CS, Chopp M (2003) Statins induce angiogenesis, neurogenesis, and synaptogenesis after stroke. Ann Neurol 53(6):743–751
3. Prinz V, Laufs U, Gertz K, Kronenberg G, Balkaya M, Leithner C, Lindauer U, Endres M (2008) Intravenous rosuvastatin for acute stroke treatment: an animal study. Stroke 39(2):433–438
4. Biffi A, Devan WJ, Anderson CD, Cortellini L, Furie KL, Rosand J, Rost NS (2011) Statin treatment and functional outcome after ischemic stroke: case-control and meta-analysis. Stroke 42(5):1314–1319
5. Chen PS, Cheng CL, Kao Yang YH, Yeh PS, Li YH (2014) Impact of early statin therapy in patients with ischemic stroke or transient ischemic attack. Acta Neurol Scand 129(1):41–48
6. Goldstein LB, Amarenco P, Zivin J, Messig M, Altafullah I, Callahan A, Hennerici M, MacLeod MJ, Sillesen H, Zweifler R, Michael K, Welch A, Stroke Prevention by Aggressive Reduction in Cholesterol Levels Investigators (2009) Statin treatment and stroke outcome in the Stroke Prevention by Aggressive Reduction in Cholesterol Levels (SPARCL) trial. Stroke 40(11):3526–3531
7. Cougo-Pinto PT, Santos BL, Dias FA, Fabio SR, Werneck IV, Camilo MR, Abud DG, Leite JP, Pontes-Neto OM (2012) Frequency and predictors of symptomatic intracranial hemorrhage after intravenous thrombolysis for acute ischemic stroke in a Brazilian public hospital. Clinics (Sao Paulo) 67(7):739–743
8. Engelter ST, Soinne L, Ringleb P, Sarikaya H, Bordet R, Berrouschot J, Odier C, Arnold M, Ford GA, Pezzini A, Zini A, Rantanen K, Rocco A, Bonati LH, Kellert L, Strbian D, Stoll A, Meier N, Michel P, Baumgartner RW, Leys D, Tatlisumak T, Lyrer PA (2011) IV thrombolysis and statins. Neurology 77(9):888–895
9. Martinez-Ramirez S, Delgado-Mederos R, Marin R, Suarez-Calvet M, Sainz MP, Alejaldre A, Vidal-Jordana A, Marti-Vilalta JL, Marti-Fabregas J (2012) Statin pretreatment may increase the risk of symptomatic intracranial haemorrhage in thrombolysis for ischemic stroke: results from a case-control study and a meta-analysis. J Neurol 259(1):111–118
10. Meseguer E, Mazighi M, Lapergue B, Labreuche J, Sirimarco G, Gonzalez-Valcarcel J, Lavallee PC, Cabrejo L, Guidoux C, Klein IF, Olivot JM, Rouchaud A, Desilles JP, Amarenco P (2012) Outcomes after thrombolysis in AIS according to prior statin use: a registry and review. Neurology 79(17):1817–1823
11. Rocco A, Sykora M, Ringleb P, Diedler J (2012) Impact of statin use and lipid profile on symptomatic intracerebral haemorrhage, outcome and mortality after intravenous thrombolysis in acute stroke. Cerebrovasc Dis 33(4):362–368
12. Uyttenboogaart M, Koch MW, Koopman K, Vroomen PC, Luijckx GJ, De Keyser J (2008) Lipid profile, statin use, and outcome after intravenous thrombolysis for acute ischaemic stroke. J Neurol 255(6):875–880
13. Alvarez-Sabin J, Huertas R, Quintana M, Rubiera M, Delgado P, Ribo M, Molina CA, Montaner J (2007) Prior statin use may be associated with improved stroke outcome after tissue plasminogen activator. Stroke 38(3):1076–1078
14. Miedema I, Uyttenboogaart M, Koopman K, De Keyser J, Luijckx GJ (2010) Statin use and functional outcome after tissue plasminogen activator treatment in acute ischaemic stroke. Cerebrovasc Dis 29(3):263–267
15. Cappellari M, Bovi P, Moretto G, Zini A, Nencini P, Sessa M, Furlan M, Pezzini A, Orlandi G, Paciaroni M, Tassinari T, Procaccianti G, Di Lazzaro V, Bettoni L, Gandolfo C, Silvestrelli G, Rasura M, Martini G, Melis M, Calloni MV, Chiodo-Grandi F, Beretta S, Guarino M, Altavista MC, Marcheselli S, Galletti G, Adobbati L, Del Sette M, Mancini A, Orrico D, Monaco S, Cavallini A, Sciolla R, Federico F, Scoditti U, Brusaferri F, Grassa C, Specchio L, Bongioanni MR, Sparaco M, Zampolini M, Greco G, Colombo R, Passarella B, Adami A, Consoli D, Toni D (2013) The THRombolysis and STatins (THRaST) study. Neurology 80(7):655–661
16. Cappellari M, Deluca C, Tinazzi M, Tomelleri G, Carletti M, Fiaschi A, Bovi P, Moretto G (2011) Does statin in the acute phase of ischemic stroke improve outcome after intravenous thrombolysis? A retrospective study. J Neurol Sci 308(1–2):128–134
17. Ni Chroinin D, Asplund K, Asberg S, Callaly E, Cuadrado-Godia E, Diez-Tejedor E, Di Napoli M, Engelter ST, Furie KL, Giannopoulos S, Gotto AM Jr, Hannon N, Jonsson F, Kapral MK, Marti-Fabregas J, Martinez-Sanchez P, Milionis HJ, Montaner J, Muscari A, Pikija S, Probstfield J, Rost NS, Thrift AG, Vemmos K, Kelly PJ (2013) Statin therapy and outcome after ischemic stroke: systematic review and meta-analysis of observational studies and randomized trials. Stroke 44(2):448–456
18. Scheitz JF, Seiffge DJ, Tutuncu S, Gensicke H, Audebert HJ, Bonati LH, Fiebach JB, Tranka C, Lyrer PA, Endres M, Engelter ST, Nolte CH (2014) Dose-related effects of statins on symptomatic intracerebral hemorrhage and outcome after thrombolysis for ischemic stroke. Stroke 45(2):509–514
19. Dowlatshahi D, Demchuk AM, Fang J, Kapral MK, Sharma M, Smith EE, Registry of the Canadian Stroke Network (2012) Association of statins and statin discontinuation with poor outcome and survival after intracerebral hemorrhage. Stroke 43(6): 1518–1523
20. Hacke W, Kaste M, Fieschi C, von Kummer R, Davalos A, Meier D, Larrue V, Bluhmki E, Davis S, Donnan G, Schneider D, Diez-Tejedor E, Trouillas P (1998) Randomised double-blind placebo-controlled trial of thrombolytic therapy with intravenous alteplase in acute ischaemic stroke (ECASS II). Second European-Australasian Acute Stroke Study Investigators. Lancet 352(9136): 1245–1251
21. Hacke W, Kaste M, Bluhmki E, Brozman M, Davalos A, Guidetti D, Larrue V, Lees KR, Medeghri Z, Machnig T, Schneider D, von

Kummer R, Wahlgren N, Toni D, Investigators E (2008) Thrombolysis with alteplase 3 to 4.5 hours after acute ischemic stroke. N Engl J Med 359(13):1317–1329
22. Brott T, Adams HP Jr, Olinger CP, Marler JR, Barsan WG, Biller J, Spilker J, Holleran R, Eberle R, Hertzberg V et al (1989) Measurements of acute cerebral infarction: a clinical examination scale. Stroke 20(7):864–870
23. Adams HP Jr, del Zoppo G, Alberts MJ, Bhatt DL, Brass L, Furlan A, Grubb RL, Higashida RT, Jauch EC, Kidwell C, Lyden PD, Morgenstern LB, Qureshi AI, Rosenwasser RH, Scott PA, Wijdicks EF, American Heart Association/American Stroke Association Stroke Council, American Heart Association/American Stroke Association Clinical Cardiology Council, American Heart Association/American Stroke Association Cardiovascular Radiology and Intervention Council, Atherosclerotic Peripheral Vascular Disease Working Group, Quality of Care Outcomes in Research Interdisciplinary Working Group (2007) Guidelines for the early management of adults with ischemic stroke: a guideline from the American Heart Association/American Stroke Association Stroke Council, Clinical Cardiology Council, Cardiovascular Radiology and Intervention Council, and the Atherosclerotic Peripheral Vascular Disease and Quality of Care Outcomes in Research Interdisciplinary Working Groups: The American Academy of Neurology affirms the value of this guideline as an educational tool for neurologists. Circulation 115(20):e478–e534
24. Patkar AA, Hill K, Batra V, Vergare MJ, Leone FT (2003) A comparison of smoking habits among medical and nursing students. Chest 124(4):1415–1420
25. Adams HP Jr, Bendixen BH, Kappelle LJ, Biller J, Love BB, Gordon DL, Marsh EE 3rd (1993) Classification of subtype of acute ischemic stroke. Definitions for use in a multicenter clinical trial. TOAST. Trial of Org 10172 in Acute Stroke Treatment. Stroke 24(1):35–41
26. van Swieten JC, Koudstaal PJ, Visser MC, Schouten HJ, van Gijn J (1988) Interobserver agreement for the assessment of handicap in stroke patients. Stroke 19(5):604–607
27. Elkind MS, Flint AC, Sciacca RR, Sacco RL (2005) Lipid-lowering agent use at ischemic stroke onset is associated with decreased mortality. Neurology 65(2):253–258
28. Sacco RL, Elkind M, Boden-Albala B, Lin IF, Kargman DE, Hauser WA, Shea S, Paik MC (1999) The protective effect of moderate alcohol consumption on ischemic stroke. JAMA 281(1): 53–60
29. Wang S, Lee SR, Guo SZ, Kim WJ, Montaner J, Wang X, Lo EH (2006) Reduction of tissue plasminogen activator-induced matrix metalloproteinase-9 by simvastatin in astrocytes. Stroke 37(7): 1910–1912
30. Zhang L, Zhang ZG, Ding GL, Jiang Q, Liu X, Meng H, Hozeska A, Zhang C, Li L, Morris D, Zhang RL, Lu M, Chopp M (2005) Multitargeted effects of statin-enhanced thrombolytic therapy for stroke with recombinant human tissue-type plasminogen activator in the rat. Circulation 112(22):3486–3494
31. Owens AP 3rd, Passam FH, Antoniak S, Marshall SM, McDaniel AL, Rudel L, Williams JC, Hubbard BK, Dutton JA, Wang J, Tobias PS, Curtiss LK, Daugherty A, Kirchhofer D, Luyendyk JP, Moriarty PM, Nagarajan S, Furie BC, Furie B, Johns DG, Temel RE, Mackman N (2012) Monocyte tissue factor-dependent activation of coagulation in hypercholesterolemic mice and monkeys is inhibited by simvastatin. J Clin Invest 122(2):558–568
32. Laumen H, Skurk T, Hauner H (2008) The HMG-CoA reductase inhibitor rosuvastatin inhibits plasminogen activator inhibitor-1 expression and secretion in human adipocytes. Atherosclerosis 196(2):565–573
33. The National Institute of Neurological Disorders and Stroke rt-PA Stroke Study Group (1995) Tissue plasminogen activator for acute ischemic stroke. N Engl J Med 333(24):1581–1587
34. Kidwell CS, Chalela JA, Saver JL, Starkman S, Hill MD, Demchuk AM, Butman JA, Patronas N, Alger JR, Latour LL, Luby ML, Baird AE, Leary MC, Tremwel M, Ovbiagele B, Fredieu A, Suzuki S, Villablanca JP, Davis S, Dunn B, Todd JW, Ezzeddine MA, Haymore J, Lynch JK, Davis L, Warach S (2004) Comparison of MRI and CT for detection of acute intracerebral hemorrhage. JAMA 292(15):1823–1830
35. Neumann-Haefelin T, Hoelig S, Berkefeld J, Fiehler J, Gass A, Humpich M, Kastrup A, Kucinski T, Lecei O, Liebeskind DS, Rother J, Rosso C, Samson Y, Saver JL, Yan B, Group MRS (2006) Leukoaraiosis is a risk factor for symptomatic intracerebral hemorrhage after thrombolysis for acute stroke. Stroke 37(10):2463–2466

TBI and SBI Section

Decreasing the Cerebral Edema Associated with Traumatic Intracerebral Hemorrhages: Use of a Minimally Invasive Technique

Jeff W. Chen, Michelle R. Paff, Daniella Abrams-Alexandru, and Sean W. Kaloostian

Introduction

Traumatic brain injury (TBI) encompasses a myriad of pathologies, including extra-axial blood clots and intraparenchymal hemorrhages. Whereas there is general agreement on the surgical removal of epidural or subdural hematomas, there is debate on the utility and efficacy of removing traumatic intracerebral hemorrhages (tICHs). This is particularly true of deep-seated subcortical hemorrhages. The argument against surgery is that the traditional craniotomy and dissection through the brain to remove the blood clot leads to further collateral damage. Furthermore, decompressive craniectomies alone may control ICP but do not necessarily address the focal edema around the hemorrhage. Several studies have been done on spontaneous intracerebral hemorrhages (sICH). The STITCH trials did not demonstrate improved outcomes with surgical treatment of the deep subcortical hemorrhages [1, 2]. Other studies using stereotactic minimally invasive techniques have suggested improved outcomes when the hematoma volume is reduced to 15 cc or less [3, 4]. However, it is clear that peri-hematoma edema can lead to increased ICP, dysautoregulation, and cerebral ischemia. Hematoma enlargement typically occurs within the first 12 h and perihematoma edema peaks around 5–6 days after the injury and lasts up to 14 days [5].

The situation with tICH is more complex than that with sICH. In addition to the mass effect and edema from the hemorrhage, there are also the effects of the TBI and any secondary insults such as hypoxia and hypotension. All of these contribute to cerebral edema and ICP issues throughout the entire brain. Thus, removal of the tICH addresses one component of this rather heterogeneous injury. Some have advocated treating TBI with uncontrollable ICP with decompressive craniectomy. Technical aspects have improved to avoid complications such as venous infarcts at the edges of the craniectomy [6, 7]. However, one of the drawbacks is the lack of neurologic improvement and the creation of patients in persistent vegetative states [8, 9]. Mathiesen et al. [10] found that patients with an admission Glasgow Coma Score of at least 6 and a lesion volume of at least 20 ml who had surgery without previous neurological deterioration had significantly better outcomes than those who did not have surgery or had surgery after deterioration. But overall, surgical practice in the treatment of tICH varies widely. The failure of the recent DECRA trial for TBI to demonstrate improved neurologic outcomes has raised the question of whether the decompression that treats the ICP also treats the underlying injury, whether it be from contusions or cerebral edema [11, 12]. There is variation in the types of decompressive craniectomies utilized and reported by neurosurgeons [13, 14]. The typical craniectomy that we employ is depicted in Fig. 1. Note the careful application of the patulous graft to allow a controlled expansion of the brain.

It is our thought that there is a role for the removal of tICH to prevent secondary brain injury from mass effect and cerebral edema. In this retrospective study, we discuss our experience using a minimally invasive tubular technique to reach subcortical tICH. This was done in an abbreviated manner from the Mi Space technique. These modifications were necessary because of patient acuity. These did not impact the overall ability to rapidly and safely remove the tICH.

Presented in Part at the International Symposium of Cerebral Edema
September 27, 2014
Huntington Beach, California

The Authors declare that they have no potential financial conflicts.
Author contributions:
JC: writing and design of article, evaluation of data, critical appraisal of manuscript
MP: Drawing of Fig. 1, critical appraisal of manuscript
DA: Drawing of Fig. 2, critical appraisal of manuscript
SK: design of article, evaluation of data, critical appraisal of manuscript

J.W. Chen (✉) • M.R. Paff • D. Abrams-Alexandru
S.W. Kaloostian
Department of Neurological Surgery,
The University of California, Irvine, CA, USA
e-mail: jeffewc1@uci.edu

R.L. Applegate et al. (eds.), *Brain Edema XVI: Translate Basic Science into Clinical Practice*, Acta Neurochirurgica Supplement, Vol. 121,
DOI 10.1007/978-3-319-18497-5_48, © Springer International Publishing Switzerland 2016

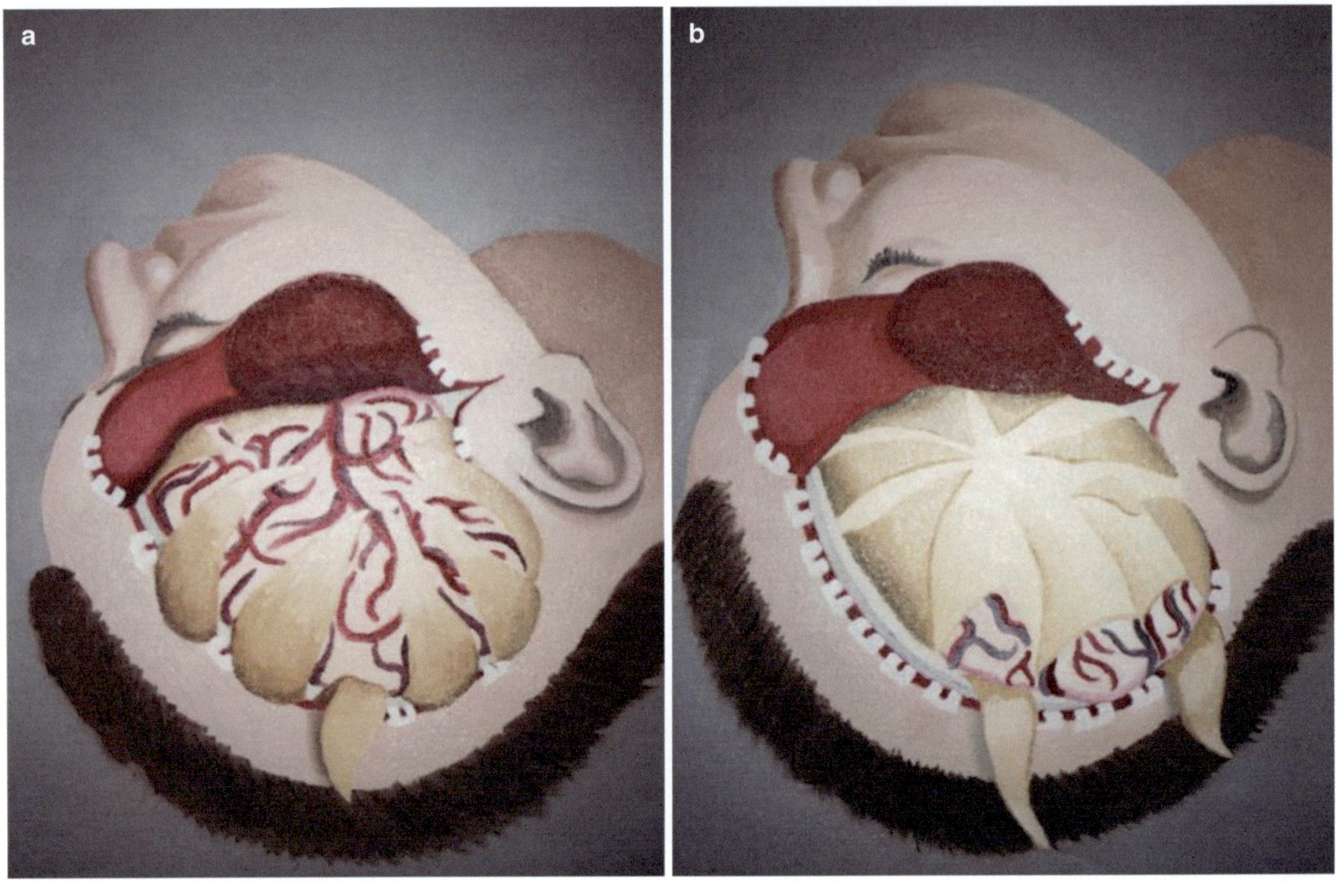

Fig. 1 The traditional decompressive craniectomy. (**a**) Large right-sided fronto-temporal-parietal decompressive craniectomy is done and the bone is removed. Additional bone is removed for the subtemporal decompression. The dura is opened in a stellate fashion to allow the brain to protrude outward. (**b**) A patulous graft is placed (i.e. bovine pericardium) under the leaves of the stellated dura. The leaves of the dura are sutured to the graft to "tent" down the leaves against the patcth. Thus, the brain is allowed to expand out in a controlled manner. Note the prominent veins at the craniectomy edge. The dural patch is designed to prevent pinching of the veins that can exacerbate the situation by leading to venous congestion, increased cerebral edema, and cerebral infarction.

Methods and Materials

We retrospectively reviewed our experience utilizing the modified Mi SPACE technique [15] to treat tICH. The BrainPath access system was used in all cases to reach the hematoma; it is a cylindrical tube with a fixed 13.5 mm diameter with built-in ventilation along the transition point, which allows for existing increased ICP from the bleed to be dissipated during cannulation per Ritsma et al. [15]. This along with the Myriad, a motor-driven instrument that mimics the function of suction and microscissors, are US Food and Drug Administration (FDA)-cleared devices that were obtained from NICO Corp. (Indianapolis, IN, USA). Neuronavigation was performed using the Stryker navigation system (Stryker Corp., Kalamazoo, MI, USA). Visualization was accomplished with the Zeiss Pentaro operating microscope rather than using the Video Telescopic Assisted Microscopy (VTOM) (Storz Corp., Culver City, CA, USA) described as part of the Mi SPACE technique [15].

The craniotomy was performed over the sulcus overlying the tICH. The craniotomy was typically about 3 cm in diameter. A trans-sulcal approach was utilized to reach the epicenter of the blood clot. In planning the trajectory to the clot, the pathway was taken to preserve the surrounding white matter tracks and to follow the long axis of the hemorrhage. Figure 2 depicts the principle of the trans-sulcal approach to reach a deep basal ganglia region hemorrhage. This is a coronal view. The actual trajectory is via a more anterior approach.

The volumes of the tICH were calculated using the axbxc/2 methodology [16, 17]. The Glasgow Outcome Score (GOS) [18] for these patients was reported at 3 months as they had not yet had their 6-month evaluation.

Results

We identified 6 patients with 8 tICHs that were evacuated using the modified Mi SPACE technique during the time period from August 2014 to December 2014 (see Table 1). There were two patients who had two tICHs evacuated via

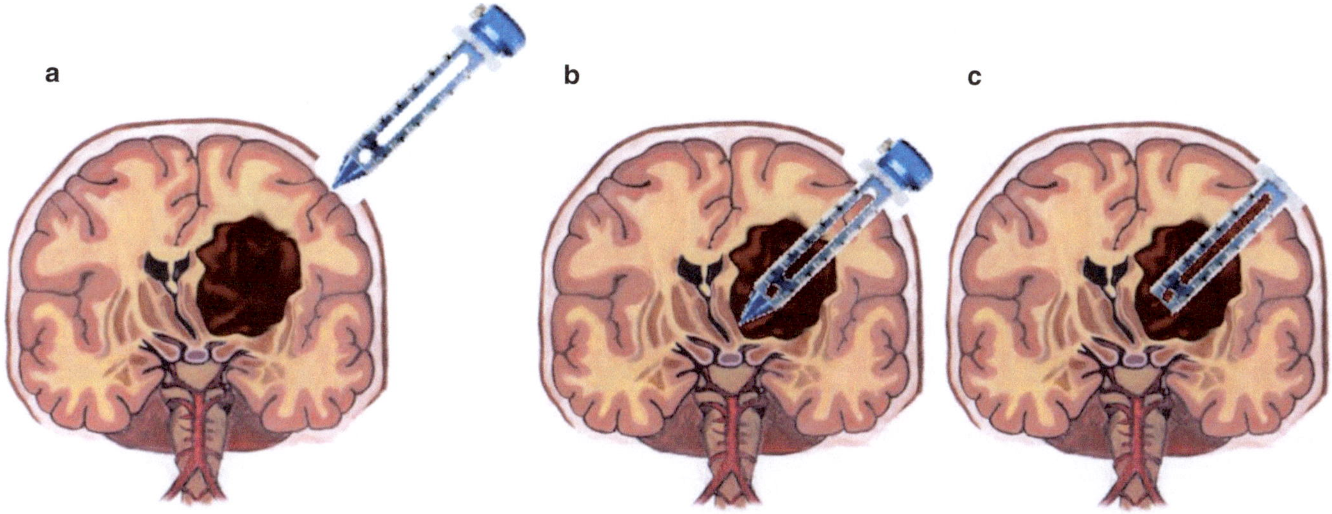

Fig. 2 Use of the trans-sulcal BrainPath approach to deep subcortical hemorrhages. Diagram depicting the trans-sulcal BrainPath approach to the deep seated hemorrhage (**a**). The trajectory is selected to follow the long axis of the ICH. For a basal ganglia region hemorrhage, an approach anterior to the coronal suture that angles back is effective in reaching the epicenter (**b**). Once the sheath is docked (**c**) in position, the tICH frequently delivers itself because of the surrounding increased ICP. It may also be aspirated out using the NICO Myriad aspirator that has a specially designed foot pedal that allows fine regulation of the aspiration force

Table 1 Characteristics of patients undergoing BrainPath evacuation of tICH

Patient #	Age (years)	Gender	Mechanism of injury	Coagulopathy	Location	Volume (ml)	GCS	GOS	Time to BrainPath
1	26	M	Assault	N	R subfrontal	19			3 days
					L subfrontal	27	4 T	3	
2	41	M	Fall	Y: renal failure	Bifrontal intraventricular	165	3 T	5	18 h
3	54	F	Fall	Y: ETOH liver	R frontal	25	4 T	2	3 days
					R temporal	32			
4	55	M	Peds vs. motor vehicle	N	L temporal	38	11 T	3	3 days
5	57	F	Fall	Y: ETOH liver	R frontal	85	11 T	5	3 h
6	65	M	High-speed MVC	N	Left BG	56	7 T	5	2 h

This table summarizes the characteristics of the patients who underwent evacuation of tICH using the BrainPath technique. The best GCS after the initial stabilization and prior to the tICH evacuation is noted. The Glasgow Outcome Score (GOS) was done at 3 months as the 3 surviving patients are awaiting their 6-month follow-up. The $a \times b \times c/2$ method was used to approximate the volume of the tICH as described in *Materials and Methods*. Patients 2, 5, and 6 underwent BrainPath evacuation of the tICH acutely (<24 h) because of the large mass effect and neurological deterioration. Patient 2 improved to GCS = 6 T and expired 10 days later because of multisystem organ failure. Patient 5 improved to GCS = 11 T but expired 14 days later after a cardio-pulmonary arrest during the ventilator wean. Patient 6 underwent urgent decompression of a large traumatic BG (basal ganglia) hemorrhage that evolved during the initial resuscitation. This surgery was done without the use of Stryker neuronavigation. The delay for patients 1, 3, and 4 was due to treatment of ICPs with other modalities (i.e., ventriculostomy, hyperosmolar therapy). Patient 3 had a right-sided decompressive craniectomy and other ICP-lowering therapies prior to the BrainPath evacuation of the tICH (see Fig. 3)

two separate mini-craniotomies because the clots were in different lobes or different hemispheres of the brain. All of the hemorrhages were supratentorial and located as follows: right frontal-basal ganglia region = 3, right temporal = 1, left temporal = 1, bilateral ventricles = 1, right subfrontal = 1, left subfrontal = 1. The age range was 26–65. The mean age was 50. The male-to-female ratio was 2:1. Mechanisms of injury were as follows: motor vehicle related = 2, falls = 3, assault = 1. Seven out of eight hemorrhages were evacuated with the use of the Stryker neuronavigation system; one was evacuated based on anatomical landmarks because there was not sufficient time to organize the navigation scan and system as the patient had an evolving tICH with rapidly increasing ICP after a high-speed motor vehicle collision. One

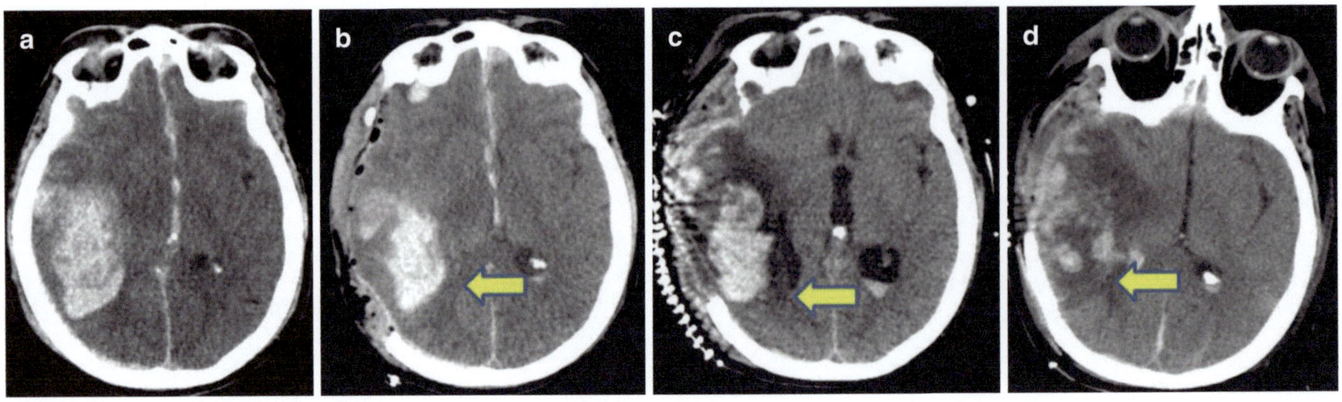

Fig. 3 Large subcortical traumatic intracerebral hemorrhage (tICH) treated first with decompressive craniectomy then with the BrainPath subcortical removal technique. Evolution of the cerebral edema around a tICH. This patient suffered a ground level fall and had a coagulopathy from alcohol. The initial CT scan demonstrated the large right temporal tICH and the patient had a declining Glascow Coma Score (GCS) of 5 (**a**). She underwent urgent right-sided decompressive craniectomy and her postoperative scan on postoperative day #1 is seen in (**b**). The *arrow* is pointing to the zone of edema extending into the white matter tracks. This edema increases on postoperative day 3 (*arrow* **c**) to involve the white matter tracks. Because of the increased edema and trapping of the ventricles as well as increased ICP and decline in wakefulness, the patient underwent evacuation of the tICH via the Mi SPACE technique. Her immediate postoperative CT scan is seen in (**d**). The zone of edema is less pronounced but still present. At 3 months, the patient made an excellent recovery and was independent with activities of daily living

patient had previously undergone a decompressive craniectomy for the tICH (see Fig. 3).

Discussions

Numerous animal and human studies have demonstrated that the reaction of the brain to an ICH leads to edema, mass effect, and ischemic brain damage [19–21]. In addition to the compression and mass effect, there is also the effect of the breakdown products of the hemorrhage, including iron, which is a neurotoxin [22]. sICH has been studied extensively and, to date, the surgical treatment of the deep subcortical sICHs continues to be debated [2, 23]. Siddique et al. [24] examined their experience with both sICH and tICH and found that, although there were different demographics and outcomes, the role and influence of surgery on both types of ICH was poorly defined. The STICH trial for sICH suggested a slight benefit for the evacuation of superficial hemorrhages [1, 2]. The results from a randomized trial for the surgical treatment of tICH has not been published to date [25, 26].

Patients with tICH have edema from the TBI as well as that incited by the hematoma. As such, the brain is more sensitive to any manipulation and outcomes are poor. There is a reluctance to operate on these unless there are signs of neurological compromise or there are ICP problems. Francis et al. [27] found, in 76 % of neurosurgeons surveyed, that ICP was routinely monitored in patients with tICH. Additionally, the clear preference for treatment was via a ventriculostomy and mannitol. The use of the BrainPath technique to reach a subcortical tICH necessitates the passage of the 13-mm-diameter tube through brain that has already been traumatized by the TBI. A concern about increasing the trauma to the brain and worsening the edema is legitimate.

One of the key principles of the Mi SPACE technique with the BrainPath cannula and sheath is using a stereotactic-guided approach to select a trajectory to the target that spares the white matter tracks and fibers [15]. By traveling along a pathway that is parallel to the key fiber tracks rather than perpendicular, trauma is decreased because there is less division of the fibers. By targeting the epicenter of the tICH, the working port is "protected" by the surrounding clot, which delivers itself with little manipulation because the surrounding edematous white matter serves to drive the clot out the BrainPath sheath. We routinely used the NICO Myriad aspirator, which has a controlled suction device with a side port. This allows one to dissect with the tip of the aspirator and at the same time protect the white matter. This is in contrast to the traditional fluted suction system, which is open at the tip. Another key principle of the Mi SPACE technique is the use of an articulated Mitaka arm (Mitaka USA, Inc., Park City, UT, USA) combined with the VIATOM light and visualization source (Storz Corp., Culver City, CA, USA). We did not use this but found instead that the standard operating room microscope was quite adequate. This did not have the improved ergonomics or degrees of freedom afforded by the Mitaka, particularly for parietal or occipital approaches. Nonetheless, the operating room microscope was more familiar to the hospital staff and was easily and rapidly deployed. This was particularly important during the weekend and night shifts.

Our series is small and preliminary. However, we do demonstrate that the principles of the Mi SPACE methodology

[15] may be used with tICH. With all eight tICHs we found that we were able to achieve >90 % removal of the tICH by targeting the epicenter. However, as seen in Fig. 3, there are small contusions in the surrounding brain that are best left alone. Attempting to remove all of these would result in surrounding damage to the adjacent white matter tracks. There were no rebleeds into the clot bed after the evacuation of the tICH. This was the case even in those patients with a chronic coagulopathy (patients # 2, 3, 5). The fact that the surrounding brain was generally swollen and edematous may have helped to tamponade any potential bleeding.

The timing of the surgery may affect the outcome. Patients 1, 3, and 4 had their BrainPath surgeries 3 days after the trauma. This allowed us to perform these surgeries in a more controlled manner and to optimize medical factors. The question is whether earlier surgery decreases the brain ischemia and edema. Figure 3 demonstrates the progression of the cerebral edema around the tICH despite the decompressive craniectomy that was done first. The cerebral edema is likely the result of both the ischemia from the compression as well as the edema generated from the blood break-down products [22, 28]. Although patients 2 and 5 expired, they actually made reasonable neurological recoveries before dying of other organ dysfunctions. We were able to treat patients with a wide range of hemorrhage volumes. Generally, patients with tICHs that were <50 ml had better outcomes.

Conclusions

We introduce the concept of using a minimally invasive approach for the evacuation of tICH. This has the advantage of targeting the epicenter of the clot and minimizing damage to the surrounding white matter tracks by respecting the directionality of these tracks. This may be effectively and safely deployed in a rapid manner. The removal of the tICH may decrease cerebral edema by decreasing the local mass effect and response to the breakdown products of the hemorrhage. Further studies need to be done to determine the optimum time for surgery as well as the optimal use of other edema-lowering measures after the BrainPath procedure.

References

1. Mendelow AD, Gregson BA, Fernandes HM et al (2005) Early surgery versus initial conservative treatment in patients with spontaneous supratentorial intracerebral haematomas in the International Surgical Trial in Intracerebral Haemorrhage (STICH): a randomised trial. Lancet 365:387–397
2. Mendelow AD, Unterberg A (2007) Surgical treatment of intracerebral haemorrhage. Curr Opin Crit Care 13:169–174
3. Barnes B, Hanley DF, Carhuapoma JR (2014) Minimally invasive surgery for intracerebral haemorrhage. Curr Opin Crit Care 20: 148–152
4. Morgan T, Zuccarello M, Narayan R, Keyl P, Lane K, Hanley D (2008) Preliminary findings of the minimally-invasive surgery plus rtPA for intracerebral hemorrhage evacuation (MISTIE) clinical trial. Acta Neurochir Suppl 105:147–151
5. Monteith SJ, Harnof S, Medel R et al (2013) Minimally invasive treatment of intracerebral hemorrhage with magnetic resonance-guided focused ultrasound. J Neurosurg 118:1035–1045
6. Huang X, Wen L (2010) Technical considerations in decompressive craniectomy in the treatment of traumatic brain injury. Int J Med Sci 7:385–390
7. Chibbaro S, Di Rocco F, Mirone G et al (2011) Decompressive craniectomy and early cranioplasty for the management of severe head injury: a prospective multicenter study on 147 patients. World Neurosurg 75:558–562
8. Ahmad FU, Bullock R (2011) Decompressive craniectomy for severe head injury. World Neurosurg 75:451–453
9. Lund-Johansen M (2011) Decompressive craniectomy for traumatic brain injury-when and how? World Neurosurg 75: 454–455
10. Mathiesen T, Benediktsdottir K, Johnsson H, Lindqvist M, von Holst H (1995) Intracranial traumatic and non-traumatic haemorrhagic complications of warfarin treatment. Acta Neurol Scand 91:208–214
11. Chi JH (2011) Craniectomy for traumatic brain injury: results from the DECRA trial. Neurosurgery 68:N19–N20
12. Cooper DJ, Rosenfeld JV, Murray L et al (2011) Decompressive craniectomy in diffuse traumatic brain injury. N Engl J Med 364:1493–1502
13. Bor-Seng-Shu E, Figueiredo EG, Amorim RL et al (2012) Decompressive craniectomy: a meta-analysis of influences on intracranial pressure and cerebral perfusion pressure in the treatment of traumatic brain injury. J Neurosurg 117:589–596
14. Sahuquillo J, Martinez-Ricarte F, Poca MA (2013) Decompressive craniectomy in traumatic brain injury after the DECRA trial. Where do we stand? Curr Opin Crit Care 19:101–106
15. Ritsma B, Kassam A, Dowlatshahi D, Nguyen T, Stotts G (2014) Minimally invasive subcortical parafascicular transsulcal access for clot evacuation (Mi SPACE) for intracerebral hemorrhage. Case Rep Neurol Med 2014:102307
16. Broderick JP, Brott TG, Duldner JE, Tomsick T, Huster G (1993) Volume of intracerebral hemorrhage. A powerful and easy-to-use predictor of 30-day mortality. Stroke 24:987–993
17. Newman GC (2007) Clarification of abc/2 rule for ICH volume. Stroke 38:862
18. Jennett B, Snoek J, Bond MR, Brooks N (1981) Disability after severe head injury: observations on the use of the Glasgow Outcome Scale. J Neurol Neurosurg Psychiatry 44: 285–293
19. Inaji M, Tomita H, Tone O, Tamaki M, Suzuki R, Ohno K (2003) Chronological changes of perihematomal edema of human intracerebral hematoma. Acta Neurochir Suppl 86:445–448
20. Siddique MS, Fernandes HM, Wooldridge TD, Fenwick JD, Slomka P, Mendelow AD (2002) Reversible ischemia around intracerebral hemorrhage: a single-photon emission computerized tomography study. J Neurosurg 96:736–741
21. Butcher KS, Baird T, MacGregor L, Desmond P, Tress B, Davis S (2004) Perihematomal edema in primary intracerebral hemorrhage is plasma derived. Stroke 35:1879–1885
22. Xi G, Keep RF, Hoff JT (2006) Mechanisms of brain injury after intracerebral haemorrhage. Lancet Neurol 5:53–63
23. Mitchell P, Gregson BA, Vindlacheruvu RR, Mendelow AD (2007) Surgical options in ICH including decompressive craniectomy. J Neurol Sci 261:89–98

24. Siddique MS, Gregson BA, Fernandes HM et al (2002) Comparative study of traumatic and spontaneous intracerebral hemorrhage. J Neurosurg 96:86–89
25. Francis R, Rowan EN, Gregson BA, Mendelow AD (2011) Traumatic intracerebral hemorrhage–to operate or not? World Neurosurg 76:484–485
26. Gregson BA, Rowan EN, Mitchell PM et al (2012) Surgical trial in traumatic intracerebral hemorrhage (STITCH(Trauma)): study protocol for a randomized controlled trial. Trials 13:193
27. Francis R, Gregson BA, Mendelow AD (2014) Attitudes to intracranial pressure monitoring of traumatic intracerebral haemorrhage. Br J Neurosurg 28:663–665
28. Keep RF, Hua Y, Xi G (2012) Intracerebral haemorrhage: mechanisms of injury and therapeutic targets. Lancet Neurol 11: 720–731

Reduction of Cerebral Edema via an Osmotic Transport Device Improves Functional Outcome after Traumatic Brain Injury in Mice

Devin W. McBride, Virginia Donovan, Mike S. Hsu, Andre Obenaus, V.G.J. Rodgers, and Devin K. Binder

Introduction

Traumatic brain injury (TBI) is the foremost cause of morbidity and mortality in persons under 45 years of age worldwide. Approximately 200,000 TBI victims in the United States require hospitalization annually, resulting in about 52,000 deaths [13]. TBI has a primary injury phase, caused by the direct external mechanical force, and a secondary injury phase, caused by a myriad of delayed deleterious physiological events. Secondary injury, characterized by cerebral edema, is a major contributor to the morbidity and mortality after TBI [10]. Cerebral edema, an increase in brain tissue water content, is classically identified as either vasogenic edema, water accumulation in the extracellular space after blood-brain barrier (BBB) disruption, or cytotoxic edema, intracellular water accumulation [10, 13].

Cerebral edema resulting from TBI includes both cytotoxic and vasogenic edema mechanisms. After TBI, glial cells swell due to shifts in the extracellular pH and ion concentrations, such as potassium, sodium, and chloride [10]. Vasogenic edema, caused by direct BBB injury, combines with the resulting cytotoxic edema. Ultimately, both types of edema cause a vicious cycle that can culminate in uncontrollable brain swelling, resulting in permanent brain damage or death.

In recent years, advances in diagnostic imaging allow for treatment and surgical intervention of severe brain edema to be performed more rapidly following TBI [3]. Severe TBI management requires a combinatorial approach of surgeries and therapies including osmotherapy, ventriculostomy, and decompressive craniectomy. Although these three treatments are standard practice for severe brain edema, even combinations of them may have limited success in treating patients [5, 16, 18]. Osmotherapy may be effective at acutely reducing intracranial pressure (ICP), but its disadvantages are clinical variability, transient duration of its effects, and possible deleterious systemic effects [2, 4, 8, 11, 17]. Ventriculostomy alone is often ineffective at reducing brain edema because removing the total volume of cerebrospinal fluid (CSF), approximately 150 ml for adults, only accounts for about 10 % of brain volume. Performing decompressive craniectomy surgery for severe TBI reduces ICP elevations, however, it does not treat cerebral edema directly. Recently, the therapeutic benefits of decompressive craniectomy have been debated; the DECRA trial results suggest that performing a decompressive craniectomy for diffuse TBI may not alter patient outcomes [5].

The ideal treatment for severe cerebral edema should be capable of directly removing water from injured tissue in a controlled manner that does cause harm to healthy tissue. An osmotic transport device (OTD) is one such intervention that directly extracts water from brain tissue via direct osmotherapy. We have developed an OTD using a hollow-fiber membrane module embedded in a hydratable material for osmotic therapy. Treatment by direct osmotherapy requires direct contact with the injured, edematous tissue for water extraction. An OTD was recently shown to enhance survival rate of water intoxicated mice [14] and reduce brain water

D.W. McBride
Department of Physiology and Pharmacology, Loma Linda University School of Medicine, Loma Linda, CA, USA

V. Donovan
Cell, Molecular and Developmental Biology Program, University of California, Riverside, CA, USA

M.S. Hsu • D.K. Binder, MD, PhD (✉)
Division of Biomedical Sciences, School of Medicine, University of California, 1247 Webber Hall, Riverside, CA 92521, USA
e-mail: dbinder@ucr.edu

A. Obenaus
Cell, Molecular and Developmental Biology Program, University of California, Riverside, CA, USA

Department of Pediatrics, Loma Linda University School of Medicine, Loma Linda, CA, USA

V.G.J. Rodgers
Department of Bioengineering, University of California, Riverside, CA, USA

R.L. Applegate et al. (eds.), *Brain Edema XVI: Translate Basic Science into Clinical Practice*, Acta Neurochirurgica Supplement, Vol. 121,
DOI 10.1007/978-3-319-18497-5_49,

content in mice after TBI [15]. The purpose of this study was to evaluate the effect of direct osmotherapy using an OTD for improving neurobehavior in mice after TBI.

Materials and Methods

All experiments were approved by the Institutional Animal Care and Use Committee (IACUC) at Loma Linda University. Adult female C57/BL6 mice, 10–12 weeks old, were used in all experiments.

Traumatic Brain Injury Model

Animals were anesthetized with 3 % isoflurane in O_2 (2.5 l/min initial, 1.5 l/min sustained). Anesthetized animals were placed into a standard rodent stereotactic frame, a midline skin incision was made, and a right-sided craniectomy (5 mm diameter) was performed (1 mm posterior to the bregma and 1 mm lateral to midline). TBI was induced via controlled cortical impact. Briefly, a 3-mm impactor tip was discharged at a 20° angle with a velocity of 5.0 m/s, a 200 ms dwell time, and an impact depth of 1.5 mm. After TBI, the craniectomy was left open, the skin was sutured, and the animal was allowed to recover.

Treatment

One day following TBI, animals were anesthetized with 3 % isoflurane in O_2 (2.5 l/min initial, 1.5 l/min sustained). Sutures were removed to expose the injury site. One group of animals ($n=3$) continued to be treated with a craniectomy for 2 more hours (craniectomy lasted 26 h in total). The other group of animals ($n=3$) was treated with a craniectomy and an OTD for 2 h (craniectomy for 24 h followed by 2 h of craniectomy plus OTD). After 2 h treatment, the craniectomy was sealed with bone wax, skin was sutured, and the animal was allowed to recover.

OTD treatment was previously described [14, 15]. Briefly, the lumen solution (350 g/l bovine serum albumin in artificial CSF at pH 7.4) was passed through hollow fibers (regenerated cellulose, 13 kDa molecular weight cut-off; Spectrum Laboratories, Inc., Rancho Dominguez, CA, USA) embedded in an agar hydrogel (0.3 % agar in artificial CSF, pH 7.4) with a Reynolds number between 50 and 100.

Neurobehavior Testing

One day before surgical procedures, all animals were subjected to neurobehavioral testing. The foot fault test was used to evaluate sensorimotor response and proprioception. The beam balance test was used to evaluate proprioception and balance. Animals were also subjected to post-TBI neurobehavior testing 1 day after treatment (2 days post TBI). Additionally, naïve animals ($n=6$) were subjected to the neurobehavior tests.

A rectangular grid (3 ft×1 ft, 0.6 in grid spacing, 7.5° from horizontal) was used for the foot fault test. Each animal was allowed to freely move on the grid for 60 s per trial and a total of two trials (30 min between each trial). Each trial was video recorded for post-test analysis. A foot fault was defined as the misplacement of a fore or hind limb, such that the paw fell completely through the bars. The number of hind limb foot faults per active time were analyzed by an investigator blinded to experimental conditions. Active time was defined as the time spent exploring the grid. Number of hind limb foot faults per active time is presented as the mean ± standard error of the mean (SEM). Intergroup comparisons were analyzed using one-way analysis of variance (ANOVA) with Tukey post hoc tests.

The beam balance test used a Plexiglas beam (2 ft×0.2 in, 2 ft tall) to measure the time to fall, distance traveled, and number of turns. The animals were placed perpendicular to the beam in the center. Each animal was allowed to walk unrestricted in either direction for up to 60 s per trial (time to fall or 60 s, whichever came first) and a total of two trials (30 min between each trial). Each trial was video recorded for post-test analysis. The time to fall (s), distance traveled (recorded in 5 cm ticks), and number of turns (left, right, total) were analyzed by an investigator blinded to experimental conditions. The time to fall data for each trial was included in the analysis. The average distance traveled (between the two trials) was normalized to the average distance traveled in the pretest performance (pre-injury). The average number of turns was normalized to the average number of turns in the pretest performance for the number of left, right, and total turns. Each measure is presented as the mean ± SEM. Intergroup comparisons were analyzed using one-way ANOVA with Tukey post hoc tests for time to fall and ANOVA on ranks for normalized distance traveled and normalized number of turns (left, right, and total turns analyzed independently).

Results

Foot Fault Test

Naïve animals (Naïve, $n=6$) performing the foot fault test were able to traverse the grid having only 0.08 ± 0.018 hind limb foot faults per second. Injured animals treated with only a craniectomy (TBI+C, $n=3$) had a significantly higher number of hind limb foot faults per second (0.55 ± 0.294) compared with those of naïve animals ($p<0.05$). When TBI-injured animals are treated with a craniectomy and an OTD (TBI+C+OTD, $n=3$), the number of hind limb foot faults per second (0.19±0.038) were reduced to a level comparable to those of naïve animals ($p>0.05$) but not statistically different from injured animals treated with craniectomy only ($p>0.05$) (Fig. 1).

Beam Balance Test

Naïve animals (Naïve, $n=6$) subjected to the beam balance test were all able to walk on the beam for the entire time allotted, so the time to fall was 60±0.0 s. However, injured animals treated with a craniectomy only (TBI+C, $n=3$) had more difficulty remaining on the beam (time to fall: 43±10.6 s); time to fall for injured animals treated with a craniectomy only was significantly lower than that of naïve animals ($p<0.05$). Treatment with a craniectomy plus an OTD (TBI+C+OTD) improved their proprioception (no animals fell, time to fall: 60±0.0 s) to that of the naïve group ($p>0.05$) (Fig. 2a).

In the 60 s given to naïve animals for walking on the beam, the distance traveled was 115±65 cm. When normalized to the baseline distance traveled for each animal, the naïve group had a normalized distance traveled of 1.0±0.08. Injured animals treated with a craniectomy only had a significantly lower normalized distance traveled (0.5±0.12) compared with naïve animals ($p<0.05$). But when injured animals are treated with a craniectomy and an OTD, the normalized distance traveled (1.2±0.25) was significantly higher than injured animals treated with only a craniectomy ($p<0.05$) and indistinguishable from naïve animals ($p>0.05$) (Fig. 2b).

The number of turns, normalized to naïve values, for the naïve animals were 1.0±0.26, 1.0±0.21, and 1.0±0.13 for the left, right, and total turns, respectively. Normalized number of turns for injured animals treated with a craniectomy only were 0.0±0.00, 0.3±0.16, and 0.2±0.11 for the left, right, and total turns, respectively. Normalized number of turns for injured animals treated with a craniectomy only were 1.0±0.58, 0.3±0.33, and 0.4±0.29 for the left, right, and total turns, respectively. Statistical significance was observed between the normalized number of turns for naïve animals and injured animals treated with craniectomy only for left and total turns ($p<0.05$). All other intergroup comparisons were not statistically significant ($p>0.05$) (Fig. 2c).

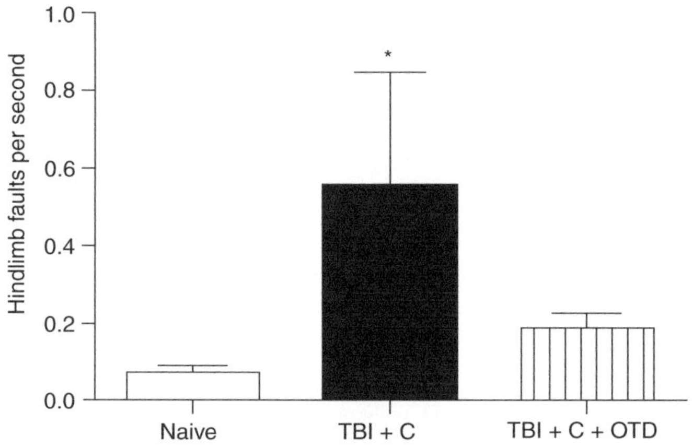

Fig. 1 Hind limb foot faults per second. Injured animals treated with a craniectomy only (*TBI+C*) have significantly more hind limb foot faults per second than naïve animals (Naïve). Injured animals treated with a craniectomy plus OTD (*TBI+C+OTD*) have a reduced number of hind limb foot faults per second, such that the foot faults are comparable (not statistically significant) to the number of foot faults per second by naïve animals. * $p<0.05$ vs Naïve

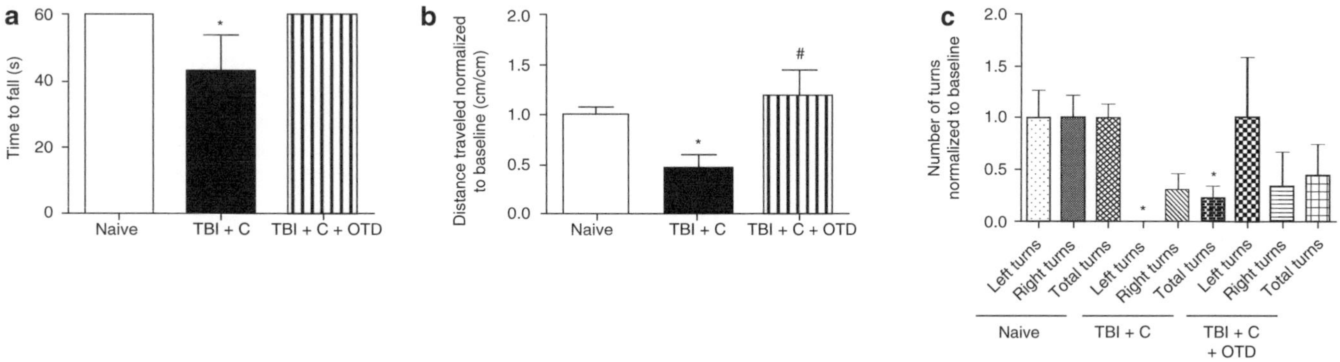

Fig. 2 Beam balance test. (**a**) Time to fall (s) was significantly lower for injured animals treated with a craniectomy (*TBI+C*) compared with naïve animals (Naïve). Injured animals treated with a craniectomy plus OTD (*TBI+C+OTD*) had a time to fall similar to naïve animals. (**b**) Distance traveled (normalized to the pretest baseline distance traveled, cm/cm) was significantly reduced in injured animals treated with a craniectomy only (*TBI+C*) compared with naïve animals. Treatment with a craniectomy plus OTD (*TBI+C+OTD*) significantly improved the distance traveled compared with animals treated with a craniectomy only. (**c**) Number of turns (normalized to the pretest baseline values) was significantly reduced in injured animals treated with a craniectomy only (*TBI+C*) for the number of left and total turns. Injured animals treated with a craniectomy plus OTD (*TBI+C+OTD*) improved the number of turns such that no significant difference was observed between naïve animals for the number of left and total turns. No difference was observed between the numbers of right turns between any of the groups. * $p<0.05$ vs Naïve, # $p<0.05$ vs TBI+C

Discussion

The effect of craniectomy treatment for severe TBI on patient outcomes has been debated. Experimental evidence for the therapeutic benefits, including functional recovery, for craniectomy treatment of severe TBI in animal models has been thoroughly examined and primarily indicates that craniectomy is neuroprotective [6, 20]. However, the study by Floyd et al. [6] examined the effect of craniectomy position and found that slight differences in the position of the craniectomy can produce changes in cognitive performance in a rat TBI model. The results of Floyd et al. were mimicked in the study by Lee et al. [12], which also observed a correlation between the location of craniectomy and functional recovery. Clinical reports are also inconsistent on the effect of craniectomy and patient outcome; whereas several reports observed improved patient outcome after decompressive craniectomy [1, 9, 19], the HeADDFIRST [7] and DECRA [5] clinical trials found conflicting and/or inconclusive results of craniectomy treatment on patient outcome. While we wait for the results of the RESCUEicp trial, the need for a treatment of cerebral edema remains of the utmost importance. An OTD has been shown to improve survival rates of water intoxicated mice [14] and reduce brain edema in mice with TBI [15]. Herein, we hypothesized that direct osmotherapy via an OTD is more neuroprotective than craniectomy alone, improving functional outcomes after TBI in mice.

The neurological function of mice after TBI was examined via testing of sensorimotor, proprioception, and balance. The foot fault test found TBI to be associated with functional deficits in the hind limbs of injured animals treated with a craniectomy only compared with those of naïve animals. When injured animals are treated with a craniectomy and an OTD, the number of hind limb faults decreased such that it was not statistically different from the naïve animals. The beam balance test identified that TBI was associated with balance (time to fall) and motor deficits (reduced distance traveled and turning) in animals treated with a craniectomy only compared with naïve animals. When injured animals are treated with a craniectomy plus an OTD, balance is improved and motor deficits are reduced. These tests supported our hypothesis that craniectomy plus OTD (combined therapy) improves functional outcome better than craniectomy alone and further support the therapeutic benefits of direct osmotherapy.

Although the efficacy of surgical decompressive craniectomy for brain swelling treatment is debated [5], in the most severe cases of cerebral edema it is still performed because it reduces elevated ICP to prevent to occurrence of transtentorial herniation. However, decompressive craniectomy does not directly treat cerebral edema. Yet, direct osmotherapy via an OTD is capable of direct water removal and reduction of brain swelling [15]. The combination of a craniectomy and an OTD is more advantageous than a craniectomy only inasmuch as, not only will ICP be reduced, but water will be directly removed from edematous tissue.

In conclusion, a craniectomy plus an OTD is capable of providing more functional recovery compared with craniectomy alone. Future studies are needed to examine the effect of the craniectomy plus OTD treatment on long-term functional recovery, including sensorimotor, anxiety, and memory neurobehavior tests.

Acknowledgments This work was supported by National Institutes of Health K08 grant NS-059674 (DKB). Devin McBride was supported by a National Science Foundation IGERT Video Bioinformatics Fellowship (Grant DGE 0903667).

Disclosure This device and its applications are described in a patent application titled Compositions and Methods for Reducing Edema (# 20,130,115,267) submitted by the authors and the University of California, Riverside on November 1, 2012. There is no commercial support at this time. The authors have no conflicts of interest to report.

References

1. Adamo MA, Drazin D, Waldman JB (2009) Decompressive craniectomy and postoperative complication management in infants and toddlers with severe traumatic brain injuries. J Neurosurg Pediatr 3:334–339
2. Bingaman WE, Frank JI (1995) Malignant cerebral edema and intracranial hypertension. Neurol Crit Care 13:479–509
3. Bullock MR, Povlishock JT, Carney NA, Ghajar J, Bratton SL, Chestnut RM, McConnell Hammond FF, Harris OA, Hartl R, Manley GT, Nemecek A, Newell DW, Rosenthal G, Schouten J, Shutter L, Timmons SD, Ullman JS, Videtta W, Wilberger JE, Wright DW (2007) Guidelines for the management of severe traumatic brain injury. J Neurotrauma 24:S1–S106
4. Castillo LB, Bugedo GA, Paranhos JL (2009) Mannitol or hypertonic saline for intracranial hypertension? A point of view. Crit Care Resusc 11:151–154
5. Cooper DJ, Rosenfeld JV, Murray L, Arabi YM, Davies AR, D'Urso P, Kossman T, Ponsford J, Seppelt I, Reilly P, Wolfe R, DECRA Trial Investigators, Australian and New Zealand Intensive Care Society Clinical Trials Group (2011) Decompressive craniectomy in diffuse traumatic brain injury. N Engl J Med 364:1493–1502
6. Floyd CL, Golden KM, Black RT, Hamm RJ, Lyeth BG (2002) Craniectomy position affects Morris water maze performance and hippocampal cell loss after parasagittal fluid percussion. J Neurotrauma 19:303–316
7. Frank JI, Schumm LP, Wroblewski K, Chyatte D, Rosengart AJ, Kordeck C, Thisted RA (2014) Hemicraniectomy and durotomy upon deterioration from infarction-related swelling trial: randomized pilot clinical trial. Stroke 45:781–787
8. Hariri RJ (1994) Cerebral edema. Neurosurg Clin N Am 5:687–706
9. Howard JL, Cipolle MD, Anderson M, Sabella V, Shollenberger D, Li PM, Pasquale MD (2008) Outcome after decompressive craniectomy for the treatment of severe traumatic brain injury. J Trauma 65:380–385; discussion 385–386

10. Kettenmann H, Ransom BR (2005) Neuroglia. Oxford University Press, London
11. Keyrouz SG, Dhar R, Diringer MN (2008) Variation in osmotic response to sustained mannitol administration. Neurocrit Care 9:204–209
12. Lee DH, Hong SH, Kim SK, Lee CS, Phi JH, Cho BK, Wang KC (2009) Reproducible and persistent weakness in adult rats after surgical resection of motor cortex: evaluation with limb placement test. Childs Nerv Syst 25:1547–1553
13. Marmarou A (2003) Pathophysiology of traumatic brain edema: current concepts. Acta Neurochir Suppl 86:7–10
14. McBride DW, Hsu MS, Rodgers VGJ, Binder DK (2012) Improved survival following cerebral edema using a novel hollow fiber-hydrogel device. J Neurosurg 116:1389–1394
15. McBride DW, Szu JI, Hale C, Hsu MS, Rodgers VGJ, Binder DK (2014) Reduction of cerebral edema after traumatic brain injury using an osmotic transport device. J Neurotrauma 31:1948–1954
16. Rabinstein AA (2006) Treatment of cerebral edema. Neurologist 12:59–73
17. Suarez JI, Qureshi AI, Bhardwaj A, Williams MA, Schnitzer MS, Mirski M, Hanley DF, Ulatowski JA (1998) Treatment of refractory intracranial hypertension with 23.4% saline. Crit Care Med 26:1118–1122
18. Timofeev I, Dahyot-Fizelier C, Keong N, Norje J, Al-Rawi PG, Czosnyka M, Menon DK, Kirkpatrick PJ, Gupta AK, Hutchinson PJ (2009) Ventriculostomy for control of raised ICP in acute traumatic brain injury. Acta Neurochir Suppl 102:99–104
19. Vahedi K, Vicaut E, Mateo J, Kurtz A, Orabi M, Guichard JP, Boutron C, Couvreur G, Rouanet F, Touze E, Guillon B, Carpentier A, Yelnik A, George B, Payen D, Bousser MG (2007) Sequential-design, multicenter, randomized, controlled trial of early decompressive craniectomy in malignant middle cerebral artery infarction (DECIMAL Trial). Stroke 38:2506–2517
20. Zweckberger K, Stoffel M, Baethmann A, Plesnila N (2003) Effect of decompression craniotomy on increase of contusion volume and functional outcome after controlled cortical impact in mice. J Neurotrauma 20:1307–1314

Deferoxamine Attenuated the Upregulation of Lipocalin-2 Induced by Traumatic Brain Injury in Rats

Jinbing Zhao, Guohua Xi, Gang Wu, Richard F. Keep, and Ya Hua

Introduction

Traumatic brain injury (TBI) is one of the main causes of morbidity and mortality in adolescents and children. Intracranial bleeding is a common consequence of TBI. Thus, 56 % of TBI patients had at least one intracranial bleed according to one report [11]. Our previous studies in intracerebral hemorrhage (ICH) and subarachnoid hemorrhage (SAH) demonstrated that iron and iron-handling proteins were elevated [8, 10, 15, 17], indicating enhanced iron accumulation after hemorrhage in the brain.

Lipocalin-2 (LCN-2) is a member of the lipocalin family, which is a group of secreted proteins that can bind and transport a wide variety of small hydrophobic molecules [7]. LCN-2 is a 25 kDa protein associated with gelatinase/MMP9 from human neutrophils, and is also known as 24p3 (mouse homolog) and neutrophil gelatinase-associated lipocalin (NGAL, human homolog). LCN-2 can bind to siderophores, which are secreted by microorganisms to scavenge environmental iron for bacterial survival [1]. There is also evidence that LCN-2 is involved in iron transport in mammalian cells [4]. In the central nervous system, LCN-2 is present in astrocytes in various parts of normal rat brain and upregulated after kainite-induced neuronal injury [3]. LCN-2 has been reported in astrocytes and neurons after contusion injury of the spine, and LCN-2-deficient mice showed better neurological recovery [13].

Deferoxamine (DFX) is an iron chelator, which reduces brain injuries induced by ICH [8, 12], intraventricular hemorrhage (IVH) [2], SAH [10], and TBI [18]. In this study, we investigated whether TBI induced upregulation of LCN-2 in cortex and hippocampus, and the effect of DFX on that expression.

J. Zhao • G. Xi • G. Wu • R.F. Keep • Y. Hua, MD (✉)
Department of Neurosurgery, University of Michigan, R5018 Biomedical Science Research Building, 109 Zina Pitcher Place, Ann Arbor, MI 48109-2200, USA
e-mail: yahua@umich.edu

Methods

Animal Preparation

Adult male Sprague-Dawley rats (weight 280–320 g) were purchased from Charles River Laboratories (Portage, MI, USA). All animal use protocols were approved by the University of Michigan Committee on the Use and Care of Animals. Rats were fasted but with free access to water for 2 h before surgery.

Lateral Fluid-Percussion-Induced Traumatic Brain Injury

TBI was induced by lateral fluid-percussion (2.5–3.5 atm) as described previously [18]. Isoflurane was used for anesthesia induction (v/v 5 %) and maintenance (2.5–3.0 %) with a rodent mechanical ventilator (tidal volume: 2–2.5 ml, rate: 55–60/min; Harvard Apparatus, Holliston, MA, USA). Rectal temperature was kept at 37.5±0.2 °C using a heating pad. General blood parameters including blood pressure, pH, PaO_2, $PaCO_2$, blood glucose, and hematocrit were monitored and kept in normal ranges. Rats were then placed in a prone position on the stereotactic frame. Both bregma and lambda sutures were exposed by midline longitudinal incision of scalp. A 5-mm-diameter right parietal craniotomy, centered at 3 mm lateral and 4 mm posterior of the bregma, was then performed using a dental drill without dura laceration. A plastic female Luer Lock hub was then attached to the craniotomy site using cyanoacrylate adhesive followed by dental cement and that hub was used to attach the fluid percussion devise. After the fluid percussion, the female hub was removed, the skull flap fixed back in place, and the scalp incision sutured closed. Temporary apnea after the fluid percussion was observed, and ventilation was maintained until recovery of spontaneous respiration. Rats in the sham operation group had the same surgical procedures except the fluid percussion.

R.L. Applegate et al. (eds.), *Brain Edema XVI: Translate Basic Science into Clinical Practice*, Acta Neurochirurgica Supplement, Vol. 121,
DOI 10.1007/978-3-319-18497-5_50,

Experimental Groups

The study was divided into two parts. In the first part, rats underwent a sham operation ($n=12$) or a TBI (euthanized at day 1 ($n=19$), day 3 ($n=17$) and day 7 ($n=11$)). They were then perfused with phosphate-buffered saline (PBS; 0.1 mol/L, pH 7.4) and the brains used for Western blot analysis and immunohistochemistry. In the second part, rats were treated with vehicle ($n=8$ per time point) or DFX (100 mg/kg, intramuscular; $n=10$ per time point) at 2 h and then every 12 h after TBI. Rats were euthanized at days 1 or 3, and the brains were perfused and used for Western blotting.

Western Blot Analysis

Western blot was performed according to a standard protocol [9, 16]. Briefly, 30 µg of total tissue protein was loaded and separated by SDS-polyacrylamide gel electrophoresis (SDS-PAGE) and transferred to nitrocellulose membrane. The primary antibody was goat anti-rat LCN-2 (1:400 dilution, R&D Systems).

Immunohistochemistry

The avidin-biotin complex technique was used for immunohistochemistry as described previously [9, 16]. The primary antibody was goat anti-rat LCN-2 (1:200 dilution). Sections incubated in the absence of primary antibodies were used as negative controls.

Statistical Analysis

KaleidaGraph (Version 4.0) was used for statistical analysis. Differences among groups and subgroups were assessed by one-way analysis of variance (ANOVA) with Student-Newman-Keuls post hoc test. All data are expressed as mean ± SE, and $p<0.05$ was set as statistical significance.

Results

FPI Parameters, Mortality, and General Physiological Parameters

There was no significant difference of the recorded pressure of Fluid Percussion Injury (2.5 ± 0.10 vs. 2.43 ± 0.18 atm) between the groups. Total mortality after TBI was 15 % (15/102). Of these, 87 % (13/15) died immediately after TBI because of respiratory failure. Physiological parameters, including hematocrit, mean arterial blood pressure, blood pH, PaO_2, $PaCO_2$, and blood glucose, were controlled within normal ranges. Body weight loss was higher in the TBI groups compared with sham-operated rats ($p<0.05$) but was similar in DFX- and vehicle-treated groups.

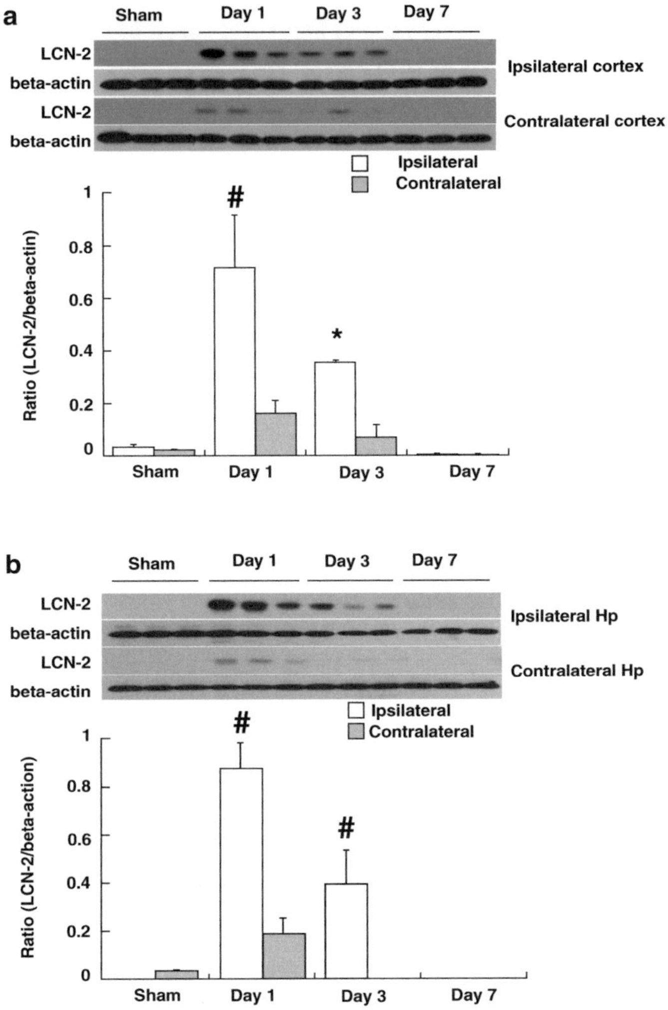

Fig. 1 LCN-2 protein levels in cortex (**a**) and hippocampus (**b**) after a sham operation (at day 1) or a TBI (at days 1, 3, and 7). Values are means ± SE, $n=3$ for each group; * $p<0.05$, # $p<0.01$ vs. sham and contralateral tissues

LCN-2 protein levels (expressed as a ratio to beta-actin) were increased in both cortex (0.72 ± 0.19 vs. 0.03 ± 0.01 in sham-operated rats, $p<0.01$; Fig. 1a) and hippocampus (0.87 ± 0.11 vs. 0.002 ± 0.001 in shams, $p<0.001$; Fig. 1b) at day 1 after TBI. Peak LCN-2 protein levels after TBI were at day 1, with a decrease at day 3 ($p<0.05$) and almost no LCN-2 expression at 7 days after TBI (Fig. 1). LCN-2 positive cells were found in ipsilateral cortex and hippocampus at

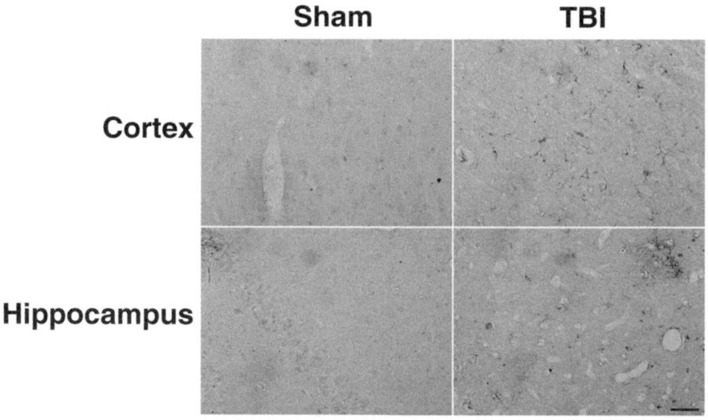

Fig. 2 LCN-2 immunoreactivity in cortex and hippocampus after a sham operation or a TBI at day 1. Scale bar=50 μm

day 1 after TBI but not in sham-operated rats. Most of the positive cells were glial-like (Fig. 2).

DFX treatment (100 mg/kg, intramuscularly, at 2 and 14 h after TBI) attenuated LCN-2 protein levels in both ipsilateral cortex (0.75±0.24 vs. 1.23±0.11 in vehicle, $p<0.05$, Fig. 3a) and hippocampus (0.56±0.14 vs. 0.93±0.08 in vehicle, $p<0.01$, Fig. 3b) at day 1 after TBI.

Discussion

The major findings of the present study were (1) enhanced expression of LCN-2 in cortex and hippocampus after TBI and (2) systemic treatment with DFX attenuated the TBI-induced LCN-2 upregulation.

Lateral fluid percussion has been widely used to induce TBI since the 1980s. In the present study, TBI increased LCN-2 protein levels in the ipsilateral cortex and hippocampus with a peak at day 1. There was almost no LCN-2 expression in sham-operated groups or in the contralateral samples from the TBI groups. In our previous research in this TBI model, we have found hemorrhage in multiple locations, including subdural, subarachnoid, intraparenchymal, and intraventricular [18]. We have also found that LCN-2 is induced by an intracerebral injection of blood (100 μl), an ICH model, in rats [5]. In combination, these results suggest that the upregulation in LCN-2 after TBI is, at least in part, a response to the hemorrhage that occurs. It should be noted that LCN-2 upregulation in the ICH model was greater and longer lasting than found after TBI, and this may reflect the different size of hemorrhage in the two models.

After a cerebral hemorrhage, hemoglobin is released from lysed extravascular erythrocytes and degraded into heme, which is then further degraded into three components by heme oxygenase: ferric iron, carbon monoxide, and biliverdin. Our previous research reported iron levels in CSF

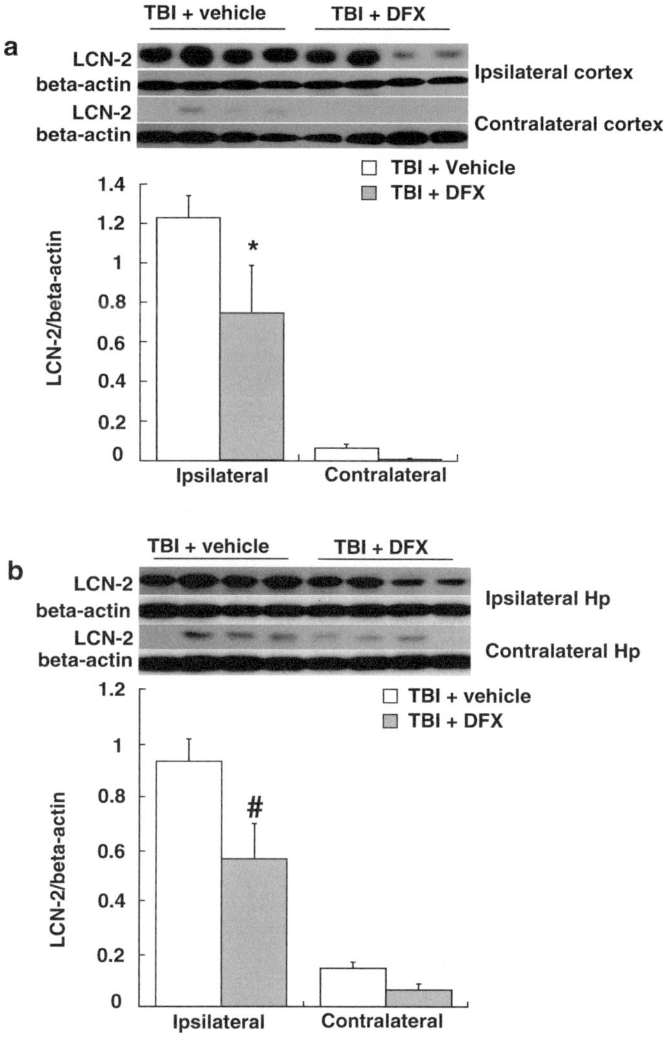

Fig. 3 LCN2 protein levels in the ipsi- and contralateral cortex (**a**) and hippocampus (**b**) at day 1 after TBI. Rats were treated with DFX (100 mg/kg) or vehicle. Values are means±SE, $n=4$ for each group; * $p<0.05$, # $p<0.01$ vs. vehicle group

increased on the first day, peaked on the third day, and remained high for at least 1 month after experimental ICH [14]. We have previously found that iron plays an important role in ICH-induced LCN-2 upregulation [5]. In the current study, the decrease in TBI-induced LCN-2 upregulation with DFX also suggests that iron is an important inducer of LCN-2 after TBI.

Evidence suggests that LCN-2 is involved in iron uptake into cells expressing the LCN-2 cell surface receptor, LCN2R [4]. Thus, the increase in LCN-2 after TBI may be involved in clearing hemorrhage-derived iron. However, whether LCN-2 has a beneficial or detrimental role in TBI has yet to be investigated. In spinal cord injury, LCN-2-deficient mice showed better neurological recovery [13]. Similarly, we have recently found that the absence of LCN-2 reduces SAH-induced white matter injury [6]. Further studies are needed to explore the effects of LCN-2 in TBI, whether it is detrimental, whether it may be involved in cellular iron overload, and whether it is involved in the post-TBI inflammatory response because LCN-2 is an acute phase protein.

Acknowledgment This study was supported by the Joyce & Don Massey Family Foundation, and grants NSFC81301049 and NSFC81271374, 973 Program-2014CB541600, and an UMHS-PUHSC Joint Institute grant.

References

1. Barasch J, Mori K (2004) Cell biology: iron thievery. Nature 432:811–813
2. Chen Z, Gao C, Hua Y, Keep RF, Muraszko K, Xi G (2010) Role of iron in brain injury after intraventricular hemorrhage. Stroke 42:465–470
3. Chia WJ, Dawe GS, Ong WY (2011) Expression and localization of the iron-siderophore binding protein lipocalin 2 in the normal rat brain and after kainate-induced excitotoxicity. Neurochem Int 59:591–599
4. Devireddy LR, Gazin C, Zhu X, Green MR (2005) A cell-surface receptor for lipocalin 24p3 selectively mediates apoptosis and iron uptake. Cell 123:1293–1305
5. Dong M, Xi G, Keep RF, Hua Y (2013) Role of iron in brain lipocalin 2 upregulation after intracerebral hemorrhage in rats. Brain Res 1505:86–92
6. Egashira Y, Hua Y, Keep RF, Xi G (2014) Acute white matter injury after experimental subarachnoid hemorrhage: potential role of lipocalin 2. Stroke 45:2141–2143
7. Flower DR, North AC, Sansom CE (2000) The lipocalin protein family: structural and sequence overview. Biochim Biophys Acta 1482:9–24
8. Hatakeyama T, Okauchi M, Hua Y, Keep RF, Xi G (2013) Deferoxamine reduces neuronal death and hematoma lysis after intracerebral hemorrhage in aged rats. Transl Stroke Res 4:546–553
9. Jin H, Xi G, Keep RF, Wu J, Hua Y (2013) DARPP-32 to quantify intracerebral hemorrhage-induced neuronal death in basal ganglia. Transl Stroke Res 4:130–134
10. Lee JY, Keep RF, He Y, Sagher O, Hua Y, Xi G (2010) Hemoglobin and iron handling in brain after subarachnoid hemorrhage and the effect of deferoxamine on early brain injury. J Cereb Blood Flow Metab 30:1793–1803
11. Maas AI, Stocchetti N, Bullock R (2008) Moderate and severe traumatic brain injury in adults. Lancet Neurol 7:728–741
12. Okauchi M, Hua Y, Keep RF, Morgenstern LB, Schallert T, Xi G (2010) Deferoxamine treatment for intracerebral hemorrhage in aged rats: therapeutic time window and optimal duration. Stroke 41:375–382
13. Rathore KI, Berard JL, Redensek A, Chierzi S, Lopez-Vales R, Santos M, Akira S, David S (2011) Lipocalin 2 plays an immunomodulatory role and has detrimental effects after spinal cord injury. J Neurosci 31:13412–13419
14. Wan S, Hua Y, Keep RF, Hoff JT, Xi G (2006) Deferoxamine reduces CSF free iron levels following intracerebral hemorrhage. Acta Neurochir Suppl 96:199–202
15. Wu J, Hua Y, Keep RF, Nakamura T, Hoff JT, Xi G (2003) Iron and iron-handling proteins in the brain after intracerebral hemorrhage. Stroke 34:2964–2969
16. Xi G, Keep RF, Hua Y, Xiang J, Hoff JT (1999) Attenuation of thrombin-induced brain edema by cerebral thrombin preconditioning. Stroke 30:1247–1255
17. Xi G, Strahle J, Hua Y, Keep RF (2014) Progress in translational research on intracerebral hemorrhage: is there an end in sight? Prog Neurobiol 115C:45–63
18. Zhao J, Chen Z, Xi G, Keep RF, Hua Y (2014) Deferoxamine attenuates acute hydrocephalus after traumatic brain injury in rats. Transl Stroke Res 5:586–594

Cerebrovascular Time Constant in Patients with Head Injury

Alex Trofimov, George Kalentiev, Alexander Gribkov, Oleg Voennov, and Vera Grigoryeva

Introduction

The basic principle of brain damage therapy is to maintain adequate perfusion and oxygenation, which is impossible without the evaluation of these parameters and the timely correction of detected disorders [12]. It is believed that neuromonitoring should not be limited to monitoring of single parameters of homeostasis but should tend to determine and monitor the state of various organs and systems based on integral analysis with the calculation of derivative (surrogate) indices and values, which reflect the state of various parts of homeostasis for further correction of any detected disorders [16]. This approach enables us to determine the functional state of those structures for which direct study is either impossible or only accessible experimentally, such as the microvasculature [18].

However, in clinical practice, the determination of these values has had, until recently, some significant technical constraints associated with the necessity of the lifetime assessment of pulse changes in the area of the main vessel under study during one cardiac cycle [3, 14]. There are no such constraints when determining τ, cerebrovascular time constant, which characterizes the time for complete filling with blood of the cerebral pial bed during one cardiac cycle [5]. Hence, cerebrovascular time constant can be evaluated, by analogy with an resistor-capacitor circuit, product of compliance of the cerebral arterial bed (Ca) [1] and cerebrovascular resistance (CVR) [5]. This index is independent of the pulse difference of the blood transfer vessel area [7]. Although the term "time constant" is used, the values of the time constants vary widely with different cerebral pathology, such as subarachnoid hemorrhage, carotid stenosis, and hypoxic brain injury [6, 8, 17]. In a broad sense, τ changes reflect the brain's ability to maintain continuous perfusion of the cerebral microcirculation under conditions of spontaneous variations of intracranial pressure [9]. However, τ peculiarities still remain poorly studied.

The aim of the study was to assess the time constant of the cerebral arterial bed in patients with severe traumatic brain injury (TBI) with and without intracranial hematoma.

Materials and Methods

We examined 116 polytrauma patients with severe head injury who were treated at the Nizhny Novgorod Regional Trauma Center Level I in 2012–2014. The mean age of the patients with head injury was 34.5 ± 15.6 years (from 15 to 73 years). There were 53 women and 63 men. The first group included 58 patients without intracranial hematoma and the second group included 58 patients with epidural (7), subdural (48,) and multiple (3) hematomas. The wakefulness level according to GCS (Glasgow Coma Score) averaged 11.2 ± 1.4 in the first group and 10.1 ± 3.4 in the second group. The severity of their state according to ISS (Injury Severity Score) was 31 ± 12 in the first group and 28 ± 11 in the second group. Clinical outcomes are summarized in Table 1.

Perfusion Computed Tomography

All patients were subjected to perfusion computed tomography (PCT) by 64-slice tomograph (Toshiba Aquilion TSX-101A; Toshiba Medical Systems, Europe BV, Zoetermeer,

A. Trofimov (✉)
Department of Polytrauma and Critical Care, Regional Hospital named after N.A. Semashko, 190, Rodionov str, Nizhny Novgorod 603126, Russian Federation

Department of Neurosurgery, Nizhniy Novgorod State Medical Academy, Nizhniy Novgorod, Russian Federation
e-mail: xtro7@mail.ru

G. Kalentiev • A. Gribkov • O. Voennov
Department of Critical Care, Regional Hospital named after N.A. Semashko, 190, Rodionov str, Nizhniy Novgorod, Russian Federation

V. Grigoryeva
Department of Neurosurgery, Nizhniy Novgorod State Medical Academy, Nizhniy Novgorod, Russian Federation

R.L. Applegate et al. (eds.), *Brain Edema XVI: Translate Basic Science into Clinical Practice*, Acta Neurochirurgica Supplement, Vol. 121,
DOI 10.1007/978-3-319-18497-5_51,

Table 1 Clinical outcome (Glasgow Outcome Score) of polytraumatized patients

N (%)	GOS 1 Good recovery	GOS 2 Moderate disability	GOS 3 Severe disability	GOS 4 Vegetative state	GOS 5 Death	Total
Group 1	27	16	11	3	1	58 (100 %)
Group 2	25	14	8	8	3	58 (100 %)

The Netherlands). PCT was performed 1–12 days after TBI in the first group and 2–8 days after surgical evacuation of the hematoma in the second group. The perfusion examination report included an initial contrast-free CT of the brain [15]. The so-called "area of interest" was established based on areas of middle cerebral artery.

Extended scanning was further performed of four such "areas of interest," 32 mm in thickness, within 55 s with a contrast agent administered (the brain perfusion mode). The scanning parameters were 120 kVp, 70 mA, 70 mAs, and 1,000 ms. The contrast agent (Ultravist 370, Schering AG, Germany) was administered with an automatic syringe injector (Stellant, Medrad, Indianola, PA, USA) into a peripheral vein through a standard catheter (20 G) at a rate of 4–5 ml/s in a dose of 30–50 ml per one examination.

After scanning, the data volume was transferred to a workstation (Vitrea 2, Vital Imaging, Inc., ver. 4.1.8.0). Artery and vein marks were automatically recorded, followed by the manual control of indices in the time-concentration diagram.

The so-called "area of interest" was established based on subcortical areas of middle cerebral artery. Arteriovenous amplitude of regional cerebral blood volume oscillation (delta cerebral blood volume, ΔCBV) was calculated as the difference between arterial and venous blood volume in the "region of interest" of 1 cm^2 [9].

Cerebral blood flow velocity of the middle cerebral artery was recorded bilaterally using transcranial Doppler ultrasound with 2-MHz probes attached with a headband (Sonomed 300 M, Spectromed, Moscow, Russia). Arterial blood pressure was measured noninvasively (MAP 03, Cardex, Moscow, Russia) after PCT.

Statistical Analysis

For the calculation of the time constant, we used the formula proposed by Kasprowicz et al. [9], amended by Czosnyka et al. [4]:

$$\mathbf{t} = \text{ampCaBV} \times \text{MAP} / \text{Vmean} \times \text{ampABP}$$

where ampCaBV is the arteriovenous amplitude of regional cerebral blood volume, MAP is mean arterial pressure, Vmean is mean flow velocity rate of middle cerebral artery, and ampABP is amplitude arterial blood pressure. Reference range τ was chosen according Kasprowicz et al. [7] as 0.22±0.06 sec.

The *t*-test for dependent samples was utilized to analyze differences in means of parameters between the ipsilateral and contralateral sides of the temporal lobes. The program Statistica 7.0 (StatSoft Inc., Tulsa, OK, USA) was used for the analysis. A significance level of $p < 0.05$ was determined.

Results

Mean values and standard deviations of the data are summarized in Table 2. The cerebrovascular time constant was shorter ($p = 0.05$) in both the first and second group (with or without traumatic hematomas) in comparison with normal data ($p < 0.05$). The time constant in the second group was shorter than in the first group, both on the side of the former hematoma ($p = 0.012$) and on the contralateral side ($p = 0.044$). Moreover, there was no significant difference in τ between the perifocal zone of the former hematoma and the same locus of the contralateral hemisphere. Also, no significant effects of patient age on the τ value were found ($p > 0.05$).

Discussion

Microcirculatory disorders play a key role in the development of hypoperfusion and secondary brain ischemia [4, 11]. One of the factors, which enables simultaneous estimation of both the capacitive and resistive characteristics of the cerebral pial bed, is cerebrovascular time constant, which is calculated as the product of cerebrovascular arterial compliance and cerebrovascular resistance [17].

In our opinion, there may be a few reasons for the τ reduction, but all of them seem to be associated with brain edema: first, development of combined (vasogenic and cytotoxic) edema resulting from a drop in arterial compliance [1, 2], and, second, brain edema may cause pial compression and reduce the total volume of capacitive vessels, thus changing the value of resistivity [13]. The τ shortening by hematoma on the side of the eliminated cortical compression may be explained by the vasodilation of vessels resulting from the vascular wall tone dysautoregulation [13]. This is indirectly confirmed by the fact of remaining τ variations even after the compression factor elimination. The failure of microcirculatory autoregulation may result in disturbed blood outflow from the channel and in the long stagnation of some blood in

Table 2 Comparison of the analyzed parameters

		MAP (mm Hg)	ampABP (mm Hg)	Vmean (sm/s)	ΔCBV (sm^3)	τ (sec)
1	Group 1	99.1 ± 13.6	63.9 ± 11.7	41.1 ± 13.3	2.6 ± 0.8	0.10 ± 0.02
2	Group 2 (ipsilateral sides)	97.9 ± 14.6	65.3 ± 12.2	46.5 ± 16.4	2.6 ± 1.8	0.08 ± 0.08
3	Group 2 (contralateral sides)	97.9 ± 14.6	65.3 ± 12.2	41.7 ± 13.8	2.9 ± 1.4	0.09 ± 0.07
	p (1–2)	0.701	0.541	0.086	0.772	0.012[a]
	p (1–3)	0.225	0.428	0.821	0.355	0.044[a]
	p (2–3)	0.231	0.166	0.284	0.62	0.399

[a]Difference is statistically significant

resistive vessels, whereby the pial bed may be filled much faster [10].

Limitations of the Study

It is probably impossible to carry out the dynamic assessment of τ without a repeated PCT. We failed to completely eliminate a mathematical error associated with the measurement of the "area of interest" space.

We believe that the results of our study provide conditions for a differentiated approach to solving the question of timing of orthopedic correction of extracranial injuries in polytraumatized patients, which is during the period of microcirculatory normalization and minimal risk of the secondary brain injury.

Conclusion

The cerebrovascular time constant was shorter ($p = 0.05$) in both the first and second groups in comparison with normal data. The cerebrovascular time constant in the second group was shorter than in the first group, both on the side of the former hematoma (p = 0.012) and on the contralateral side (p = 0.044). The results indicate severe dysregulation of cerebral blood flow in severe TBI, which increases in patients with polytrauma and traumatic hematomas.

Conflicts of Interest We declare that we have no conflicts of interest.

References

1. Avezaat CJ, Eijndhoven JH (1984) Cerebrospinal fluid pulse pressure and craniospatial dynamics. A theoretical, clinical and experimental study. Erasmus University, Rotterdam
2. Avezaat CJ, van Eijndhoven JH (1986) Clinical observations on the relationship between cerebrospinal fluid pulse pressure and intracranial pressure. Acta Neurochir 79:13–29
3. Carrera E, Kim D, Castellani G (2010) Cerebral arterial compliance in patients with internal carotid artery disease. Eur J Neurol 18:711–718
4. Czosnyka M, Richards H, Reinhard M (2012) Cerebrovascular time constant: dependence on cerebral perfusion pressure and end-tidal carbon dioxide concentration. Neurol Res 34:17–24
5. Dewey R, Pierer H, Hunt WE (1974) Experimental cerebral hemodynamics. Vasomotor tone, critical closing pressure, and vascular bed resistance. J Neurosurg 41:597–606
6. Howlett J, Northington F (2013) Cerebrovascular autoregulation and neurologic injury in neonatal hypoxic-ischemic encephalopathy. Pediatr Res 74(5):525–535
7. Kasprowicz M, Diedler J, Reinhard M (2012) Time constant of the cerebral arterial bed. Acta Neurochir Suppl 114:17–21
8. Kasprowicz M, (2012) Assessment of cerebral hemodynamics based on pulse waveform analysis of intracranial pressure, arterial blood pressure and crerebral blood flow. Thesis, Vroclaw University, with a summary in Polish and Enlish
9. Kasprowicz M, Diedler J, Reinhard M (2012) Time constant of the cerebral arterial bed in normal subjects. Ultrasound Med Biol 38:1129–1137
10. Lassen NA (1964) Autoregulation of cerebral blood flow. Circ Res 15:201–204
11. ter Laan M (2014) Neuromodulation of cerebral blood flow. Proefschrift ter verkrijging van de graad van doctor, Groningen, p 125
12. Lewis P, Rosenfeld J (2012) Monitoring of the association between cerebral blood flow velocity and intracranial pressure. Acta Neurochir 114:147–152
13. Marmarou A (2007) A review of progress in understanding the pathophysiology and treatment of brain edema. Neurosurg Focus 22(5):E1
14. Riva N, Budohoski K, Smielewski P (2012) Transcranial Doppler Pulsatility Index: what it is and what it isn't. Neurocrit Care 17:58–66
15. Shin BJ, Anumula N (2014) Does the location of the arterial input function affect quantitative CTP in patients with vasospasm? AJNR Am J Neuroradiol 35:49–54
16. Ursino M, Lodi C (1997) A simple mathematical model of the interaction between intracranial pressure and cerebral hemodynamics. J Appl Physiol 82:1256–1269
17. Varsos GV, Richards H, Kasprowicz M (2013) Cessation of diastolic cerebral blood flow velocity: the role of critical closing pressure. Neurocrit Care 20(1):40–48
18. Varsos GV, Richards H, Kasprowicz M (2013) Critical closing pressure determined with a model of cerebrovascular impedance. J Cereb Blood Flow Metab 33:235–243

Thrombin Preconditioning in Surgical Brain Injury in Rats

Michael Benggon, Hank Chen, Richard L. Applegate II , and John Zhang

Introduction

Preserving neurological function and decreasing perioperative morbidity associated with intracranial neurosurgery is of utmost importance to patients and their physicians. Study depends on a reliable animal model of brain injury resulting from the surgical procedure itself. The model of surgical brain injury (SBI) in rats provides a consistent platform to study the negative effects of manipulating brain tissue. Major pathological changes found via this method are predominantly caused by increased brain edema surrounding the damaged tissue [8, 11].

Preconditioning brain tissue through several small ischemic events preceding a larger event has been shown to improve outcomes in stroke models [9]. Further studies demonstrated neuroprotection associated with using only the protein components associated with ischemic episodes, such as thrombin, in small pretreatment doses [6, 10, 17]. Thrombin preconditioning has been shown to attenuate ischemic stroke-induced brain edema through early induction of heat shock protein 27 and aquaporin 4 proteins [6, 17]. These changes enable the affected cell to remodel its shape and allow for transcellular movement of excess water, which is likely important for diminishing vasogenic edema [13].

Intranasal administration of neurotrophic factors circumvents the blood-brain barrier and avoids invasive procedures needed to deliver therapies to brain parenchyma. Pathways to the cerebral spinal fluid from the nose include transcellular transport across or pericellular diffusion around olfactory epithelium [7, 16]. Proteins as large as albumin have been shown to effectively cross into cerebral spinal fluid via intranasal routes. The protein nerve growth factor (approximately 37 kDa), which is similar in molecular weight to thrombin (approximately 36 kDa), has been found in the central nervous system after only 20–60 min following intranasal administration [2, 16].

In this study, we hypothesized that thrombin pretreatment and/or preconditioning delivered via intranasal or intracerebral ventricular routes would decrease brain edema and improve postoperative neurological function in surgical brain injury in rats.

Methods

All procedures were approved by the Loma Linda University Institutional Animal Care and Use Committee and conform to the United States Public Health Service Policy on Humane Care and Use of Laboratory Animals and the Guide for the Care and Use of Laboratory Animals. A total of 77 adult male Sprague-Dawley rats weighing 285–355 g were used.

Surgical Brain Injury

SBI was obtained as described in previous studies [1, 11]. Animals were anesthetized with an intraperitoneal injection of ketamine 100 mg/kg and xylazine 10 mg/kg. A

M. Benggon, MD
Department of Anesthesiology, Loma Linda University, School of Medicine, 11234 Anderson Street, Loma Linda, CA, USA

H. Chen, MD
Department of Basic Science, Division of Physiology, Loma Linda School of Medicine, Loma Linda, CA, USA

R.L. Applegate II, MD (✉)
Department of Anesthesiology, Loma Linda University, School of Medicine, Room 2532 LLUMC, 11234 Anderson Street, Loma Linda, CA 92374, USA
e-mail: rapplegate@llu.edu

J. Zhang, MD, PhD
Department of Basic Science, Division of Physiology, Loma Linda School of Medicine, Loma Linda, CA, USA

Department of Anesthesiology, Loma Linda University, School of Medicine, Room 2532 LLUMC, 11234 Anderson Street, Loma Linda, CA 92374, USA

R.L. Applegate et al. (eds.), *Brain Edema XVI: Translate Basic Science into Clinical Practice*, Acta Neurochirurgica Supplement, Vol. 121, DOI 10.1007/978-3-319-18497-5_52,

midline scalp incision was made and the skull exposed. Using a micro drill, a 5-mm × 5-mm craniotomy starting at the bregma was made. Puncture and reflection of the dura mater marked initial brain injury time. Sharp dissection and removal of the entire right frontal lobe 2 mm lateral and 1 mm anterior to the bregma was then achieved. The remaining surfaces of adjacent brain tissue were then briefly electrocauterized for approximately 2 s, and hemostasis obtained with gentle direct pressure with tissue applicators. The removed skull was then replaced and the scalp closed with suture before recovering the animal in a temperature-controlled environment. Animals were observed closely for signs of pain after the procedure, and every animal received 1 mL of 0.9 % saline subcutaneously for hydration. Sham animals received craniotomy without dura mater puncture, with the skull being immediately replaced and the procedure continuing on from there as described above.

Treatment Groups

Study arms were divided into three treatment time courses: one-time pretreatment 1 or 5 days prior to SBI, or once-daily preconditioning for 5 days prior to SBI. Time courses were further subdivided by either intranasal (IN) or intracerebral ventricular (ICV) treatment routes, and finally grouped by either vehicle or thrombin (thrombin from rat plasma, Sigma-Aldrich, St. Louis, MO, USA) therapies, for a total of 13 treatment groups when including the sham group (see Figures). Thrombin was dosed as 0.1 unit/10 μL 0.9 % saline ICV, and 5 units/50 μL 0.9 % saline IN. Pretreatment times and intracerebral ventricular dosing was chosen to be similar to previous studies [4–6, 14]. Vehicle doses of 0.9 % saline were matched for volume (i.e., 10 μL ICV and 50 μL IN).

Intracerebral Ventricular Injection

ICV injections were performed as described in previous studies [4–6, 14]. Animals were anesthetized with the same intraperitoneal injection of ketamine and xylazine used for SBI above. The animal's head was shaved with an electric razor and a midline scalp incision was made prior to fixation of the rat onto a stereotaxic frame with an attached syringe pump. The injection point was located and drilled at −1.1 mm lateral and −1.5 mm posterior to the zero point at the bregma. Injection of thrombin or vehicle was made at −3.2 mm from the outer surface of the skull at a rate no more than 0.5 μL/min. Once the treatment was completed, the scalp was sutured closed and the animal observed closely in a temperature-controlled environment until fully recovered.

Intranasal Injection

IN injections were also performed according to previous study protocols [2]. Anesthesia was obtained as described above with a ketamine/xylazine intraperitoneal injection. Thrombin and vehicle doses were administered in 5-μL drops every 2 min, alternating between nares, until the full dose was administered with the animals lying supine on a heating pad. Each rat was observed throughout the recovery process in a controlled environment.

Exclusion Criteria

Animals that died any time before outcomes were measured were excluded. Otherwise, all surviving rats were tested and their data included in analysis.

Neurological Testing

A blinded observer performed a modified 21-point sensorimotor test that scores for spontaneous activity, body proprioception, response to vibrissae touch, limb symmetry, lateral turning ability, forepaw outstretching, and climbing ability [3]. The same observer also obtained a vibrissae-elicited forelimb placement test, where the animal's vibrissae were brushed by a table edge while watching for a reflex placement of the ipsilateral forepaw on the table or lack thereof. The number of correctly elicited forepaw placements was recorded out of 10 attempts for each side and a percentage calculated [15]. Both of these tests were administered 24 h after initial brain injury.

Brain Water Content

Immediately after neurologic testing, the animals were killed under isoflurane-induced anesthesia and their brains promptly removed. These were then sectioned into ipsilateral and contralateral frontal and parietal lobes, cerebellum, and brain stem, and then placed into a 100 °C oven for 48 h after being weighed. After dehydration in the oven, the brain sections were weighed once more and the percentage of brain water content calculated by subtracting the dry weight from the wet weight and multiplying by 100 [8, 11].

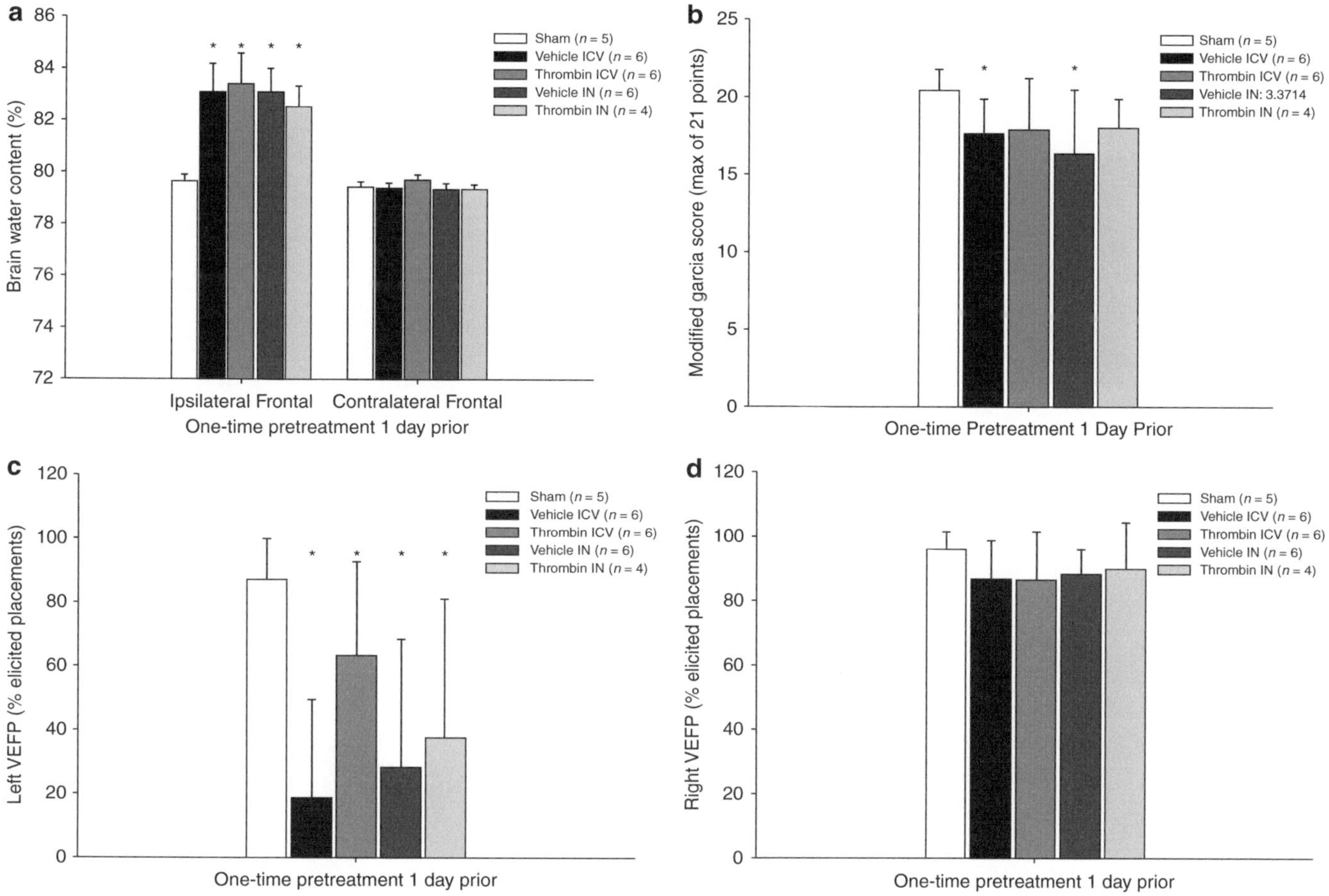

Fig. 1 One-time pretreatment, 1 day prior to surgical brain injury: (**a**) postoperative brain water content; (**b**) modified 21-point sensorimotor score; (**c**) left-sided (contralateral to injured area) percentage of correct vibrissae-elicited forelimb placements, from total attempts; (**d**) right-sided percentage of correct vibrissae-elicited forelimb placements, from total attempts. *$p<0.05$ when compared with sham group. Thrombin intracerebral ventricular (*ICV*) or intranasal (*IN*) administration did not differ significantly from vehicle

Statistical Analysis

One-way analysis of variance was used to test for significance between groups, and the Tukey method was used for all pairwise multiple comparisons. Statistical significance was achieved with a $p<0.05$. All statistical analyses were made using SigmaStat 3.5 (Aspire Software International, Ashburn, VA, USA).

Results

Mortality

A total of six animals (7.7 %) died prior to data collection and therefore were excluded from the study. Three animals died instantly after attempted intraperitoneal injection of anesthetic prior to SBI (one thrombin intranasal 1 day prior group, one vehicle ICV daily preconditioning group, and one vehicle IN daily preconditioning group), presumably from accidental intravascular injection. Three animals died shortly after SBI (one thrombin IN daily preconditioning group from uncontrolled intracranial hemorrhage 1 h later, and one thrombin IN 1 day prior and one vehicle IN 5 days prior died from possible pulmonary congestion with subsequent respiratory failure during recovery). Data from a total of 71 animals was analyzed in this study (please see figures for number of animals per group).

Pretreatment or Preconditioning with Thrombin Does Not Reduce Brain Water Content

There was a statistically significant difference in ipsilateral frontal brain water content among all groups ($p<0.001$), and between sham animals and all treatment groups ($p<0.05$). Thrombin-treated animals, however, did not differ significantly from vehicle-treated animals regardless of therapy administration route or timing (Figs. 1, 2, and 3; $p>0.05$).

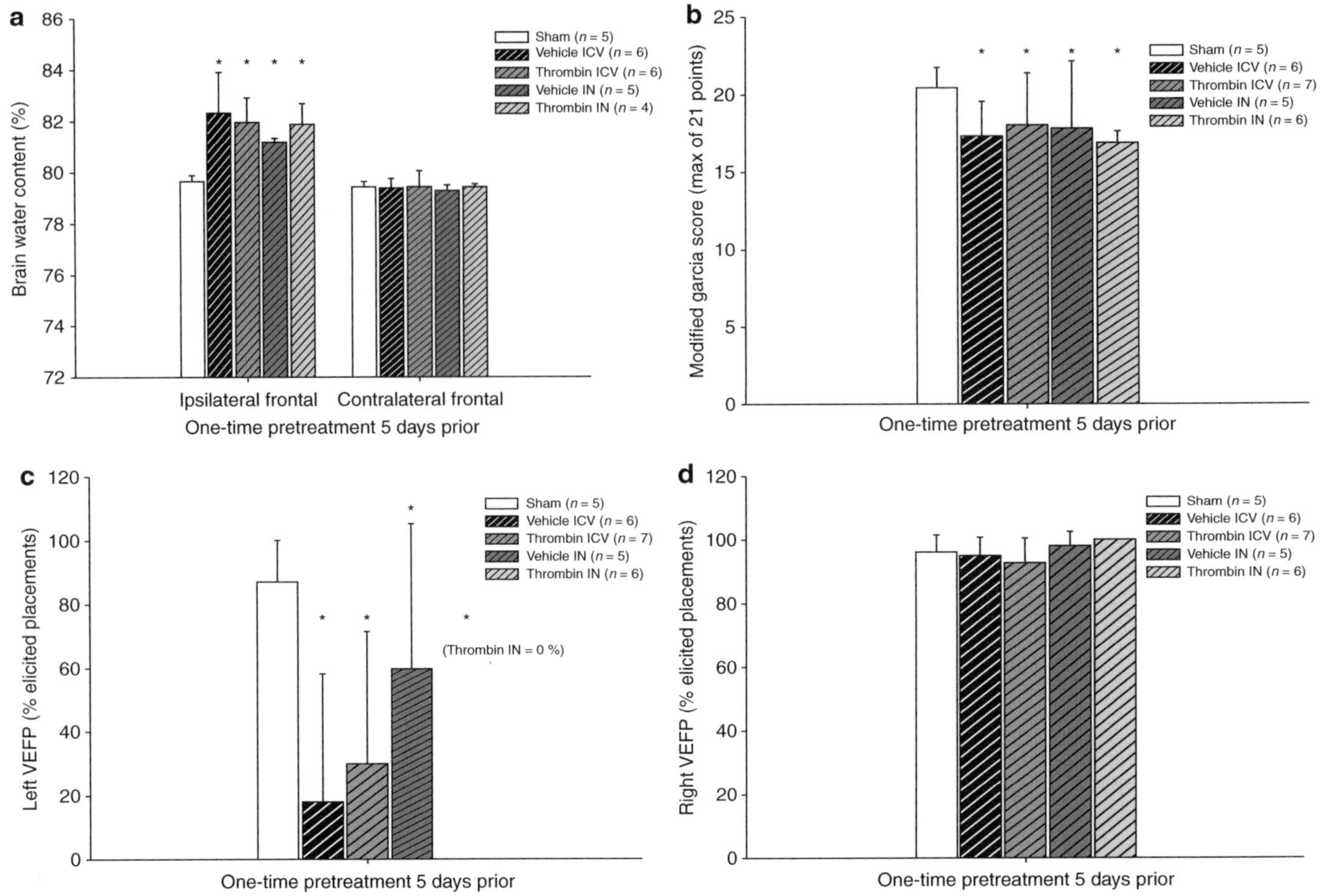

Fig. 2 One-time pretreatment, 5 days prior to surgical brain injury: (**a**) postoperative brain water content; (**b**) modified 21-point sensorimotor score; (**c**) left-sided (contralateral to injured area) percentage of correct vibrissae-elicited forelimb placements, from total attempts; (**d**) right-sided percentage of correct vibrissae-elicited forelimb placements, from total attempts. $*p<0.05$ when compared with sham group. Thrombin intracerebral ventricular (*ICV*) or intranasal (*IN*) administration did not differ significantly from vehicle. Thrombin IN left vibrissae-elicited forelimb placement had zero correct placements

Pretreatment or Preconditioning with Thrombin Does Not Improve Neurological Scores

There also was a significant difference between all groups of animals in the vibrissae-elicited forelimb placement test ($p<0.001$). Sham and treatment groups were significantly different ($p<0.05$), but thrombin- and vehicle-treated animals were not, regardless of route or timing of administration (Figs. 1, 2, and 3; $p>0.05$). Statistical analysis of the modified 21-point sensorimotor test results showed no difference between all groups ($p=0.8$).

Discussion

This study was designed to assess the outcome impact of thrombin pretreatment and preconditioning via intranasal and ICV administration routes in a model of surgical brain injury in rats as either reduction in brain edema or improvement in neurological function 24 h after surgical brain injury. Although thrombin preconditioning via ICV or intracerebral injection has been shown to effectively decrease brain edema in models of ischemic brain injury in rodents [6, 17], in the present study pretreatment or preconditioning with thrombin did not change any of these outcomes in comparison with control groups. Several factors could have contributed to this.

In addition to testing whether the benefit of thrombin pretreatment could be obtained in a surgical brain injury model, this study was designed to find a clinically relevant way to deliver the therapy. We chose the intranasal route to the cerebral spinal fluid (CSF) paired with ICV injections to compare the two methods of delivery for efficacy. However, because no significant result was seen from deliberate placement of thrombin into the CSF via the ICV route, or by presumed transport to the CSF via the IN route, we found it unnecessary to ascertain whether IN administration of thrombin was as effective as ICV. The fact that no improvement in outcomes was found likely is attributable to the type

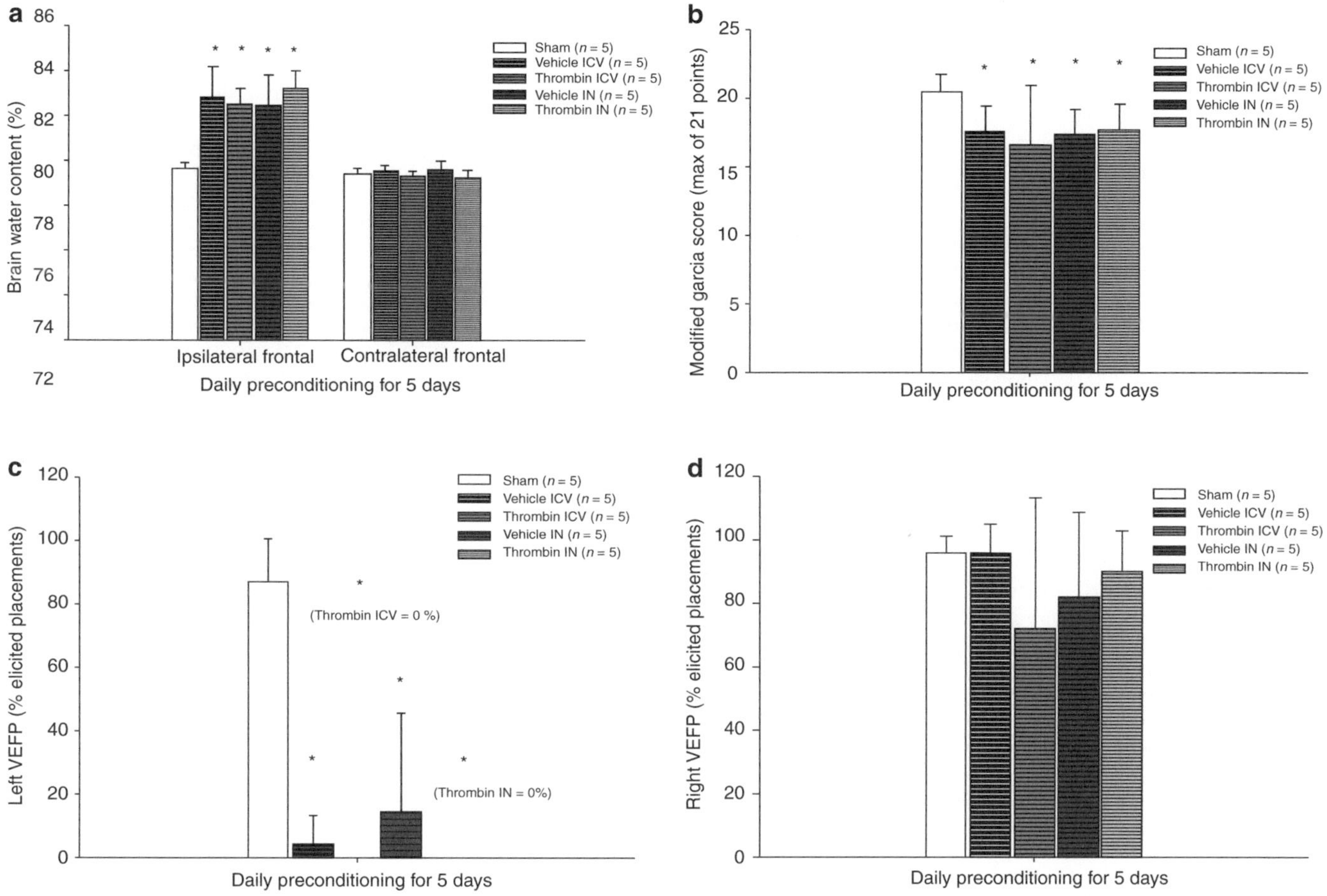

Fig. 3 Daily preconditioning for 5 days prior to surgical brain injury: (**a**) postoperative brain water content; (**b**) modified 21-point sensorimotor score; (**c**) left-sided (contralateral to injured area) percentage of correct vibrissae-elicited forelimb placements, from total attempts; (**d**) right-sided percentage of correct vibrissae-elicited forelimb placements, from total attempts. *$p<0.05$ when compared with sham group. Thrombin intracerebral ventricular (*ICV*) or intranasal (*IN*) administration did not differ significantly from vehicle. Thrombin ICV and IN left vibrissae-elicited forelimb placements had zero placements

of injury. The injured area in the surgical brain injury model is very large, and areas further away from the cerebral ventricles may never interact with the thrombin. In this model, the blood-brain barrier is mechanically disrupted, exposing brain parenchyma directly to blood and irrigation fluids across a sizable area. Any intracellular change that may improve localized disease from edema could be masked by the magnitude of injury caused in this model. Our goal was to find a clinically relevant therapy, and therefore the cohort size was powered to find only large treatment effects as in previous studies [1].

The lack of a significant difference between any of the treatment groups and the sham group in the modified 21-point sensorimotor exam was a confounding result. This test has been shown to give consistent results even between different observers, which correlate to the amount of diseased tissue [12]. Two experienced observers were used for this test and both were blinded to the groups, so it is unlikely that bias could have been inadvertently introduced. There were several outlying scores in the 1 day prior thrombin ICV and IN pretreatment groups that could have distorted the data. Also, although all the other treatment groups show a significant difference when compared with sham in the sensorimotor exam, that difference is still relatively small. In a previous study, it was shown that increased brain water content in this model correlated with worsened neurological outcome [1]. The vibrissae-elicited forelimb placement test demonstrated that in this study, and it may be better suited for demonstrating the degree of injury for comparison.

In conclusion, this study showed no improvement in 24 h post-injury brain water content or neurological function after one-time thrombin pretreatment 1 or 5 days prior, or with once-daily thrombin preconditioning for 5 days prior to surgical brain injury in rats.

Disclosure This study was supported in part by National Institutes of Health grant NS084921. All authors attest they have no conflicts of interest to disclose.

References

1. Benggon M, Chen H, Applegate R, Martin R, Zhang JH (2012) Effect of dexmedetomidine on brain edema and neurological outcomes in surgical brain injury in rats. Anesth Analg 115:154–159
2. De Rosa R, Garcia AA, Braschi C, Capsoni S, Maffei L, Berardi N, Cattaneo A (2005) Intranasal administration of nerve growth factor (NGF) rescues recognition memory deficits in AD11 anti-NGF transgenic mice. Proc Natl Acad Sci U S A 102:3811–3816
3. Garcia JH, Wagner S, Liu KF, Hu XJ (1995) Neurological deficit and extent of neuronal necrosis attributable to middle cerebral artery occlusion in rats. Statistical validation. Stroke 26:627–634
4. Granziera C, Thevenet J, Price M, Wiegler K, Magistretti PJ, Badaut J, Hirt L (2007) Thrombin-induced ischemic tolerance is prevented by inhibiting c-jun N-terminal kinase. Brain Res 1148:217–225
5. Henrich-Noack P, Striggow F, Reiser G, Reymann KG (2006) Preconditioning with thrombin can be protective or worsen damage after endothelin-1-induced focal ischemia in rats. J Neurosci Res 83:469–475
6. Hirt L, Ternon B, Price M, Mastour N, Brunet JF, Badaut J (2009) Protective role of early aquaporin 4 induction against postischemic edema formation. J Cereb Blood Flow Metab 29:423–433
7. Illum L (2000) Transport of drugs from the nasal cavity to the central nervous system. Eur J Pharm Sci 11:1–18
8. Jadhav V, Matchett G, Hsu FP, Zhang JH (2007) Inhibition of Src tyrosine kinase and effect on outcomes in a new in vivo model of surgically induced brain injury. J Neurosurg 106:680–686
9. Kato H, Liu Y, Araki T, Kogure K (1991) Temporal profile of the effects of pretreatment with brief cerebral ischemia on the neuronal damage following secondary ischemic insult in the gerbil: cumulative damage and protective effects. Brain Res 553:238–242
10. Masada T, Xi G, Hua Y, Keep RF (2000) The effects of thrombin preconditioning on focal cerebral ischemia in rats. Brain Res 867:173–179
11. Matchett G, Hahn J, Obenaus A, Zhang J (2006) Surgically induced brain injury in rats: the effect of erythropoietin. J Neurosci Methods 158:234–241
12. Pantoni L, Bartolini L, Pracucci G, Inzitari D (1998) Interrater agreement on a simple neurological score in rats. Stroke 29:871–872
13. Papadopoulos MC, Manley GT, Krishna S, Verkman AS (2004) Aquaporin-4 facilitates reabsorption of excess fluid in vasogenic brain edema. FASEB J 18:1291–1293
14. Price M, Badaut J, Thevenet J, Hirt L (2010) Activation of c-Jun in the nuclei of neurons of the CA-1 in thrombin preconditioning occurs via PAR-1. J Neurosci Res 88:1338–1347
15. Schallert T, Fleming SM, Leasure JL, Tillerson JL, Bland ST (2000) CNS plasticity and assessment of forelimb sensorimotor outcome in unilateral rat models of stroke, cortical ablation, parkinsonism and spinal cord injury. Neuropharmacology 39:777–787
16. Thorne RG, Frey WH 2nd (2001) Delivery of neurotrophic factors to the central nervous system: pharmacokinetic considerations. Clin Pharmacokinet 40:907–946
17. Xi G, Keep RF, Hua Y, Xiang J, Hoff JT (1999) Attenuation of thrombin-induced brain edema by cerebral thrombin preconditioning. Stroke 30:1247–1255

Valproic Acid Pretreatment Reduces Brain Edema in a Rat Model of Surgical Brain Injury

Lei Huang, Wendy Woo, Prativa Sherchan, Nikan H. Khatibi, Paul Krafft, William Rolland, Richard L. Applegate II, Robert D. Martin, and John Zhang

Introduction

Surgical brain injury (SBI) often occurs to brain tissue at the edge of surgical resection and results from direct trauma, hemorrhage, retraction, and electrocautery [1, 6, 16]. It is a well-recognized and important clinical problem, but no specific treatments have been developed. Blood-brain barrier (BBB) disruption is one important neuropathology underlying brain injury. While a leaky BBB increases brain edema, it also favors peripheral immune cells infiltration, both of which exacerbate neural injury [8, 11, 14, 21]. Our previous studies have demonstrated that therapeutic interventions targeting BBB preservation were neuroprotective in the rodent model of surgical brain injury [7, 10, 20].

Valproic acid (VA), a histone deacetylase (HDAC), is widely used as a mood stabilizer for bipolar disorder and as an anticonvulsant in epileptics [18]. VA has been shown to be neuroprotective in several animal models of brain diseases, including ischemic reperfusion brain injury, traumatic brain injury, and intracerebral hemorrhage [4, 12, 15, 17–19]. This clinically available medicine may offer a promising therapeutic approach to ameliorate brain edema associated with SBI. Different from other brain injury, the delivery of this neuroprotective intervention presurgically would be a rational and practical way to minimize SBI in patients undergoing planned neurosurgery. In the present study, we investigated the effects of VA using a rat model of SBI, hypothesizing that VA pretreatment would decrease brain edema and improve neurological outcome.

Materials and Methods

Animals

All procedures in this study were approved by the Institutional Animal Care and Use Committee at Loma Linda University and complied with the National Institutes of Health Guide for the Care and Use of Laboratory Animals.

A total of 57 Sprague-Dawley rats weighing 280–350 g were randomized into the following studies. Twenty-four of these rats were used for 24-h studies: sham ($n=6$), SBI + vehicle ($n=6$), SBI + low-dose VA ($n=6$), and SBI + high-dose VA ($n=6$). Given that a low dose but not a high dose of VA was effective in the 24-h studies, 18 of the 57 rats were used for 72-h studies subsequently: sham ($n=6$), SBI + vehicle ($n=6$), and SBI + low-dose VA ($n=6$). The last 15 rats were used for 24-h zymography studies: sham ($n=5$), SBI + vehicle ($n=5$), and SBI + low-dose VA ($n=5$). All rats were housed in a climate-controlled environment with a 12-h light/dark cycle prior to surgeries.

L. Huang
Department of Anesthesiology, Loma Linda University, Room 2532 LLUMC, 11234 Anderson Street, Loma Linda, CA 92374, USA

Division of Physiology, Department of Basic Science, Loma Linda University, Loma Linda, CA, USA

W. Woo • P. Sherchan • P. Krafft • W. Rolland
Division of Physiology, Department of Basic Science, Loma Linda University, Loma Linda, CA, USA

N.H. Khatibi • R.L. Applegate II, MD (✉) • R.D. Martin
Department of Anesthesiology, Loma Linda University, Room 2532 LLUMC, 11234 Anderson Street, Loma Linda, CA 92374, USA
e-mail: rapplegate@llu.edu

J. Zhang
Department of Anesthesiology, Loma Linda University, Room 2532 LLUMC, 11234 Anderson Street, Loma Linda, CA 92374, USA

Division of Physiology, Department of Basic Science, Loma Linda University, Loma Linda, CA, USA

Department of Neurosurgery, Loma Linda University, Loma Linda, CA, USA

R.L. Applegate et al. (eds.), *Brain Edema XVI: Translate Basic Science into Clinical Practice*, Acta Neurochirurgica Supplement, Vol. 121,
DOI 10.1007/978-3-319-18497-5_53,

Surgical Procedure

Anesthesia was induced via induction chamber with 4 % isoflurane, and maintained with 2.5 % via nasal mask. Rats were placed prone in a stereotactic frame under a surgical operating microscope. SBI was induced as previously described [20]. Briefly, a midline incision was made with a No. 11 surgical blade to dissect the skin and connective tissue. The periosteum was reflected to expose the bregma and the right frontal skull. A 5×5-mm square craniotomy with the lower left corner at the bregma was made by a microdrill on the right frontal skull, Care was taken to keep the dura intact. For SBI animals, the dura was incised and a dissection of brain tissue was made to create a right frontal partial lobectomy. The margins of the brain tissue cut were 2 mm lateral to the sagittal suture and 1 mm proximal to the coronal suture, with the depth extending to the base of the skull. Electrocautery was used for 2 s along the coronal and sagittal borders to simulate electrocautery use in the operating room. Intraoperative packing and normal saline irrigation were used until hemostasis was obtained. Sham surgeries underwent the same surgical procedure without craniotomy and brain resection. Skin was sutured with 3.0 silk suture. Vital signs were monitored throughout surgery and recovery. At 24 or 72 h after surgery, neurobehavior was assessed, after which animals were sacrificed for brain water content or zymography as described below.

Treatment Groups

VA was administered subcutaneously 30 min prior to surgery. The low and high doses were selected based on previous studies of brain ischemia and traumatic brain injury [4, 18]. VA dilutions were freshly prepared on the day of surgery. For the low-dose group (100 mg/kg), VA was diluted to 30 mg/ml with 0.9 % sodium chloride. For the high-dose group (300 mg/kg), VA was diluted to 90 mg/ml with 0.9 % sodium chloride. SBI control was only pretreated with vehicle of 0.9 % sodium chloride in similar volumes.

Brain Water Content

Under deep anesthesia, the rat brain was quickly removed and dissected into six parts on ice: right frontal, left frontal, right parietal, left parietal, cerebellum, and brain stem. The wet weights of tissue samples were then measured immediately and dry weights were obtained after drying in an oven at 105 °C for 48 h. The percentage of water content in each part was calculated as {(wet weight − dry weight)/wet weight} × 100 %.

Matrix Metalloproteinase (MMP) Zymograph

MMP-9 and MMP-2 gelatinase activities in right frontal lobes were assessed by the zymography method as previously described [13]. Briefly, the dissected brain was homogenized in lysis buffer on ice. Following centrifugation, total supernatant protein concentrations were measured using the Bradford assay (Bio-Rad, Hercules, CA, USA). Equal protein extracts of 50 μg were loaded and separated by 10 % Tris-Glycine gel with 0.1 % gelatin as substrate (Bio-Rad). After separation, the gel was renatured and incubated in developing buffer at 37 °C for 24 h. The gel was further stained with 0.5 % Coomassie Blue R-250 for 30 min. Gelatinolytic activity was determined as clear zones or bands at the appropriate molecular weights.

Neurobehavioral Test

Before sacrificing animals, each animal had neurological assessments using modified Garcia and beam balance tests [20]. Tests were performed by an examiner (PS) kept blinded to the treatment information. The modified Garcia test involves a 21-point sensorimotor assessment that includes seven tests. Each test has a score ranging from 0 to 3, with a maximum score of 21. The tests evaluate spontaneous activity, side stroking, vibrios touch, limb symmetry, climbing, lateral turning, and forelimb walking. The beam balance test involves a beam held in place by platforms at either side. Rats were observed for behavior and time to reach either platform. Scores ranged from 0 to 5, 5 being the best.

Statistics

Quantitative data was expressed as the mean ± SEM. One-way analysis of variance (ANOVA) for multiple comparisons was used to determine differences of brain water content and MMP activities among all the groups at each time point. One-way ANOVA on ranks was used for modified Garcia and beam balance test analysis between median ranks due to failure of data normality test. A p-value less than 0.05 was considered statistically significant.

Results

Low-Dose VA Reduced SBI-Induced Brain Edema

At 24 and 72 h post surgery, brain water contents in right frontal lobes were significantly higher in all SBI animals compared with shams (80.07±0.38 %), as shown in Fig. 1. Among all the experimental groups, brain water contents were not significantly different within other brain regions, including left frontal, right parietal, left parietal, cerebellum, and brain stem.

At 24 h post surgery, VA pretreatment at the low dose significantly reduced brain edema in the right frontal lobe (81.88±1.12 %) when compared with the vehicle-pretreated SBI (83.73±1.21 %) and high-dose VA pretreatment SBI (83.30±0.3 %). The high-dose pretreatment group did not significantly decrease right frontal lobe edema compared with vehicle-pretreated SBI (Fig. 1a).

At 72 h post surgery, there was a trend that low-dose VA pretreatment reduced brain water content within the right frontal lobe in comparison with the vehicle-pretreated SBI group (82.57±1.1 % vs 83.32±1.05 %), but this was not statistically significant (Fig. 1b).

MMP Enzymatic Activity in Brain after SBI

At 24 h post surgery, MMP-9 significantly increased in vehicle-pretreated SBI animals compared with shams (Fig. 2). However, pretreatment with low-dose VA did not significantly reduce the elevation of MMP-9 enzymatic activity. There was no significant difference in MMP-2 activity among sham, vehicle-pretreated SBI, and low-dose VA-pretreated SBI groups.

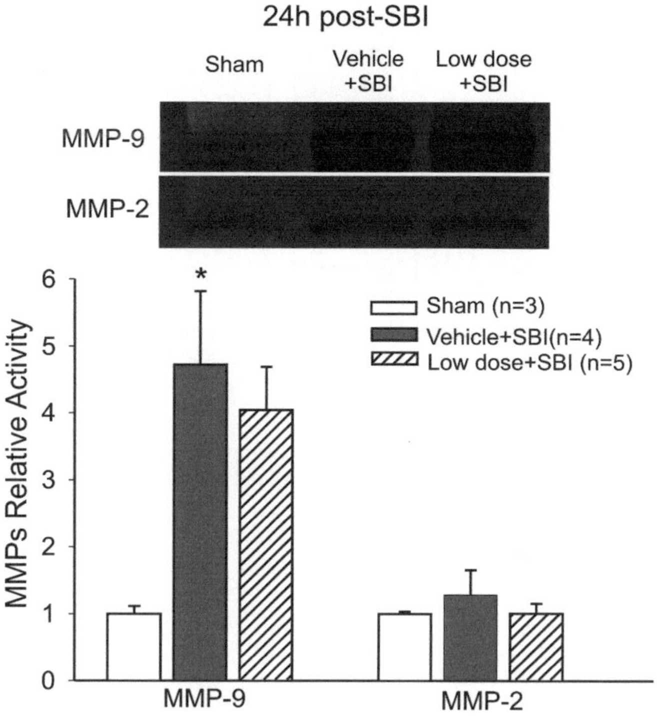

Fig. 2 MMP activities at 24 h post SBI. There was significantly increased MMP-9 but not MMP-2 activity in vehicle-pretreated SBI animals compared with sham. Low-dose valproic acid pretreatment did not significantly attenuate the elevation. *$p<0.05$ vs sham

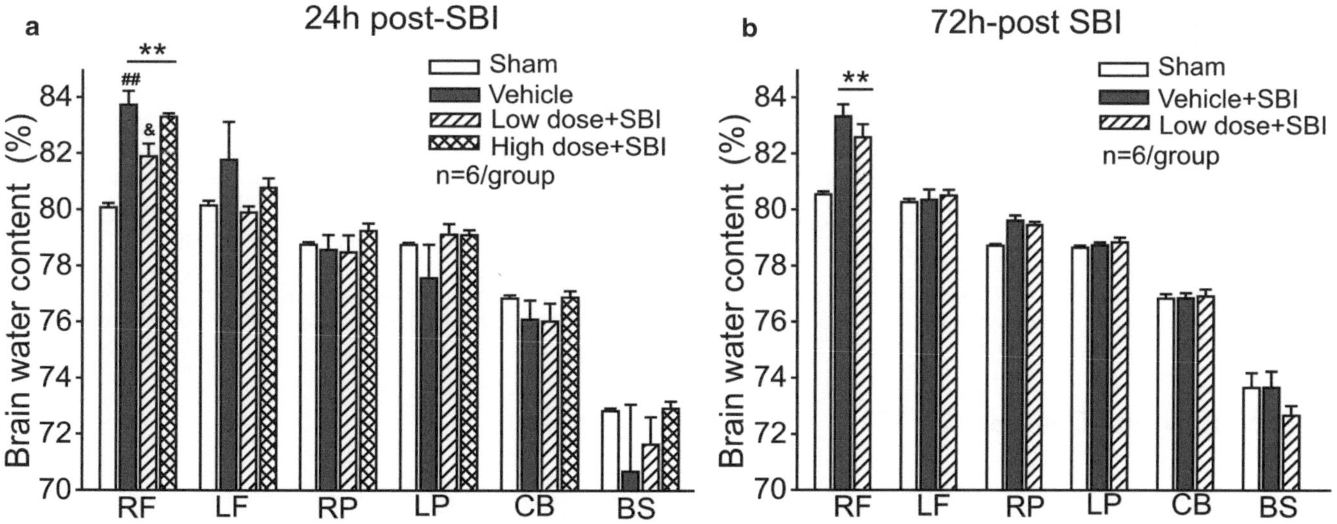

Fig. 1 Brain water content at 24 and 72 h post SBI. Brain water content was significantly higher in the ipsilateral frontal lobe (RF) of SBI animals than in shams at 24 h (**a**) and 72 h (**b**) post injury. Low-dose valproic acid (VA) pretreatment significantly reduced the brain water content increase within RF compared with vehicle-pretreated SBI animals at 24 h (**a**) post injury but not at 72 h (**b**). **$p<0.01$ vs sham, ##$p<0.01$ vs low-dose VA pretreatment, &$p<0.05$ vs low-dose VA pretreatment. *RF* right frontal lobe, *LF* left frontal lobe, *RP* right parietal lobe, *LP* left parietal lobe, *CB* cerebellum, *BS* brain stem

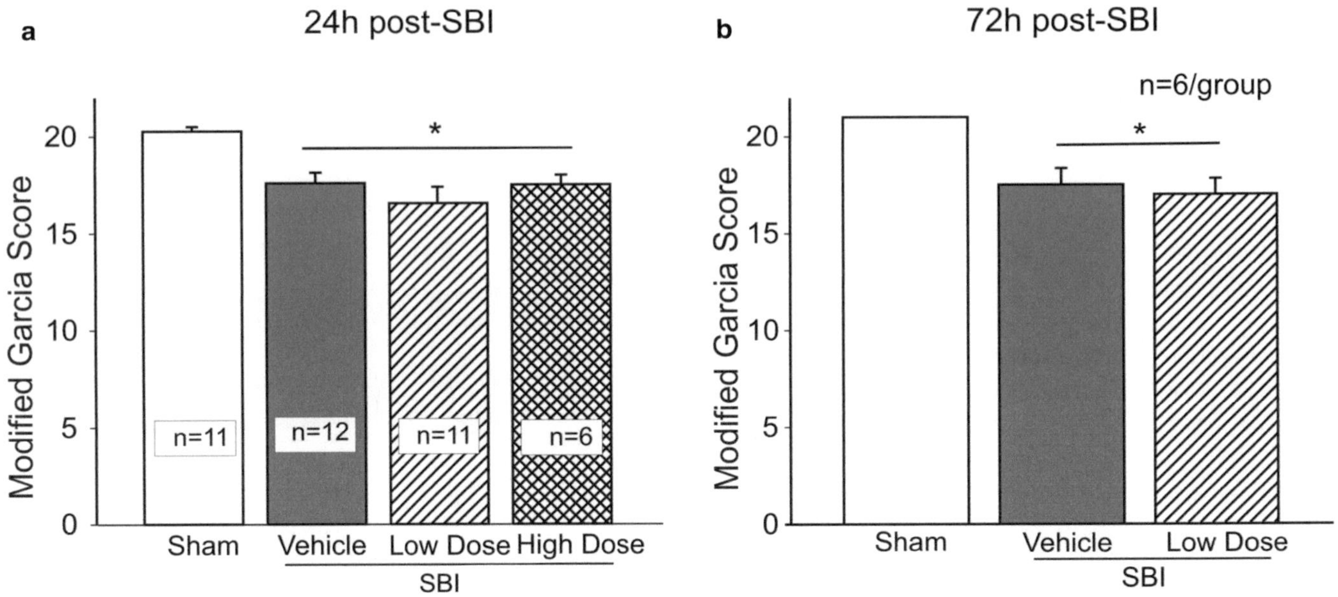

Fig. 3 Modified Garcia test at 24 and 72 h post SBI. SBI animals were associated with lower Garcia scores than shams at 24 h (**a**) and 72 h (**b**) post injury. Valproic acid pretreatment did not significantly improve Garcia scores at either time point. $*p<0.05$ vs sham

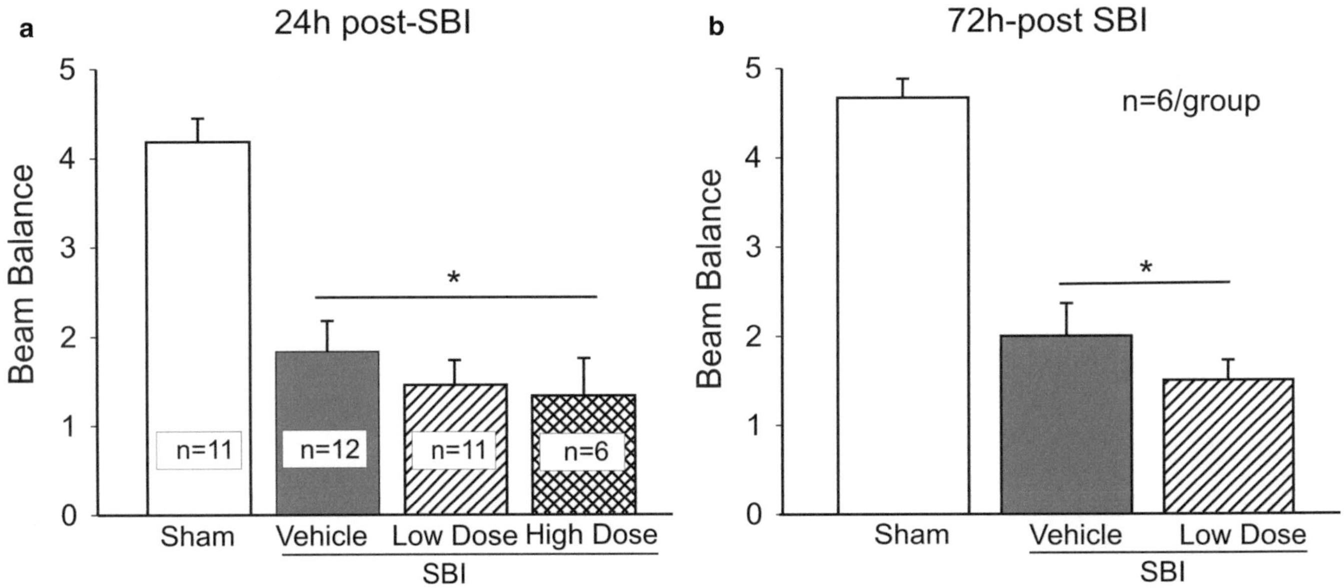

Fig. 4 Beam balance test at 24 and 72 h post SBI. SBI animals were associated with lower beam balance scores than shams at 24 h (**a**) and 72 h (**b**) post injury. Valproic acid pretreatment did not significantly improve beam balance performance at either time point. $*p<0.05$ vs sham

Neurobehavioral Deficits after SBI

At 24 and 72 h post surgery, modified Garcia and beam balance scores were significantly less in all SBI animals than shams, suggesting SBI-induced neurological deficit. Neither the low dose nor high dose of VA pretreatment significantly improved the impaired neurological function compared with vehicle-pretreated SBI (Figs. 3 and 4).

Discussion

In the present study, we demonstrated the neuroprotective effect of single-dose (100 mg/kg) VA against brain edema in a rat model of SBI. Our findings were that (1) VA pretreatment significantly attenuated brain edema at 24 h after SBI; (2) there were not significant suppressions of MMP activities associated with VA pretreatment; and (3) neurological deficits following SBI were not significantly improved by a single dose of VA pretreatment.

A rodent model of SBI introduced by our group has been shown to mimic the clinical human neurosurgery situation in that it results in the most typical postoperative consequences [7, 20]. It offers us a clinically relevant platform to study the basic pathophysiological mechanisms of SBI and to evaluate specific treatment strategies. In the right frontal lobe where brain tissue surrounds the resection site, there was a significant 3.3 % increase in water content compared with sham. Brain water content is a good indicator of brain swelling resulting from the edema. A 1 % increase in brain water content, equivalent to approximately a 4.3 % increase in tissue swelling, can lead to intracranial pressure elevation [9]. Our finding suggested the important role of brain edema associated with BBB disruption in the pathophysiology of SBI [7, 10, 20]. Neuroprotective strategies targeting brain edema would promise to limit postoperative complications; enabling more aggressive surgical approaches. The advantages and feasibility of preoperative treatment strategies rather than postoperative interventions for planned neurosurgical procedures have not been fully realized. In the present study, we demonstrated the efficacy of VA pretreatment against brain edema induced by SBI. When VA was administered 30 min before brain resection, it significantly reduced brain edema compared with vehicle-pretreated animals at 24 h after SBI. This result echoes studies in both transient and permanent middle cerebral artery occlusion (MCAO) models that show VA pretreatment attenuated ischemic brain damage and brain edema associated with BBB disruption [12, 18]. Similarly, 30 min post-injury administration of VA has also been shown to improve BBB integrity in a rodent model of traumatic brain injury [4]. The lack of protection persistent to 72 h implies that enhanced long-term neuroprotective effects may be achieved by multiple VA interventions before and after SBI.

MMPs are proteases that cleave the extracellular matrix, causing disruption of BBB, and play a critical role in brain injury associated with a variety of brain diseases [2, 3, 5]. In the current study, there was significantly higher MMP-9 activity at 24 h after SBI. It was consistent with our findings earlier using the SBI model that MMP-9 enzymatic activity was greatly elevated in the vulnerable peri-resection brain regions over the first 3 days post surgery [20]. VA pretreatment was associated with a lower level of MMP-9 activity, but this was not significantly different from that of vehicle-pretreated animals. The statistical insignificance may the result of the small sample size. On the other hand, it is possible that anti-inflammation and antioxidative effects also constitute the neuroprotective mechanisms of VA [17]. Following traumatic brain injury, BBB protection by VA may involve HDAC inhibition-mediated suppression of NF-κB and tight junction degradation in addition to MMP-9 suppression [18]. Additional research will help elucidate the underlying mechanism of VA against brain edema in the setting of SBI.

Compared with shams, modified Garcia test identified mild motor deficits in all SBI animals at 24 h post SBI and persistent to 72 h, accordant with the previous findings in the SBI model [7, 10, 20]. Along with brain edema, partial loss of frontal lobe premotor cortex or/and hemorrhage and cell death within the peri-resection frontal lobe tissue could contribute to neurological deficits. The effect of single injections of valproic acid against brain edema appeared not to be sufficient for functional protection in this study.

We conclude that VA pretreatment attenuates brain edema at 24 h after SBI in the absence of significant MMP inhibitions. Such BBB protection provided by a single intervention of VA appears to be neither long term nor associated with neurobehavioral benefits.

Acknowledgments This study is partially supported by grants from National Institute of Health (NIH) NS081740, NS043338 to J. Zhang.

Conflict of Interest Statement All authors have no conflicts of interest to disclose.

References

1. Andrews RJ, Muto RP (1992) Retraction brain ischaemia: cerebral blood flow, evoked potentials, hypotension and hyperventilation in a new animal model. Neurol Res 14:12–18
2. Aoki T, Sumii T, Mori T, Wang X, Lo EH (2002) Blood–brain barrier disruption and matrix metalloproteinase-9 expression during reperfusion injury: mechanical versus embolic focal ischemia in spontaneously hypertensive rats. Stroke 33:2711–2717
3. Badaut J, Bix GJ (2014) Vascular neural network phenotypic transformation after traumatic injury: potential role in long-term sequelae. Transl Stroke Res 5:394–406
4. Dash PK, Orsi SA, Zhang M, Grill RJ, Pati S, Zhao J, Moore AN (2010) Valproate administered after traumatic brain injury provides neuroprotection and improves cognitive function in rats. PLoS One 5:e11383
5. Gasche Y, Copin JC, Sugawara T, Fujimura M, Chan PH (2001) Matrix metalloproteinase inhibition prevents oxidative stress-associated blood–brain barrier disruption after transient focal cerebral ischemia. J Cereb Blood Flow Metab 21:1393–1400
6. Hellwig D, Bertalanffy H, Bauer BL, Tirakotai W (2003) Pontine hemorrhage. J Neurosurg 99:796; author reply 796–797
7. Jadhav V, Matchett G, Hsu FPK, Zhang JH (2007) Inhibition of Src tyrosine kinase and effect on outcomes in a new in vivo model of surgically induced brain injury. J Neurosurg 106: 680–686
8. Khanna A, Kahle KT, Walcott BP, Gerzanich V, Simard JM (2014) Disruption of ion homeostasis in the neurogliovascular unit underlies the pathogenesis of ischemic cerebral edema. Transl Stroke Res 5:3–16
9. Marmarou A, Signoretti S, Aygok G, Fatouros P, Portella G (2006) Traumatic brain edema in diffuse and focal injury: cellular or vasogenic? Acta Neurochir Suppl 96:24–29
10. Matchett G, Hahn J, Obenaus A, Zhang J (2006) Surgically induced brain injury in rats: the effect of erythropoietin. J Neurosci Methods 158:234–241
11. Pennypacker KR (2014) Targeting the peripheral inflammatory response to stroke: role of the spleen. Transl Stroke Res 5: 635–637

12. Qian YR, Lee MJ, Hwang S, Kook JH, Kim JK, Bae CS (2010) Neuroprotection by valproic acid in mouse models of permanent and transient focal cerebral ischemia. Korean J Physiol Pharmacol 14:435–440
13. Romanic AM, White RF, Arleth AJ, Ohlstein EH, Barone FC (1998) Matrix metalloproteinase expression increases after cerebral focal ischemia in rats: inhibition of matrix metalloproteinase-9 reduces infarct size. Stroke 29:1020–1030
14. Seifert HA, Pennypacker KR (2014) Molecular and cellular immune responses to ischemic brain injury. Transl Stroke Res 5: 543–553
15. Sinn DI, Kim SJ, Chu K, Jung KH, Lee ST, Song EC, Kim JM, Park DK, Kun Lee S, Kim M, Roh JK (2007) Valproic acid-mediated neuroprotection in intracerebral hemorrhage via histone deacetylase inhibition and transcriptional activation. Neurobiol Dis 26:464–472
16. Solaroglu I, Beskonakli E, Kaptanoglu E, Okutan O, Ak F, Taskin Y (2004) Transcortical-transventricular approach in colloid cysts of the third ventricle: surgical experience with 26 cases. Neurosurg Rev 27:89–92
17. Suda S, Katsura KI, Kanamaru T, Saito M, Katayama Y (2013) Valproic acid attenuates ischemia-reperfusion injury in the rat brain through inhibition of oxidative stress and inflammation. Eur J Pharmacol 707:26–31
18. Wang Z, Leng Y, Tsai LK, Leeds P, Chuang DM (2011) Valproic acid attenuates blood–brain barrier disruption in a rat model of transient focal cerebral ischemia: the roles of HDAC and MMP-9 inhibition. J Cereb Blood Flow Metab 31:52–57
19. Xuan A, Long D, Li J, Ji W, Hong L, Zhang M, Zhang W (2012) Neuroprotective effects of valproic acid following transient global ischemia in rats. Life Sci 90:463–468
20. Yamaguchi M, Jadhav V, Obenaus A, Colohan A, Zhang JH (2007) Matrix metalloproteinase inhibition attenuates brain edema in an in vivo model of surgically-induced brain injury. Neurosurgery 61:1067–1075
21. Zhao X, Sun G, Zhang H, Ting SM, Song S, Gonzales N, Aronowski J (2014) Polymorphonuclear neutrophil in brain parenchyma after experimental intracerebral hemorrhage. Transl Stroke Res 5:554–561

Epsilon Aminocaproic Acid Pretreatment Provides Neuroprotection Following Surgically Induced Brain Injury in a Rat Model

Esther S. Komanapalli, Prativa Sherchan, William Rolland II, Nikan Khatibi, Robert D. Martin, Richard L. Applegate II, Jiping Tang, and John H. Zhang

Introduction

Neurosurgical procedures can damage viable brain tissue unintentionally through a wide range of mechanisms. This surgically induced brain injury (SBI) can be a result of direct surgical trauma, intraoperative bleeding, thermal injury from electrocautery, or stretch damage from tissue retraction [1, 6]. The concern with these injuries is the escalated inflammatory response that mounts in an attempt to combat the effects of brain tissue damage. Propagation of this local response may result in direct cell death, enhanced disruption of the blood-brain barrier (BBB) causing an increase in brain edema formation, and subsequent deterioration in neurobehavioral function [7, 8, 14]. Therefore, some studies have looked into targeting specific anti-inflammatory mediators that may be more effective at reducing cell death and brain edema while improving neurobehavioral outcome following surgical brain injury [14]. Unfortunately, current therapies such as steroids and diuretics are relatively nonspecific and focus mostly on reducing the postoperative edema that has already developed [7].

Plasmin is a serine protease that acts to dissolve fibrin blood clots. It is released from the liver into the systemic circulation as a zymogen called plasminogen [13]. Upon binding to cell surfaces, plasminogen can be converted to plasmin by a variety of enzymes, including tissue plasminogen activator (tPA). A growing body of animal-based studies provides evidence to suggest that tPA-activated plasmin may orchestrate the disruption of the BBB by enhancing matrix metalloproteinase activity and nuclear factor kB [2, 9, 15]. Additionally, clinical studies have shown that re-hemorrhage following subarachnoid hemorrhage can be significantly reduced by plasmin inhibition [5, 11]. Thus, it is possible that blockade of plasmin may provide a level of neuroprotection.

Epsilon aminocaproic acid (EAA) is a well-recognized lysine antifibrinolytic analogue. It works primarily by competitively inhibiting the conversion of plasminogen to plasmin in the bloodstream [3]. By doing so, EAA can reduce the levels of active plasmin and potentially preserve the neurovascular unit of the brain. Consequently, in the present study, we investigated the role of EAA in SBI, specifically determining its role in reducing brain edema and neurobehavioral deficits. We hypothesized that pretreatment with EAA will attenuate brain edema formation and, in turn, preserve neurobehavioral function in a rat SBI model.

Materials and Methods

Animals

The Institutional Animal Care and Use Committee (IACUC) of Loma Linda University approved all procedures for this study. Twenty-eight Sprague-Dawley rats weighing 280–350 g (Charles River, Wilmington, MA, USA) were housed in a 12-h light/dark cycle at a controlled temperature and

E.S. Komanapalli • N. Khatibi • R.D. Martin
R.L. Applegate II, MD
Department of Anesthesiology, Loma Linda University School of Medicine, Loma Linda, CA, USA

P. Sherchan • W. Rolland II • J. Tang
Department of Physiology and Pharmacology, Loma Linda University School of Medicine, Loma Linda, CA, USA

J.H. Zhang, MD, PhD (✉)
Department of Anesthesiology, Loma Linda University School of Medicine, Loma Linda, CA, USA

Department of Physiology and Pharmacology, Loma Linda University School of Medicine, Loma Linda, CA, USA

Departments of Anesthesiology, Physiology and Neurosurgery, Loma Linda University School of Medicine, 11234 Anderson Street, Room 2562B, Loma Linda, CA 92354, USA

Department of Neurosurgery, Loma Linda University School of Medicine, Loma Linda, CA, USA
e-mail: johnzhang3910@yahoo.com

R.L. Applegate et al. (eds.), *Brain Edema XVI: Translate Basic Science into Clinical Practice*, Acta Neurochirurgica Supplement, Vol. 121,
DOI 10.1007/978-3-319-18497-5_54,

humidity with free access to food and water. During surgery, body temperature was monitored and kept constant. Rats were divided into four groups: sham ($n=7$), SBI ($n=7$), SBI + low-dose EAA ($n=7$), and SBI + high-dose EAA ($n=7$).

SBI Rat Model

Anesthesia was induced in an induction chamber with 4 % isoflurane concentration, and maintained with 2.5 % concentration via nasal mask. Rats were placed prone in a stereotactic frame under a surgical operating microscope. A midline incision was made with a No. 11 surgical blade to dissect the skin and connective tissue. The periosteum was reflected to expose the bregma and the right frontal skull. A square operating area with a 5-mm edge was identified, with the lower left corner at the bregma. A microdrill was used to thin out the cranium to translucency, being careful not to penetrate the skull and underlying dura. A bone lifter and forceps were then used to lift the piece of square bone. Dura overlying brain tissue was exposed. Sham surgeries were stopped at this point. For the SBI and treatment groups, a 22-gauge needle was then used to incise the dura and underlying brain tissue. A dissection of brain tissue was made to create a partial right frontal lobe resection. The margins of the brain tissue cut were 2 mm lateral to the sagittal suture and 1 mm proximal to the coronal suture, with the depth extending to the base of the skull. Electrocautery was used for 2 s along the coronal and sagittal borders to simulate electrocautery use in the operating room. Intraoperative packing and normal saline irrigation were used until hemostasis was obtained. The overlying connective tissue was replaced and skin was sutured with 3.0 silk sutures. Vital signs were monitored throughout surgery and recovery. Animals were recovered and maintained until 24 h after surgery for neurobehavioral tests. Animals were sacrificed after neurobehavioral testing to measure brain water content was performed as described below.

Treatment Methods

EAA was administered 30 min prior to surgery. The doses for low- and high-dose groups were based on previous studies on subarachnoid hemorrhage models [5]. For the low-dose group (150 mg/kg), EAA was diluted to 30 mg/ml with 0.9 % sodium chloride and given through an intraperitoneal injection 30 min prior to SBI. For the high-dose group (450 mg/kg), EAA was diluted to 90 mg/ml with 0.9 % sodium chloride and given through an intraperitoneal injection 30 min prior to SBI. The EAA dilutions were freshly prepared on the day of surgery. Control was provided by normal saline injections administered in similar volumes given through an intraperitoneal injection 30 min before surgery to sham and or SBI animals.

Assessment of Neurobehavioral Deficits

Neurological outcomes were assessed by an observer blinded to group at 24 h post SBI using the modified Garcia score [4]. The modified Garcia score is a 21-point sensorimotor assessment system consisting of seven tests with scores of 0–3 for each test (maximum score = 21). The seven tests are (1) spontaneous activity, (2) side stroking, (3) vibrissae touch, (4) limb symmetry, (5) climbing (6) lateral turning, and (7) forelimb walking.

Brain Water Content

Brain water content was measured at 24 h after surgery. At the time of sacrifice, the rat brain was immediately removed and divided into six parts: right frontal, left frontal, right parietal, left parietal, cerebellum, and brain stem. The tissue samples were weighed on an electronic digital balance (APX-60, Denver Instrument, Arvada, CO, USA) then placed in an oven at 105° centigrade for 48 h. The percentage of water content was calculated as [(wet weight – dry weight)/wet weight] × 100 %.

Statistical Methods

Quantitative data were expressed as the mean ± SEM for brain water content and Garcia test. One-way analysis of variance (ANOVA) was used to determine brain water content differences between the means and expressed with 95 % confidence intervals of the means. One-way ANOVA on ranks was used for modified Garcia test analysis, and data were expressed as median (25–75 % interquartile range) because they were not normally distributed. Statistical analysis was performed using computerized statistical software (Sigma Plot 10.0, Systat Software, San Jose, CA, USA). A p-value of <0.05 was considered statistically significant.

Results

EAA Therapy Reduced Brain Water Content Following SBI in Rats

Brain water content was measured 24 h post SBI. Low-dose EAA (150 mg/kg) significantly reduced brain water content (79.83 ± 1.12 %) compared with the vehicle-treated SBI group

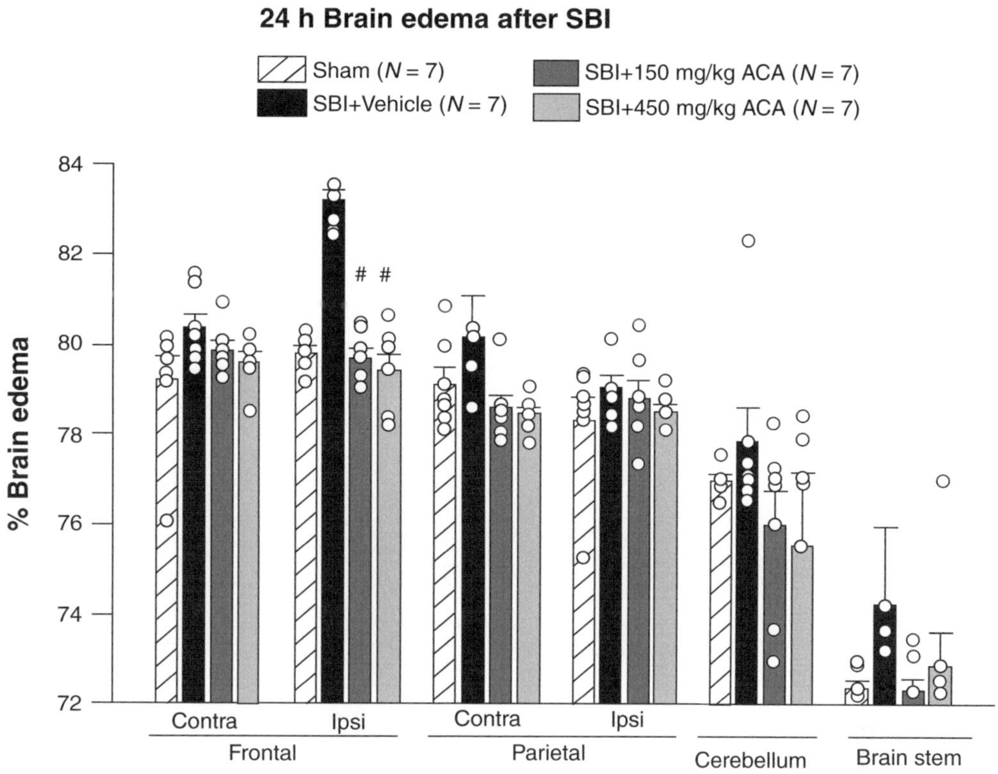

Fig. 1 Brain water content at 24 h after surgery. Brain water content was increased in the right frontal lobe at 24 h after SBI. This increase was significantly reduced with both high-dose and low-dose EAA therapy: sham group (79.71 ± 0.38 %); SBI group (82.76 ± 1.21 %); low-dose EAA (79.83 ± 1.12 %); high-dose EAA (450 mg/kg) (79.71 ± 0.38 %). $^{\#}p<0.05$ compared with vehicle group

(82.76 ± 1.21 %; $p<0.05$). This water content was comparable with the sham group (79.71 ± 0.38 %). High-dose EAA (450 mg/kg) rats showed a significant reduction in brain water content at 24 h (79.46 ± 1.5 %) compared with the vehicle-treated SBI group (82.76 ± 1.21 %; $p<0.05$) and was again comparable with the sham group (79.71 ± 0.38 %) (Fig. 1).

EAA Therapy Improved Neurobehavioral Function Following SBI in Rats

The modified Garcia test was performed to evaluate sensorimotor deficits at 24 h post SBI. Vehicle-treated SBI rats (14.50 ± 1.23) showed significant neurobehavioral deficit compared with the sham group (19.83 ± 0.88; $p<0.05$). Low-dose EAA (150 mg/kg) rats showed a significant improvement in neurobehavioral function at 24 h (18.33 ± 0.85) compared with the vehicle-treated SBI group (14.50 ± 1.23; $p<0.05$). High-dose EAA (450 mg/kg) rats showed a significant improvement in neurobehavioral function (18.50 ± 0.76) compared with the vehicle-treated SBI group (14.50 ± 1.23; $p<0.05$) (Fig. 2).

Discussion

Neurosurgical procedures can lead to postoperative cerebral damage at the margins of the operative site. This SBI can damage viable brain tissue unintentionally by a wide range of methods used during neurosurgical interventions. The concern with these injuries is the heightened inflammatory response that can propagate direct cell death that, in turn, can enhance BBB disruption, with subsequent increase in brain edema and deterioration in neurobehavioral function. Even if patients survive the insult, currently there are limited effective treatment options to help them recover afterwards. Similarly, effective pretreatment therapies to help prevent and/or reduce SBI damage are also limited. In the present study, we investigated the effects of EAA therapy on SBI, including the potential of this therapy to reduce brain edema and thus prevent the development of sensorimotor behavioral deficits.

Structural brain damage manifesting as cell death and edema following SBI is not an uncommon phenomenon. Previous work in SBI has shown massive neuronal degeneration and death in the area of injury [12], along with findings of increased expression of proapoptotic factors, inflammatory mediators, and proteolytic enzymes throughout the brain and in circulation. Furthermore, BBB integrity can be compromised through matrix metalloproteinase upregulation [2, 9, 15], which leads to propagation of inflammatory cell-mediated cerebral damage and worsening of cerebral edema. One of the orchestrators of BBB disruption is plasmin.

EAA acid is a well-recognized lysine antifibrinolytic analogue. It works primarily by competitively inhibiting the conversion of plasminogen to plasmin in the bloodstream [3]. By doing so, EAA can reduce the levels of active plasmin and potentially preserve the neurovascular unit of the brain.

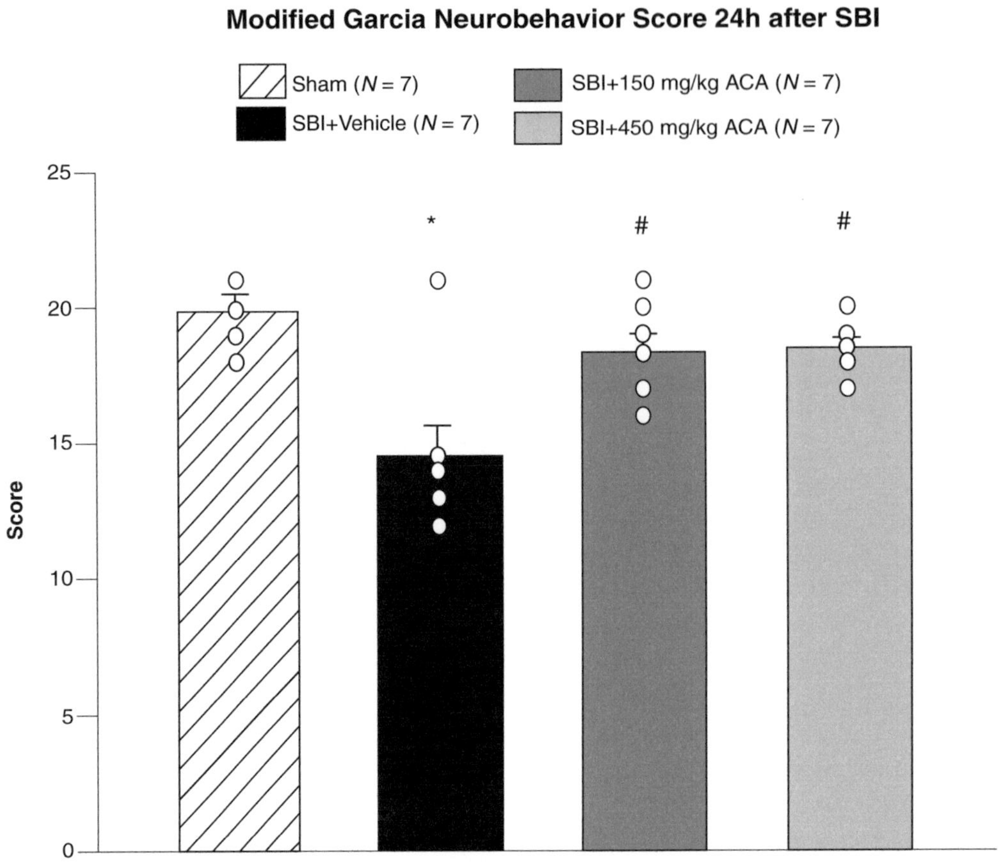

Fig. 2 Neurobehavioral function at 24 h after surgery. Vehicle rats had significant neurobehavioral deficits compared with sham rats. Both low- and high-dose EAA treatment significantly improved neurobehavioral testing scores at 24 h post SBI: sham group (19.83 ± 0.88); SBI group (14.50 ± 1.23); low-dose EAA (150 mg/kg) (18.33 ± 0.85); high-dose EAA (450 mg/kg) (18.50 ± 0.76). *$p<0.05$ compared with sham group; #$p<0.05$ compared with vehicle group

Previous studies in the pediatric extracorporeal membrane oxygenation patient population found that EAA significantly reduced the incidence of intracerebral hemorrhage through BBB preservation, possibly through plasmin inhibition. In the spontaneous intracerebral hemorrhagic stroke population, research suggests that EAA could decrease hematoma sizes in stroke victims by reducing plasmin-mediated neuronal damage [10]. Other studies showed that re-hemorrhage following subarachnoid hemorrhage was significantly reduced, in part because of plasmin inhibition [5, 11]. These studies suggest a role for EAA therapy to block the effects of plasmin on BBB disruption and, in doing so, improve the neurological outcome of subject populations. We found that EAA therapy before surgery resulted in reduced cerebral edema and with the apparent structural protection, neurobehavioral function was well preserved. This is similar to previous work, suggesting that EAA may provide a therapeutic regimen necessary to block plasmin-mediated neurovascular and neurologic damage. Our study had limitations in that we did not study the potential mechanism of EAA-induced reduction in brain edema following SBI. Further studies are warranted to determine how EAA mediates preservation of the neurovascular unit following SBI.

In conclusion, this study implies that morphologic changes in the brain, including brain edema, are affected positively by EAA pretreatment, and, through this protection, neurobehavioral function can be preserved. Consequently, further studies are needed to explore the use of EAA therapy in the clinical setting of SBI.

Sources of Funding This study is partially supported by National Institutes of Health grant NS084921.

Disclosures All authors attest they have no conflicts of interest to disclose.

References

1. Andrews RJ, Muto RP (1992) Retraction brain ischaemia: cerebral blood flow, evoked potentials, hypotension and hyperventilation in a new animal model. Neurol Res 14:12–18

2. Aoki T, Sumii T, Mori T, Wang X, Lo EH (2002) Blood–brain barrier disruption and matrix metalloproteinase-9 expression during reperfusion injury: mechanical versus embolic focal ischemia in spontaneously hypertensive rats. Stroke 33:2711–2717
3. Deysine M, Cliffton EE (1964) Mechanism of action of epsilon aminocaproic acid in the control of hemorrhage. Ann N Y Acad Sci 115:291–297
4. Garcia JH, Wagner S, Liu KF, Hu XJ (1995) Neurological deficit and extent of neuronal necrosis attributable to middle cerebral artery occlusion in rats. Statistical validation. Stroke 26:627–634
5. Harrigan MR, Rajneesh KF, Ardelt AA, Fisher WS 3rd (2010) Short-term antifibrinolytic therapy before early aneurysm treatment in subarachnoid hemorrhage: effects on rehemorrhage, cerebral ischemia, and hydrocephalus. Neurosurgery 67:935–939
6. Hernesniemi J, Leivo S (1996) Management outcome in third ventricular colloid cysts in a defined population: a series of 40 patients treated mainly by transcallosal microsurgery. Surg Neurol 45:2–14
7. Jadhav V, Solaroglu I, Obenaus A, Zhang JH (2007) Neuroprotection against surgically induced brain injury. Surg Neurol 67:15–20
8. Khatibi NH, Jadhav V, Matus B, Fathali N, Martin R, Applegate R, Tang J, Zhang JH (2011) Prostaglandin E2 EP1 receptor inhibition fails to provide neuroprotection in surgically induced brain-injured mice. Acta Neurochir Suppl 111:277–281
9. Lee SR, Guo SZ, Scannevin RH, Magliaro BC, Rhodes KJ, Wang X, Lo EH (2007) Induction of matrix metalloproteinase, cytokines and chemokines in rat cortical astrocytes exposed to plasminogen activators. Neurosci Lett 417:1–5
10. Piriyawat P, Morgenstern LB, Yawn DH, Hall CE, Grotta JC (2004) Treatment of acute intracerebral hemorrhage with epsilon-aminocaproic acid: a pilot study. Neurocrit Care 1:47–51
11. Starke RM, Kim GH, Fernandez A, Komotar RJ, Hickman ZL, Otten ML, Ducruet AF, Kellner CP, Hahn DK, Chwajol M, Mayer SA, Connolly ES Jr (2008) Impact of a protocol for acute antifibrinolytic therapy on aneurysm rebleeding after subarachnoid hemorrhage. Stroke 39:2617–2621
12. Sulejczak D, Grieb P, Walski M, Frontczak-Baniewicz M (2008) Apoptotic death of cortical neurons following surgical brain injury. Folia Neuropathol 46:213–219
13. Weitz JI, Stewart RJ, Fredenburgh JC (1999) Mechanism of action of plasminogen activators. Thromb Haemost 82:974–982
14. Yamaguchi M, Jadhav V, Obenaus A, Colohan A, Zhang JH (2007) Matrix metalloproteinase inhibition attenuates brain edema in an in vivo model of surgically-induced brain injury. Neurosurgery 61:1067–1075; discussion 1075–1066
15. Zhang X, Polavarapu R, She H, Mao Z, Yepes M (2007) Tissue-type plasminogen activator and the low-density lipoprotein receptor-related protein mediate cerebral ischemia-induced nuclear factor-kappaB pathway activation. Am J Pathol 171:1281–1290

Correlation Between Subacute Sensorimotor Deficits and Brain Edema in Rats after Surgical Brain Injury

Devin W. McBride, Yuechun Wang, Loic Adam, Guillaume Oudin, Jean-Sébastien Louis, Jiping Tang, and John H. Zhang

Introduction

No matter how carefully a neurosurgical procedure is performed, it is intrinsically linked to postoperative deficits resulting in delayed healing caused by direct trauma, hemorrhage, and brain edema, termed surgical brain injury (SBI) [1, 3, 7, 11]. Cerebral edema and hemorrhage are major postoperative complications of SBI and are major contributors to patient morbidity, resulting in increased postoperative care.

Although there are several interventions utilized to minimize bleeding and damage to healthy tissue surrounding the retraction site, there is still significant burden placed on the US health-care system for postoperative recovery of neurosurgical patients [2]. Although novel therapies are being developed in preclinical models, translation of these therapies is limited, possibly because of the inadequate use of neurobehavioral testing [16, 21].

The SBI rodent model [11] mimics clinical SBI pathophysiology, including intraoperative hemorrhage, brain edema, neuroinflammation, and postoperative hematoma [10, 11]. Although numerous behavioral tests are available to assess functional recovery after injury [14, 15, 17, 18], many of them have not been examined for the SBI rodent model. Furthermore, the choice of behavioral test depends on the neurological disease of interest; SBI significantly impairs the sensorimotor function.

The most common sensorimotor tests for rodents are the composite Garcia neuroscore and beam walking test. Although these tests were first utilized for assessing function in rodents after ischemic brain injury [21], they have also been utilized in the rat SBI model [11]. However, a variety of alternative sensorimotor tests exist and have not been the focus of functional assessment after SBI [4, 12]. Furthermore, no publication has yet examined whether a correlation between brain water content and functional deficits exists after SBI in rats. Thus, herein we examine the correlation between neurological function and brain water content in rats 24 h after SBI.

Materials and Methods

All experiments were approved by the Institutional Animal Care and Use Committee at Loma Linda University. Adult male Sprague-Dawley (SD) rats (290–320 g) were used in all experiments.

Surgical Brain Injury Model

SBI was induced in male SD rats via partial unilateral frontal lobectomy as previously described [11]. Briefly, animals were anesthetized with 3 % isoflurane in O_2 mixed with medical gas (4.5 L/min initial, 2.5 L/min sustained). Anesthetized animals were placed into a standard rodent stereotactic frame, a midline skin incision was made, and a right-sided craniectomy (5×5 mm) was performed (1 mm posterior to the bregma and 2 mm lateral to midline). The right frontal lobe was sharply dissected to the base of the brain. Hemostasis was achieved using a combination of electrocautery, direct pressure with hemostatic dressings, and normal saline irrigation. Once intraoperative hemorrhage stopped, the cranial window was sealed with bone wax, the skin was sutured, and animals were allowed

D.W. McBride • Y. Wang • L. Adam • G. Oudin
J.-S. Louis • J. Tang
Department of Physiology and Pharmacology, Loma Linda University School of Medicine, Loma Linda, CA, USA

J.H. Zhang, MD, PhD (✉)
Department of Physiology and Pharmacology, Loma Linda University School of Medicine, Loma Linda, CA, USA

Department of Neurosurgery, Loma Linda University School of Medicine, Loma Linda, CA, USA
e-mail: jhzhang@llu.edu

R.L. Applegate et al. (eds.), *Brain Edema XVI: Translate Basic Science into Clinical Practice*, Acta Neurochirurgica Supplement, Vol. 121,
DOI 10.1007/978-3-319-18497-5_55, © Springer International Publishing Switzerland 2016

to recover. Animals received subcutaneous injections of 0.9 % normal saline (1 mL) and buprenorphine (0.03 mg/kg).

Neurobehavior Testing

Twenty-four hours after injury, neurobehavior was assessed using the composite Garcia neuroscore ($n = 10$), beam walking test ($n = 10$), corner turn test ($n = 10$), and beam balance test ($n = 35$) as previously described [5, 8, 13, 21].

Briefly, composite Garcia neuroscore [5] consists of seven independent subtests (spontaneous activity, axial sensation, vibrissae proprioception, limb movement symmetry, lateral turning, forelimb walking, and climbing), each scored between 0 (completely impaired function) and 3 (retained complete function). The neuroscore for sham versus SBI animals was analyzed using the Mann–Whitney test and presented as mean ± standard error of the mean (SEM).

Assessment of beam walking ability [21] was conducted by placing rats midway on a horizontal round beam (90 × 2 cm) connected to two platforms at the beam ends. Rats were given 40 s to move along the beam. Scoring was as follows: 0 (worst performance) if animals fell off the beam in less than 40 s, 1 if animals stayed on the beam for at least 40 s, 2 if animals moved less than halfway to a platform (in less than 40 s) and stayed on the beam at least 25 s, 3 if animals moved more than halfway to a platform and stayed on the beam at least 25 s, 4 if animals reached a platform in less than 40 s, 5 if animals reached a platform in less than 25 s. The beam walking score for sham versus SBI animals was analyzed using the Mann–Whitney test and presented as the mean ± SEM.

The corner turn test [9] examined preference for left versus right turning. Rats approached a 30° corner, and to exit, animals had to turn around along the corner, turning to the left or right. The choice of turning side was recorded for 20 trials with at least 30 s between each trial. Corner turn test score was calculated ((as number of left turns)/(total turns)) × 100.

The beam balance test [6] examines proprioception and balance using a horizontal Plexiglas beam (2 × 80 cm, 25 cm tall). The animals were placed midway on the beam, and with an innate tendency to avoid falling, animals walked along the beam. A total of 3 min was given for the beam balance test. The distance traveled during the 3 min was scored in 1-cm ticks.

After neurological testing, animals were sacrificed for right frontal lobe brain water content evaluation using the wet-dry method [20]. Under deep anesthesia, animals were decapitated and brain samples quickly removed. Dissected brains were separated into frontal and parietal lobes for the ipsilateral (right) and contralateral (left) hemispheres, then weighed for wet weights. The samples were dried at 100 °C for 24 h before measuring the dry weights. Brain water content was calculated as ((wet weight − dry weight)/(wet weight)) × 100. Brain water content was analyzed using unpaired t-test and presented as the mean ± SEM.

All behavioral data are presented as the individual data points and corresponding brain water content. Correlation between brain water content and neurological deficits was analyzed with the Spearman's rank correlation coefficients (ρ) and best-fit linear regressions were determined.

Results

The brain water content of animals subjected to SBI (82.57 ± 0.313 %) is significantly elevated compared with sham-operated animals (80.27 ± 0.178 %) ($p < 0.05$, Fig. 1a).

Neurobehavior

Twenty-four hours after SBI, before euthanasia, animals were subjected to four neurobehavioral tests: composite Garcia neuroscore (neuroscore), beam walking test, corner turn test, and beam balance test.

Composite Garcia Neuroscore

The neuroscore of injured animals (15.8 ± 0.52) was statistically lower than that of sham animals (19.71 ± 0.18) ($p < 0.05$, Fig. 1b) 24 h after SBI. However, while statistically lower than SBI-injured animals, the neuroscore did not significantly correlate with the brain water content of the right-frontal lobe 24 h post-ictus ($\rho = -0.02$, $p > 0.05$, Fig. 2a).

Beam Walking

Beam walking score for SBI-injured animals (1.4 ± 0.36) was significantly lower than sham animals (4.3 ± 0.36) ($p < 0.05$, Fig. 1c). Yet, no significant correlation was observed between the beam walking score and right-frontal lobe brain water content 24 h after SBI ($\rho = -0.33$, $p > 0.05$, Fig. 2b).

Corner Turn Test

The number of left turns in the corner turn test significantly correlated with the brain water content of the right-frontal lobe 24 h following SBI ($\rho = -0.70$, $p < 0.05$, Fig. 2c).

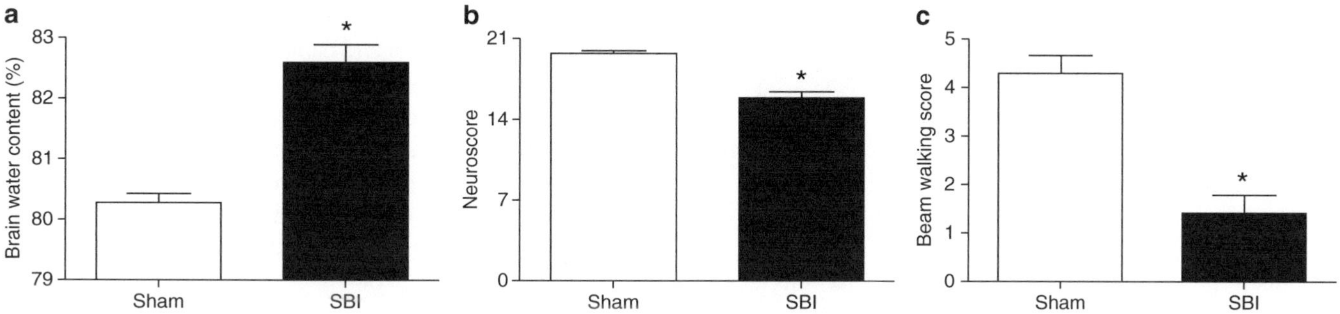

Fig. 1 Brain water content and neurobehavior differences after SBI. (**a**) Brain water content (sham $n=7$, SBI $n=12$). (**b**) Composite Garcia neuroscore (sham $n=7$, SBI $n=12$). (**c**) Beam walking score (sham $n=7$, SBI $n=12$) *p < 0.05 vs Sham

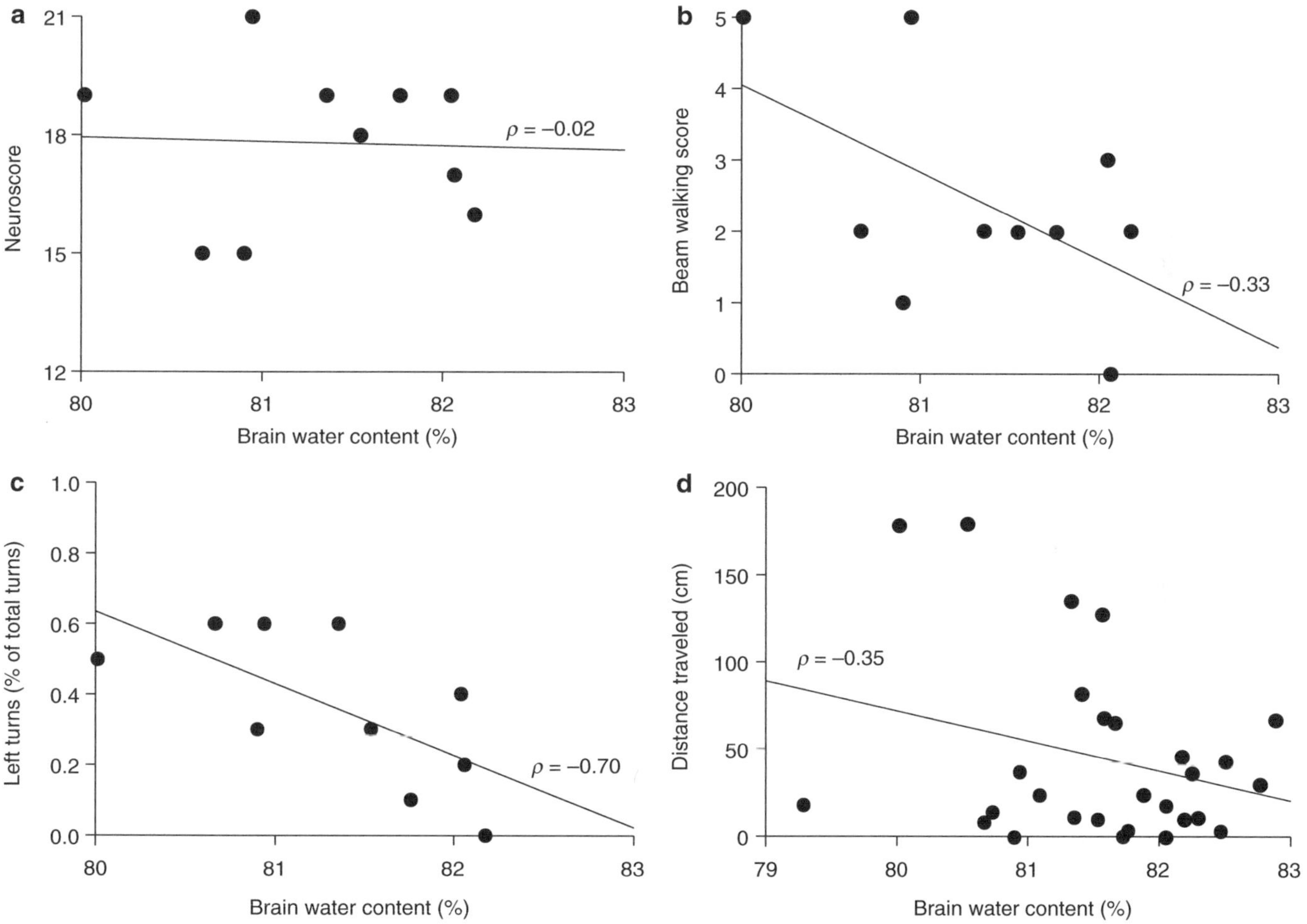

Fig. 2 Neurobehavior correlation with brain water content in animals subjected to SBI. (**a**) Composite Garcia neuroscore ($n=10$). (**b**) Beam walking score ($n=10$). (**c**) Corner turn test ($n=10$). (**d**) Beam balance test ($n=35$). All correlations were tested for correlation using Spearman's rank correlation coefficient (ρ) and statistical significance (p-value)

Beam Balance Test

The distance traveled for the beam balance test also significantly correlated with brain water content ($\rho=-0.35$, $p<0.05$, Fig. 2d).

Discussion

SBI pathophysiology develops over several hours after the initial insult. The primary injury consists of the initial lobectomy and intraoperative hemorrhage [11]. Secondary injury occurs within hours of resection and includes brain edema, neuroinflammation, and postoperative hematoma [10, 11]. As with most neurological diseases, brain edema is a predictor of poor outcome in patients. Therefore, development of novel therapies for reducing or preventing cerebral edema is key to lowering the costs of SBI.

The rat model of SBI, developed by Vikram et al. [11], mimics the damage to healthy tissue that is unavoidable during many neurosurgical procedures. Post SBI, rats experience an increase of 4–5 % in brain water content of the right-frontal lobe, causing tissue swelling [11]. The current study utilized the rat SBI model to identify the appropriate sensorimotor tests for evaluating drug efficacy after SBI.

Herein, four common and inexpensive sensorimotor tests were examined for their ability to predict the magnitude of cerebral edema after SBI. The composite Garcia neuroscore is a combination of several subtests evaluating sensorimotor function [5, 13]. Furthermore, the composite Garcia neuroscore has the benefit of identifying deficits caused by unilateral injury because a number of the tests examine left versus right function, such as axial sensation and limb movement symmetry [5, 13]. Despite the fact that statistically significant functional deficits are found between SBI-injured animals and sham animals (Fig. 1b), they did not correlate with the brain water content. This is likely due, in part, to the inclusion of neuroscore subtests that do not identify unilateral injury but rather the presence of an injury, such as spontaneous movement. It is important to note that the vast majority of SBI-injured animals scored perfectly on the spontaneous activity subtest, which has previously been observed for unilateral injuries [13].

The beam walking test examined motor coordination and balance. Although the beam walking test found a difference in the ability of injured animals to cross to a platform compared with sham animals (Fig. 1c), no correlation was observed between beam walking score and brain water content. Despite the lack of correlation for the beam walking test, a trend is apparent, suggesting that an injury is present, but the uninjured side was likely able to compensate for the deficits in an animal's ability to complete the beam walking test. Our results for the beam walking test are similar to other unilateral injuries, specifically intracerebral hemorrhage, which found that brain water content did not correlate with the function of rodents on the beam walking test [13].

The corner turn test was first used to examine functional deficits after focal cerebral ischemia in mice [22]. The animal's tendency to turn in a particular direction is measured using the corner turn test, and after a unilateral injury, such as SBI, animals are expected to turn toward the ipsilateral side due to functional deficits in the contralateral limbs [19]. The nature of the SBI rodent model argues for use of the corner turn test, and is supported by the significant correlation between corner turn functional deficits and brain water content in rats after SBI. The beam balance test, which examines proprioception and balance deficits, has many variations, increasing sensitivity for finding marked differences in the performance of injured versus noninjured animals. Herein, we utilized the standard horizontal plane and used the distance traveled as the measure of injury. Although the beam balance test is not inherently a test used to identify unilateral injury, we observed that the functional deficits correlated with brain water content. Similar to the beam walking test, animals may be able to compensate for unilateral deficits, preferring to use the uninjured side. However, the amount of time allotted for testing with the beam balance test (3 min) may have increased sensitivity, making the neurobehavioral deficits apparent in the analysis of distance traveled during this task.

In conclusion, the brain water content of SBI-injured rats was found to significantly correlate to the functional deficits in the corner turn and beam balance tests. No correlation was found for the neuroscore and beam walking score and brain water content. This study suggests that the most appropriate neurofunctional tests for post-SBI behavioral analysis are the corner turn and beam balance tests. Further studies include examining additional cost-effective neurobehavior tests for correlation between functional deficits and brain edema.

Acknowledgments This work was supported by National Institutes of Health grants R01 NS043338 and NS084921 (JHZ).

Disclosure The authors have no conflicts of interest to report.

References

1. Andrews RJ, Muto RP (1992) Retraction brain ischaemia: cerebral blood flow, evoked potentials, hypotension and hyperventilation in a new animal model. Neurol Res 14:12–18
2. Dautremont JF, Rudmik LR, Yeung J, Asante T, Nakoneshny SC, Hoy M, Lui A, Chandarana SP, Matthews TW, Schrag C, Dort JC (2013) Cost-effectiveness analysis of a postoperative clinical care pathway in head and neck surgery with microvascular reconstruction. J Otolaryngol Head Neck Surg 42:59
3. Deletis V, Sala F (2001) The role of intraoperative neurophysiology in the protection or documentation of surgically induced injury to the spinal cord. Annals of the New York Academy of Sciences 939:137–144
4. Eckermann JM, Wanqiu C, Jadhav V, Hsu FPK, Colohan ART, Tang J, Zhang JH (2011) Hydrogen is neuroprotective against surgically induced brain injury. Med Gas Res 1:7
5. Garcia JH, Wagner S, Liu KF, Hu XJ (1995) Neurological deficit and extent of neuronal necrosis attributable to middle cerebral artery occlusion in rats – statistical validation. Stroke 26:627–634
6. Goldstein LB, Davis JN (1990) Beam-walking in rats: studies towards developing an animal model of functional recovery after brain injury. J Neurosci Methods 31:101–107
7. Hellwig D, Bertalanffy H, Bauer BL, Tirakotai W (2003) Pontine hemorrhage. J Neurosurg 99:796; auther reply: 796–797

8. Hua Y, Schallert T, Keep RF, Wu JM, Hoff JT, Xi GH (2002) Behavioral tests after intracerebral hemorrhage in the rat. Stroke 33:2478–2484
9. Hua Y, Xi GJ, Keep RF, Wu JM, Jiang YJ, Hoff JT (2002) Plasminogen activator inhibitor-1 induction after experimental intracerebral hemorrhage. J Cereb Blood Flow Metab 22:55–61
10. Hyong A, Jadhav V, Lee S, Tong W, Rowe J, Zhang JH, Tang J (2008) Rosiglitazone, a PPAR gamma agonist, attenuates inflammation after surgical brain injury in rodents. Brain Res 1215:218–224
11. Jadhav V, Matchett G, Hsu FPK, Zhang JH (2007) Inhibition of Src tyrosine kinase and effect on outcomes in a new in vivo model of surgically induced brain injury. J Neurosurg 106:680–686
12. Jadhav V, Ostrowski RP, Tong W, Matus B, Jesunathadas R, Zhang JH (2009) Cyclo-oxygenase-2 mediates hyperbaric oxygen preconditioning-induced neuroprotection in the mouse model of surgical brain injury. Stroke 40:3139–3142
13. Krafft PR, McBride DW, Lekic T, Rolland WB, Mansell CE, Ma Q, Tang J, Zhang JH (2014) Correlation between subacute sensorimotor deficits and brain edema in two mouse models of intracerebral hemorrhage. Behav Brain Res 264:151–160
14. Kunze A, Zierath D, Drogomiretskiy O, Becker K (2014) Strain differences in fatigue and depression after experimental stroke. Transl Stroke Res 5:604–611
15. Kunze A, Zierath D, Drogomiretskiy O, Becker K (2014) Variation in behavioral deficits and patterns of recovery after stroke among different rat strains. Transl Stroke Res 5:569–576
16. Lapchak PA, Zhang JH, Noble-Haeusslein LJ (2013) RIGOR guidelines: escalating STAIR and STEPS for effective translational research. Transl Stroke Res 4:279–285
17. Nobile CW, Palmateer JM, Kane J, Hurn PD, Schallert T, Adkins DL (2014) Impaired limb reaction to displacement of center of gravity in rats with unilateral striatal ischemic injury. Transl Stroke Res 5:562–568
18. Rosell A, Agin V, Rahman M, Morancho A, Ali C, Koistinaho J, Wang X, Vivien D, Schwaninger M, Montaner J (2013) Distal occlusion of the middle cerebral artery in mice: are we ready to assess long-term functional outcome? Transl Stroke Res 4: 297–307
19. Schallert T (2006) Behavioral tests for preclinical intervention assessment. NeuroRx 3:497–504
20. Tang JP, Liu J, Zhou CM, Alexander JS, Nanda T, Granger DN, Zhang JH (2004) MMP-9 deficiency enhances collagenase-induced intracerebral hemorrhage and brain injury in mutant mice. J Cereb Blood Flow Metab 24:1133–1145
21. Zausinger S, Hungerhuber E, Baethmann A, Reulen HJ, Schmid-Elsaesser R (2000) Neurological impairment in rats after transient middle cerebral artery occlusion: a comparative study under various treatment paradigms. Brain Res 863:94–105
22. Zhang L, Schallert T, Zhang ZG, Jiang Q, Arniego P, Li QJ, Lu M, Chopp M (2002) A test for detecting long-term sensorimotor dysfunction in the mouse after focal cerebral ischemia. J Neurosci Methods 117:207–214

Propofol Pretreatment Fails to Provide Neuroprotection Following a Surgically Induced Brain Injury Rat Model

Colleen Pakkianathan, Michael Benggon, Nikan H. Khatibi, Hank Chen, Suzzanne Marcantonio, Richard Applegate II, Jiping Tang, and John Zhang

Introduction

Neurosurgical procedures unintentionally damage viable brain tissue by a wide range of methods. These surgically induced brain injuries (SBI) can be a result of direct surgical trauma, intraoperative bleeding, thermal injury from electrocautery, or stretch damage from tissue retraction [2, 6]. The concern with these injuries is the heightened inflammatory response that mounts in an attempt to combat the effects of brain tissue damage. Propagation of this local response may result in direct cell death, enhanced disruption of the blood-brain barrier (BBB), causing an increase in brain edema formation, and subsequent deterioration in neurobehavioral function [10, 17]. Unfortunately, current therapies such as steroids and diuretics are relatively nonspecific and focus mostly on reducing the postoperative edema that has already transpired [10]. Further, evidence from human randomized controlled trials does not yet allow firm conclusions regarding clinical practice [4]. Therefore, studies have investigated targeting specific anti-inflammatory mediators before surgery, as this pretreatment may be more effective at reducing cell death and brain edema while improving neurobehavior.

C. Pakkianathan • M. Benggon • N.H. Khatibi
R. Applegate II, MD (✉)
Department of Anesthesiology, Loma Linda School of Medicine, Room 2532 LLUMC, 11234 Anderson Street, Loma Linda, CA 92354, USA
e-mail: rapplegate@llu.edu

H. Chen • J. Tang
Division of Physiology, Department of Basic Science, Loma Linda School of Medicine, Loma Linda, CA, USA

S. Marcantonio • J. Zhang
Department of Anesthesiology, Loma Linda School of Medicine, Room 2532 LLUMC, 11234 Anderson Street, Loma Linda, CA 92354, USA

Division of Physiology, Department of Basic Science, Loma Linda School of Medicine, Loma Linda, CA, USA

Propofol (2,6-diisopropylphenol) is a short-acting, intravenous hypnotic agent widely used for the induction and maintenance of general anesthesia in the perioperative setting, for intensive care unit patient sedation, and for short-term sedation during interventional procedures [11]. The favorable pharmacokinetic characteristics and neurologic profiles of propofol have resulted in its popularity among health-care professionals. Propofol post-treatment following transient cerebral ischemia has been suggested to provide brain protection against direct and indirect inflammatory damages through scavenging reactive oxygen species, potentiation of GABA-A-mediated inhibition of synaptic transmission, and/or inhibition of glutamate release [12, 19].

In the present study, we investigated the potential for pretreatment with propofol to confer a neuroprotective effect in SBI rats. We hypothesized that pretreatment would preserve structural integrity of the brain with reductions in brain edema formation and reduced neurobehavioral deficits.

Materials and Methods

Animals

The Loma Linda University Institutional Animal Care and Use Committee approved all procedures for this study. Twenty-four adult male Sprague-Dawley rats weighing 280–350 g (Charles River, Wilmington, MA, USA) were housed in a controlled temperature and humidity environment with a 12-h light/dark cycle and given free access to food and water. During surgery, body temperature was monitored and kept constant. The rats were randomly assigned to one of four groups: sham ($n=6$), SBI+ vehicle ($n=6$), SBI+ 20 mg/kg propofol ($n=6$), and SBI+ 60 mg/kg propofol ($n=6$).

R.L. Applegate et al. (eds.), *Brain Edema XVI: Translate Basic Science into Clinical Practice*, Acta Neurochirurgica Supplement, Vol. 121, 323
DOI 10.1007/978-3-319-18497-5_56,

SBI Rat Model

Anesthesia was induced in an induction chamber with 4 % isoflurane concentration and maintained with 2.5 % concentration via nasal mask. Rats were placed prone in a stereotactic frame under a surgical operating microscope. A midline incision was made with a No. 11 surgical blade to dissect the skin and connective tissue. The periosteum was reflected to expose the bregma and the right frontal skull. A square operating area with a 5-mm edge was identified, with the lower left corner at the bregma. A microdrill was used to thin out the cranium to translucency, being careful not to penetrate the skull and underlying dura. A bone lifter and forceps were then used to lift the piece of square bone. Dura overlying brain tissue was exposed. Sham surgeries were stopped at this point. For the SBI and treatment groups, a 22-gauge needle was used to incise the dura and underlying brain tissue. A dissection of brain tissue was made to create a right frontal lobectomy. The margins of the brain tissue cut were 2 mm lateral to the sagittal suture and 1 mm proximal to the coronal suture, with the depth extending to the base of the skull. Electrocautery was used for 2 s along the coronal and sagittal borders to simulate electrocautery use in the operating room. Intraoperative packing and normal saline irrigation was used until hemostasis was obtained. The overlying connective tissue was replaced and skin was sutured with 3.0 silk sutures. Vital signs were monitored throughout surgery and recovery. Animals were recovered and maintained 24 h after surgery for neurobehavioral tests. Animals were sacrificed after neurobehavioral testing for brain water content as described below.

Treatment Methods

Propofol was administered 30 min before surgery via intraperitoneal injections. The doses for low- and high-dose groups were based on previous studies in transient ischemic models [3, 9, 18]. Control was provided by administering 10 % intralipid intraperitoneal injections in similar volumes 30 min before surgery to sham and SBI animals.

Assessment of Neurobehavioral Deficits

An observer who was blinded to group assignment assessed neurological outcomes at 24 h after SBI using the modified Garcia score, vibrissae-elicited forelimb placement, and adhesive bilateral tactile stimulation tests [5, 13, 15]. The modified Garcia score is a 21-point sensorimotor assessment system consisting of seven tests with scores of 0–3 for each test (maximum score=21). These seven tests included (1) spontaneous activity, (2) side stroking, (3) vibrissae touch, (4) limb symmetry, (5) climbing, (6) lateral turning, and (7) forelimb walking.

For the vibrissae-elicited forelimb placement test, rats were held by their torsos, allowing the forelimb to hang free. The rats were gently moved up and down before testing to facilitate muscle relaxation and eliminate any struggling movement. Trials during which extreme muscle tension, struggling, or placing of any of the limbs onto the experimenter's hand occurred were not counted. Independent testing of each forelimb was induced by brushing the respective vibrissae on the corner edge of a countertop. Intact rats place the forelimb ipsilateral to the stimulated vibrissae quickly onto the countertop. Depending on the extent of injury, placement of the forelimb contralateral to the injury in response to contralateral vibrissae contact with the countertop may be impaired. Each rat was tested 10 times for each forelimb, and the percentage of trials in which the rat placed the appropriate forelimb on the edge of the countertop in response to the vibrissae stimulation was determined. Testers were highly experienced and blind to the treatment group of the animal [13].

The adhesive bilateral tactile stimulation test measures somatosensory deficit. Briefly, two small pieces of adhesive-backed paper dots (of equal size, 113.1 mm^2) were used as bilateral tactile stimuli occupying the distal-radial region on the wrist of each forelimb. The time required to remove the stimuli from each limb was recorded. Each rat received five trials at 24 h after injury and the mean time required to remove both stimuli from limbs was recorded [15].

Brain Water Content

Brain water content was measured 24 h after surgery. At the time of sacrifice, the rat brain was immediately removed and divided into six parts: right frontal, left frontal, right parietal, left parietal, cerebellum, and brain stem. The tissue samples were weighed on an electronic digital balance (APX-60, Denver Instrument, Arvada, CO, USA). Samples were then placed in an oven at 105° centigrade for 48 h. The percentage of water content was calculated as [(wet weight − dry weight)/wet weight] × 100 %.

Statistical Methods

Quantitative data were expressed as the mean ± standard error of the mean (SEM) for brain water content. One-way analysis of variance (ANOVA) was used to determine brain water content differences between the means and expressed with 95 % confidence intervals of the means. One-way ANOVA on ranks was used for the neurobehavioral tests analysis and data were expressed as median (25–75 % interquartile range) because these were not normally distributed. Analysis was performed using computerized software, with a p-value < 0.05 considered statistically significant.

Results

Propofol Therapy Fails to Reduce Brain Water Edema Following SBI in Rats

Brain water content was measured at 24 h post-injury using the established model noted above. As shown in Fig. 1, neither propofol dose demonstrated a statistically significant reduction in brain water content at 24 h (high-dose: 82.5 ± 1.0 %; low-dose: 83 ± 1.0 %) compared with the SBI rat group (82.5 ± 1.0 %; p-value >0.05).

Propofol Therapy Fails to Reduce Neurobehavioral Deficits Following SBI in Rats

Results of modified Garcia test, vibrissae-elicited forelimb placement, and adhesive bilateral tactile stimulation tests conducted at 24 h after SBI showed that vehicle rats presented with severe neurobehavioral deficits compared with sham rats (Fig. 2). However, pretreatment with low- or high-dose propofol failed to reduce neurobehavioral deficits following SBI at 24 h after injury (p > 0.05).

Discussion

Surgically induced brain injuries can damage viable brain tissue unintentionally by a wide range of methods. The concern with these injuries is that heightened inflammatory response can propagate direct cell death, enhance disruption of the BBB, and subsequently worsen deterioration in

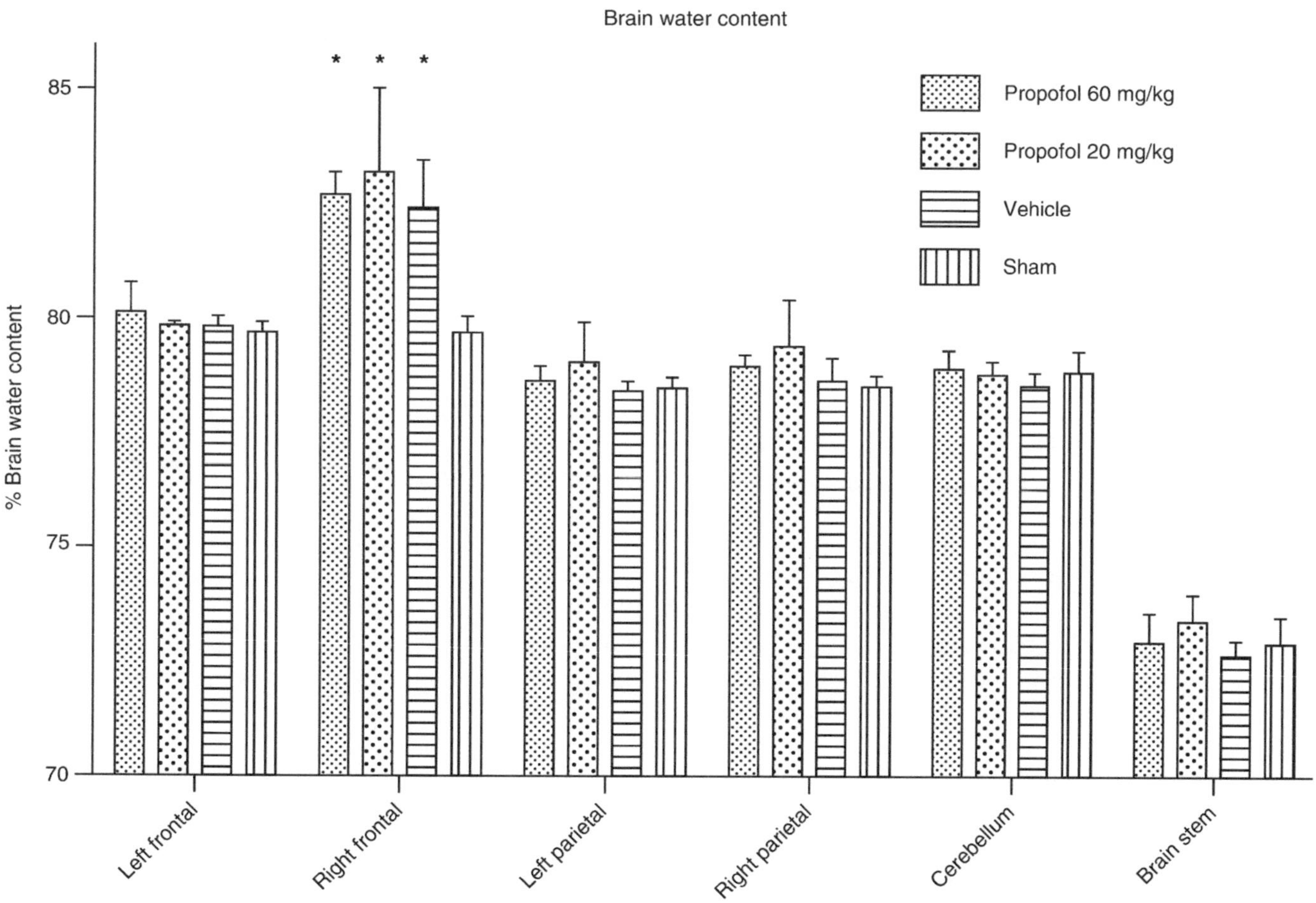

Fig. 1 Brain water content at 24 h; brain water content increased significantly in the right frontal lobe at 24 h post SBI injury. This increase was not reduced following propofol therapy (p > 0.05)

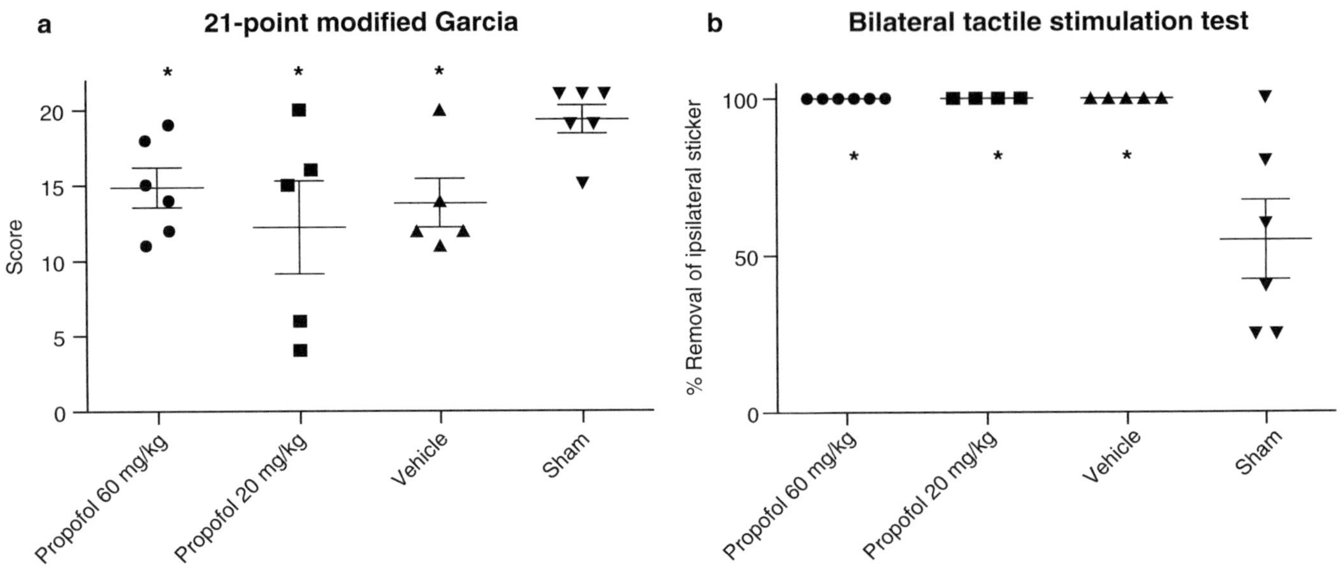

Fig. 2 Neurobehavioral function. Neurobehavioral deficits were present in all vehicle rats compared with sham rats. Following propofol treatment, there was no significant improvement in either (**a**) the 21-point Garcia or (**b**) the bilateral tactile stimulation test at 24 h post SBI ($p > 0.05$)

neurobehavioral function. Even if patients survive the insult, effective treatment options that improve recovery are limited. Further, no established presurgery therapies are available to help prevent or reduce these collateral damages. In the present study, we investigated the effects of propofol pretreatment therapy on SBI in hopes of demonstrating the potential for this therapy to reduce structural damage at the site of injury and, in doing so, lessen the subsequent sensorimotor behavioral deficits.

Structural brain damage manifesting as cell death and edema following SBI is not an uncommon phenomenon. Previous work in SBI demonstrates massive neuronal degeneration and death in the area of injury [16], including increased expression of proapoptotic factors in cortical neurons and inflammatory cytokines. Study of propofol therapy post-injury using a traumatic brain injury model in rats found that a protective effect can develop through suppression of microglia cell activation and inhibition of a number of inflammatory markers in the ischemic brain [8, 14]. This was echoed in a study that found propofol could reduce lipopolysaccharide-induced inflammatory mediators [7]. Similarly, propofol was shown to reduce cerebral infarct volume by over 30 % using an in vitro model of focal ischemia [1], suggesting preservation of brain structure could occur if inflammatory mediators were attenuated.

Interpretation of our findings is limited by several factors. In our study, vehicle SBI rats had significant damage to their brain structure, as evidenced by a statistically significant increase in brain water content. However propofol pretreatment failed to demonstrate a reduction in brain water content following surgery. The lack of structural preservation was associated with a similar reduction in neurobehavioral deficits following brain injury compared with vehicle treatment, suggesting propofol therapy may not provide neuroprotection as a pretreatment modality in SBI models. However, the timing of treatment could have impacted this result. We chose to inject propofol 30 min prior to the insult to mimic the usual anesthetic course during neurosurgery as closely as possible. However, given the pharmacokinetics of propofol, it is possible there is a need for multiple treatments during and after the injury to demonstrate neuroprotection. To activate and/or amplify targets involved in the plasticity process and improve neurobehavioral deficits, additional propofol doses may be needed after the initial injury. Alternatively, the sheer magnitude of injury caused by this particular established SBI model may be greater than the degree of neuroprotection provided by propofol, thus potentially masking potential impacts on outcome measures.

The results of this study imply that SBI-related morphologic changes in the brain are not affected by propofol pretreatment. Consequently, further studies will be needed to explore the use of propofol therapy in the clinical setting of SBI.

Sources of Funding This study is partially supported by National Institutes of Health grant NS084921.

Disclosure All authors attest they have no conflicts of interest to disclose.

References

1. Adembri C, Venturi L, Tani A, Chiarugi A, Gramigni E, Cozzi A, Pancani T, De Gaudio RA, Pellegrini-Giampietro DE (2006) Neuroprotective effects of propofol in models of cerebral ischemia: inhibition of mitochondrial swelling as a possible mechanism. Anesthesiology 104:80–89
2. Andrews RJ, Muto RP (1992) Retraction brain ischaemia: cerebral blood flow, evoked potentials, hypotension and hyperventilation in a new animal model. Neurol Res 14:12–18
3. Arcadi FA, Rapisarda A, De Luca R, Trimarchi GR, Costa G (1996) Effect of 2,6-diisopropylphenol on the delayed hippocampal cell loss following transient forebrain ischemia in the gerbil. Life Sci 58:961–970
4. Bilotta F, Gelb AW, Stazi E, Titi L, Paoloni FP, Rosa G (2013) Pharmacological perioperative brain neuroprotection: a qualitative review of randomized clinical trials. Br J Anaesth 110(Suppl 1): i113–i120
5. Garcia JH, Wagner S, Liu KF, Hu XJ (1995) Neurological deficit and extent of neuronal necrosis attributable to middle cerebral artery occlusion in rats. Statistical validation. Stroke 26:627–634
6. Hernesniemi J, Leivo S (1996) Management outcome in third ventricular colloid cysts in a defined population: a series of 40 patients treated mainly by transcallosal microsurgery. Surg Neurol 45:2–14
7. Hsing CH, Lin MC, Choi PC, Huang WC, Kai JI, Tsai CC, Cheng YL, Hsieh CY, Wang CY, Chang YP, Chen YH, Chen CL, Lin CF (2011) Anesthetic propofol reduces endotoxic inflammation by inhibiting reactive oxygen species-regulated Akt/IKKbeta/NF-kappaB signaling. PLoS One 6:e17598
8. Hsu BG, Yang FL, Lee RP, Peng TC, Chen HI (2005) Effects of post-treatment with low-dose propofol on inflammatory responses to lipopolysaccharide-induced shock in conscious rats. Clin Exp Pharmacol Physiol 32:24–29
9. Ito H, Watanabe Y, Isshiki A, Uchino H (1999) Neuroprotective properties of propofol and midazolam, but not pentobarbital, on neuronal damage induced by forebrain ischemia, based on the GABAA receptors. Acta Anaesthesiol Scand 43:153–162
10. Jadhav V, Solaroglu I, Obenaus A, Zhang JH (2007) Neuroprotection against surgically induced brain injury. Surg Neurol 67:15–20
11. Kotani Y, Shimazawa M, Yoshimura S, Iwama T, Hara H (2008) The experimental and clinical pharmacology of propofol, an anesthetic agent with neuroprotective properties. CNS Neurosci Ther 14:95–106
12. Lee JH, Cui HS, Shin SK, Kim JM, Kim SY, Lee JE, Koo BN (2013) Effect of propofol post-treatment on blood–brain barrier integrity and cerebral edema after transient cerebral ischemia in rats. Neurochem Res 38:2276–2286
13. Lekic T, Ani C (2012) Posterior circulation stroke: animal models and mechanism of disease. J Biomed Biotechnol 2012: 587590
14. Luo T, Wu J, Kabadi SV, Sabirzhanov B, Guanciale K, Hanscom M, Faden J, Cardiff K, Bengson CJ, Faden AI (2013) Propofol limits microglial activation after experimental brain trauma through inhibition of nicotinamide adenine dinucleotide phosphate oxidase. Anesthesiology 119:1370–1388
15. Schallert T, Upchurch M, Lobaugh N, Farrar SB, Spirduso WW, Gilliam P, Vaughn D, Wilcox RE (1982) Tactile extinction: distinguishing between sensorimotor and motor asymmetries in rats with unilateral nigrostriatal damage. Pharmacol Biochem Behav 16:455–462
16. Sulejczak D, Grieb P, Walski M, Frontczak-Baniewicz M (2008) Apoptotic death of cortical neurons following surgical brain injury. Folia Neuropathol 46:213–219
17. Yamaguchi M, Jadhav V, Obenaus A, Colohan A, Zhang JH (2007) Matrix metalloproteinase inhibition attenuates brain edema in an in vivo model of surgically-induced brain injury. Neurosurgery 61:1067–1075
18. Yamaguchi S, Hamaguchi S, Mishio M, Okuda Y, Kitajima T (2000) Propofol prevents lipid peroxidation following transient forebrain ischemia in gerbils. Can J Anaesth 47:1025–1030
19. Zhou R, Yang Z, Tang X, Tan Y, Wu X, Liu F (2013) Propofol protects against focal cerebral ischemia via inhibition of microglia-mediated proinflammatory cytokines in a rat model of experimental stroke. PLoS One 8:e82729

Hydrocephalus Section

Intraventricular Injection of Noncellular Cerebrospinal Fluid from Subarachnoid Hemorrhage Patient into Rat Ventricles Leads to Ventricular Enlargement and Periventricular Injury

Peiliang Li, Neeraj Chaudhary, Joseph J. Gemmete, B. Gregory Thompson, Ya Hua, Guohua Xi, and Aditya S. Pandey

Introduction

Aneurysmal subarachnoid hemorrhage (SAH) is a life-threatening condition leading to significant morbidity and mortality and affecting nearly 35,000 patients on a yearly basis [1, 2]. SAH patients can present with acute hydrocephalus (HCP) leading to increase in intracranial pressure (ICP) and thus reduced cerebral perfusion pressure [3], leading to significant secondary early brain injury (EBI) [4]. Acute HCP development post SAH could be explained by several mechanisms: cerebrospinal fluid (CSF) flow obstruction secondary to blood products, CSF dynamic changes, and CSF absorption deficit [5]. Interestingly, one study has shown that intraventricular fibrinolysis aimed at lysing intraventricular blood neither reduced permanent shunt dependency nor influenced functional outcome [6]. Our previous animal studies revealed that not only lysed red blood cell and iron could induce HCP but that HCP could also be induced by intraventricular injection of thrombin [7, 8]. Thus, the metabolic products of blood seem to play a role in the development of HCP after hemorrhage. Nonetheless, the mechanisms of developing acute HCP and EBI post SAH are not well understood. We aimed to document the development of HCP and subependymal injury after injecting CSF from human SAH patients into rat ventricles with the goal of determining the mechanism of such injuries.

P. Li
Department of Neurosurgery, University of Michigan, Ann Arbor, MI, USA

Department of Neurosurgery, Huashan Hospital, Fudan University, Shanghai, China

N. Chaudhary • J.J. Gemmete • B.G. Thompson
Y. Hua • G. Xi • A.S. Pandey, MD (✉)
Department of Neurosurgery, University of Michigan, Ann Arbor, MI, USA
e-mail: adityap@med.umich.edu

Materials and Methods

Animal use protocols were approved by the University of Michigan Committee on the Use and Care of Animals. A total of seven male Sprague-Dawley rats (3 months old, Charles River Laboratories, Portage, MI, USA), weighing 250–300 g, were used in this study and randomly enrolled in the CSF injection group ($n=4$) or control group ($n=3$). Informed consents were obtained from SAH patients whose CSF was collected for this study.

Model Establishment

Rats were anesthetized with pentobarbital (50 mg/kg, intraperitoneally) and the right femoral artery was catheterized to monitor arterial blood pressure, blood pH, PaO_2, $PaCO_2$, hematocrit, and glucose levels. Core body temperature was maintained at 37.5 °C with a feedback-controlled heating pad. Rats were positioned in a stereotaxic frame (Kopf Instruments, Tujunga, CA, USA). A cranial burr hole (1 mm) was drilled and a 26-gauge needle was inserted stereotaxically into the right lateral ventricle (coordinates: 0.6 mm posterior, 4.5 mm ventral, and 1.6 mm lateral to the bregma). Two-hundred microliters of SAH patient's noncellular CSF or control CSF was injected with 0.04 mg/mL propidium iodide (PI), an indicator of necrotic cell death, using a micro-infusion pump (World Precision Instruments, Sarasota, FL, USA). After injection, the needle was removed, the burr hole was filled with bone wax, and the skin incision was closed with sutures. The rats were kept on a warm pad separately until fully awake. Rats that had intraventricular injection with patient SAH CSF were called the experimental group as compared with the rats injected with control patient non-SAH CSF, denoted as the control group.

R.L. Applegate et al. (eds.), *Brain Edema XVI: Translate Basic Science into Clinical Practice*, Acta Neurochirurgica Supplement, Vol. 121, 331
DOI 10.1007/978-3-319-18497-5_57, © Springer International Publishing Switzerland 2016

Ventricle Area Measurement and PI-Positive Cell Density

Brain sections were dehydrated with ethanol at graded concentrations of 50–100 %(v/v) and then stained with hematoxylin and eosin (H&E staining). Three brain sections (50 μm anterior and posterior to the bregma level) were scanned and the ventricle was outlined on a computer by a blinded observer. The ventricular areas were measured using NIH Image J software (Image Version 1.63, National Institutes of Health). The mean of the three measurements was regarded as the ventricular area at the bregma level. PI-positive cell density was meanwhile analyzed on the same section.

Immunohistochemistry

Rats were anesthetized with pentobarbital (100 mg/kg, intraperitoneally) and perfused with 4 % paraformaldehyde in 0.1 mol/L phosphate-buffered saline (pH 7.4). The brains were removed and kept in 4 % paraformaldehyde for 24 h and then immersed in 30 % sucrose for 2–3 days at 4 °C. Brains were embedded in optimal cutting temperature compound (Sakura Finetek, Torrance, CA, USA) and 18-mm-thick slices cut using a cryostat. Immunohistochemical studies were performed using the avidin–biotin complex technique as previously described [9]. The primary antibody was rabbit anti-HO-1 (1:400 dilution; Abcam, Cambridge, MA, USA). The numbers of HO-1–positive cells in each tissue sample were counted in three fields of view and expressed as the mean of the positive cells per square millimeter.

Statistical Analysis

All data in this study are presented as mean ± standard deviation (SD). Data from different animal groups were analyzed using analysis of variance with a Student *t*-test. Differences were considered significant at probability values less than 0.05.

Results

Physiologic parameters, including mean arterial blood pressure, arterial blood gases, pH, hematocrit, and glucose, were within normal range. All rats within the study survived.

There was overall enlargement of the lateral ventricles in the rats that had patient SAH CSF injection as compared with control patient CSF injection. This was objectively appreciated as rats with patient SAH CSF injection had much larger ventricles as compared with rats with control patient CSF injection (3.1 ± 0.3 mm² vs 1.9 ± 0.2, $p<0.05$, Fig. 1). More severe periventricular injury was documented in the experimental rats as compared with control rats as evident by the greater periventricular PI staining within the experimental group (0.192 ± 0.083 vs 0.008 ± 0.002, $p<0.05$, Fig. 2). Increasing periventricular injury was also appreciated in the experimental group as compared with the control group as evident by the greater oxidative injury based on elevated HO-1 expression (HO-1–positive cell intensity, 0.589 ± 0.170 vs 0.044 ± 0.018, $p<0.05$, Fig. 3).

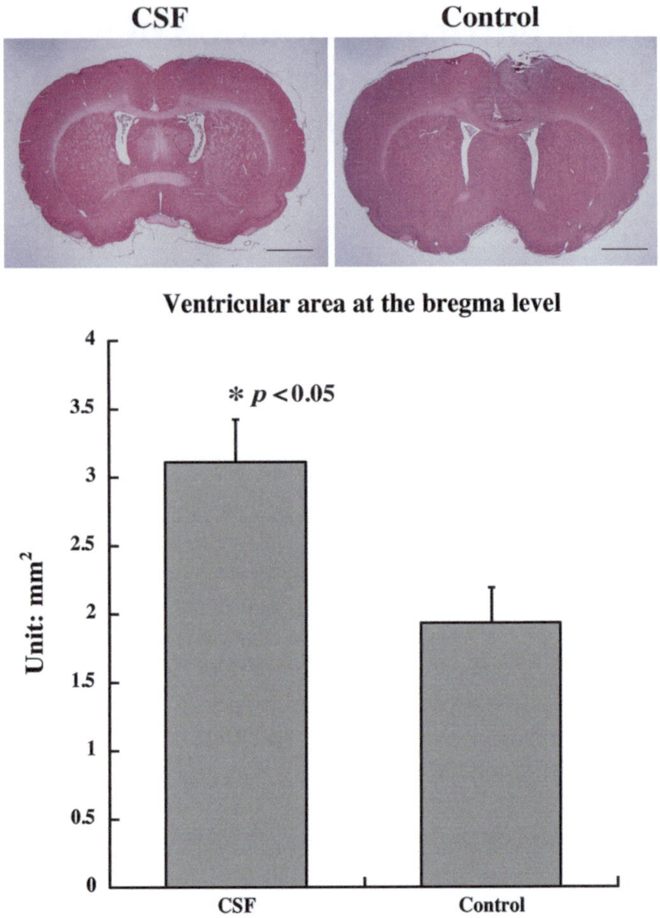

Fig. 1 Brain sections at the bregma level show enlarged lateral ventricle area within experimental rats compared with control rats

Discussion

We aim to understand the role of human SAH noncellular CSF in causing hydrocephalus and periventricular cellular injury toward the goal of understanding the underlying mechanisms. We were able to show that the experimental

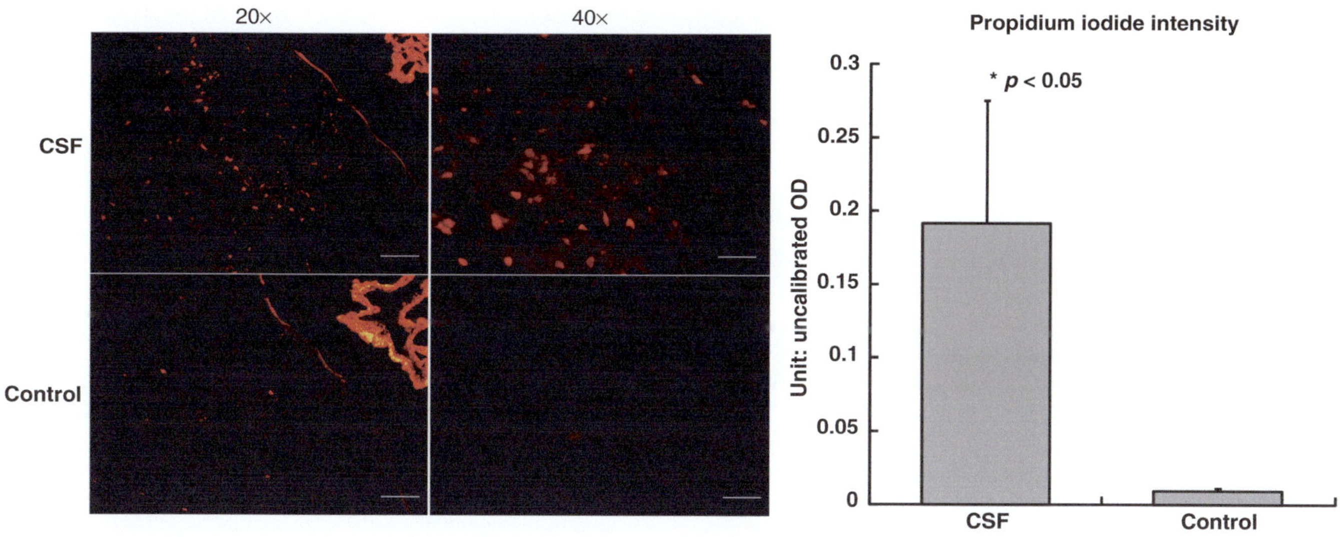

Fig. 2 Greater cellular necrotic death as evident by propidium iodide staining within the experimental group compared with the control group of rats

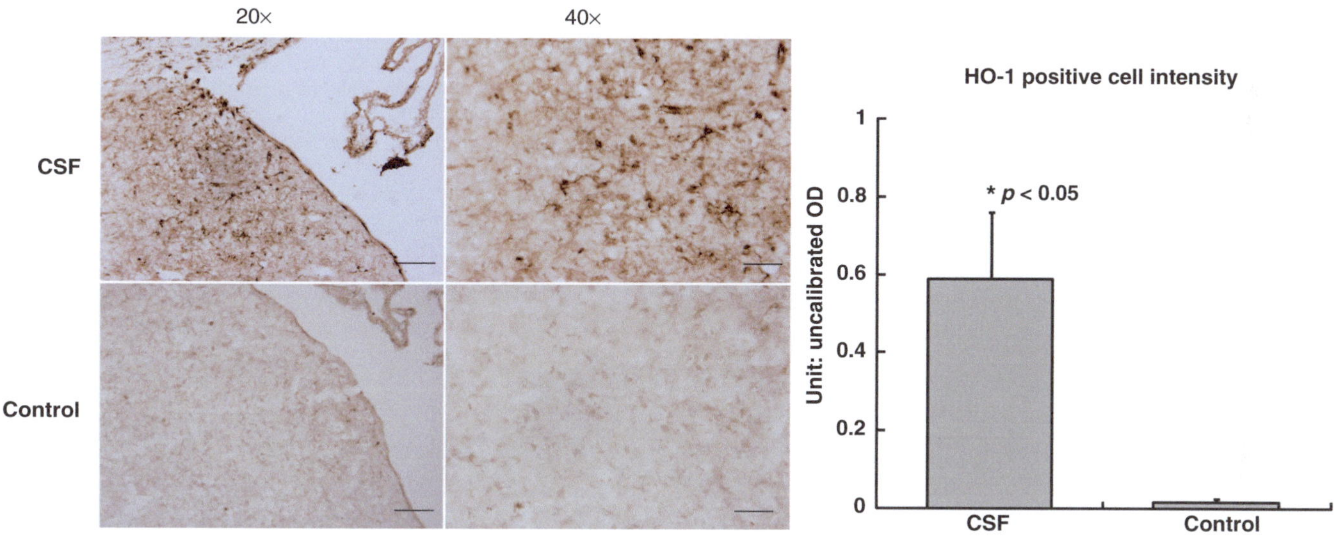

Fig. 3 Periventricular HO-1 expression, a marker of oxidative injury, was much greater in the experimental group compared with the control group of rats

group of rats, intraventricular injection of SAH CSF, had larger ventricles as compared with control rats, intraventricular injection of control patient CSF. Although this outcome could be related to immune or inflammatory reactions related to cross-species reaction, we controlled for this by having the control group also have intraventricular injection with human CSF. Thus, any inflammatory changes should also be present within the control rats.

Our previous studies [7, 8, 10] successfully proved that different solutions, such as iron, thrombin, and lysed red blood cells, have the possibility to induce a hydrocephalus regardless of the real concentration of these content in CSF. Shim et al. [11] analyzed the concentration of vascular endothelial growth factor (VEGF) in the CSF from patients with hydrocephalus and injected a VEGF solution with similar concentration into the lateral ventricle of rats and also succeeded in establishing a hydrocephalus model. Nonetheless, numerous biochemical components are present within the SAH CSF and, most likely, have a complex interplay in causing hydrocephalus. We aim to evaluate this mechanism by mixing inhibitors of certain pathways to understand whether SAH CSF injection will continue to cause hydrocephalus.

Propidium iodide is an intercalating and fluorescent agent, which is impermeable to membrane and excluded from viable cells. However, PI is able to penetrate necrotic cells and is incorporated into the nucleic acid [12]. The experimental group of rats had increased PI and HO-1 staining within the periventricular region, thus representing greater cellular death as well as oxidative injury in rats injected with SAH CSF.

Our study is limited by the fact that human CSF was injected within rats, thus immune reactions are to be expected and could be contributing to the changes observed. In addition, our current study represents rats that were only injected with one patient's SAH CSF and thus injection with more patients' SAH CSF will increase the power and reliability of the results.

Acknowledgment This study was supported by grants NS073959, NS079157, and NS084049 from the National Institutes of Health and 973 Program-2014CB541600.

Conflict of Interest Statement None of the authors have any conflict of interest.

References

1. Van Gijn J, Kerr RS, Rinkel GJ (2007) Subarachnoid haemorrhage. Lancet 369:306–318
2. Ferro JM, Canhao P, Peralta R (2008) Update on subarachnoid haemorrhage. J Neurol 255:465–479
3. Van Asch CJ, van der Schaaf IC, Rinkel GJ (2010) Acute hydrocephalus and cerebral perfusion after aneurysmal subarachnoid hemorrhage. AJNR Am J Neuroradiol 31:67–70
4. Milhorat TH (1987) Acute hydrocephalus after aneurysmal subarachnoid hemorrhage. Neurosurgery 20:15–20
5. Dorai Z, Hynan LS, Kopitnik TA, Samson D (2003) Factors related to hydrocephalus after aneurysmal subarachnoid hemorrhage. Neurosurgery 52:763–769; discussion 769–71
6. Gerner ST, Kuramatsu JB, Abel H (2014) Intraventricular fibrinolysis has no effects on shunt dependency and functional outcome in endovascular-treated aneurysmal SAH. Neurocrit Care 21: 435–443
7. Gao C, Du H, Hua Y, Keep RF, Strahle J, Xi G (2014) Role of red blood cell lysis and iron in hydrocephalus after intraventricular hemorrhage. J Cereb Blood Flow Metab 34:1070–1075
8. Gao F, Liu F, Chen Z, Hua Y, Keep RF, Xi G (2014) Hydrocephalus after intraventricular hemorrhage: the role of thrombin. J Cereb Blood Flow Metab 34:489–494
9. Wu J, Hua Y, Keep RF, Nakamura T, Hoff JT, Xi G (2003) Iron and iron-handling proteins in the brain after intracerebral hemorrhage. Stroke 34:2964–2969
10. Okubo S, Strahle J, Keep RF, Hua Y, Xi G (2013) Subarachnoid hemorrhage-induced hydrocephalus in rats. Stroke 44:547–550
11. Shim JW, Sandlund J, Han CH (2013) VEGF, which is elevated in the CSF of patients with hydrocephalus, causes ventriculomegaly and ependymal changes in rats. Exp Neurol 247:703–709
12. Jin H, Xi G, Keep RF, Wu J, Hua Y (2013) DARPP-32 to quantify intracerebral hemorrhage-induced neuronal death in basal ganglia. Transl Stroke Res 4:130–134

The Effect of Gender on Acute Hydrocephalus after Experimental Subarachnoid Hemorrhage

Hajime Shishido, Haining Zhang, Shuichi Okubo, Ya Hua, Richard F. Keep, and Guohua Xi

Introduction

Subarachnoid hemorrhage (SAH) is a subtype of stroke with high mortality and morbidity. Studies suggest that early brain injury following SAH could be a primary therapeutic target [7, 20]. Studies also have indicated that there is a 19–63 % incidence of acute hydrocephalus within 3 days of SAH [1, 6, 10, 19]. Our previous study demonstrated that frequency of hydrocephalus reached 44 % in an endovascular perforation SAH model in male rats [15]. Acute hydrocephalus is a predictor of poor outcome after SAH [6]. However, the mechanisms of SAH-induced hydrocephalus have not been fully elucidated.

Women have higher risk of SAH than men [11, 13, 17] and an increased risk for SAH-induced hydrocephalus. It is important to identify why women are at higher risk for SAH and initiate appropriate prevention strategies [2, 4]. In this study, we hypothesized the gender influences the initial impact of an SAH and investigated gender differences in hydrocephalus development following SAH in rats.

H. Shishido, MD • S. Okubo, MD
Department of Neurosurgery, University of Michigan, Ann Arbor, MI, USA

Department of Neurosurgery, Kagawa University, Kagawa, Japan

H. Zhang, MD, PhD
Department of Neurosurgery, University of Michigan, Ann Arbor, MI, USA

Department of Neurology, 1st Affiliated Hospital, Jilin University, Changchun, China

Y. Hua, MD • R.F. Keep, PhD • G. Xi, MD (✉)
Department of Neurosurgery, University of Michigan, Ann Arbor, MI, USA
e-mail: guohuaxi@umich.edu

Materials and Methods

Animal Preparation and SAH Induction

Animal use protocols were approved by the University of Michigan Committee on the Use and Care of Animals. Animals were housed under standard 12:12 light–dark conditions and allowed free access to water and food. A total of 52 male and 52 female adult Sprague-Dawley rats were used in this study (body weight: 250–350 g; Charles River Laboratories Portage, MI). SAH induction was performed using an endovascular perforation technique ($n = 41$ per gender group) as previously described [12, 15]. In brief, rats were anesthetized with 5 % isoflurane. After intubation and initiation of mechanical ventilation, isoflurane was maintained at 2.5–3 %. After this, the left external carotid artery was identified under a surgical microscope, transected distally, and reflected caudally in line with the internal carotid artery. A 4-0 nylon monofilament suture was inserted into the stump of the external carotid artery through the common carotid artery bifurcation and into the internal carotid artery. The filament was advanced distally into the intracranial internal carotid artery to cause a vascular perforation. The filament was then withdrawn. Sham rats underwent the same procedure without perforation ($n = 11$ per each gender).

MRI and Ventricular Volume Measurement

MRI was performed at 24 h after surgery in a 7.0-T Varian MR scanner (Varian Inc Palo Alto, CA) with acquisition of T2 fast spin-echo and T2* gradient-echo sequences using a field of view of 35 × 35 mm, matrix of 256 × 256 mm, and 25 coronal slices (0.5-mm thick). All ventricular volumes from the frontal horn of the lateral ventricle to the foramen of

R.L. Applegate et al. (eds.), *Brain Edema XVI: Translate Basic Science into Clinical Practice*, Acta Neurochirurgica Supplement, Vol. 121, DOI 10.1007/978-3-319-18497-5_58, © Springer International Publishing Switzerland 2016

Luschka were outlined and the areas were measured by Image J software by a blinded observer. The combined ventricular areas over all slices was multiplied by section thickness to calculate ventricle volume. The volume of intraventricular hemorrhage was measured as the hypointensity lesion volume in T2*-weighted images. Acute hydrocephalus was defined as a ventricular volume at 24 h after SAH that was more than 3 standard deviations (SD) greater than the mean in sham animals, as previously described [15, 21].

Grading of SAH

The extent of SAH was assessed using a modified grading system as previously described [18]. The basal brain, including brain stem, was divided into six segments. Each segment was assigned a grade from 0 to 3, depending on the amount of blood, as follows: Grade 0, no SAH; Grade 1, minimal subarachnoid blood; Grade 2, moderate blood clot with recognizable arteries; and Grade 3, massive hemorrhage covering the cerebral arteries. The minimum SAH scale is 0 and the maximum is 18.

Behavior Score

Neurological deficits were evaluated at 24 h after SAH using the modified Garcia's scoring system as previously described [8, 16]. The neurobehavioral study consisted of the following six tests: (1) spontaneous activity, (2) symmetry in the movement of four limbs, (3) forepaw outstretching, (4) climbing, (5) body proprioception, and (6) response to vibrissae touch. Each test was assigned a score from 0 to 3. The minimum neurological score is 2 and the maximum is 18.

Statistical Analysis

All data in this study are presented as means ± SD. Statistical differences among groups were analyzed using Student's *t*-test and Spearman rank correlation test. Statistical significance was set at $p<0.05$.

Results

No rats died after the sham operation. Ventricular volumes in male rats (12.8 ± 3.8 mm^3; $n=11$) and in female rats (11.4 ± 1.6 mm^3; $n=11$) were similar after the sham operation ($p>0.05$).

In female rats, SAH resulted in significant ventricular enlargement at 24 h (33.4 ± 17.2 mm^3; $n=32$) compared with sham-operated rats (11.4 ± 1.6 mm^3, $p<0.001$, Fig. 1a–c). SAH also resulted in larger T2* hypointensity volumes (2.2 ± 2.0 mm^3 vs 0.60 ± 0.41 mm^3 in shams) in female rats ($p<0.001$). The ventricular T2* hypointensity volume (degree of ventricular hemorrhage) correlated with ventricular volume ($r=0.34$, $p<0.05$, Fig. 1d).

After SAH, there was no significant difference between genders in mortality rate (females 11/41, 27 %; males 9/41, 22 %; 9/41; $p>0.05$), SAH severity grade (females 13 ± 4, $n=32$; males 11 ± 5, $n=27$; $p>0.05$, Fig. 2a) and modified Garcia score (females 14 ± 3, $n=32$; males14 ± 3, $n=25$; $p>0.5$). In addition, the size of ventricular T2* hypointensity lesions (intraventricular hemorrhage) was not different in females (2.2 ± 2.0 mm^3; $n=32$) and males (1.4 ± 2.2 mm^3; $n=30$) after SAH ($p>0.05$, Fig. 2b).

In male rats, ventricular volume after SAH (27.7 ± 16.3 mm^3; $n=30$) was also larger than those in sham-operated animals (12.8 ± 3.8 mm^3; $n=11$; $p<0.01$) as previously described (15). Thus, in both male and female rats, SAH caused ventricular enlargement. However, the relative change in ventricular volume (compared with sham-operated rats) at 24 h was significantly greater in females (292 ± 150 %, $n=32$) than males (216 ± 127 %, $n=30$; $p<0.05$, Fig. 2c). Similarly, the occurrence of acute hydrocephalus (ventricular volume>+3 SD above the mean in sham rats) was markedly greater in females (75 %; 24/32) than in males (47 %; 14/30, $p<0.05$, Fig. 2d). These results indicate that gender plays a role in the development of acute hydrocephalus after SAH.

Discussion

Acute hydrocephalus is associated with poor outcome after SAH [6]. Hydrocephalus develops within 72 h (acute hydrocephalus) in 20–63 % of SAH patients but rarely occurs in SAH patients at 3–7 days (2–3 %; subacute hydrocephalus) [9, 10]. It is generally accepted that fibrosis of the leptomeninges and arachnoid granulations cause impaired cerebrospinal flow and decreased absorption, resulting in hydrocephalus development. However, the exact mechanisms of hydrocephalus development after SAH remain poorly understood. In a clinical study, the presence of an intraventricular hemorrhage had a high statistical correlation with hydrocephalus [9] and we found that the degree of hydrocephalus correlated with the amount of intraventricular blood in a rat SAH model [15].

In addition to SAH incidence being higher in women than in men [13], more female patients develop acute hydrocephalus after SAH [19]. Female gender was also one of the parameters associated with the likelihood of needing a permanent shunt [3]. In this study, we examined the effect of gender in

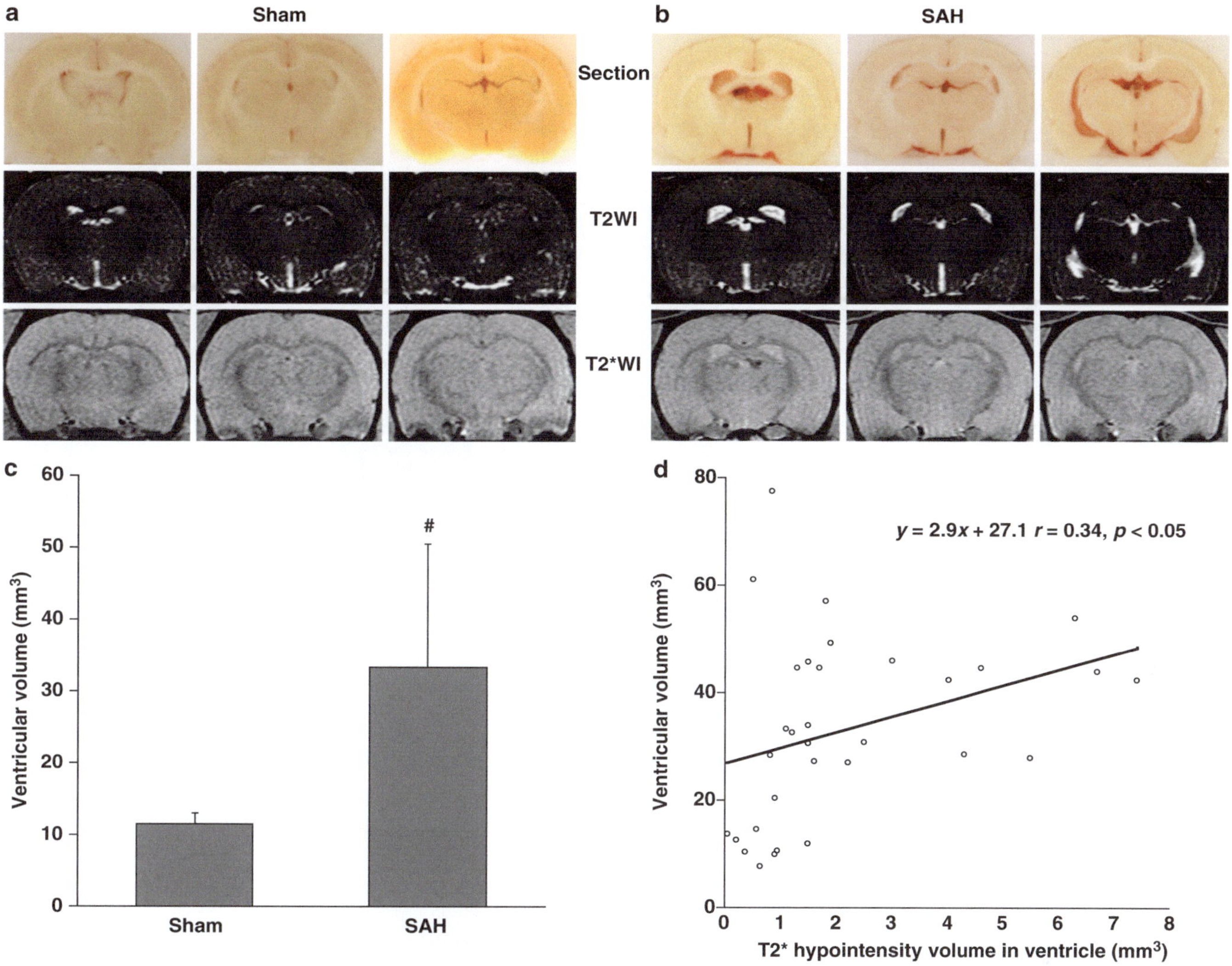

Fig. 1 (**a**, **b**) Coronal frozen brain sections and T2- and T2*-weighted magnetic resonance images from rats that had (**a**) sham operation or (**b**) SAH at 24 h after the procedures. (**c**, **d**) Measurement of ventricular volume in T2-weighted MRIs at 24 h after SAH or sham procedure (**c**) and the correlation between ventricular volume and ventricular T2* hypointensity volume at 24 h after SAH (**d**). Values are mean ± SD, $n = 11–32$, $^{\#}p < 0.001$ vs sham group

experimental rat SAH and found that acute hydrocephalus occurs more frequently in females. In a clinical study, acute hydrocephalus after SAH occurred 2.2-fold more frequently in women compared with men [14]. In another study, female gender was one factor associated with shunt-dependent hydrocephalus [5]. These results all suggest that the gender is the factor in the development of acute hydrocephalus after SAH.

There are some limitations to this study: (1) the time course of SAH-induced hydrocephalus in different genders after SAH was not determined and (2) it is still unknown whether estrogen has a role in hydrocephalus development.

Conclusion

The present study demonstrated that gender impacts acute hydrocephalus development in a rat model of SAH. Future studies should determine the role of estrogen in SAH-induced hydrocephalus.

Acknowledgment This study was supported by grants NS-073595, NS-079157 and NS-084049 from the National Institutes of Health (NIH). The content is solely the responsibility of the authors and does not necessarily represent the official views of the NIH.

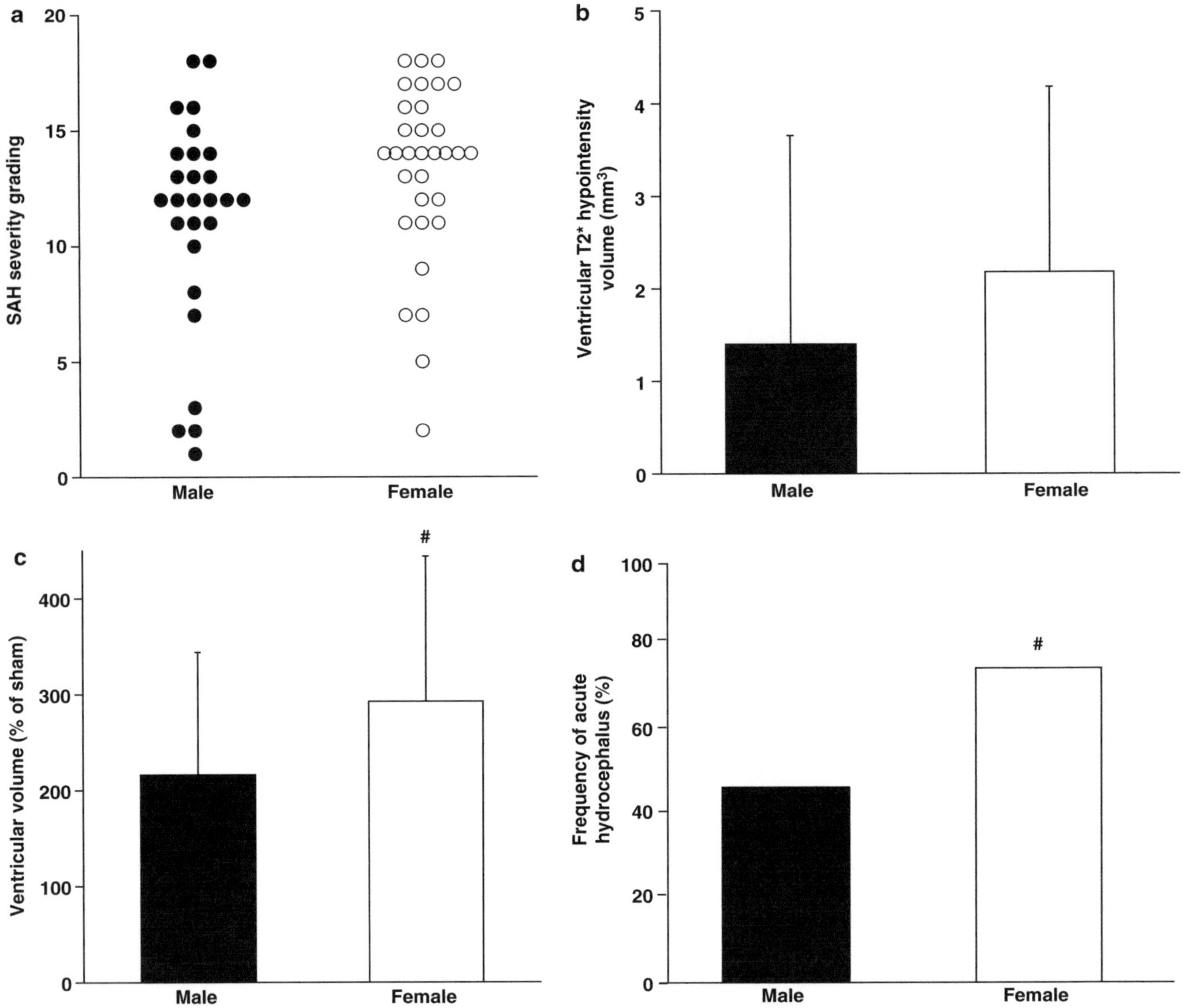

Fig. 2 (**a**) SAH severity grades, (**b**) ventricular T2* hypointensity volumes, (**c**) ventricular volumes (as a percentage of values in sham-operated animals), and (**d**) frequency of acute hydrocephalus in male and female rats at 24 h after SAH. Values are mean ± SD, $n = 27–32$, $^{\#}p < 0.05$ vs male group

References

1. Black PM (1986) Hydrocephalus and vasospasm after subarachnoid hemorrhage from ruptured intracranial aneurysms. Neurosurgery 18:12–16
2. Bushnell C, McCullough LD, Awad IA, Chireau MV, Fedder WN, Furie KL, Howard VJ, Lichtman JH, Lisabeth LD, Pina IL, Reeves MJ, Rexrode KM, Saposnik G, Singh V, Towfighi A, Vaccarino V, Walters MR (2014) Guidelines for the prevention of stroke in women: a statement for healthcare professionals from the American Heart Association/American Stroke Association. Stroke 45:1545–1588
3. Chan M, Alaraj A, Calderon M, Herrera SR, Gao W, Ruland S, Roitberg BZ (2009) Prediction of ventriculoperitoneal shunt dependency in patients with aneurysmal subarachnoid hemorrhage. J Neurosurg 110:44–49
4. Davis CM, Fairbanks SL, Alkayed NJ (2013) Mechanism of the sex difference in endothelial dysfunction after stroke. Transl Stroke Res 4:381–389
5. Dorai Z, Hynan LS, Kopitnik TA, Samson D (2003) Factors related to hydrocephalus after aneurysmal subarachnoid hemorrhage. Neurosurgery 52:763–769; discussion 769–771
6. Dupont S, Rabinstein AA (2013) Extent of acute hydrocephalus after subarachnoid hemorrhage as a risk factor for poor functional outcome. Neurol Res 35:107–110
7. Fujii M, Yan J, Rolland WB, Soejima Y, Caner B, Zhang JH (2013) Early brain injury, an evolving frontier in subarachnoid hemorrhage research. Transl Stroke Res 4:432–446
8. Garcia JH, Wagner S, Liu KF, Hu XJ (1995) Neurological deficit and extent of neuronal necrosis attributable to middle cerebral artery occlusion in rats. Statistical validation. Stroke 26:627–634; discussion 635

9. Germanwala AV, Huang J, Tamargo RJ (2010) Hydrocephalus after aneurysmal subarachnoid hemorrhage. Neurosurg Clin N Am 21:263–270
10. Hasan D, Vermeulen M, Wijdicks EF, Hijdra A, van Gijn J (1989) Management problems in acute hydrocephalus after subarachnoid hemorrhage. Stroke 20:747–753
11. Kongable GL, Lanzino G, Germanson TP, Truskowski LL, Alves WM, Torner JC, Kassell NF (1996) Gender-related differences in aneurysmal subarachnoid hemorrhage. J Neurosurg 84:43–48
12. Lee JY, Keep RF, He Y, Sagher O, Hua Y, Xi G (2010) Hemoglobin and iron handling in brain after subarachnoid hemorrhage and the effect of deferoxamine on early brain injury. J Cereb Blood Flow Metab 30:1793–1803
13. Longstreth WT Jr, Koepsell TD, Yerby MS, van Belle G (1985) Risk factors for subarachnoid hemorrhage. Stroke 16:377–385
14. Mirsad HMM, Zlatko E, Harun B (2007) Extent of subarachnoid hemorrhage and development of hydrocephalus. Acta Media Academica 36:70–75
15. Okubo S, Strahle J, Keep RF, Hua Y, Xi G (2013) Subarachnoid hemorrhage-induced hydrocephalus in rats. Stroke 44:547–550
16. Park S, Yamaguchi M, Zhou C, Calvert JW, Tang J, Zhang JH (2004) Neurovascular protection reduces early brain injury after subarachnoid hemorrhage. Stroke 35:2412–2417
17. Rothwell PM, Coull AJ, Silver LE, Fairhead JF, Giles MF, Lovelock CE, Redgrave JN, Bull LM, Welch SJ, Cuthbertson FC, Binney LE, Gutnikov SA, Anslow P, Banning AP, Mant D, Mehta Z (2005) Population-based study of event-rate, incidence, case fatality, and mortality for all acute vascular events in all arterial territories (Oxford Vascular Study). Lancet 366:1773–1783
18. Sugawara T, Ayer R, Jadhav V, Zhang JH (2008) A new grading system evaluating bleeding scale in filament perforation subarachnoid hemorrhage rat model. J Neurosci Methods 167:327–334
19. van Asch CJ, van der Schaaf IC, Rinkel GJ (2010) Acute hydrocephalus and cerebral perfusion after aneurysmal subarachnoid hemorrhage. AJNR Am J Neuroradiol 31:67–70
20. Zhang JH (2014) Vascular neural network in subarachnoid hemorrhage. Transl Stroke Res 5:423–428
21. Zhao J, Chen Z, Xi G, Keep RF, Hua Y (2014) Deferoxamine attenuates acute hydrocephalus after traumatic brain injury in rats. Transl Stroke Res 5:586–594

Effects of Gender and Estrogen Receptors on Iron-Induced Brain Edema Formation

Qing Xie, Guohua Xi, Richard F. Keep, and Ya Hua

Introduction

The mechanism of intracerebral hemorrhage (ICH)-induced brain injury has focused on the role of the coagulation cascade- and iron-induced brain injury [29]. Iron has a key role and is capable of causing lipid peroxidation and free radical formation, thus contributing to delayed edema along with oxidative stress after ICH [12, 23, 25, 28, 31]. These processes can lead to brain cell degeneration and death [13].

A number of studies have shown that outcome from experimental brain injury is clearly sex-linked [3, 11, 15, 26]. Our previous study showed that female mice have less brain edema and a faster recovery of behavioral deficits after ICH. In addition, 17β-estradiol treatment in male mice markedly reduced ICH-induced brain edema [21]. Moreover, Culmsee et al. [2] found that estrogen protected against iron-induced neurotoxicity in vitro.

The mechanisms underlying the effects of gender and estrogen have yet to be fully elucidated. Many studies have focused on the role of estrogen receptors (ERs). Such studies have suggested effects of ER-β in behavior, learning and memory, neural development, feeding, and sexual differentiation of the brain, but that it is not essential to neuroprotection against ischemia [8, 9, 16, 22, 24, 27]. In contrast, ER-α can be dramatically induced after injury and it has a role in protecting against delayed cell death after ischemia [6, 7]. However, their roles in ICH are less clear.

The current study examined the effects of ERs in iron-induced neurotoxicity. In addition to determining the impact of gender, it examined the effects of ICI 182, 780, a high-affinity estrogen receptor antagonist, and tamoxifen, a selective estrogen receptor modulator, and a high-affinity ligand at GPR-30 [18].

Materials and Methods

Animal Preparation and Intracerebral Infusion

The animal use protocols were approved by the University of Michigan Committee of the Use and Care of Animals. In this study, C57BL/6 mice (Jackson Laboratory, Bar Harbor, ME, USA) at the age of 8–12 weeks were used. The animals were anesthetized with mixture of ketamine (90 mg/kg, intraperitoneally (IP)) and xylazine (5 mg/kg, IP). The mice were positioned in a stereotactic frame (Model 500, Kopf Instruments, Tujunga, CA, USA), and a cranial burr hole (1 mm) was drilled on the right coronal suture 2.5 mm lateral to the midline. All mice received an injection of 10 μL of either saline or $FeCl_2$ into the right basal ganglia at a rate of 1 μL per minute through a 30-gauge needle (coordinates 0.2 mm anterior, 3.5 mm ventral, and 2.5 mm lateral to the bregma) with the use of a microinfusion pump. Then the needle was removed and the skin incision sutured closed [1].

Experimental Groups

There were three experimental groups in this study. First, either male ($n=8$) or female ($n=14$) mice received an injection of 10 μL $FeCl_2$ (1 mM in 10 μL saline) into the right caudate. Second, female mice received an intracaudate injection of saline with ICI 182, 780 ($n=6$), or $FeCl_2$ (1 mM) with

Q. Xie
Departments of Neurosurgery, University of Michigan, Ann Arbor, MI, USA

Department of Neurosurgery, Huashan Hospital, Fudan University, Shanghai, China

G. Xi • R.F. Keep • Y. Hua, MD (✉)
Departments of Neurosurgery, University of Michigan, Ann Arbor, MI, USA
e-mail: yahua@umich.edu

R.L. Applegate et al. (eds.), *Brain Edema XVI: Translate Basic Science into Clinical Practice*, Acta Neurochirurgica Supplement, Vol. 121,
DOI 10.1007/978-3-319-18497-5_59, © Springer International Publishing Switzerland 2016

ICI 182, 780 ($n=11$), or vehicle ($n=9$). Third, male mice were treated with tamoxifen (5 mg/kg, IP, $n=5$) or vehicle (DMSO, IP, $n=5$) 1 h after receiving an intracaudate injection of $FeCl_2$ (1 mM). All mice were euthanized 24 h after intracerebral injection and the brains used to determine brain water content and ion levels.

Brain Water and Ion Contents Measurement

Mice were anesthetized (ketamine 120 mg/kg and xylazine 5 mg/kg, IP). Brains were removed immediately and a coronal brain slice (approximately 3 mm thick) 4 mm from the frontal pole was cut with a blade. The brain slice was divided into ipsilateral and contralateral hemisphere along the midline. The cerebellum served as a control. Brain samples were weighed on an electronic analytical balance to obtain the wet weight (WW) and then dried in a gravity oven (Blue M. Electric Co.) at 100 °C for 24 h to obtain the dry weight (DW). Brain water content was calculated as (WW – DW)/WW. The dehydrated samples were digested in 0.5 mL of 1 mol/L nitric acid for 7–10 days and sodium and potassium contents measured by a flame photometer (Model IL 943, Instrumentation Laboratory, Inc., Lexington, MA, USA). The ion content was expressed in microequivalents per gram of dehydrated brain tissue (μEq/g dry weight) [30].

Statistical Analysis

All data in this study are presented as mean ± standard deviation (SD). Data were analyzed with Student's t-test and analysis of variance (ANOVA). Significance levels were set at $p<0.05$.

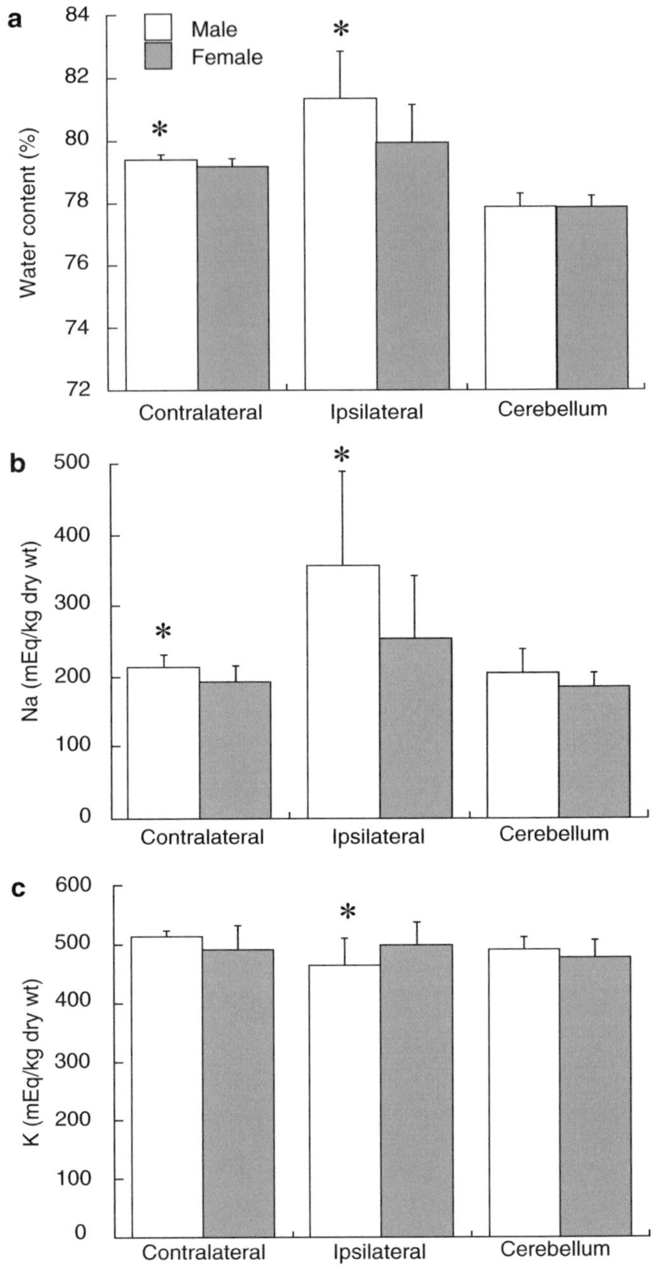

Fig. 1 Brain water content (**a**), sodium (**b**), and potassium (**c**) concentrations in brains of female and male mice at 24 h after intracaudate injection of $FeCl_2$ (1 mM in 10 μL saline). Values are mean ± SD, $n=8$ or 14, $^*p<0.05$

Results

Twenty-four hours after $FeCl_2$ injection, brain water content in the ipsilateral hemisphere was lower in female mice than in males (79.9 ± 1.2 vs 81.4 ± 1.5 %, $p<0.05$, Fig. 1a). There was no difference in water content of cerebellum with gender. Also, the female mice had lower sodium accumulation (253 ± 88 vs 356 ± 132 μEq/g in males, $p<0.05$, Fig. 1b) and potassium loss (499 ± 39 vs 464 ± 47μEq/g dry weight in males, $p<0.05$, Fig. 1c).

Co-injection of ICI 182, 780 enhanced $FeCl_2$-induced brain edema (80.3 ± 1.3 vs 79.3 ± 0.4 % in vehicle, $p<0.05$, Fig. 2a), sodium accumulation (269 ± 66 vs 220 ± 28 μEq/g in vehicle, $p<0.05$, Fig. 2b), and potassium loss (470 ± 48 vs 522 ± 29 μEq/g dry weight in vehicle, $p<0.01$, Fig. 2c) in the ipsilateral hemisphere in females. Intracaudate injection of ICI 182, 780 (1 μg) did not induce brain edema formation (79.0 ± 0.2 vs. 79.1 ± 0.2 % in the contralateral hemisphere, $p>0.05$).

Systemic treatment with tamoxifen (5 mg/kg, IP) in males significantly reduced $FeCl_2$-induced brain edema (78.7 ± 0.4 vs 81.1 ± 1.8 % in vehicle, $p<0.05$, Fig. 3a). This reduced edema was associated with a reduction in sodium accumulation (188 ± 7 vs 331 ± 130 μEq/g dry weight, $p<0.05$, Fig. 3b) and a tendency for reduced potassium loss (474 ± 18 vs 448 ± 34 μEq/g dry weight, $p>0.05$, Fig. 3c) in the ipsilateral hemisphere.

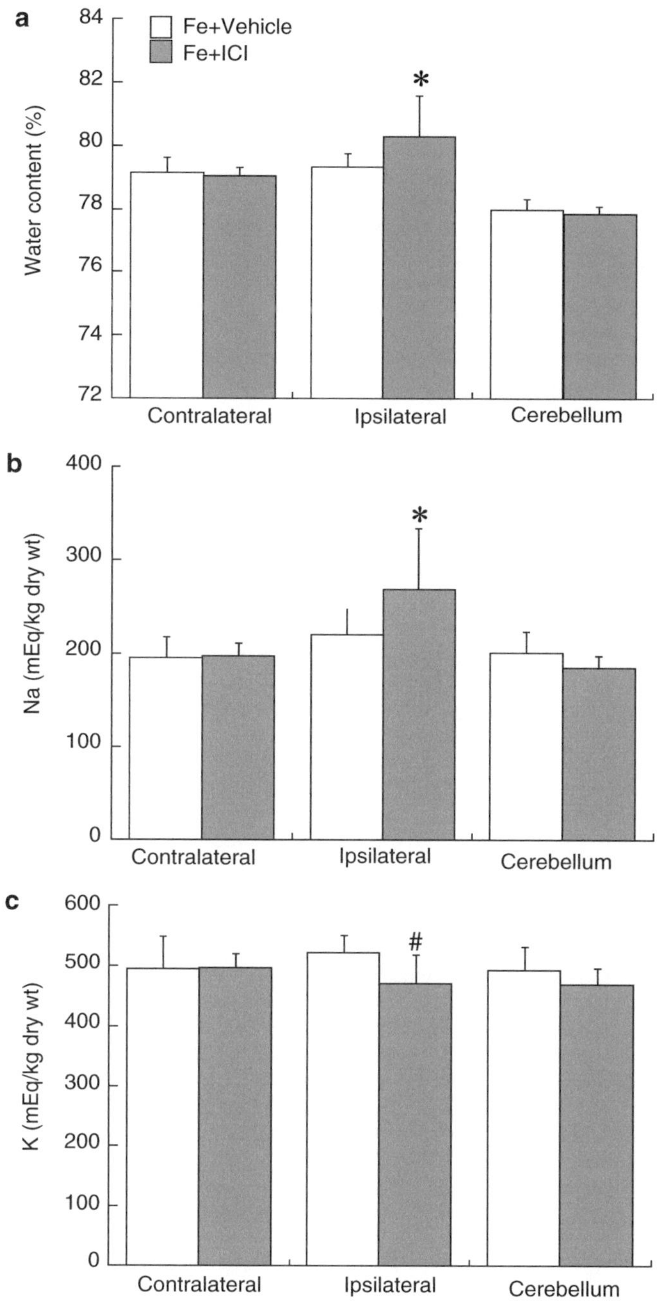

Fig. 2 Brain water content (**a**), sodium (**b**), and potassium (**c**) concentrations in female mice 24 h after intracaudate injection with $FeCl_2$ (1 mM) mixed with ICI 182, 780 (1 μg) or vehicle. Values are mean ± SD, $n = 9$ to 11, *$p < 0.05$ and #$p < 0.01$

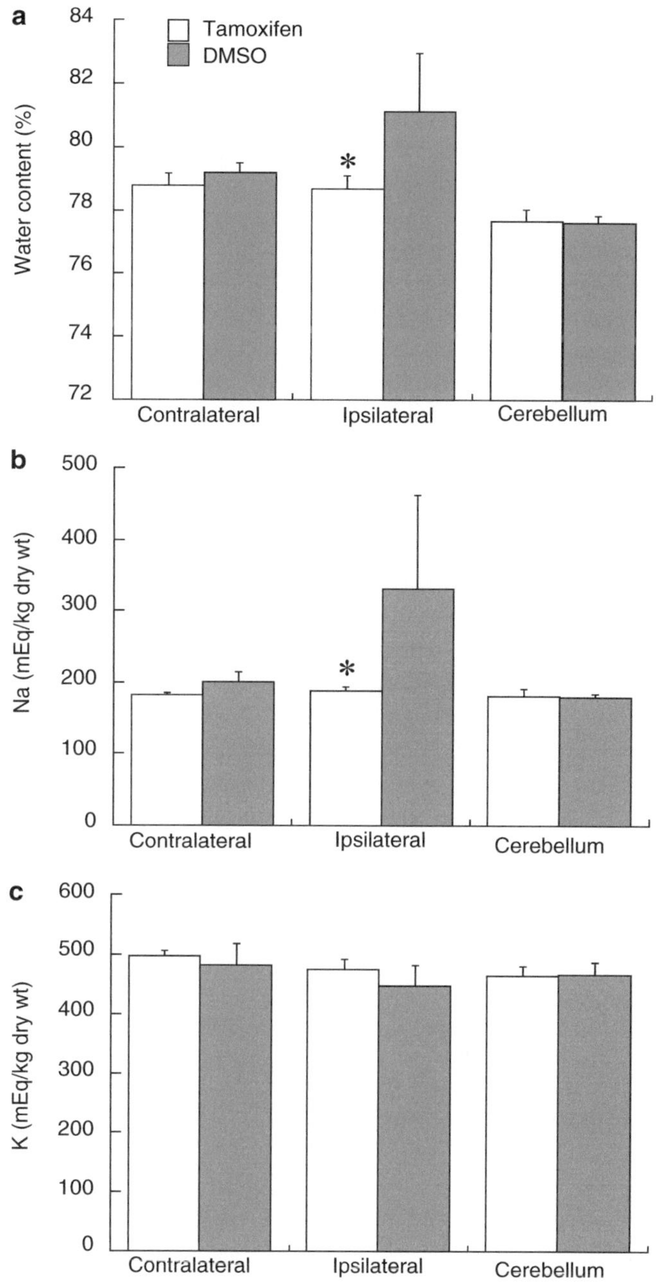

Fig. 3 Brain water content, sodium, and potassium concentrations of male mice 24 h after intracaudate injection with $FeCl_2$ (1 mM, 10 μL) into right caudate. Mice were treated with tamoxifen (5 mg/kg) or DMSO intraperitoneally at 1 h after the injection. Values are mean ± SD, $n = 5$, *$p < 0.05$

Discussion

Our previous studies showed that estrogen pretreatment reduces iron-induced brain edema and neuronal death in rats [10]. In this study, we found that iron induced less brain edema formation in female mice than in male mice. The nonspecific ER antagonist, ICI 182, 780, enhanced iron-induced brain edema formation in females. We have previously shown that ICI 182, 780 exacerbates ICH-induced brain edema in female but not in male rats [20]. In addition, one systemic treatment once with a high dose of tamoxifen (5 mg/kg) at 1 h post could reduce iron-induced brain edema in males. These results all suggest a role of ER in reducing iron-induced brain injury (a component of ICH-induced injury).

Since Kimelberg et al. [14] reported a neuroprotective effect of tamoxifen in males after stroke, tamoxifen has been shown to have neuroprotective effects in females and in other diseases such as Parkinson's disease [5, 14, 19]. We have shown that tamoxifen (5 mg/kg) is neuroprotective in male rats after ICH [32]. Estrogen-receptor modulators may have effects via genomic and non-genomic signaling and antioxidant mechanisms [4]. In support of a direct antioxidant action, tamoxifen has been shown to have direct superoxide scavenging abilities in vitro [17]. However, whether the direct antioxidant action of tamoxifen involves activation of the estrogen receptors remains unclear. Iron induces lipid peroxidation and free radical formation, which contributes to delayed edema along with oxidative stress after ICH [12, 25, 28, 31]. The effects of tamoxifen on iron-induced brain edema may have similar mechanisms to those inducing neuroprotection in cerebral ischemia, but this needs further investigation. It should be noted that there was a study showing that ICI 182, 780 administered did not block the effect of high-dose tamoxifen on infarct size, which suggests that tamoxifen may act in an estrogen receptor-independent manner [33].

In conclusion, there are remarkable gender differences in iron-induced brain edema. This protection in female mice can be blocked by a nonspecific estrogen receptor antagonist, ICI 182,780. In addition, the estrogen receptor modulator tamoxifen attenuated iron-induced brain edema in male mice. The results from this study suggest a role of estrogen receptors in reducing iron-induced brain edema.

This study was supported by grants NS-073595, NS-079157, and NS-084049 from the National Institutes of Health (NIH); and NSFC30901549 from National Science Foundation of China.

References

1. Cheng Y, Xi G, Jin H, Keep RF, Feng J, Hua Y (2014) Thrombin-induced cerebral hemorrhage: role of protease-activated receptor-1. Transl Stroke Res 5:472–475
2. Culmsee C, Vedder H, Ravati A, Junker V, Otto D, Ahlemeyer B, Krieg JC, Krieglstein J (1999) Neuroprotection by estrogens in a mouse model of focal cerebral ischemia and in cultured neurons: evidence for a receptor-independent antioxidative mechanism. J Cereb Blood Flow Metab 19:1263–1269
3. Davis CM, Fairbanks SL, Alkayed NJ (2013) Mechanism of the sex difference in endothelial dysfunction after stroke. Transl Stroke Res 4:381–389
4. Dhandapani KM, Brann DW (2002) Protective effects of estrogen and selective estrogen receptor modulators in the brain. Biol Reprod 67:1379–1385
5. Dluzen DE, McDermott JL, Anderson LI (2001) Tamoxifen diminishes methamphetamine-induced striatal dopamine depletion in intact female and male mice. J Neuroendocrinol 13:618–624
6. Dubal DB, Rau SW, Shughrue PJ, Zhu H, Yu J, Cashion AB, Suzuki S, Gerhold LM, Bottner MB, Dubal SB, Merchanthaler I, Kindy MS, Wise PM (2006) Differential modulation of estrogen receptors (ERs) in ischemic brain injury: a role for ERalpha in estradiol-mediated protection against delayed cell death. Endocrinology 147:3076–3084
7. Dubal DB, Shughrue PJ, Wilson ME, Merchenthaler I, Wise PM (1999) Estradiol modulates bcl-2 in cerebral ischemia: a potential role for estrogen receptors. J Neurosci 19:6385–6393
8. Dubal DB, Zhu H, Yu J, Rau SW, Shughrue PJ, Merchenthaler I, Kindy MS, Wise PM (2001) Estrogen receptor alpha, not beta, is a critical link in estradiol-mediated protection against brain injury. Proc Natl Acad Sci U S A 98:1952–1957
9. Geary N, Asarian L, Korach KS, Pfaff DW, Ogawa S (2001) Deficits in E2-dependent control of feeding, weight gain, and cholecystokinin satiation in ER-alpha null mice. Endocrinology 142:4751–4757
10. Gu Y, Xi G, Liu W, Keep RF, Hua Y (2010) Estrogen reduces iron-mediated brain edema and neuronal death. Acta Neurochir Suppl 106:159–162
11. Herson PS, Koerner IP, Hurn PD (2009) Sex, sex steroids, and brain injury. Semin Reprod Med 27:229–239
12. Huang FP, Xi G, Keep RF, Hua Y, Nemoianu A, Hoff JT (2002) Brain edema after experimental intracerebral hemorrhage: role of hemoglobin degradation products. J Neurosurg 96:287–293
13. Jin H, Xi G, Keep RF, Wu J, Hua Y (2013) DARPP-32 to quantify intracerebral hemorrhage-induced neuronal death in basal ganglia. Transl Stroke Res 4:130–134
14. Kimelberg HK, Feustel PJ, Jin Y, Paquette J, Boulos A, Keller RW Jr, Tranmer BI (2000) Acute treatment with tamoxifen reduces ischemic damage following middle cerebral artery occlusion. Neuroreport 11:2675–2679
15. Koellhoffer EC, McCullough LD (2013) The effects of estrogen in ischemic stroke. Transl Stroke Res 4:390–401
16. Kudwa AE, Bodo C, Gustafsson JA, Rissman EF (2005) A previously uncharacterized role for estrogen receptor beta: defeminization of male brain and behavior. Proc Natl Acad Sci U S A 102:4608–4612
17. Kuo YM, Chen HH, Shieh CC, Chuang KP, Cherng CG, Yu L (2003) 4-Hydroxytamoxifen attenuates methamphetamine-induced nigrostriatal dopaminergic toxicity in intact and gonadetomized mice. J Neurochem 87:1436–1443
18. Lin BC, Suzawa M, Blind RD, Tobias SC, Bulun SE, Scanlan TS, Ingraham HA (2009) Stimulating the GPR30 estrogen receptor with a novel tamoxifen analogue activates SF-1 and promotes endometrial cell proliferation. Cancer Res 69:5415–5423
19. Mehta SH, Dhandapani KM, De Sevilla LM, Webb RC, Mahesh VB, Brann DW (2003) Tamoxifen, a selective estrogen receptor modulator, reduces ischemic damage caused by middle cerebral artery occlusion in the ovariectomized female rat. Neuroendocrinology 77:44–50
20. Nakamura T, Hua Y, Keep RF, Park JW, Xi G, Hoff JT (2005) Estrogen therapy for experimental intracerebral hemorrhage in rats. J Neurosurg 103:97–103
21. Nakamura T, Xi G, Hua Y, Schallert T, Hoff JT, Keep RF (2004) Intracerebral hemorrhage in mice: model characterization and application for genetically modified mice. J Cereb Blood Flow Metab 24:487–494
22. Ogawa S, Eng V, Taylor J, Lubahn DB, Korach KS, Pfaff DW (1998) Roles of estrogen receptor-alpha gene expression in reproduction-related behaviors in female mice. Endocrinology 139:5070–5081
23. Pandey AS, Xi G (2014) Intracerebral hemorrhage: a multimodality approach to improving outcome. Transl Stroke Res 5:313–315
24. Rissman EF, Heck AL, Leonard JE, Shupnik MA, Gustafsson JA (2002) Disruption of estrogen receptor beta gene impairs spatial learning in female mice. Proc Natl Acad Sci U S A 99:3996–4001
25. Siesjo BK, Agardh CD, Bengtsson F (1989) Free radicals and brain damage. Cerebrovasc Brain Metab Rev 1:165–211

26. Vagnerova K, Koerner IP, Hurn PD (2008) Gender and the injured brain. Anesth Analg 107:201–214
27. Wang L, Andersson S, Warner M, Gustafsson JA (2003) Estrogen receptor (ER)beta knockout mice reveal a role for ERbeta in migration of cortical neurons in the developing brain. Proc Natl Acad Sci U S A 100:703–708
28. Wu J, Hua Y, Keep RF, Schallert T, Hoff JT, Xi G (2002) Oxidative brain injury from extravasated erythrocytes after intracerebral hemorrhage. Brain Res 953:45–52
29. Xi G, Hua Y, Bhasin RR, Ennis SR, Keep RF, Hoff JT (2001) Mechanisms of edema formation after intracerebral hemorrhage: effects of extravasated red blood cells on blood flow and blood–brain barrier integrity. Stroke 32:2932–2938
30. Xi G, Keep RF, Hoff JT (1998) Erythrocytes and delayed brain edema formation following intracerebral hemorrhage in rats. J Neurosurg 89:991–996
31. Xi G, Keep RF, Hoff JT (2002) Pathophysiology of brain edema formation. Neurosurg Clin N Am 13:371–383
32. Xie Q, Guan J, Wu G, Xi G, Keep RF, Hua Y (2011) Tamoxifen treatment for intracerebral hemorrhage. Acta Neurochir Suppl 111:271–275
33. Zhang Y, Milatovic D, Aschner M, Feustel PJ, Kimelberg HK (2007) Neuroprotection by tamoxifen in focal cerebral ischemia is not mediated by an agonist action at estrogen receptors but is associated with antioxidant activity. Exp Neurol 204: 819–827

Elevated Cytoplasmic Free Zinc and Increased Reactive Oxygen Species Generation in the Context of Brain Injury

Christian J. Stork and Yang V. Li

Introduction

Although zinc (zinc(II), the zinc ion; Zn^{2+}) is not itself redox active due to its stable electron configuration, there is nonetheless mounting and compelling evidence that intracellular free zinc accumulation promotes the generation of reactive oxygen species (ROS) and reactive nitrogen species (RNS) by multiple mechanisms under "excitotoxic" conditions. Much work has shed light on the molecular and cellular injury sequelae in cerebral ischemia [1, 10, 16, 40, 42], and prolonged seizures [41]; yet approved cell protective therapies in such conditions remain elusive. This review is intended to summarize recent evidence regarding the mechanisms by which the consistently observed phenomenon of intracellular zinc elevation during neuronal injury scenarios results in the production of ROS/RNS, as well as zinc elevation leading to increased ROS/RNS production and the hastening of cell death. Evidence will be presented regarding the sources of intracellular zinc, mechanisms of its release, and the interaction of intracellular free zinc accumulation and the generation of ROS/RNS under conditions promoting neuronal injury and death such as in ischemia.

Overview of Normal Zinc Neurophysiology

Zinc serves an array of necessary biological roles. Zinc ion is found in the catalytically active site of hundreds of biological enzymes [68]. Proteins with catalytic zinc activity are found in all six major functional enzyme categories [3]. Zinc serves integral structural roles in numerous proteins without known catalytic activity, including the ubiquitous zinc finger protein motif. Evidence indicates that up to 10 % of the human proteome (about 2,800 proteins) are expected to be zinc binding in vivo [2]. The virtual omnipresence of zinc in cellular proteins and the redox sensitivity of many protein zinc binding residues represents an important potential source of zinc liberation during neuronal injury. Important to the proposed mechanisms of intracellular zinc liberation and ROS/RNS generation is oxidant-induced release of zinc from proteins such as the cytosolic metallothionein-III (MT-III) [69]. Under physiological conditions of oxidant-induced zinc release from MT-III, the released zinc itself has been shown to initiate transcription of metal ion binding proteins and maintain homeostasis [37, 38].

Normal brain function shows a critical dependence on zinc ion availability, where nutritional zinc deficiency was shown to lead to impaired cognition in rats [9, 24]. Zinc deficiency was also associated with the development of abnormal electrophysiological responses from hippocampal mossy fibers [25]. The average intracellular zinc concentration is considered to be about 250 μM, which agrees with the calculated whole brain zinc average of 150 μM [14, 18]. In agreement with the estimation of Eide [18] the vast majority of this cellular zinc has been demonstrated to be protein bound and/or sequestered into organelles [14]. Nonetheless, in situations of oxidative stress-induced intracellular zinc release, it is apparent that when even a fraction of the total cellular zinc becomes liberated, the effects are highly cytotoxic.

The actual availability of free intracellular zinc is tightly regulated by protein binding and organelle sequestration, such that free zinc is markedly lower than total zinc. Thus, free cytosolic zinc concentrations have been reliably demonstrated to be in the picomolar to nanomolar range [14]. Among the intracellular proteins that maintain free zinc at such low concentrations are the metallothioneins, capable of sequestering as many as seven zinc ions per monomer [47].

C.J. Stork, MD (✉) • Y.V. Li
Department of Biomedical Sciences, Ohio University Heritage College of Osteopathic Medicine,
Irvine Hall, Athens, OH 45701, USA
e-mail: storkc@ohio.edu; liy1@ohio.edu

R.L. Applegate et al. (eds.), *Brain Edema XVI: Translate Basic Science into Clinical Practice*, Acta Neurochirurgica Supplement, Vol. 121,
DOI 10.1007/978-3-319-18497-5_60,

Roles of Zinc in Physiological Neuronal Communication

Zinc has been repeatedly observed to be co-stored with glutamate in synaptic vesicles, where zinc is also co-released with synaptic glutamate into the extracellular space in response to neural stimulation. Activity of the zinc-specific transporter ZnT3 is required for zinc uptake into synaptic vesicles, where ZnT3 knockout mice showed a complete absence of vesicular zinc [12], yet still showed cytosolic zinc accumulation with injury.

The physiological role of synaptic zinc release was largely speculative until it was shown that synaptic zinc release was necessary for the induction of long-term potentiation (LTP) between hippocampus mossy fibers (MF) and CA3 neuron synapses [43]. Further insight into the mechanism of how zinc promotes MF-CA3 LTP was gained by experiments demonstrating zinc activation of Trk signaling in a neurotrophin-independent manner [26, 27]. Deletion of the TrkB receptor, inhibition of TrkB kinase activity, and selective zinc chelation with CaEDTA all resulted in selective impairment of MF-CA3 LTP [27]. These results suggest a physiological reason for vesicular co-release of zinc and glutamate, where zinc secreted during high-frequency MF activity enters the postsynaptic membrane through ionotropic glutamate receptors and transactivates TrkB receptors to enhance synaptic transmission. Another means by which zinc was shown to promote TrkB signaling was suggested by experiments showing zinc promoted the maturation of pro-BDNF to BDNF to thereby result in TrkB activation [28]. Further work has shown zinc release from MT-III by ROS to be necessary for the activation of TrkB [26].

Zinc has been shown to modulate the activity of postsynaptic NMDA receptors through interaction with low- and high-affinity binding sites [30, 53, 54]. Zinc has also been shown to interact with and block the activity of $GABA_A$ receptors [56]. Synaptic zinc has been shown to also specifically trigger metabotropic signaling in addition to the well-documented effects of zinc on ionotropic receptors. In hippocampal CA3 neurons, it was shown that synaptically released zinc interacted with a putative zinc-sensing receptor (ZnR) and resulted in activation of both mitogen-activated protein kinase (MAPK) and CaMKII pathways [6].

Physiological Intracellular Zinc Storage and Release

Eukaryotic cells contain total zinc concentrations in the range of 180–250 μM, whereas the localization of endogenous intracellular metal ion binding agents results in free zinc levels in the picomolar range [14, 37, 52]. Chief among the intracellular proteins that maintain free zinc at such low concentrations are the metallothionein (MT) proteins, capable of sequestering up to seven zinc ions per monomer [38]. Zinc is accumulated inside eukaryotic cells and extruded from the cell by the action of two families of zinc transport proteins, the ZIPs (SLC39) and the ZnTs (SLC30) [18]. ZIPs function to transport zinc and/or other metal ions from the extracellular space or from the lumen of cellular organelles to the cell's cytoplasm [14, 18].

A key physiological function of zinc transport proteins is the accumulation of zinc into cellular organelles to promote the loading of zinc-dependent proteins [13]. Work with $ZnT5^{-/-}$ $ZnT7^{-/-}$ (double knockout) cells showed that the catalytic activity of the zinc-dependent alkaline phosphatase enzyme was significantly reduced compared with wild type controls [29], demonstrating that zinc sequestration within the secretory pathway was a physiological mechanism in the basal state and that organelle zinc sequestration was necessary for normal function.

Evidence shows the sequestration of intracellular zinc into the endoplasmic reticulum (ER) [66], where cultured cortical neurons demonstrated TPEN-sensitive ER zinc localization in the basal state. Further, in a manner strikingly similar to intracellular calcium storage, this ER-localized zinc pool was mobilized by both thapsigargin and IP_3 administration [66]. An additional organelle with zinc-sequestering activity is the mitochondrion. Zinc accumulation within mitochondria was demonstrated to occur through mechanisms involving the calcium-uniporter and by uniporter-independent means [46]. While it has been established that isolated mitochondria can take up exogenous zinc, data from untreated intact neurons show that resting mitochondria do contain endogenous zinc [15, 21], and zinc sequestered in mitochondria can be stimulated for release [21].

Zinc and Mitochondrial ROS Production

Oxidant-induced endogenous zinc release disrupts mitochondrial function [7, 58]. Zinc, like Ca^{2+}, can be taken up by the mitochondrial uniporter [57] but also enters the organelle by an alternative pathway [46]. Intracellular free zinc accumulation has been shown to be devastating to mitochondrial function itself, even apart from the production of ROS [31, 71]. In one mechanism, MT-III has also been shown to translocate to mitochondria and release zinc into the intramembranous space, resulting in the inhibition of respiration [72]. In addition to the block of mitochondrial respiration, elevated zinc has also been shown to result in the loss of mitochondrial membrane potential and the development of the permeability transition leading to the release of proapoptotic factors, including cytochrome *c* [7], ultimately leading to cell death.

Even early investigations into the effects of zinc on mitochondrial function indicated that zinc inhibited respiration [62]. More recent reports have described specific targets, where submicromolar zinc was shown to inhibit mitochondrial respiration by inhibition of the α-ketoglutarate dehydrogenase complex [8]. Further investigation showed that zinc interaction with the lipoamide dehydrogenase (LADH) subunit of the α-ketoglutarate dehydrogenase complex strongly inhibited the enzyme's lipoamide dehydrogenase reaction [8, 20]. Zinc inhibits the LADH reaction to inhibit mitochondrial respiration, and accelerates by fivefold an alternative catalytic activity of LADH that produces hydrogen peroxide and superoxide radical [20]. In addition to the stimulation of ROS generation, these effects of zinc deplete ATP production and lead to cellular energy loss [19, 31]. In the presence of exogenous extracellular zinc, neuronal zinc entry through Ca^{2+}-permeable AMPA/kainate channels triggers prolonged mitochondrial ROS production [59].

In a brain slice oxygen glucose deprivation (OGD) model of neuronal ischemia, the observed cytosolic zinc accumulation was rapidly taken up by mitochondria and contributed to the loss of mitochondrial potential [48]. In the model suggested, intracellular zinc increases early after the start of OGD, where mitochondrial zinc uptake initially functioned to buffer the cytosolic zinc increase but then rapidly resulted in mitochondrial deregulation and cytosolic zinc elevation [48, 49].

Relationship of Calcium and Zinc and ROS

The clear relationship between ion dyshomeostasis, including zinc as well as Ca^{2+}, and neuronal injury is widely reported [33, 51, 67]. An interesting relationship between Ca^{2+} and zinc release was observed during OGD, with the early zinc elevation contributing to the later deregulation of Ca^{2+} [48, 49]. Further insight into the respective consequences of elevated mitochondrial zinc and/or Ca^{2+} was gained by experiments showing that increased zinc triggered strong and rapid mitochondrial ROS production, whereas the majority of Ca^{2+}-induced ROS production occurred outside the mitochondria [11]. Zinc-dependent increases in Ca^{2+} were shown to be key to neuroprotection from glutamate-induced excitotoxicity elicited by a preconditioning mechanism [32]. Clearly, the precise relationships between zinc and Ca^{2+} elevations in excitotoxic neuronal injury largely remain unclear and represent an important future target of investigation.

Work from multiple labs using brain slice OGD models showed fluorescent calcium indicators detect zinc elevation during in vitro ischemia (a scenario of increased ROS generation), which can easily be interpreted solely as a Ca^{2+} transient [48, 64]. Chelation of the increased zinc during ischemia and reperfusion resulted in significantly reduced cellular death [64]. These results show that both zinc and Ca^{2+} appear to be "overloaded" in ischemia and reperfusion. One is compelled to ask why there are two such similar signals and what the relationship is between these ions in ischemia and reperfusion? When hippocampal slices were loaded with cell-permeable Calcium Green-1, as expected, a steady increase in fluorescence intensity was detected during OGD and reperfusion [64]. Application of the selective zinc chelator TPEN diminished the Calcium Green-1 fluorescence during OGD and reperfusion [64], and treatments designed to limit intracellular elevation of zinc were significantly more protective than those designed to limit Ca^{2+} elevation [65]. These data strongly suggest that zinc contributes predominantly to the rising fluorescence intensity measured with Ca^{2+} indicators during OGD and reperfusion of hippocampal slices. Furthermore, the data from zinc chelation revealed that Ca^{2+} signals detected with fluorescent Ca^{2+} indicators are less significant than previously thought. If results previously attributed to Ca^{2+} could, in part, be attributed to zinc, then the "calcium-overload" that has been described in the past, using Ca^{2+}-sensitive indicators, needs to be reexamined to determine whether Ca^{2+} signals are, in fact, a major cause of neuronal damage under these scenarios. Such evidence shows the urgent need for the development of truly selective fluorescent Ca^{2+} indicators.

Non-mitochondrial Zinc-Induced ROS Production

Outside mitochondria, elevated free zinc has been demonstrated to be the activator of a number of ROS- and RNS-generating activities. In turn, ROS and RNS generation have been shown to result in zinc liberation from cellular protein sites including metallothionein, to further exacerbate oxidative and nitrative injury leading to cell death. The interplay between increased free zinc and ROS and/or RNS generation by NADPH oxidase (NOX), nitric oxide synthase (NOS), and 12-lipoxygenase (12-LOX) will be discussed.

NADPH oxidase is expressed in neurons [60, 70] and catalyzes the formation of superoxide. Extracellular zinc application has been shown to promote production of ROS by the activation of NOX by means of protein kinase C activation [36, 50]. CaEDTA application (a zinc chelator) blocks the activation of NOX in a model of hypobaric hypoxia-induced neuroinflammation, demonstrating the zinc-induced activation of this powerful ROS-producing system [44]. Concerning the effects of zinc in chemically induced hypoxia of neurons, recent work has shown that zinc can be either protective or injurious depending on the type of chemical used to induce hypoxia [34].

Elevated zinc was also seen to increase the activity of another free radical-producing enzyme, the neuronal form of nitric oxide synthase (nNOS) [5, 35, 36], resulting in increased nitric oxide (NO) production. In vitro work has shown NO to be capable of interacting with metallothionein to result in the NO-mediated release of zinc [4, 5, 39, 73], highlighting the positive feedback interplay between

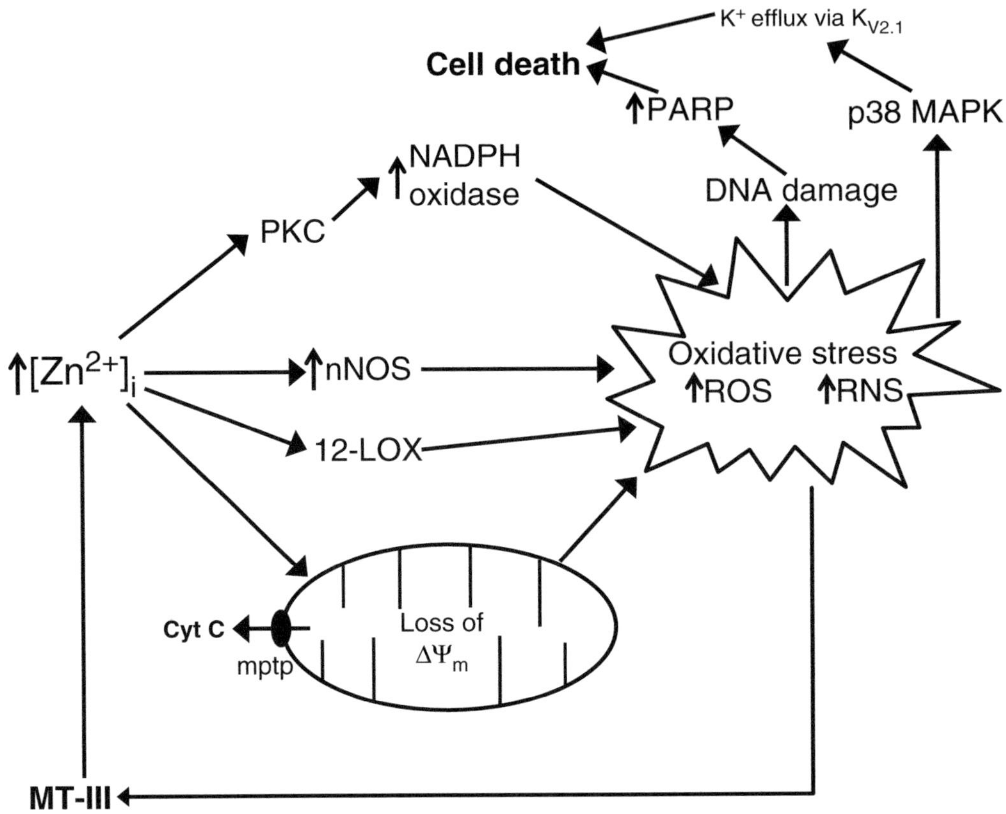

Fig. 1 Intracellular zinc accumulation, as occurs early in excitotoxic conditions, results in the activation of multiple ROS- and RNS-generating mechanisms; which in turn result in further zinc accumulation, leading to cell death. Mitochondrial zinc accumulation leads to the loss of $\Delta\Psi_m$, inhibition of respiration, ROS production, and the development of the mitochondrial permeability transition pore and the promotion of apoptosis through cytochrome c release. NADPH activation by zinc acting through protein kinase C (PKC) represents a particularly robust source of excitotoxic ROS. The direct activation of nNOS and 12-LOX by zinc also represent important sources of oxidative stress and further zinc liberation. DNA damage induced by ROS and RNS generation results in PARP activation and cell death. ROS/RNS elevation induced by zinc can also activate p38 MAPK, which promotes K^+ efflux through $K_{V2.1}$, leading to cell shrinkage and cell death. See text for details

increased zinc and elevations of ROS/RNS. Through such mechanisms, elevated intracellular free zinc promotes both NO production by nNOS and superoxide generation by NOX. Zinc-induced NOX activation, and zinc-induction of NOS activity, resulted in free radical-induced DNA damage and poly(ADP-ribose) polymerase-1 (PARP) activation with the depletion of NAD^+ and ATP followed by cell death [36]. The reaction product of NO and superoxide is peroxynitrite ($ONOO^-$), a free radical shown to be both potently neurotoxic and also a trigger of zinc release. Peroxynitrite liberates zinc from metallothionein to result in elevated intracellular zinc, p38 MAP kinase activation, K^+ efflux via $K_{V2.1}$, and cell death [7, 61].

In addition to the activation of p38 by zinc leading to the $K_{V2.1}$-mediated K^+ current, evidence shows that zinc also promotes enhanced K^+ currents through $K_{V2.1}$ by inhibiting Y124 dephosphorylation [55]. Thus, increased free zinc not only promotes injurious $K_{V2.1}$-mediated K^+ efflux through activation of p38, but also inhibits $K_{V2.1}$ dephosphorylation, thereby increasing injurious K^+ efflux by $K_{V2.1}$ by two independent mechanisms. These enhancements of K^+ currents contribute to cell volume changes and death after ischemic stroke [63], among other neuronal injury scenarios [61].

A further means by which increased intracellular zinc has been shown to result in increased ROS production is the zinc-induced activation of 12-LOX and subsequent ROS generation [75]. Products of 12-LOX from arachidonic acid include a C-12 aldehyde [22]. The observation that aldehydes release zinc from cellular proteins [23] suggests the involvement of zinc-induced 12-LOX activation with further zinc release and the exacerbation of cellular injury.

In addition to the effects in neurons, oxidative and nitrative stress induce zinc release from astrocytes [45] and oligodendrocytes [17, 74]. Peroxynitrite causes activation of ERK1/2 and 12-LOX and the generation of ROS in primary cultures of oligodendrocytes [74]. These data suggest that under conditions of increased oxidative stress, such as in ischemia and reperfusion, a positive feedback cycle between elevated intracellular free zinc and increased ROS/RNS production occurs not only in neurons but also in their supporting glia (Fig. 1).

A striking feature of free zinc-induced ROS and RNS generation is that these reactive species interact with cellular targets to oxidatively liberate further zinc. In this way, increased free zinc induces the formation of ROS and RNS that subsequently induce further intracellular zinc release leading to cell death, showing a neurotoxic mechanism of positive feedback between free zinc and ROS/RNS.

Summary

Zinc has many indispensable roles in cellular and neuronal function. Levels of free zinc are tightly regulated by intracellular metal binding proteins and zinc transporters. While assiduously regulated under normal conditions, free zinc levels can rise rapidly under conditions of oxidative stress, wherein ROS and RNS liberate zinc from proteins, and the elevated zinc induces further ROS and RNS generation. Questions on the precise relationship between ROS/RNS, zinc, and calcium elevation remain, where the clarification of the ions' respective roles in injury represent important future paths of investigation.

The neurotoxic relationship between increased intracellular zinc levels and the generation of ROS has many implications. Important among them is that the reactive species can induce zinc release and increased intracellular free zinc. This elevated zinc can then promote further elevation of ROS and RNS, demonstrating positive-feedback signaling that ultimately leads to cell death under an array of injury scenarios. Therapeutic interventions in these deleterious signaling cascades represent novel approaches at reducing the ROS/RNS and zinc accumulation-induced cell injury under a variety of excitotoxic scenarios.

Declaration of Conflict of Interest The authors have no conflict of interest to declare.

References

1. An C, Shi Y, Li P, Hu X, Gan Y, Stetler RA, Leak RK, Gao Y, Sun BL, Zheng P, Chen J (2014) Molecular dialogs between the ischemic brain and the peripheral immune system: dualistic roles in injury and repair. Prog Neurobiol 115:6–24
2. Andreini C, Banci L, Bertini I, Rosato A (2006) Counting the zinc-proteins encoded in the human genome. J Proteome Res 5:196–201
3. Andreini C, Bertini I (2012) A bioinformatics view of zinc enzymes. J Inorg Biochem 111:150–156
4. Aravindakumar CT, Ceulemans J, De Ley M (1999) Nitric oxide induces Zn2+ release from metallothionein by destroying zinc-sulphur clusters without concomitant formation of S-nitrosothiol. Biochem J 344(Pt 1):253–258
5. Berendji D, Kolb-Bachofen V, Meyer KL, Grapenthin O, Weber H, Wahn V, Kroncke KD (1997) Nitric oxide mediates intracytoplasmic and intranuclear zinc release. FEBS Lett 405:37–41
6. Besser L, Chorin E, Sekler I, Silverman WF, Atkin S, Russell JT, Hershfinkel M (2009) Synaptically released zinc triggers metabotropic signaling via a zinc-sensing receptor in the hippocampus. J Neurosci Off J Soc Neurosci 29:2890–2901
7. Bossy-Wetzel E, Talantova MV, Lee WD, Scholzke MN, Harrop A, Mathews E, Gotz T, Han J, Ellisman MH, Perkins GA, Lipton SA (2004) Crosstalk between nitric oxide and zinc pathways to neuronal cell death involving mitochondrial dysfunction and p38-activated K+ channels. Neuron 41:351–365
8. Brown AM, Kristal BS, Effron MS, Shestopalov AI, Ullucci PA, Sheu KF, Blass JP, Cooper AJ (2000) Zn2+ inhibits alpha-ketoglutarate-stimulated mitochondrial respiration and the isolated alpha-ketoglutarate dehydrogenase complex. J Biol Chem 275: 13441–13447
9. Caldwell DF, Oberleas D, Clancy JJ, Prasad AS (1970) Behavioral impairment in adult rats following acute zinc deficiency. Proceedings of the Society for Experimental Biology and Medicine. Soc Exp Biol Med 133:1417–1421
10. Chen F, Qi Z, Luo Y, Hinchliffe T, Ding G, Xia Y, Ji X (2014) Non-pharmaceutical therapies for stroke: mechanisms and clinical implications. Prog Neurobiol 115:246–269
11. Clausen A, McClanahan T, Ji SG, Weiss JH (2013) Mechanisms of rapid reactive oxygen species generation in response to cytosolic Ca2+ or Zn2+ loads in cortical neurons. PLoS One 8, e83347
12. Cole TB, Wenzel HJ, Kafer KE, Schwartzkroin PA, Palmiter RD (1999) Elimination of zinc from synaptic vesicles in the intact mouse brain by disruption of the ZnT3 gene. Proc Natl Acad Sci U S A 96:1716–1721
13. Coleman JE (1992) Zinc proteins: enzymes, storage proteins, transcription factors, and replication proteins. Annu Rev Biochem 61:897–946
14. Colvin RA, Bush AI, Volitakis I, Fontaine CP, Thomas D, Kikuchi K, Holmes WR (2008) Insights into Zn2+ homeostasis in neurons from experimental and modeling studies. Am J Physiol Cell Physiol 294:C726–C742
15. Colvin RA, Fontaine CP, Laskowski M, Thomas D (2003) Zn2+ transporters and Zn2+ homeostasis in neurons. Eur J Pharmacol 479:171–185
16. Deng J, Lei C, Chen Y, Fang Z, Yang Q, Zhang H, Cai M, Shi L, Dong H, Xiong L (2014) Neuroprotective gases – fantasy or reality for clinical use? Prog Neurobiol 115:210–245
17. Domercq M, Mato S, Soria FN, Sanchez-gomez MV, Alberdi E, Matute C (2013) Zn2+ –induced ERK activation mediates PARP-1-dependent ischemic-reoxygenation damage to oligodendrocytes. Glia 61:383–393
18. Eide DJ (2006) Zinc transporters and the cellular trafficking of zinc. Biochim Biophys Acta 1763:711–722
19. Gazaryan IG, Krasinskaya IP, Kristal BS, Brown AM (2007) Zinc irreversibly damages major enzymes of energy production and antioxidant defense prior to mitochondrial permeability transition. J Biol Chem 282:24373–24380
20. Gazaryan IG, Krasnikov BF, Ashby GA, Thorneley RN, Kristal BS, Brown AM (2002) Zinc is a potent inhibitor of thiol oxidoreductase activity and stimulates reactive oxygen species production by lipoamide dehydrogenase. J Biol Chem 277:10064–10072
21. Gee KR, Zhou ZL, Ton-That D, Sensi SL, Weiss JH (2002) Measuring zinc in living cells. A new generation of sensitive and selective fluorescent probes. Cell Calcium 31:245–251
22. Glasgow WC, Harris TM, Brash AR (1986) A short-chain aldehyde is a major lipoxygenase product in arachidonic acid-stimulated porcine leukocytes. J Biol Chem 261:200–204
23. Hao Q, Maret W (2006) Aldehydes release zinc from proteins. A pathway from oxidative stress/lipid peroxidation to cellular functions of zinc. FEBS J 273:4300–4310
24. Hesse GW (1979) Chronic zinc deficiency alters neuronal function of hippocampal mossy fibers. Science 205:1005–1007

25. Hesse GW, Hesse KA, Catalanotto FA (1979) Behavioral characteristics of rats experiencing chronic zinc deficiency. Physiol Behav 22:211–215
26. Huang YZ, McNamara JO (2012) Neuroprotective effects of reactive oxygen species mediated by BDNF-independent activation of TrkB. J Neurosci Off J Soc Neurosci 32:15521–15532
27. Huang YZ, Pan E, Xiong ZQ, McNamara JO (2008) Zinc-mediated transactivation of TrkB potentiates the hippocampal mossy fiber-CA3 pyramid synapse. Neuron 57:546–558
28. Hwang JJ, Park MH, Choi SY, Koh JY (2005) Activation of the Trk signaling pathway by extracellular zinc. Role of metalloproteinases. J Biol Chem 280:11995–12001
29. Ishihara K, Yamazaki T, Ishida Y, Suzuki T, Oda K, Nagao M, Yamaguchi-Iwai Y, Kambe T (2006) Zinc transport complexes contribute to the homeostatic maintenance of secretory pathway function in vertebrate cells. J Biol Chem 281:17743–17750
30. Izumi Y, Auberson YP, Zorumski CF (2006) Zinc modulates bidirectional hippocampal plasticity by effects on NMDA receptors. J Neurosci Off J Soc Neurosci 26:7181–7188
31. Jiang D, Sullivan PG, Sensi SL, Steward O, Weiss JH (2001) Zn(2+) induces permeability transition pore opening and release of pro-apoptotic peptides from neuronal mitochondria. J Biol Chem 276:47524–47529
32. Johanssen T, Suphantarida N, Donnelly PS, Liu XM, Petrou S, Hill AF, Barnham KJ (2015) PBT2 inhibits glutamate-induced excitotoxicity in neurons through metal-mediated preconditioning. Neurobiol Dis
33. Khanna A, Kahle KT, Walcott BP, Gerzanich V, Simard JM (2014) Disruption of ion homeostasis in the neurogliovascular unit underlies the pathogenesis of ischemic cerebral edema. Transl Stroke Res 5:3–16
34. Kim S, Seo JW, Oh SB, Kim SH, Kim I, Suh N, Lee JY (2015) Disparate roles of zinc in chemical hypoxia-induced neuronal death. Front Cell Neurosci 9:1
35. Kim YH, Kim EY, Gwag BJ, Sohn S, Koh JY (1999) Zinc-induced cortical neuronal death with features of apoptosis and necrosis: mediation by free radicals. Neuroscience 89:175–182
36. Kim YH, Koh JY (2002) The role of NADPH oxidase and neuronal nitric oxide synthase in zinc-induced poly(ADP-ribose) polymerase activation and cell death in cortical culture. Exp Neurol 177:407–418
37. Krezel A, Maret W (2006) Zinc-buffering capacity of a eukaryotic cell at physiological pZn. J Biol Inorg Chem JBIC 11:1049–1062
38. Krezel A, Maret W (2008) Thionein/metallothionein control Zn(II) availability and the activity of enzymes. J Biol Inorg Chem JBIC 13:401–409
39. Kroncke KD, Fehsel K, Schmidt T, Zenke FT, Dasting I, Wesener JR, Bettermann H, Breunig KD, Kolb-Bachofen V (1994) Nitric oxide destroys zinc-sulfur clusters inducing zinc release from metallothionein and inhibition of the zinc finger-type yeast transcription activator LAC9. Biochem Biophys Res Commun 200:1105–1110
40. Lai TW, Zhang S, Wang YT (2014) Excitotoxicity and stroke: identifying novel targets for neuroprotection. Prog Neurobiol 115:157–188
41. Lees GJ, Cuajungco MP, Leong W (1998) Effect of metal chelating agents on the direct and seizure-related neuronal death induced by zinc and kainic acid. Brain Res 799:108–117
42. Leng T, Shi Y, Xiong ZG, Sun D (2014) Proton-sensitive cation channels and ion exchangers in ischemic brain injury: new therapeutic targets for stroke? Prog Neurobiol 115:189–209
43. Li Y, Hough CJ, Frederickson CJ, Sarvey JM (2001) Induction of mossy fiber --> Ca3 long-term potentiation requires translocation of synaptically released Zn2+. The J Neurosci Off J Soc Neurosci 21:8015–8025
44. Malairaman U, Dandapani K, Katyal A (2014) Effect of Ca2EDTA on zinc mediated inflammation and neuronal apoptosis in hippocampus of an in vivo mouse model of hypobaric hypoxia. PLoS One 9, e110253
45. Malaiyandi LM, Dineley KE, Reynolds IJ (2004) Divergent consequences arise from metallothionein overexpression in astrocytes: zinc buffering and oxidant-induced zinc release. Glia 45:346–353
46. Malaiyandi LM, Vergun O, Dineley KE, Reynolds IJ (2005) Direct visualization of mitochondrial zinc accumulation reveals uniporter-dependent and -independent transport mechanisms. J Neurochem 93:1242–1250
47. Maret W (2008) Metallothionein redox biology in the cytoprotective and cytotoxic functions of zinc. Exp Gerontol 43:363–369
48. Medvedeva YV, Lin B, Shuttleworth CW, Weiss JH (2009) Intracellular Zn2+ accumulation contributes to synaptic failure, mitochondrial depolarization, and cell death in an acute slice oxygen-glucose deprivation model of ischemia. J Neurosci Off J Soc Neurosci 29:1105–1114
49. Medvedeva YV, Weiss JH (2014) Intramitochondrial Zn2+ accumulation via the Ca2+ uniporter contributes to acute ischemic neurodegeneration. Neurobiol Dis 68:137–144
50. Noh KM, Kim YH, Koh JY (1999) Mediation by membrane protein kinase C of zinc-induced oxidative neuronal injury in mouse cortical cultures. J Neurochem 72:1609–1616
51. O'Bryant Z, Vann KT, Xiong ZG (2014) Translational strategies for neuroprotection in ischemic stroke – focusing on acid-sensing ion channel 1a. Transl Stroke Res 5:59–68
52. Palmiter RD (1995) Constitutive expression of metallothionein-III (MT-III), but not MT-I, inhibits growth when cells become zinc deficient. Toxicol Appl Pharmacol 135:139–146
53. Paoletti P, Ascher P, Neyton J (1997) High-affinity zinc inhibition of NMDA NR1-NR2A receptors. J Neurosci Off J Soc Neurosci 17:5711–5725
54. Rachline J, Perin-Dureau F, Le Goff A, Neyton J, Paoletti P (2005) The micromolar zinc-binding domain on the NMDA receptor subunit NR2B. J Neurosci Off J Soc Neurosci 25:308–317
55. Redman PT, Hartnett KA, Aras MA, Levitan ES, Aizenman E (2009) Regulation of apoptotic potassium currents by coordinated zinc-dependent signalling. J Physiol 587:4393–4404
56. Ruiz A, Walker MC, Fabian-Fine R, Kullmann DM (2004) Endogenous zinc inhibits GABA(A) receptors in a hippocampal pathway. J Neurophysiol 91:1091–1096
57. Saris NE, Niva K (1994) Is Zn2+ transported by the mitochondrial calcium uniporter? FEBS Lett 356:195–198
58. Sensi SL, Ton-That D, Sullivan PG, Jonas EA, Gee KR, Kaczmarek LK, Weiss JH (2003) Modulation of mitochondrial function by endogenous Zn2+ pools. Proc Natl Acad Sci U S A 100:6157–6162
59. Sensi SL, Yin HZ, Carriedo SG, Rao SS, Weiss JH (1999) Preferential Zn2+ influx through Ca2+–permeable AMPA/kainate channels triggers prolonged mitochondrial superoxide production. Proc Natl Acad Sci U S A 96:2414–2419
60. Serrano F, Kolluri NS, Wientjes FB, Card JP, Klann E (2003) NADPH oxidase immunoreactivity in the mouse brain. Brain Res 988:193–198
61. Shah NH, Aizenman E (2014) Voltage-gated potassium channels at the crossroads of neuronal function, ischemic tolerance, and neurodegeneration. Transl Stroke Res 5:38–58
62. Skulachev VP, Chistyakov VV, Jasaitis AA, Smirnova EG (1967) Inhibition of the respiratory chain by zinc ions. Biochem Biophys Res Commun 26:1–6
63. Song M, Yu SP (2014) Ionic regulation of cell volume changes and cell death after ischemic stroke. Transl Stroke Res 5:17–27
64. Stork CJ, Li YV (2006) Intracellular zinc elevation measured with a "calcium-specific" indicator during ischemia and reperfusion in rat hippocampus: a question on calcium overload. J Neurosci Off J Soc Neurosci 26:10430–10437
65. Stork CJ, Li YV (2009) Rising zinc: a significant cause of ischemic neuronal death in the CA1 region of rat hippocampus. J Cereb Blood Flow Metab Off J Int Soc Cereb Blood Flow Metab 29:1399–1408

66. Stork CJ, Li YV (2010) Zinc release from thapsigargin/IP3-sensitive stores in cultured cortical neurons. J Mol Signal 5:5
67. Sun D, Kahle KT (2014) Dysregulation of diverse ion transport pathways controlling cell volume homeostasis contribute to neuroglial cell injury following ischemic stroke. Transl Stroke Res 5:1–2
68. Vallee BL, Auld DS (1990) Zinc coordination, function, and structure of zinc enzymes and other proteins. Biochemistry 29:5647–5659
69. Vallee BL, Auld DS (1995) Zinc metallochemistry in biochemistry. EXS 73:259–277
70. Vallet P, Charnay Y, Steger K, Ogier-Denis E, Kovari E, Herrmann F, Michel JP, Szanto I (2005) Neuronal expression of the NADPH oxidase NOX4, and its regulation in mouse experimental brain ischemia. Neuroscience 132:233–238
71. Wudarczyk J, Debska G, Lenartowicz E (1999) Zinc as an inducer of the membrane permeability transition in rat liver mitochondria. Arch Biochem Biophys 363:1–8
72. Ye B, Maret W, Vallee BL (2001) Zinc metallothionein imported into liver mitochondria modulates respiration. Proc Natl Acad Sci U S A 98:2317–2322
73. Zangger K, Oz G, Haslinger E, Kunert O, Armitage IM (2001) Nitric oxide selectively releases metals from the amino-terminal domain of metallothioneins: potential role at inflammatory sites. FASEB J Off Publ Fed Am Soc Exp Biol 15:1303–1305
74. Zhang Y, Wang H, Li J, Dong L, Xu P, Chen W, Neve RL, Volpe JJ, Rosenberg PA (2006) Intracellular zinc release and ERK phosphorylation are required upstream of 12-lipoxygenase activation in peroxynitrite toxicity to mature rat oligodendrocytes. J Biol Chem 281:9460–9470
75. Zhang Y, Wang H, Li J, Jimenez DA, Levitan ES, Aizenman E, Rosenberg PA (2004) Peroxynitrite-induced neuronal apoptosis is mediated by intracellular zinc release and 12-lipoxygenase activation. J Neurosc Off J Soc Neurosci 24:10616–10627

Role of Protease-Activated Receptor-1 in Glioma Growth

Qing Xie, Xuhui Bao, Zhan Hong Chen, Ying Xu, Richard F. Keep, Karin M. Muraszko, Guohua Xi, and Ya Hua

Introduction

Our previous studies have indicated an important role of thrombin in glioma development. Thus, thrombin was expressed in several kinds of glioma cells, rat gliomas and human glioblastomas [13], thrombin-enhanced glioma growth in vivo and cell proliferation in vitro [12], and thrombin-increased vascular endothelial growth factor (VEGF) levels via activating hypoxia inducible factor-1α (HIF-1α) and p44/42 mitogen-activated protein kinase (MAPK) pathways in rat gliomas [30]. Argatroban, a small molecular weight (MW 508.7) thrombin inhibitor that inhibits both free and fibrin-bound thrombin, reduced tumor mass, attenuated neurological deficits, and prolonged survival time in rat F98 gliomas [11].

Protease-activated receptors, PAR-1, -3, and -4 [5, 6], are thrombin receptors and have been found in many types of tumor cells, including rat glioma cells [18, 20, 21, 28]. Activation of PAR-1 is associated with angiogenesis [19], tumor cell proliferation [7], and invasion [8, 9]. The present study examined the effect of PAR-1 in glioma growth in a mouse model.

Q. Xie
Department of Neurosurgery, University of Michigan, 5018 BSRB, Ann Arbor, MI 48109-2200, USA

Department of Neurosurgery, Huashan Hospital, Fudan University, Shanghai, China

X. Bao • Y. Xu • R.F. Keep, PhD • K.M. Muraszko • G. Xi, MD
Y. Hua, MD (✉)
Department of Neurosurgery, University of Michigan, 5018 BSRB, Ann Arbor, MI 48109-2200, USA
e-mail: yahua@umich.edu

Z.H. Chen
Department of Neurosurgery, University of Michigan, 5018 BSRB, Ann Arbor, MI 48109-2200, USA

Department of Medical Oncology, Zhejiang Cancer Hospital, Hangzhou, Zhejiang 310022, China

Material and Methods

Cell Culture

F98 glioma cells (passage number 6–15) were obtained from American Type Culture Collection (CRL-2397 from ATCC, Manassas, VA, USA). F98 cells were grown in Dulbecco's modified Eagle's medium (DMEM, ATCC) with 10 % fetal bovine serum at 37 °C in air with 5 % CO_2.

Experimental Groups

Wild type (WT, $n=31$) and PAR-1 knockout (KO, $n=29$) mice received an injection of F98 glioma cells (2×10^7/ml in 10 μl saline) into the right caudate. Mice were used for (1) brain water content and tumor-mass weight determination at day 12 ($n=8$ for WT and 7 for KO) and (2) ELISA (enzyme-linked immunosorbent assay) assay for the protein levels of HIF-1α or VEGF day 7 ($n=5$ for each) after magnetic resonance imaging (MRI) scanning.

Animal Preparation and Tumor Cell Implantation

Animal use protocols were approved by the University of Michigan Committee on the Use and Care of Animals. Same age (4–6 months old) and gender of wild type and PAR-1 knockout (C57BL/6, Jackson Laboratory, Bar Harbor, ME, USA) mice were used in this study. Mice were anesthetized by mixture of ketamine (50 mg/kg) and xylazine (5 mg/kg) by intraperitoneal (IP) injection. Mice were lying prone with head fixed in a stereotactic frame (Kopf Instruments, Tujunga, CA, USA), and a cranial burr hole (1 mm) was drilled on the

R.L. Applegate et al. (eds.), *Brain Edema XVI: Translate Basic Science into Clinical Practice*, Acta Neurochirurgica Supplement, Vol. 121,
DOI 10.1007/978-3-319-18497-5_61,

right coronal suture 2.5 mm lateral to the midline. A microsyringe (25 μl, SGE Analytical Science, Ringwood, Victoria Australia) was inserted stereotactically into the right caudate (coordinates: 0.2 mm anterior, 3.5 mm ventral, 2.5 mm lateral to the bregma). Glioma cells (2×10^7/ml in 10 μl saline) were infused at a rate of 1 μl/min using a microinfusion pump. After injection, the needle was kept in position for another 5 min to lessen the reflux of injected tumor cells. The needle was then removed, the burr hole sealed with bone wax, and the skin incision was sutured closed.

Brain Water Content and Tumor Mass

Animals were euthanized by decapitation under deep pentobarbital anesthesia. The brains were removed immediately and separated in two hemispheres by cutting on the midline and then a coronal cut was made to separate the brain into four pieces, ipsilateral and contralateral anterior parts (Ipsi-A and Cont-A) and ipsilateral and contralateral posterior parts (Ipsi-P and Cont-P). Brain tissue samples were weighed on an electronic analytical balance (model AE 100, Mettler Instrument Co., Columbus, OH, USA) to obtain the wet weight (WW). Samples were then dried in a gravity oven at 100 °C for 24 h to obtain the dry weight (DW). Brain water content (%) was measured as ((WW – DW)/WW) × 100 %, and tumor mass was measured as (Ipsi-A + Ipsi-P) – (Cont-A + Cont-P), either in wet or dry weight.

Magnetic Resonance Imaging

Mice had head MRI scans at 7 days after glioma cell injection under anesthesia with 2 % isofluorane/air mixture. The head was fixed in a 7.0 T Varian MR scanner (183-mm horizontal bore, Varian, Palo Alto, CA, USA) with body temperature maintained at 37 °C by circulated heated air. A double-tuned volume radiofrequency coil was used to scan the head region. Following IP gadopentetate dimeglumine (Magnevist, 2 μl/mg, Bayer, Leverkusen, Germany) contrast injection, axial T_2-weighted images were acquired using a fast spin-echo sequence with the following parameters: repetition time (TR)/effective echo time (TE), 4,000/60 ms; field of view (FOV), 20 × 20 mm; matrix, 256 × 128; slice thickness, 0.5 mm; slice spacing, 0 mm; and number of slices, 25; total scan time about 2.5 min. To visualize contrast enhancement, axial T_1-weighted images were acquired using a gradient-echo sequence with the following parameters: TR/ TE, 500/15 ms; FOV, 20 × 20 mm; matrix, 128 × 128; slice thickness, 0.5 mm; slice spacing, 0 mm; and number of slices, 25; total scan time around 1.5 min [33].

Enzyme-Linked Immunosorbent Assay (ELISA)

A human/mouse total HIF-1α ELISA kit and a mouse/rat VEGF DuoSet® ELISA kit were purchased from R&D Systems (Minneapolis, MN, USA) and used. Brain samples were harvested and divided into four pieces (Cont-A, Ipsi-A, Con-P, and Ipsi-P) as described for brain water content. The samples were then homogenized with Reagent Diluent at the same ratio of weight to volume (W/V = 40 %). The supernatant was collected after centrifuge at 8,000 rpm for 5 min at 4 °C. Plates (96 wells) were coated with diluted capture antibody overnight at room temperature and were blocked with Reagent Diluent for 1 h after three washes. Brain samples (100 μl) were added into the wells and incubated for 2 h at room temperature. Detection antibody was added into the wells after three washes and incubated for 2 h at room temperature. After incubation with Streptavidin-HRP and Substrate Solution (20 min for each), stop solution was added and optical density determined at 450/540 nm using a microplate reader. Antigen quantification was measured by standard curve. All studies were repeated three times [2].

Tumor Volume Measurement

Mice were anesthetized with pentobarbital (100 mg/kg, IP). After intracardiac perfusion with 4 % paraformaldehyde in 0.1 mol/l phosphate-buffered saline (PBS, pH 7.4), the animals were decapitated. Brains were removed and kept in 4 % paraformaldehyde in 0.1 mol/l PBS (pH 7.4) for 24 h. They were then immersed in 30 % sucrose in PBS (pH 7.4) for 3–4 days at 4 °C. The brains were embedded in O.C.T. compound (Sakura Finetek, Torrance, CA, USA) and sliced consecutively as 8 μm coronal sections on a cryostat, with 30 consecutive slices. Hematoxylin and eosin staining was used for histological examination, and scanned into digital files under a microscope. Using a computerized image analysis system (NIH Image J, version 1.42), the area of tumor size on each section was measured three times to obtain an average value.

Statistics

The results are reported as mean ± standard deviation (SD). Data were analyzed by analysis of variance (ANOVA) followed by Scheffé's post hoc test, Student's *t*-test, and Trend Peto-Peto-Wilcoxon test. Differences were determined to be significant at the $p < 0.05$ levels.

Results

At day 12 after F98 cells injection, brain water content was significantly lower in the ipsilateral hemisphere of PAR-1 KO mice compared with WT mice in both anterior (79.4±1.3 % vs 81.5±1.1 % in WT mice, $p<0.05$) and posterior (77.8±0.6 % vs 78.9±1.1 % in WT mice, $p<0.05$, Fig. 1a) brain sections. Both wet (43.4±27.8 vs 11.3±23.2 mg in KO mice, $p<0.05$, Fig.1b) and dry (5.2±3.4 vs 0.3±3.4 mg in KO mice, $p<0.05$, Fig. 1c) tumor-mass weights were also higher in WT mice at that time point.

Protein levels of HIF-1α in the ipsilateral hemisphere were higher in WT mice (373±25 pg/g brain tissue) than in KO mice (333±35 pg/g brain tissue, $p<0.05$) at 7 days after F98 cells implantation. VEGF protein levels were also higher in the ipsilateral hemisphere of WT mice (219±21 vs 166±22 pg/g brain tissue in KO mice, $p<0.01$).

On T2-weighted images, the tumor showed hypointensity and isointensity compared with brain tissue, whereas peritumoral tissue was hyperintense. The brain tissue around tumor was compressed and the midline was shifted. Tumor size in WT mice was bigger than in KO mice on both T2 and T1 images. On T1-weighted images, after IP injection of Magnevist, the tumor was more obvious with its mass effect and peritumor edema. The tumor volume measured in T1 ivmages was larger in WT mice (44.0±13.0 mm^3) than in KO mice (16.9±12.5 mm^3, $p<0.05$, Fig. 2a) at day 7. Because the boundaries of the tumors were clearly demarcated, we measured the total area of tumor, which appears bigger than H&E tumor staining after tissue processing. However, H&E-stained sections also demonstrated larger tumor volumes in WT than in KO mice at day 12 (WT: 23.2±12.6 mm^3, PAR-1 KO mice: 8.6±9.7 mm^3, $p<0.05$; Fig. 2b). Tumors could be seen extending to the brain surface in WT mice but not in KO mice (Fig. 2b).

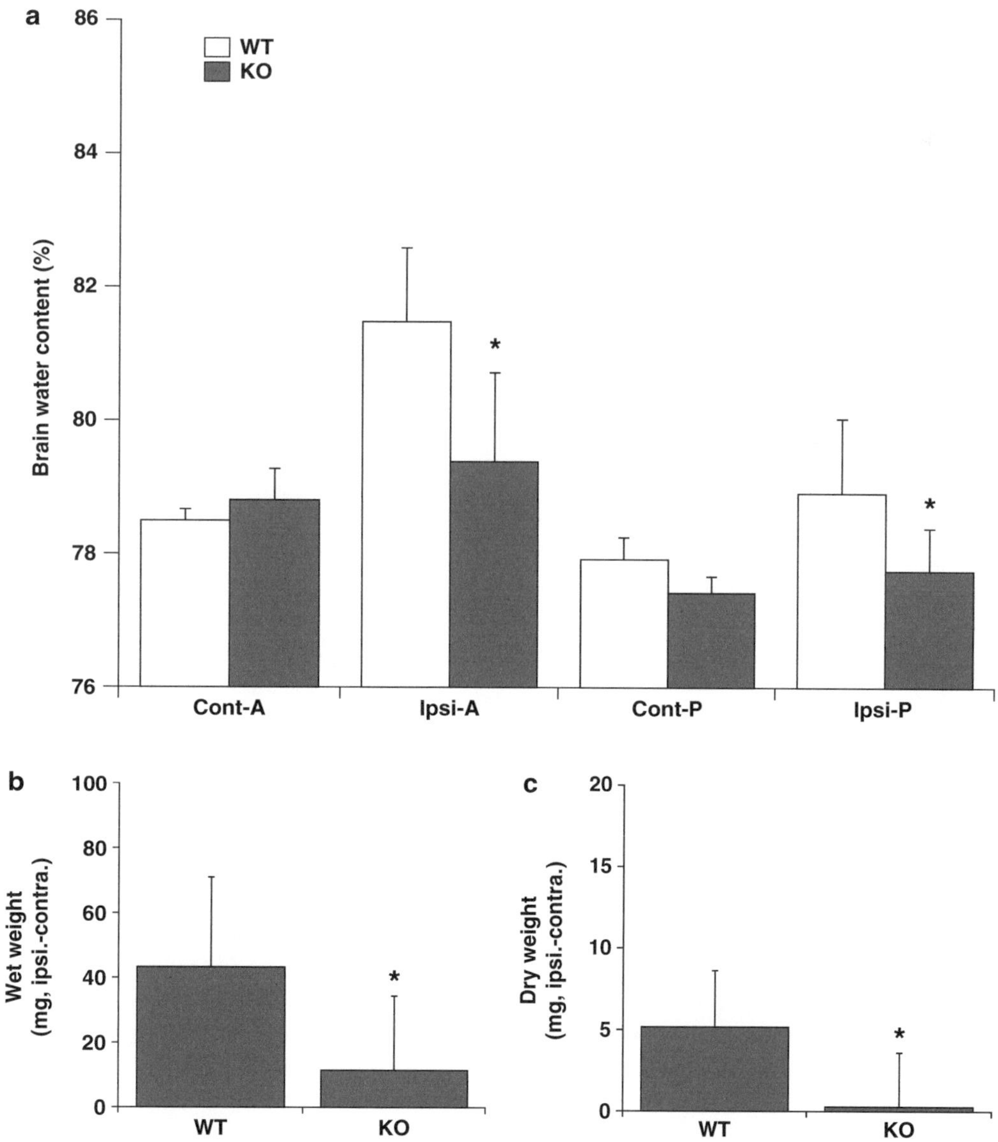

Fig. 1 Brain water content (**a**), tumor wet weight (**b**), and tumor dry weight (**c**) in the brains of WT and KO mice at day 12 after F98 cells were implanted into the right caudate. Values are mean±SD, $n=8$, $^*p<0.05$ by Student's *t*-test

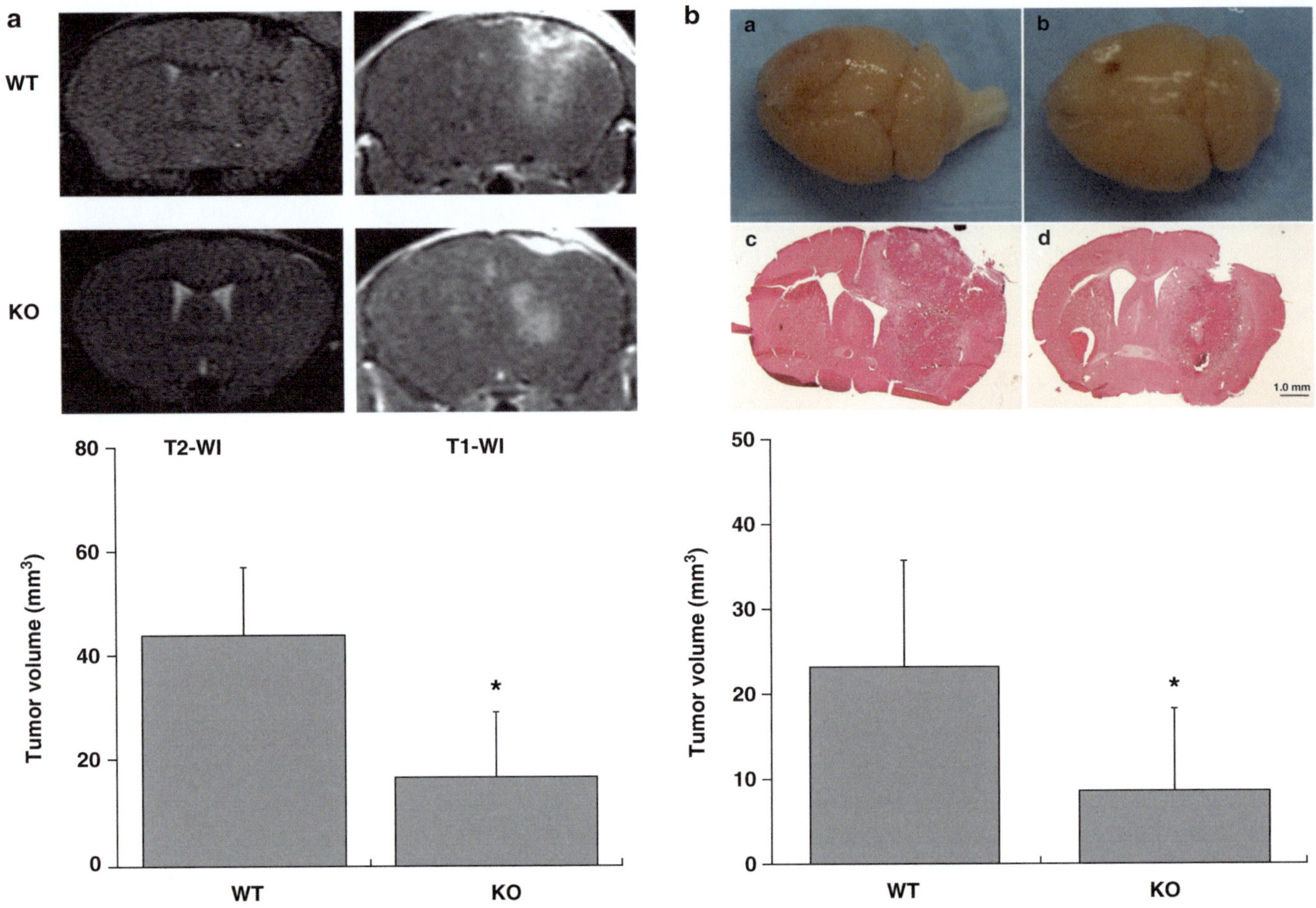

Fig. 2 (**a**) T2- and T1-weighted images and the tumor volume measured in T1 images at 7 days. (**b**) Pictures of the brain and tumor in H&E-stained sections in WT (*a*, *c*) or PAR-1 KO (*b*, *d*) mice at day 12 after F98 cells implantation. The *bar graph* shows quantification of tumor volumes. Values are mean ± SD, $n = 7–9$, $*p < 0.05$ by Student's *t*-test

Discussion

In this study, we found that F98 glioma cell implantation caused lower brain edema, less tumor mass and volume, and lower HIF-1α and VEGF expression levels in PAR-1 knockout compared with WT mice.

Thrombin is a key factor in the common pathway for activation of the coagulation system [10, 32] and may act as a growth factor for tumor cells [3]. Malignant tumors express high levels of active tissue factor, an element of the extrinsic coagulation cascade that ultimately converts prothrombin to thrombin [22, 23, 25]. In our previous studies, thrombin was detected in gliomas, and the thrombin inhibitor argatroban attenuated brain edema, tumor mass, neurological deficits, and prolonged survival time [11, 13, 14].

The tumor microenvironment is important in tumor growth and invasion [23]. Prothrombin and PAR-1 are widely distributed throughout the brain tissue (e.g., astrocytes, microglia, and neurons) [17, 29]. PAR-1 deficiency provides an opportunity to explore the role of this receptor in thrombin signaling [4] in relation to tumor biology. In the current study, PAR-1 deletion in the mouse host reduced HIF-1α and VEGF expression levels after F98 cell implantation. These two changes may be linked as VEGF is regulated by HIF-1α, which also regulates the expression of many other genes involved in the response to hypoxic environments [30]. We have previously shown that thrombin upregulates HIF-1α in brain [16] and our current results suggest that this is at least in part via PAR-1, as also suggested for colorectal cancer cells [1].

VEGF has been recognized as a major angiogenic factor [24, 31]. Angiogenesis is the process of generating new blood vessels from preexisting vessels and is considered essential for tumor growth and metastasis. The presence of vascular endothelial proliferation is significantly associated with malignancy and contributes to the extent of peritumoral edema. Thus, the decrease in VEGF levels in the KO mouse may inhibit angiogenesis and contribute to the observed reduction in tumor growth. Increased thrombin signaling, by treating glioma cells with thrombin, increased tumor growth induced by thrombin treated tumor cells [12].

Thrombin signaling may impact angiogenesis via multiple factors. Thus, thrombin also increases the expression and release of angiopoietin-2 [15] and decreases adhesion of endothelial cells to basement membrane proteins, thus facilitating their detachment and migration to distal sites and vascular remodeling [26, 27].

The current study used PAR-1 KO mice but the injected glioma cells may still express PAR-1. Thus, PAR-1 antagonists may be of benefit in glioma by downregulating VEGF production by both the tumor and peritumoral tissue.

In conclusion, the thrombin receptor PAR-1 may play an important role in glioma growth. This provides us a new strategy to treat gliomas in humans and needs further investigation.

Acknowledgment This study was supported by grants NS-073595, NS-079157, and NS-084049 from the National Institutes of Health (NIH) and NSFC30901549 from National Science Foundation of China.

References

1. Chang LH, Chen CH, Huang DY, Pai HC, Pan SL, Teng CM (2011) Thrombin induces expression of twist and cell motility via the hypoxia-inducible factor-1alpha translational pathway in colorectal cancer cells. J Cell Physiol 226:1060–1068
2. Cheng Y, Xi G, Jin H, Keep RF, Feng J, Hua Y (2014) Thrombin-induced cerebral hemorrhage: role of protease-activated receptor-1. Transl Stroke Res 5:472–475
3. Chinni C, de Niese MR, Tew DJ, Jenkins AL, Bottomley SP, Mackie EJ (1999) Thrombin, a survival factor for cultured myoblasts. J Biol Chem 274:9169–9174
4. Connolly AJ, Ishihara H, Kahn ML, Farese RV Jr, Coughlin SR (1996) Role of the thrombin receptor in development and evidence for a second receptor. Nature 381:516–519
5. Coughlin SR (2000) Thrombin signalling and protease-activated receptors. [Review] [64 refs]. Nature 407:258–264
6. Coughlin SR (2005) Protease-activated receptors in hemostasis, thrombosis and vascular biology. J Thromb Haemost 3:1800–1814
7. Darmoul D, Gratio V, Devaud H, Peiretti F, Laburthe M (2004) Activation of proteinase-activated receptor 1 promotes human colon cancer cell proliferation through epidermal growth factor receptor transactivation. Mol Cancer Res 2:514–522
8. Even-Ram S, Uziely B, Cohen P, Grisaru-Granovsky S, Maoz M, Ginzburg Y, Reich R, Vlodavsky I, Bar-Shavit R (1998) Thrombin receptor overexpression in malignant and physiological invasion processes. Nat Med 4:909–914
9. Even-Ram SC, Maoz M, Pokroy E, Reich R, Katz BZ, Gutwein P, Altevogt P, Bar-Shavit R (2001) Tumor cell invasion is promoted by activation of protease activated receptor-1 in cooperation with the alpha vbeta 5 integrin. J Biol Chem 276:10952–10962
10. Hu L, Lee M, Campbell W, Perez-Soler R, Karpatkin S (2004) Role of endogenous thrombin in tumor implantation, seeding, and spontaneous metastasis. Blood 104:2746–2751
11. Hua Y, Keep RF, Schallert T, Hoff JT, Xi G (2003) A thrombin inhibitor reduces brain edema, glioma mass and neurological deficits in a rat glioma model. Acta Neurochir Suppl 86:503–506
12. Hua Y, Tang L, Keep RF, Hoff JT, Heth J, Xi G, Muraszko KM (2008) Thrombin enhances glioma growth. Acta Neurochir Suppl 102:363–366
13. Hua Y, Tang L, Keep RF, Schallert T, Fewel M, Muraszko K, Hoff JT, Xi G (2005) The role of thrombin in gliomas. J Thromb Haemost 3:1–7
14. Hua Y, Tang LL, Fewel ME, Keep RF, Schallert T, Muraszko KM, Hoff JT, Xi GH (2005) Systemic use of argatroban reduces tumor mass, attenuates neurological deficits and prolongs survival time in rat glioma models. Acta Neurochir Suppl 95:403–406
15. Huang YQ, Li JJ, Hu L, Lee M, Karpatkin S (2002) Thrombin induces increased expression and secretion of angiopoietin-2 from human umbilical vein endothelial cells. Blood 99:1646–1650
16. Jiang Y, Wu J, Keep RF, Hua Y, Hoff JT, Xi G (2002) Hypoxia-inducible factor-1α accumulation in the brain after experimental intracerebral hemorrhage. J Cereb Blood Flow Metab 22:689–696
17. Junge CE, Sugawara T, Mannaioni G, Alagarsamy S, Conn PJ, Brat DJ, Chan PH, Traynelis SF (2003) The contribution of protease-activated receptor 1 to neuronal damage caused by transient focal cerebral ischemia. Proc Natl Acad Sci U S A 100:13019–13024
18. Kaushal V, Kohli M, Dennis RA, Siegel ER, Chiles WW, Mukunyadzi P (2006) Thrombin receptor expression is upregulated in prostate cancer. Prostate 66:273–282
19. Maragoudakis ME, Tsopanoglou NE, Andriopoulou P, Maragoudakis MM (2000) Effects of thrombin/thrombosis in angiogenesis and tumour progression. [Review] [24 refs]. Matrix Biol 19:345–351
20. Nierodzik ML, Bain RM, Liu LX, Shivji M, Takeshita K, Karpatkin S (1996) Presence of the seven transmembrane thrombin receptor on human tumour cells: effect of activation on tumour adhesion to platelets and tumor tyrosine phosphorylation. Br J Haematol 92:452–457
21. Nierodzik ML, Chen K, Takeshita K, Li JJ, Huang YQ, Feng XS, D'Andrea MR, Andrade-Gordon P, Karpatkin S (1998) Protease-activated receptor 1 (PAR-1) is required and rate-limiting for thrombin-enhanced experimental pulmonary metastasis. Blood 92:3694–3700
22. Ornstein DL, Meehan KR, Zacharski LR (2002) The coagulation system as a target for the treatment of human gliomas. Semin Thromb Hemost 28:19–28
23. Schaffner F, Ruf W (2009) Tissue factor and PAR2 signaling in the tumor microenvironment. Arterioscler Thromb Vasc Biol 29:1999–2004
24. Skobe M, Rockwell P, Goldstein N, Vosseler S, Fusenig NE (1997) Halting angiogenesis suppresses carcinoma cell invasion. Nat Med 3:1222–1227
25. Sokolova E, Reiser G (2008) Prothrombin/thrombin and the thrombin receptors PAR-1 and PAR-4 in the brain: localization, expression and participation in neurodegenerative diseases. Thromb Haemost 100:576–581
26. Tsopanoglou NE, Maragoudakis ME (2004) Role of thrombin in angiogenesis and tumor progression. Semin Thromb Hemost 30:63–69
27. Tsopanoglou NE, Papaconstantinou ME, Flordellis CS, Maragoudakis ME (2004) On the mode of action of thrombin-induced angiogenesis: thrombin peptide, TP508, mediates effects in endothelial cells via alphavbeta3 integrin. Thromb Haemost 92:846–857
28. Ubl JJ, Vohringer C, Reiser G (1998) Co-existence of two types of [Ca2+]i-inducing protease-activated receptors (PAR-1 and PAR-2) in rat astrocytes and C6 glioma cells. Neuroscience 86:597–609. [erratum appears in Neuroscience 1999;88(1):337]
29. Wang H, Ubl JJ, Stricker R, Reiser G (2002) Thrombin (PAR-1)-induced proliferation in astrocytes via MAPK involves multiple signaling pathways. Am J Physiol Cell Physiol 283:C1351–C1364
30. Xu Y, Gu Y, Keep RF, Heth J, Muraszko KM, Xi G, Hua Y (2009) Thrombin up-regulates vascular endothelial growth factor in experimental gliomas. Neurol Res 31:759–765

31. Yamahata H, Takeshima H, Kuratsu J, Sarker KP, Tanioka K, Wakimaru N, Nakata M, Kitajima I, Maruyama I (2002) The role of thrombin in the neo-vascularization of malignant gliomas: an intrinsic modulator for the up-regulation of vascular endothelial growth factor. Int J Oncol 20:921–928
32. Zacharski LR, Memoli VA, Morain WD, Schlaeppi JM, Rousseau SM (1995) Cellular localization of enzymatically active thrombin in intact human tissues by hirudin binding. Thromb Haemost 73:793–797
33. Zhao J, Chen Z, Xi G, Keep RF, Hua Y (2014) Deferoxamine attenuates acute hydrocephalus after traumatic brain injury in rats. Transl Stroke Res 5:586–594

Minocycline Attenuates Iron-Induced Brain Injury

Fan Zhao, Guohua Xi, Wenqaun Liu, Richard F. Keep, and Ya Hua

Introduction

Intracerebral hemorrhage (ICH) accounts for 10–15 % of all strokes, but it results in a disproportionately high morbidity and mortality [9, 10]. Experiments have indicated that clot lysis and iron play an important role in ICH-induced brain injury. Iron overload occurs in the brain after ICH in rats. Iron chelators like deferoxamine can reduce brain edema and improve neurological function in experimental models of ICH [4, 8, 19, 20].

A number of proteins, including ferritin, transferrin (Tf), transferrin receptor (TfR), ceruloplasmin (Cp), and heme oxygenase 1 (HO-1), are involved in maintaining brain iron homeostasis. Ferritin, a cytosolic heterodimeric protein that assembles as a 24-subunit sphere, has a dual function of iron detoxification and iron reserve [11]. Tf and TfR are involved in the transport of iron across biological membranes. Tf is the main source of iron for neurons, which express high levels of TfR. Cp is a ferroxidase necessary for the oxidation of Fe^{2+} to Fe^{3+} and subsequent binding of iron to transferrin. HO-1 is involved in the degradation of heme, which results in the production of iron (as well as biliverdin and carbon monoxide).

Minocycline, a second generation of tetracycline-based molecule, is a potent inhibitor of microglia activation [16]. It has been shown to be beneficial in several stroke models [2], presumably due to its anti-inflammatory effect. However, minocycline also has strong iron-chelating activity [3] and a previous study demonstrated it can attenuate iron neurotoxicity in cortical cell cultures, whereas two other inhibitors of microglial activation, doxycycline and macrophage/microglia inhibitory factor (MIF), were ineffective [1]. Our previous study found minocycline attenuates iron-induced brain injury, in vivo at least in part due to chelation of iron [23]. The current study further examined the effects of minocycline on the subacute brain injury induced by iron.

Materials and Methods

Animal Preparation and Intracerebral Injection

The protocols for these animal studies were approved by the University of Michigan Committee on the Use and Care of Animals. Male Sprague-Dawley rats from Charles River Laboratories (weight 275–300 g) were used in this study. Septic precautions were utilized in all surgical procedures and body temperature was maintained at 37.5 °C using a feedback-controlled heating pad. Rats were anesthetized with pentobarbital (50 mg/kg, intraperitoneally (IP)) and the right femoral artery was catheterized for continuous blood pressure monitoring and blood sampling. Blood from the catheter was used to determine pH, PaO_2, $PaCO_2$, hematocrit, and glucose. The animals were positioned in a stereotactic frame (Kopf Instruments). Minocycline was purchased from Sigma (St. Louis, MO, USA). Fifty microliters of saline, $FeCl_2$ (0.5 mM), or $FeCl_2$ mixed with minocycline (0.5 mM) was injected into the right caudate through a 26-gauge needle at a rate of 10 μl per minute using a microinfusion pump (Harvard Apparatus Inc.). The coordinates were 0.2 mm anterior to the bregma and 5.5 mm ventral and 4.0 mm lateral to midline. After intracerebral infusion, the needle was removed and the skin incision closed with suture.

F. Zhao
Department of Neurosurgery, University of Michigan, 5018 BSRB, Ann Arbor, MI 48109-2200, USA

Department of Neurosurgery, Huashan Hospital, Fudan University, Shanghai, China

G. Xi, MD • W. Liu • R.F. Keep, PhD • Y. Hua, MD (✉)
Department of Neurosurgery, University of Michigan, 5018 BSRB, Ann Arbor, MI 48109-2200, USA
e-mail: yahua@umich.edu

R.L. Applegate et al. (eds.), *Brain Edema XVI: Translate Basic Science into Clinical Practice*, Acta Neurochirurgica Supplement, Vol. 121, 361
DOI 10.1007/978-3-319-18497-5_62, © Springer International Publishing Switzerland 2016

Experiment Groups

Rats had an intracaudate injection of 50 µl of saline, $FeCl_2$ (0.5 mM), or $FeCl_2$ (0.5 mM) + minocycline (0.5 mM) and were euthanized at 72 h. Rat brains were used for immunohistochemistry ($n = 5–6$ per group) and Western blotting assay ($n = 4$ for each group).

Brain Swelling Measurements

Rats were anesthetized and underwent intracardiac perfusion with 4 % paraformaldehyde in 0.1 mol/l (pH 7.4) phosphate-buffered saline (PBS). The brains were removed and kept in 4 % paraformaldehyde for 12 h, then immersed in 30 % sucrose for 3–4 days at 4 °C. Brains were then placed in embedding OCT compound and sectioned on a cryostat (18-µm thick). Coronal sections at the blood injection site were stained with hematoxylin and eosin (H&E) and then were scanned. The bilateral caudate were outlined for area measurement using Image J (National Institutes of Health). All measurements were repeated three times and the mean value was used. Brain swelling was determined as (ipsilateral area/contralateral area) × 100 %.

Immunohistochemistry

Immunohistochemistry was performed as previously described [5, 7]. Primary antibodies were polyclonal rabbit anti-human ferritin IgG (DACO; 1:400 dilution). Normal rabbit IgG was used as negative control.

Western Blot Analysis

Western blot analysis was performed as previously described [7]. The primary antibodies were polyclonal goat anti-mouse albumin antibody (1:10,000 dilution; Bethyl Laboratories Inc. Montgomery, TX), rabbit polyclonal HO-1 antibody (1:2000 dilution; Assay Designs/Stressgen, Farmingdale, NY), polyclonal rabbit anti-human Tf (1:2000 dilution; Dako, Carpinteria, CA), monoclonal mouse anti-human TfR (1:2000 dilution; Invitrogen, Grand Island, NY), and sheep anti-ceruloplasmin antibody (1:2000 dilution; Abcam, Cambridge, MA). The antigen-antibody complexes were observed with the ECL system and exposed to Kodak X-OMAT film. The membranes were then stripped and reprobed with antibody against β-actin. The relative densities of bands were analyzed with NIH Image J [24].

Statistical Analysis

All the data in this study are presented as mean ± SD. Data were analyzed by one-way analysis of variance (ANOVA). A level of $p < 0.05$ was considered statistically significant.

Results

Brain swelling (ipsilateral caudate area as a percentage of contralateral area) was determined on H&E-stained coronal sections at 72 h after injection. $FeCl_2$ resulted in swelling of the ipsilateral caudate. Minocycline co-injection significantly reduced that swelling (104.2 % ± 3.1 % vs 112.7 % ± 5.3 % in $FeCl_2$ group, $n = 5$, $p < 0.01$, Fig. 1a)

Brain albumin, a marker of BBB disruption, was measured by Western blot analysis. Albumin levels in the ipsilateral basal ganglia were markedly increased after $FeCl_2$ injection (Fig. 1b). This increase was greatly reduced by co-injection of minocycline (1946 ± 1122 vs 6973 ± 1481 pixels in $FeCl_2$ alone group, $n = 4$, $p < 0.01$, Fig. 1b).

The protein level of heme oxygense-1 (HO-1) in the ipsilateral basal ganglia was significantly increased by $FeCl_2$ injection. The HO-1 levels in $FeCl_2$ + minocycline group (2489 ± 2022 pixels) were significantly lower than that in the $FeCl_2$ group (7668 ± 1467 pixels, $n = 4$, $p < 0.05$, Fig. 2a). Also, the immunoreactivity for ferritin (an iron storage protein) was upregulated after $FeCl_2$ injection. Ferritin-positive cells were fewer in minocycline-treated animals (510 ± 41 vs 905 ± 107 cells/mm^2 in $FeCl_2$ group, $n = 5$, $p < 0.01$, Fig. 2b).

Ceruloplasmin (CP) is involved in iron metabolism by oxidizing ferrous iron to ferric iron. Brain CP levels in the ipsilateral basal ganglia were significantly increased by $FeCl_2$ injection. This upregulation was blocked by co-injection of minocycline (2184 ± 675 vs 6629 ± 1123 pixels in $FeCl_2$ group, $n = 4$, $p < 0.01$, Fig. 3a). Tf, through binding to its receptor (TfR), is involved in the transport of iron into cells. Compared with saline control, both Tf and TfR protein levels were significantly higher in the ipsilateral basal ganglia after $FeCl_2$ injection. The co-injection of minocycline reduced that upregulation (Tf: 5574 ± 589 vs 7742 ± 1428 pixels in $FeCl_2$ group, $p < 0.05$, Fig. 3b; TfR: 3851 ± 861 vs 6702 ± 312 pixels in $FeCl_2$ group, $p < 0.01$, Fig. 3c)

Discussion

Brain iron overload occurs after ICH and can have detrimental effects [4, 5]. Intracerebral infusion of iron causes brain edema, whereas deferoxamine, an iron chelator, attenuates ICH-induced brain injury in animals, which suggests that

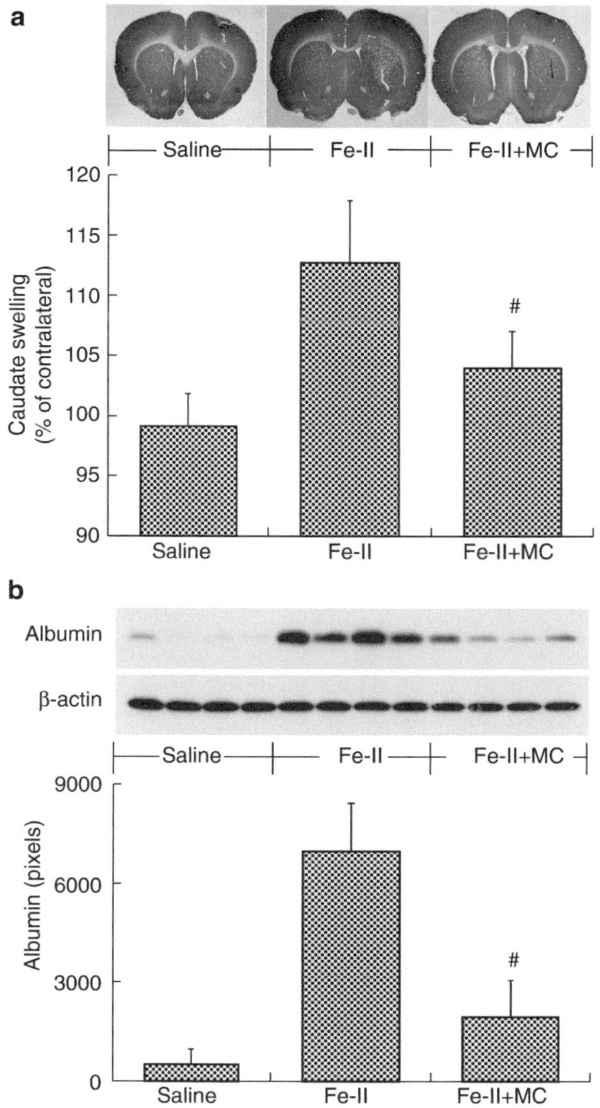

Fig. 1 (**a**) Coronal gross hematoxylin and eosin stained sections and the *bar graph* demonstrating ipsilateral caudate size expressed as a percentage of the contralateral side 72 h after injection of saline, $FeCl_2$, or $FeCl_2$+minocycline (MC; 0.5 mM). Values are expressed as means ± SD; $n = 5$, #$p < 0.01$, compared with $FeCl_2$ group. (**b**) The albumin levels in the ipsilateral basal ganglia 72 h after injection of saline, $FeCl_2$, or $FeCl_2$+MC (0.5 mM). Equal amounts 25 μg of protein were loaded. Values are means ± SD; $n = 4$, #$p < 0.01$, compared with $FeCl_2$ group

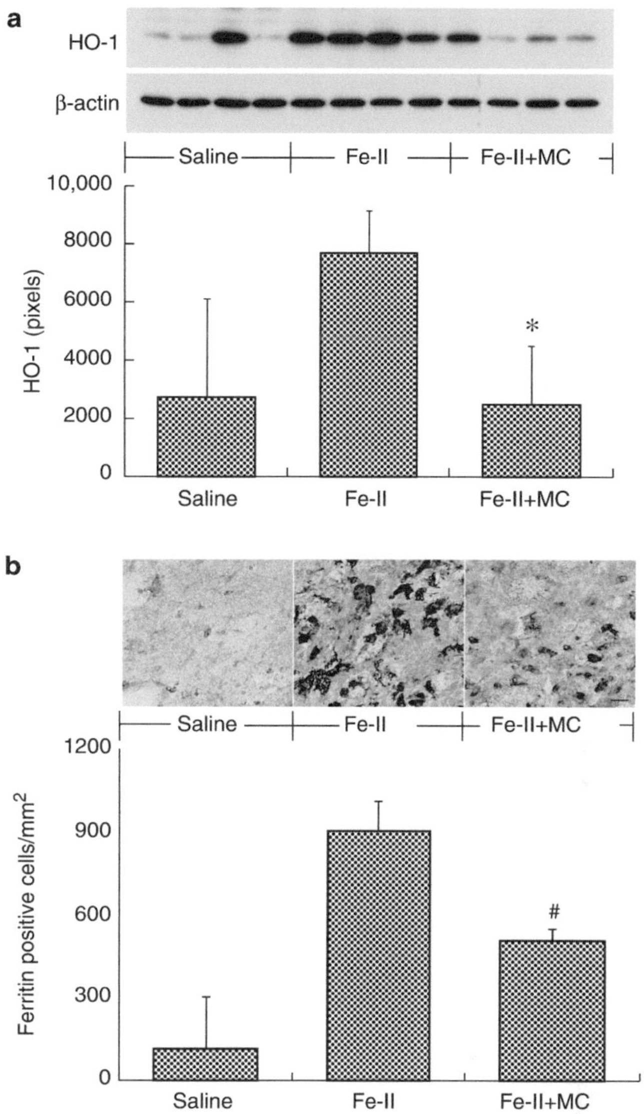

Fig. 2 (**a**) Heme oxygenase-1 (HO-1) levels in the ipsilateral basal ganglia 72 h after injection of saline, $FeCl_2$, or $FeCl_2$+ minocycline (MC; 0.5 mM). Values are means ± SD; $n = 4$, *$p < 0.05$, compared with $FeCl_2$. (**b**) Ferritin immunoreactivity in the ipsilateral basal ganglia 72 h after injection of saline, $FeCl_2$, or $FeCl_2$ + MC (0.5 mM). Values are means ± SD; $n = 6$, #$p < 0.01$, compared with $FeCl_2$. Scale bar = 20 μm

iron may contribute to brain injury after ICH [4, 6, 19]. The current study indicates that minocycline can reduce iron-induced brain injury (brain swelling, BBB disruption) and alter the expression of iron-handling proteins.

Minocycline, a tetracycline derivative, is a potent inhibitor of microglia activation [15, 16]. In vivo, minocycline reduced perihematomal brain edema, neurological deficits, and brain atrophy [18]. To date, the primary CNS mechanism implicated in minocycline neuroprotection is via a highly potent inhibitory effect on microglial activation [12, 21]. On the other hand, minocycline is a strong iron-chelator [1, 3, 23]. Recent evidence in vitro has shown that minocycline can attenuate iron neurotoxicity in cortical cell cultures. Cortical cultures treated with 10 μM ferrous sulfate for 24 h sustained loss of most neurons and an increase in malondialdehyde. Minocycline prevented this injury, with near-complete protection at 30 μM. Two other inhibitors of microglial activation, doxycycline and MIF, were ineffective. Oxidation of isolated culture membranes by iron was also inhibited by minocycline [1, 3]. Minocycline can attenuate this iron-induced brain edema, DNA damage, and neuronal death, but MIF, a microglia inhibitor, had no effect

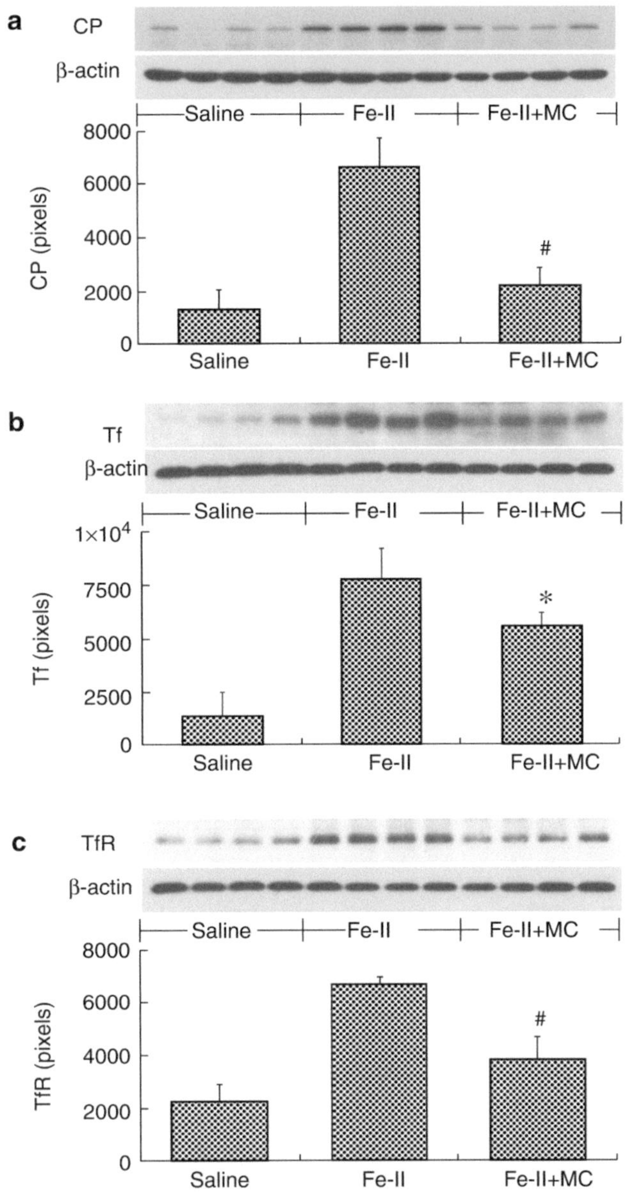

Fig. 3 Protein levels of CP (**a**), Tf (**b**) and TfR (**c**) in the ipsilateral basal ganglia 72 h after injection of saline, $FeCl_2$, or $FeCl_2$+ minocycline (MC; 0.5 mM). Values are means ± SD; $n = 4$, #$p < 0.01$, *$p < 0.05$, compared with FeCl2

[23]. In the current study, minocycline reduced iron-induced brain swelling. This confirms the ability to reduce iron neurotoxicity and indicates that the effects of minocycline on ICH-induced brain injury may at least in part be related to the effects of this drug on iron overload [23].

Multiple forms of edema are present after ICH, but the main form is vasogenic. In the present study, we found that BBB disruption occurred after intracerebral injection of ferrous iron and that minocycline greatly reduced that disruption. Preservation of BBB function by minocycline is, therefore, likely a major contributor to the reduced iron-induced brain swelling found with this drug.

Further evidence for the impact of minocycline on brain iron comes from the effects on iron handling proteins. A number of those proteins (ferritin, Tf, TfR, and CP) were markedly increased 72 h after $FeCl_2$ injection. That upregulation was significantly reduced by coinjection of minocycline. The iron chelation effect of minocycline may reduce the induction of these proteins.

Ferritin, a naturally occurring iron chelator, is involved in maintaining brain iron homeostasis. Ferritin consists of a heavy (FTH) subunit that catalyzes the rapid oxidation of ferrous to ferric iron and a light (FTL) subunit that may be involved in the nucleation of the iron core within the protein shell. Thus, ferritin has a dual function of iron detoxification and iron reserve [17], and the brain can produce ferritin. Tf and TfR are involved in the transport of iron across biological membranes. Brain endothelial cells express TfR and it is involved in transporting iron from blood to brain. However, one report indicates that there is rapid efflux of Tf from brain to blood across the BBB [22], suggesting that Tf and TfR could contribute to iron clearance when there is brain iron overload. Cp is the major copper transport protein in plasma and catalyzes the conversion of toxic ferrous iron to the safer ferric iron. Elevated brain Cp levels have been observed in patients with neurodegenerative conditions, including Alzheimer's, Parkinson's, and Huntington's diseases [14]. The upregulation of these iron handling proteins in brain in the setting of iron overload ($FeCl_2$ injection or ICH) may have important protective functions. By chelating iron, minocycline may fulfill some of the same functions (iron detoxification), but its effect on other functions (iron distribution/clearance) need to be investigated.

Heme oxygenases (HO) are key enzymes for the degradation of heme. HO-1, also called heat shock protein 32, is induced by a variety of stimuli. The biological significance of HO-1 upregulation is still uncertain. HO-1 upregulation increases free redox active iron production. Our results demonstrated that ferrous upregulated HO-1 protein levels in the brain and co-injection with minocycline reduced the upregulation of HO-1. HO-1 upregulation and reactive iron accumulation are associated with oxidative stress [13], which can be attenuated by minocycline.

In summary, systemic minocycline can alleviate iron-induced subacute brain injury. It also has a marked effect on the expression of iron-handling proteins in the brain.

Acknowledgment This study was supported by grants NS-073595, NS-079157, and NS-084049 from the National Institutes of Health (NIH), and 973 Program-2014CB541600 and NSFC81200891 from National Science Foundation of China.

References

1. Chen-Roetling J, Chen L, Regan RF (2009) Minocycline attenuates iron neurotoxicity in cortical cell cultures. Biochem Biophys Res Commun 386:322–326
2. Elewa HF, Hilali H, Hess DC, Machado LS, Fagan SC (2006) Minocycline for short-term neuroprotection. Pharmacotherapy 26:515–521
3. Grenier D, Huot MP, Mayrand D (2000) Iron-chelating activity of tetracyclines and its impact on the susceptibility of Actinobacillus actinomycetemcomitans to these antibiotics. Antimicrob Agents Chemother 44:763–766
4. Hua Y, Keep RF, Hoff JT, Xi G (2007) Brain injury after intracerebral hemorrhage: the role of thrombin and iron. Stroke 38: 759–762
5. Hua Y, Nakamura T, Keep RF, Wu J, Schallert T, Hoff JT, Xi G (2006) Long-term effects of experimental intracerebral hemorrhage: the role of iron. J Neurosurg 104:305–312
6. Huang FP, Xi G, Keep RF, Hua Y, Nemoianu A, Hoff JT (2002) Brain edema after experimental intracerebral hemorrhage: role of hemoglobin degradation products. J Neurosurg 96:287–293
7. Jin H, Xi G, Keep RF, Wu J, Hua Y (2013) DARPP-32 to quantify intracerebral hemorrhage-induced neuronal death in basal Ganglia. Transl Stroke Res 4:130–134
8. Nakamura T, Keep RF, Hua Y, Schallert T, Hoff JT, Xi G (2004) Deferoxamine-induced attenuation of brain edema and neurological deficits in a rat model of intracerebral hemorrhage. J Neurosurg 100:672–678
9. Pandey AS, Xi G (2014) Intracerebral hemorrhage: a multimodality approach to improving outcome. Transl Stroke Res 5:313–315
10. Qureshi AI, Tuhrim S, Broderick JP, Batjer HH, Hondo H, Hanley DF (2001) Spontaneous intracerebral hemorrhage. N Engl J Med 344:1450–1460
11. Salvador GA (2010) Iron in neuronal function and dysfunction. Biofactors 36:103–110
12. Stirling DP, Koochesfahani KM, Steeves JD, Tetzlaff W (2005) Minocycline as a neuroprotective agent. Neuroscientist 11:308–322
13. Suttner DM, Dennery PA (1999) Reversal of HO-1 related cytoprotection with increased expression is due to reactive iron. FASEB J 13:1800–1809
14. Texel SJ, Xu X, Harris ZL (2008) Ceruloplasmin in neurodegenerative diseases. Biochem Soc Trans 36:1277–1281
15. Tikka T, Fiebich BL, Goldsteins G, Keinanen R, Koistinaho J (2001) Minocycline, a tetracycline derivative, is neuroprotective against excitotoxicity by inhibiting activation and proliferation of microglia. J Neurosci 21:2580–2588
16. Tikka TM, Koistinaho JE (2001) Minocycline provides neuroprotection against N-methyl-D-aspartate neurotoxicity by inhibiting microglia. J Immunol 166:7527–7533
17. Vidal R, Miravalle L, Gao X, Barbeito AG, Baraibar MA, Hekmatyar SK, Widel M, Bansal N, Delisle MB, Ghetti B (2008) Expression of a mutant form of the ferritin light chain gene induces neurodegeneration and iron overload in transgenic mice. J Neurosci 28:60–67
18. Wu J, Yang S, Xi G, Fu G, Keep RF, Hua Y (2009) Minocycline reduces intracerebral hemorrhage-induced brain injury. Neurol Res 31:183–188
19. Xi G, Keep RF, Hoff JT (2006) Mechanisms of brain injury after intracerebral haemorrhage. Lancet Neurol 5:53–63
20. Xiong XY, Wang J, Qian ZM, Yang QW (2014) Iron and intracerebral hemorrhage: from mechanism to translation. Transl Stroke Res 5:429–441
21. Yrjanheikki J, Keinanen R, Pellikka M, Hokfelt T, Koistinaho J (1998) Tetracyclines inhibit microglial activation and are neuroprotective in global brain ischemia. Proc Natl Acad Sci U S A 95: 15769–15774
22. Zhang Y, Pardridge WM (2001) Rapid transferrin efflux from brain to blood across the blood-brain barrier. J Neurochem 76: 1597–1600
23. Zhao F, Hua Y, He Y, Keep RF, Xi G (2011) Minocycline-induced attenuation of iron overload and brain injury after experimental intracerebral hemorrhage. Stroke J Cereb Circ 42:3587–3593
24. Zhao J, Chen Z, Xi G, Keep RF, Hua Y (2014) Deferoxamine attenuates acute hydrocephalus after traumatic brain injury in rats. Transl Stroke Res 5:586–594

Effect of Gender on Iron-induced Brain Injury in Low Aerobic Capacity Rats

Mingzhe Zheng, Hanjian Du, Feng Gao, Lauren G. Koch, Steven L. Britton, Richard F. Keep, Guohua Xi, and Ya Hua

Introduction

Spontaneous intracerebral hemorrhage (ICH) is a common and often fatal stroke subtype [14]. Iron has a major role in brain damage following ICH [17, 20, 22]. We have shown a significant increase in brain non-heme iron after ICH in rats, and this remains high for at least 1 month [19]. Brain iron overload causes brain edema in the acute phase and brain atrophy later after ICH, with an iron chelator, deferoxamine, reducing ICH-induced brain edema, neuronal death, brain atrophy, and neurological deficits in young rats [5, 10, 16], aged rats [12, 13], and pigs [2]. Recent studies show that high levels of serum ferritin, an iron storage protein, are independently associated with poor outcome and severe brain edema in ICH patients [8, 15].

Our previous study showed that females have less brain edema and a faster recovery of behavioral deficits after ICH and 17β-estradiol treatment markedly reduced ICH-induced brain injury [1, 9, 11]. Estrogen pretreatment attenuated iron-induced brain edema and neuronal death [3, 7]. We have shown in a model that low aerobic capacity (low capacity runner rats; LCRs) had more severe ICH-induced brain injury than high capacity runners, including worse brain edema, brain atrophy, and neurological deficits, and that females were protected against ICH-induced brain edema formation in both high capacity runners and LCRs [4].

The present study examines whether gender-specific differences in iron-induced brain injury in LCR rats might contribute to the gender differences found in ICH-induced injury.

M. Zheng
Department of Neurosurgery, University of Michigan, R5018 BSRB, 109 Zina Pitcher Place, Ann Arbor, MI 48109-2200, USA

Department of Neurosurgery, Huashan Hospital, Fudan University, Shanghai, China

H. Du • F. Gao • R.F. Keep, PhD • G. Xi, MD • Y. Hua, MD (✉)
Department of Neurosurgery, University of Michigan, R5018 BSRB, 109 Zina Pitcher Place, Ann Arbor, MI 48109-2200, USA
e-mail: yahua@umich.edu

L.G. Koch • S.L. Britton
Department of Anesthesiology, University of Michigan, Ann Arbor, MI USA

Materials and Methods

Animal Preparation and Intracerebral Infusion

All animal procedures were approved by the University Committee on Use and Care of Animals, University of Michigan. A detailed description of the development of low aerobic capacity rats has been published previously [18]. Adult male ($n=7$) and female LCR rats ($n=6$) were anesthetized with pentobarbital (45 mg/kg, intraperitoneally (IP)) and the right femoral artery was catheterized to monitor arterial blood pressure, blood pH, PaO_2, $PaCO_2$, hematocrit, and glucose levels. Body temperature was maintained at 37.5 °C by a feedback-controlled heating pad. A polyethylene catheter (PE-50) was inserted into the right femoral artery to monitor arterial blood pressure and blood gases. Animals were then positioned in a stereotactic frame and injections administered into the right basal ganglia (coordinates at 0.2 mm anterior to bregma, 5.5 mm ventral, and 3.5 mm lateral to midline). All the animals had 50 μl $FeCl_2$ (0.5 mM) or saline infused into the right caudate at 5 μl/min using a microinfusion pump. After injection, the needle was removed and the skin incisions closed. T2 magnetic resonance imaging (MRI) was performed at 24 h after iron injection and the rats were then used for brain histology and Western blotting.

R.L. Applegate et al. (eds.), *Brain Edema XVI: Translate Basic Science into Clinical Practice*, Acta Neurochirurgica Supplement, Vol. 121, DOI 10.1007/978-3-319-18497-5_63,

Magnetic Resonance Imaging and Volume Measurement

Imaging was carried out in a 7.0-T Varian MR scanner (183-mm horizontal bore; Varian, Palo Alto, CA, USA) at the Center for Molecular Imaging (CMI) of the University of Michigan. Rats were anesthetized with 2 % isoflurane/air mixture throughout MRI examination. The imaging protocol for all rats included a T2 fast spin-echo sequence (TR/TE=4000/60 ms). The images were preserved as 256×256 pixels images; the lesion volumes and hemisphere volumes were measured by a blinded observer with NIH ImageJ [23]. Lesion volume was calculated by multiplying the total lesion area across all sections by the distance between the sections. Brain swelling calculation was based on 7 every other section of which the center was the anterior commissure layer. The value was ((volume of right hemisphere – volume of left hemisphere)/volume of right hemisphere)×100 %.

Immunohistochemistry

Immunohistochemistry was performed as described previously [6, 21]. Briefly, rats were anesthetized and subjected to intracardiac perfusion with 4 % paraformaldehyde in 0.1 mM phosphate-buffered saline (pH 7.4). Brains were removed and kept in 4 % paraformaldehyde for 6 h, then immersed in 30 % sucrose for 3–4 days at 4 °C. After embedding in a mixture of 30 % sucrose and OCT, 18 μm sections were cut on a cryostat. For immunohistochemistry, the primary antibodies were goat anti-albumin antibody (Bethyl Laboratories, Inc., 1:600 dilution, Montgomery, TX) and rabbit polyclonal HO-1 antibody (1:600 dilution; Assay Designs/Stressgen, Farmingdale, NY).

Western Blot Analysis

Western blot analysis was performed as previously described [21]. Briefly, brain tissue was immersed in Western sample buffer and sonicated. Protein concentration was determined by Bio-Rad protein assay kit, and 50 μg protein samples were separated by sodium dodecyl sulfate-polyacrylamide gel electrophoresis and transferred to a Hybond-C pure nitrocellulose membrane. Membranes were probed with goat anti-albumin antibody (Bethyl Laboratories, Inc., 1:10,000 dilution, Montgomery, TX), and rabbit polyclonal HO-1 antibody (1:2,000 dilution; Assay Designs/Stressgen, Farmingdale, NY). The antigen–antibody complexes were visualized with the ECL chemiluminescence system and exposed to Kodak X-OMAT film. The relative densities of bands were analyzed with NIH ImageJ.

Statistical Analysis

All the data in this study are presented as mean±standard deviation (SD). Data were analyzed by Student's *t*-test or analysis of variance (ANOVA). Differences were considered significant at $p<0.05$.

Results

The LCR rats used in this study were from generation 29–33 of the breeding program. All physiological parameters were monitored during intracerebral infusions. No rats died postoperatively.

T2 lesion volumes at 24 h after iron infusion were larger in males (120±28 mm^3) than in females (87±27 mm^3, $p<0.05$); Fig. 1a, b). There was also more severe brain swelling in males (16.6±4.1 %) compared with females (11.1±2.6 %, $p<0.05$; Fig. 1a, c).

Albumin is normally excluded from the brain by the blood-brain barrier (BBB), and entry of albumin is a marker of BBB disruption. Intracaudate $FeCl_2$ injection caused marked BBB disruption in the ipsilateral hemisphere 24 h after injection (Fig. 2) with much higher albumin protein levels in the ipsilateral basal ganglia than in the contralateral ($p<0.01$, Fig. 2). The albumin-positive area was larger in the ipsilateral hemisphere in males than females (Fig. 2) and albumin protein levels (Western blot) were significantly higher in males (7,717±1,502 vs 5,287±1,342 pixels in females, $p<0.05$; Fig. 2).

HO-1 is a marker for brain stress that is expressed at very low levels in normal brain. The number of cells immunoreactive for HO-1 at 24 h after $FeCl_2$ injection was greater in male than female LCR rats (Fig. 3). Similarly, as assessed by Western blot, HO-1 protein levels in the ipsilateral basal ganglia were higher in males than females (HO-1/β-actin: 1.31±0.44 vs 1.03±0.05, $p<0.05$; Fig. 3).

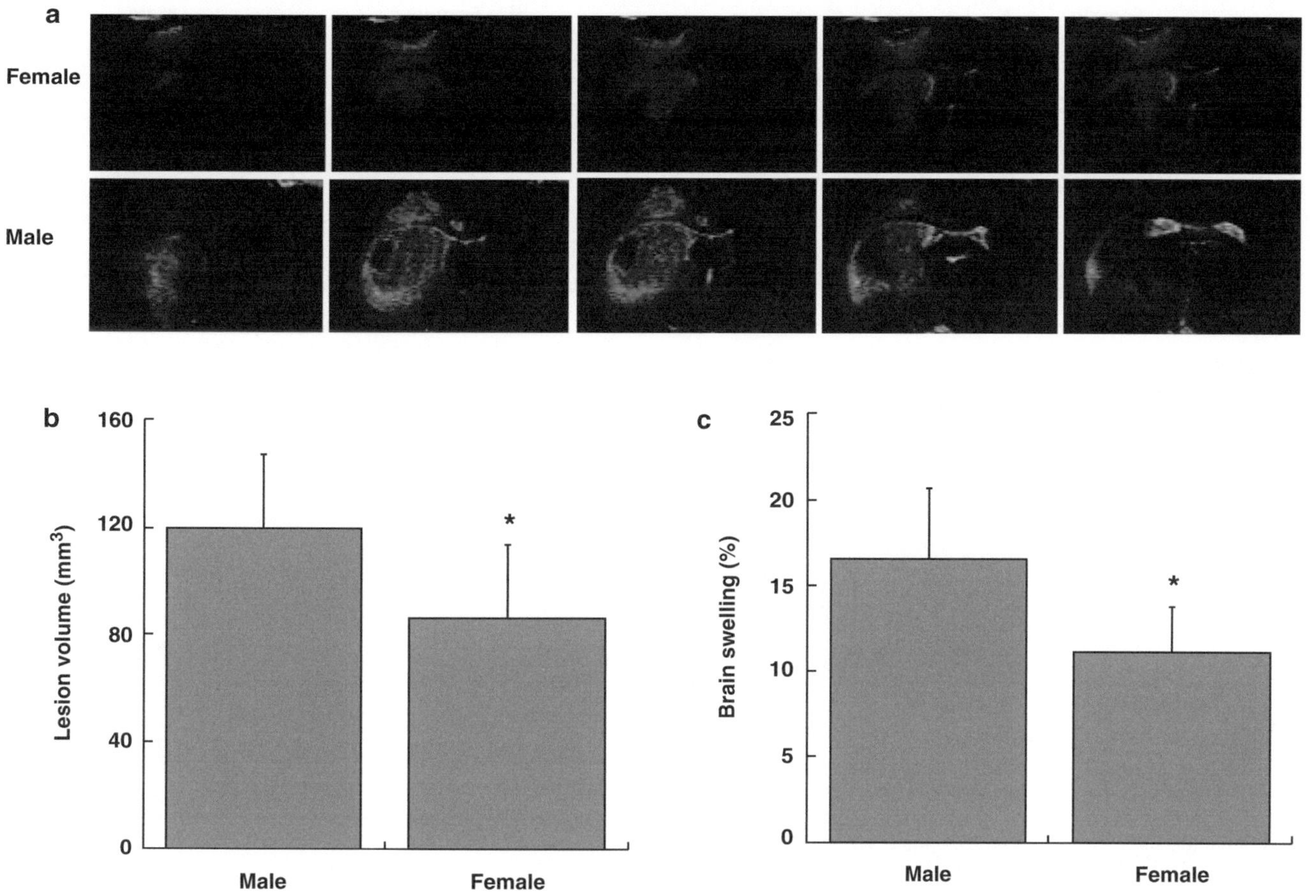

Fig. 1 (**a**) Representative T2 MRI scans of the brains of female and male LCR rats 24 h after an intracaudate injection of $FeCl_2$. (**b**) Lesion volumes calculated from such MRI scans. (**c**) Brain swelling calculated from such scans. Male LCR rats had significantly greater lesion volumes and brain swelling than females after $FeCl_2$ injection. Values are mean ± SD, $n = 6–7$, $*p < 0.05$

Discussion

In the present study, we found that male rats had comparatively more severe hemispheric swelling, BBB disruption, and larger T2 lesions after intracerebral iron injection into the caudate. In addition, iron induced much stronger expression of HO-1 in males than females.

Brain iron overload has an important role in ICH-induced brain injury. The current results suggest that differences in iron-mediated damage contribute to gender differences in ICH-induced brain injury. It is still unknown why iron-induced brain swelling is less in female LCRs. For iron-induced brain injury, most research has focused on oxidative injury. The reduction in the iron-induced upregulation of brain HO-1 expression (a cellular stress marker) in females may reflect reduced oxidative stress. This needs investigation.

Iron-induced brain edema could be vasogenic and cytotoxic. Our results showed that BBB leakage was more severe in males than females, suggesting less vasogenic brain edema in females. We have previously shown that females have less severe ICH-induced brain injury than males through an estrogen receptor-dependent mechanism [9]. More experiments are needed to determine whether estrogen and its receptors have a role in ameliorating iron-induced BBB disruption and vasogenic brain edema.

In conclusion, iron caused less brain damage, BBB leakage, and brain swelling in female LCRs compared with males. Gender differences in iron-induced injury may contribute to differences between females and males in ICH-induced brain injury.

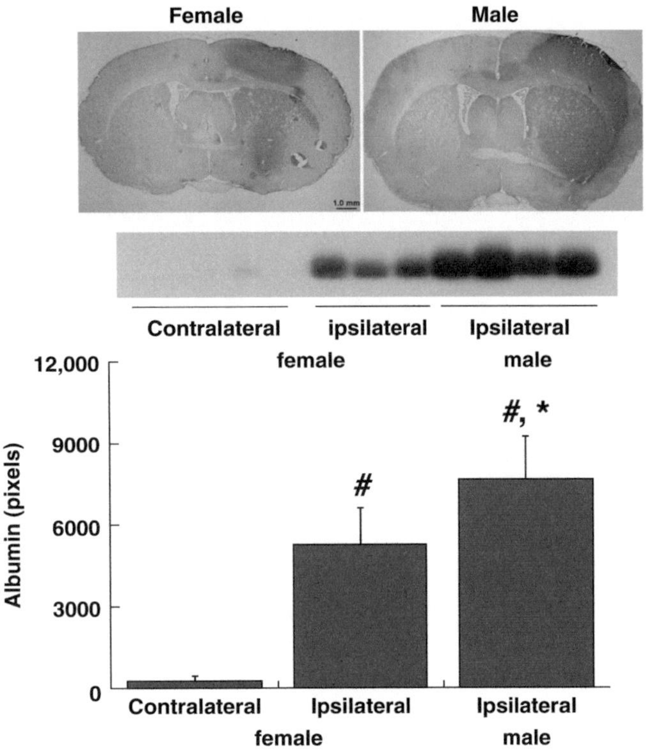

Fig. 2 Albumin immunohistochemistry and Western blot demonstrating protein extravasation into brain 24 h after intracaudate injection of $FeCl_2$ in female and male LCR rats. Albumin extravasation is a marker of BBB disruption. *Bar graph* quantifies the Western blot data. $FeCl_2$ injection caused unilateral BBB disruption that was significantly greater in male rats. Values are mean ± SD, $n = 3–4$, $^*p < 0.05$ male vs female; $\#p < 0.01$ ipsi- vs contralateral

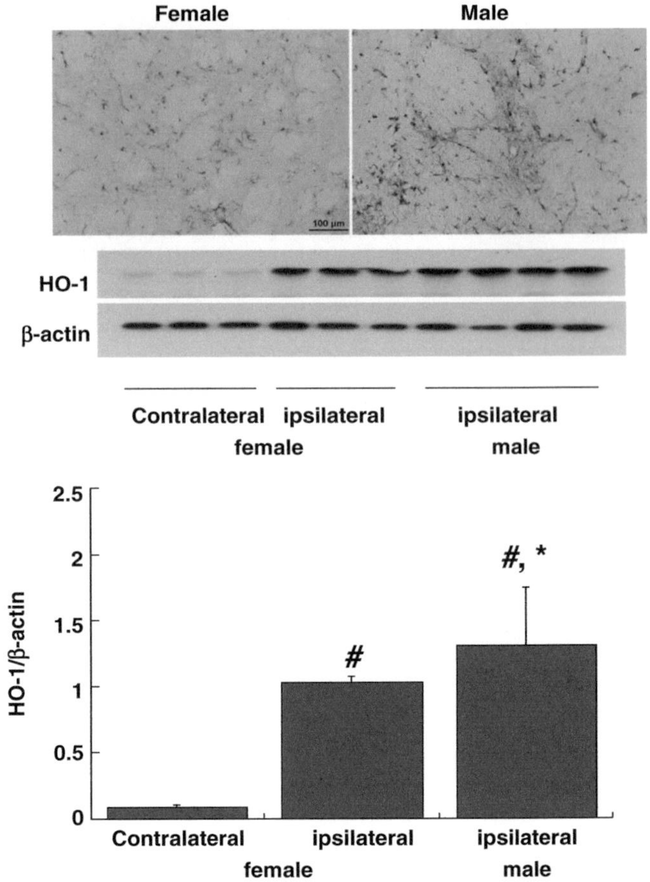

Fig. 3 Heme oxygenase 1 (*HO-1*) immunohistochemistry (ipsilateral caudate) and Western blot (basal ganglia) 24 h after intracaudate injection of $FeCl_2$ in LCR and HCR rats. The *bar graph* quantifies the Western blot normalizing the data to β-actin. $FeCl_2$ injection caused unilateral HO-1 upregulation and that upregulation was significantly greater in male rats. Values are mean ± SD, n = 3–4, $^*p < 0.05$ male vs female; $\#p < 0.01$ ipsi- vs contralateral

Acknowledgments This study was supported by grants NS-073959, NS079157, and NS-084049 from the National Institutes of Health (NIH) and 973 Program-2014CB541600. The LCR-HCR rat model system was funded by the Office of Research Infrastructure Programs/OD grant R24OD010950 and by grant R01DK099034 (to LGK and SLB) from the National Institutes of Health. SLB was also supported by National Institutes of Health grants R01DK077200 and R01GM104194. We acknowledge the expert care of the rat colony provided by Molly Kalahar and Lori Heckenkamp. Contact LGK (lgkoch@med.umich.edu) or SLB (brittons@umich.edu) for information on the LCR and HCR rats: these rat models are maintained as an international resource with support from the Department of Anesthesiology at the University of Michigan, Ann Arbor, Michigan.

References

1. Davis CM, Fairbanks SL, Alkayed NJ (2013) Mechanism of the sex difference in endothelial dysfunction after stroke. Transl Stroke Res 4:381–389
2. Gu Y, Hua Y, Keep RF, Morgenstern LB, Xi G (2009) Deferoxamine reduces intracerebral hematoma-induced iron accumulation and neuronal death in piglets. Stroke 40:2241–2243
3. Gu Y, Xi G, Liu W, Keep RF, Hua Y (2010) Estrogen reduces iron-mediated brain edema and neuronal death. Acta Neurochir Suppl 106:159–162
4. He Y, Liu W, Koch LG, Britton SL, Keep RF, Xi G, Hua Y (2012) Susceptibility to intracerebral hemorrhage-induced brain injury segregates with low aerobic capacity in rats. Neurobiol Dis 49C:22–28
5. Hua Y, Nakamura T, Keep R, Wu J, Schallert T, Hoff J, Xi G (2006) Long-term effects of experimental intracerebral hemorrhage: the role of iron. J Neurosurg 104:305–312
6. Jin H, Xi G, Keep RF, Wu J, Hua Y (2013) DARPP-32 to quantify intracerebral hemorrhage-induced neuronal death in basal Ganglia. Transl Stroke Res 4:130–134
7. Koellhoffer EC, McCullough LD (2013) The effects of estrogen in ischemic stroke. Transl Stroke Res 4:390–401
8. Mehdiratta M, Kumar S, Hackney D, Schlaug G, Selim M (2008) Association between serum ferritin level and perihematoma edema volume in patients with spontaneous intracerebral hemorrhage. Stroke J Cereb Circ 39:1165–1170
9. Nakamura T, Hua Y, Keep RF, Park JW, Xi G, Hoff JT (2005) Estrogen therapy for experimental intracerebral hemorrhage in rats. J Neurosurg 103:97–103
10. Nakamura T, Keep RF, Hua Y, Schallert T, Hoff JT, Xi G (2004) Deferoxamine-induced attenuation of brain edema and neurological deficits in a rat model of intracerebral hemorrhage. J Neurosurg 100:672–678
11. Nakamura T, Xi G, Hua Y, Schallert T, Hoff JT, Keep RF (2004) Intracerebral hemorrhage in mice: model characterization and application for genetically modified mice. J Cereb Blood Flow Metab 24:487–494
12. Okauchi M, Hua Y, Keep RF, Morgenstern LB, Schallert T, Xi G (2010) Deferoxamine treatment for intracerebral hemorrhage in aged rats: therapeutic time window and optimal duration. Stroke 41:375–382
13. Okauchi M, Hua Y, Keep RF, Morgenstern LB, Xi G (2009) Effects of deferoxamine on intracerebral hemorrhage-induced brain injury in aged rats. Stroke 40:1858–1863
14. Pandey AS, Xi G (2014) Intracerebral hemorrhage: a multimodality approach to improving outcome. Transl Stroke Res 5:313–315
15. Perez de la Ossa N, Sobrino T, Silva Y, Blanco M, Millan M, Gomis M, Agulla J, Araya P, Reverte S, Serena J, Davalos A (2010) Iron-related brain damage in patients with intracerebral hemorrhage. Stroke J Cereb Circ 41:810–813
16. Song S, Hua Y, Keep RF, Hoff JT, Xi G (2007) A new hippocampal model for examining intracerebral hemorrhage-related neuronal death: effects of deferoxamine on hemoglobin-induced neuronal death. Stroke 38:2861–2863
17. Wagner KR, Sharp FR, Ardizzone TD, Lu A, Clark JF (2003) Heme and iron metabolism: role in cerebral hemorrhage. J Cereb Blood Flow Metab 23:629–652
18. Wisloff U, Najjar SM, Ellingsen O, Haram PM, Swoap S, Al-Share Q, Fernstrom M, Rezaei K, Lee SJ, Koch LG, Britton SL (2005) Cardiovascular risk factors emerge after artificial selection for low aerobic capacity. Science 307:418–420
19. Wu J, Hua Y, Keep RF, Nakamura T, Hoff JT, Xi G (2003) Iron and iron-handling proteins in the brain after intracerebral hemorrhage. Stroke 34:2964–2969
20. Xi G, Keep RF, Hoff JT (2006) Mechanisms of brain injury after intracerebral haemorrhage. Lancet Neurol 5:53–63
21. Xi G, Keep RF, Hua Y, Xiang JM, Hoff JT (1999) Attenuation of thrombin-induced brain edema by cerebral thrombin preconditioning. Stroke 30:1247–1255
22. Xiong XY, Wang J, Qian ZM, Yang QW (2014) Iron and intracerebral hemorrhage: from mechanism to translation. Transl Stroke Res 5:429–441
23. Zhao J, Chen Z, Xi G, Keep RF, Hua Y (2014) Deferoxamine attenuates acute hydrocephalus after traumatic brain injury in rats. Transl Stroke Res 5:586–594

Acetazolamide Attenuates Thrombin-Induced Hydrocephalus

Feng Gao, Mingzhe Zheng, Ya Hua, Richard F. Keep, and Guohua Xi

Introduction

Studies have found intraventricular hemorrhage (IVH) is a predictor of poor outcome after intracerebral hemorrhage (ICH) [2, 8]. For example, the presence of IVH in patients with ICH lowered the rate of favorable outcome from 31 to 15 % and was an independent predictor of worse outcome in the International Surgical Trial in ICH [2]. That trial also showed that hydrocephalus develops in more than 50 % of patients with IVH [2]. IVH is also an independent prognostic factor for poor outcome in SAH patients and acute hydrocephalus occurs in 20–30 % of such patients [15]. However, the mechanisms of brain hemorrhage-induced hydrocephalus are not well understood.

Thrombin is a serine protease and an essential component in the coagulation cascade. Thrombin forms immediately after brain hemorrhage. Our recent study found that thrombin has a role in hydrocephalus development after IVH [6]. Acetazolamide is a carbonic anhydrase inhibitor and can reduce CSF production [3]. This study examined the effect of acetazolamide on thrombin-induced hydrocephalus.

F. Gao
Department of Neurology, The 2nd Affiliate Hospital, Zhejiang University, Zhejiang, China

Department of Neurosurgery, University of Michigan, R5018 Biomedical Science Research Building, 109 Zina Pitcher Place, Ann Arbor, MI 48109-2200, USA

M. Zheng
Department of Neurosurgery, University of Michigan, R5018 Biomedical Science Research Building, 109 Zina Pitcher Place, Ann Arbor, MI 48109-2200, USA

Department of Neurosurgery, Huashan Hospital, Fudan University, Shanghai, China

Y. Hua, MD • R.F. Keep, PhD • G. Xi, MD (✉)
Department of Neurosurgery, University of Michigan, R5018 Biomedical Science Research Building, 109 Zina Pitcher Place, Ann Arbor, MI 48109-2200, USA
e-mail: guohuaxi@umich.edu

Materials and Methods

Animal Preparation and Intraventricular Injection

Animal use protocols were approved by the University of Michigan Committee on the Use and Care of Animals. A total of 24 male Sprague-Dawley rats (Charles River Laboratories, Portage, MI, USA), at the weight of 270–300 g, were used in this study. Animals were anesthetized with pentobarbital (50 mg/kg intraperitoneally (IP)) and the right femoral artery was catheterized to monitor arterial blood pressure, blood pH, PaO_2, $PaCO_2$, hematocrit, and glucose levels. Core body temperature was maintained at 37.5 °C with a feedback-controlled heating pad. Rats were then positioned in a stereotaxic frame. A cranial burr hole (1 mm) was drilled and a 26-gauge needle was inserted stereotaxically into the right lateral ventricle (coordinates: 0.6 mm posterior, 4.5 mm ventral, and 1.6 mm lateral to the bregma). Saline or thrombin was infused using a microinfusion pump. The needle was removed after injection, the burr hole was filled with bone wax, and the skin incision was sutured closed.

Experimental Groups

There were two parts in this study. First, rats had an injection of either 50 μl saline ($n=6$) or 3 U of rat thrombin in 50 μl saline ($n=6$) into the right lateral ventricle. Second, rats had an injection of 3 U thrombin into the right lateral ventricle and were treated with either vehicle ($n=6$) or acetazolamide (30 mg/kg, IP, $n=6$) at 1 h after thrombin infusion. All rats underwent magnetic resonance imaging (MRI) 24 h after the intraventricular injection and were then euthanized. Lateral ventricle volumes were measured in T2-weighted MRI images and the brains were used for histology.

R.L. Applegate et al. (eds.), *Brain Edema XVI: Translate Basic Science into Clinical Practice*, Acta Neurochirurgica Supplement, Vol. 121, DOI 10.1007/978-3-319-18497-5_64, © Springer International Publishing Switzerland 2016

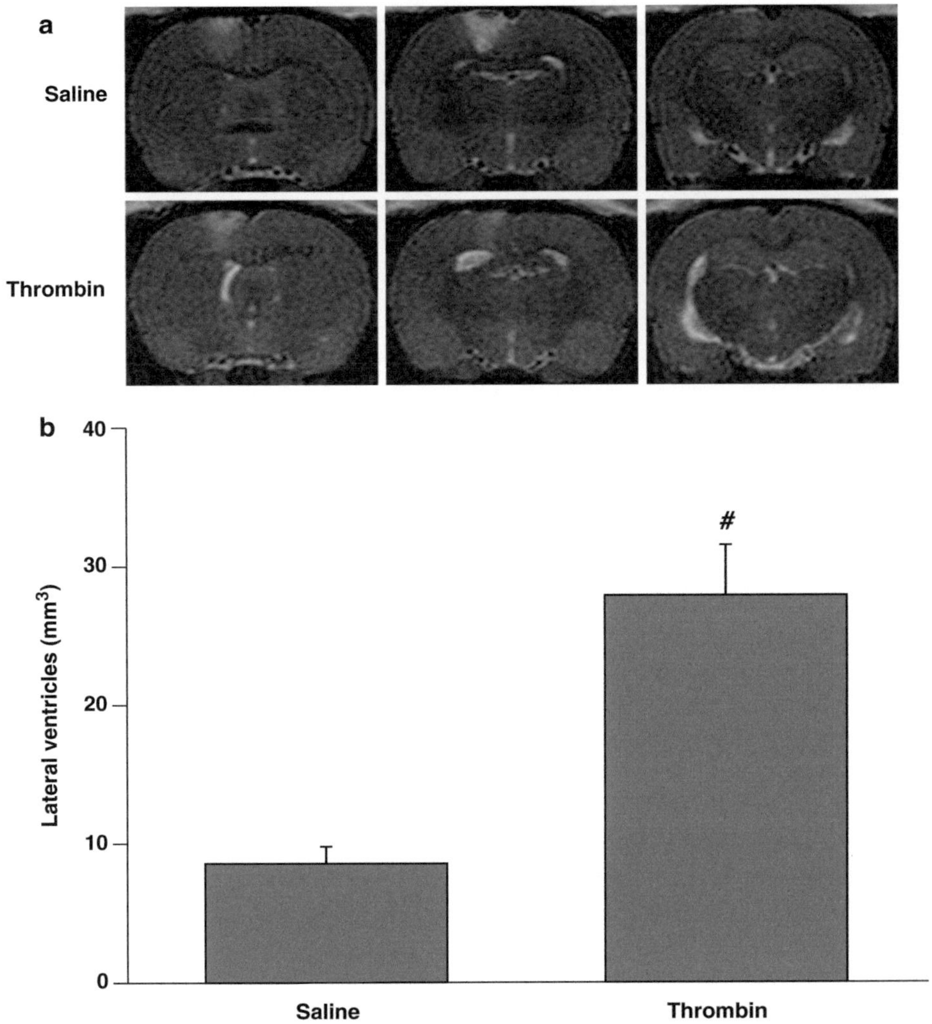

Fig. 1 T2-weighted MRI images (**a**) and lateral ventricular volume measurements (**b**) from rats 24 h after injection of 50 μl of saline or thrombin (3 U) into the right lateral ventricle. Values are means ± SD, $n=6$, # $p<0.01$ vs saline group

MRI Scanning and Ventricle Volume Measurement

Rats were anesthetized with 2 % isoflurane throughout the MRI examination. MRI scanning was performed in a 7.0-T Varian MR scanner (Varian Inc., Palo Alto, CA) with a T2 fast spin-echo sequence, using a view field of 35 × 35 mm and 25 coronal slices [17]. Ventricular volumes were measured and calculated as described previously [4, 12, 13]. Bilateral ventricles were outlined and the areas were measured. Ventricular volume was calculated by summing the ventricle areas over all slices and multiplying by the section thickness. All image analysis was performed using the ImageJ program by a blinded observer.

Ventricular Wall Damage Analysis

Ventricular wall damage was analyzed by calculating the percentage of the ependyma that was damaged, as previously described [13]. Briefly, brain sections underwent hematoxylin and eosin staining. The length of the ependyma that was disrupted or detached from the periventricular parenchyma was determined and divided by the total ventricular surface perimeter. All the analysis was performed using ImageJ software by a blinded observer.

Statistical Analysis

Values are given as means ± standard deviation (SD). Student's *t*-tests or Mann-Whitney *U* tests were used to analyze the data. Differences were considered significant at $p<0.05$.

Results

MRI showed that intraventricular injection of thrombin (3 U) resulted in hydrocephalus. Thus, lateral ventricular volume in thrombin-injected rats was significantly larger than in saline-injected rats at 24 h (27.8 ± 3.7 vs 8.5 ± 1.3 mm^3 in saline, $p<0.01$, Fig. 1). In addition, intraventricular thrombin

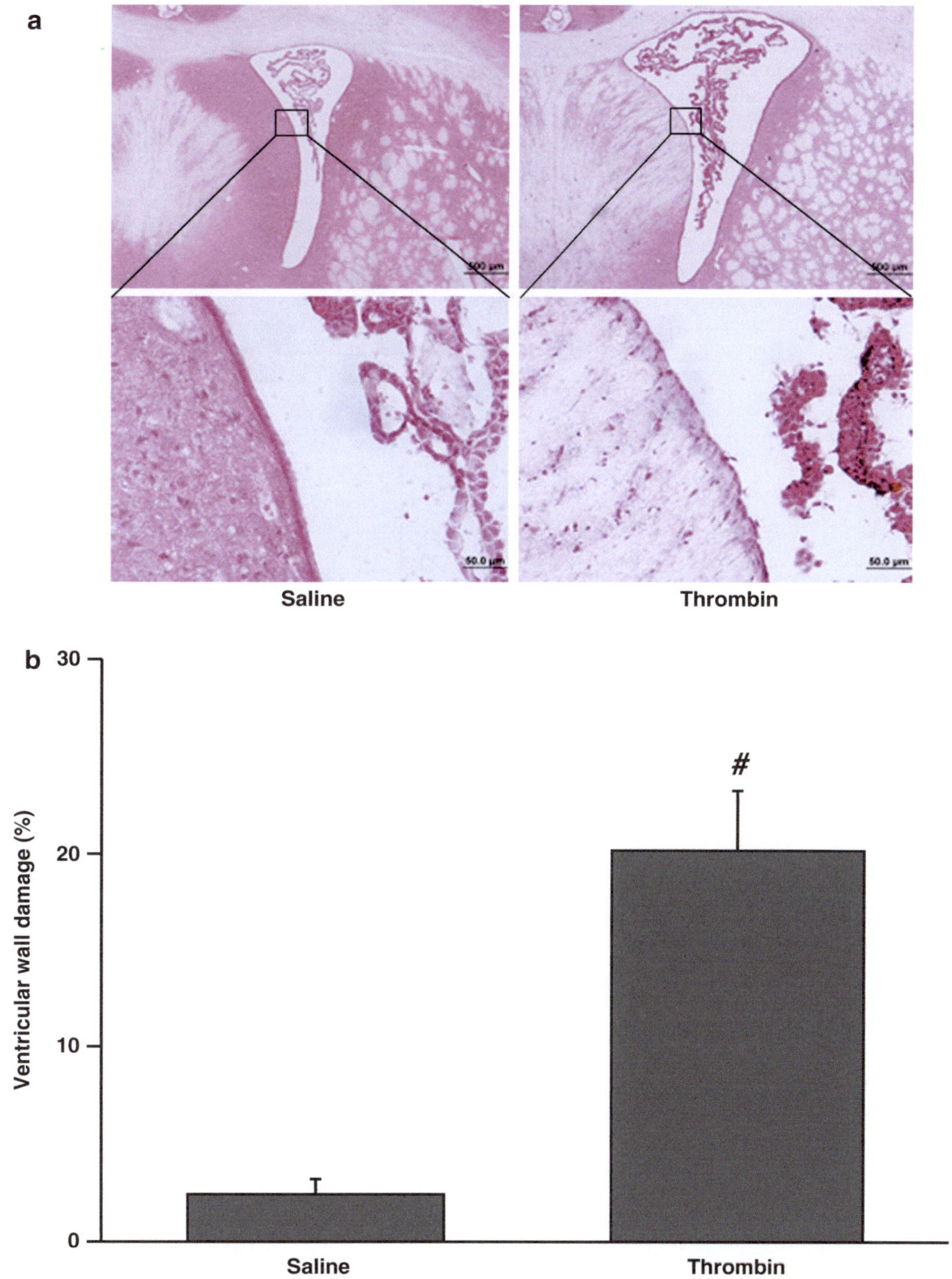

Fig. 2 The damaged ventricular wall in H&E-stained coronal sections (**a**) and the percentage of damage ventricular out of total ventricular wall (**b**) at 24 h after injection of 50 μl of saline or thrombin (3 U) into the right lateral ventricle. Values are means ± SD, $n=6$, # $p<0.01$ vs saline group

injection, but not saline injection, caused severe ventricular wall damage (20.2 ± 1.7 % vs 2.8 ± 0.4 % in saline, $p<0.01$) at 24 h (Fig. 2).

Systemic treatment with acetazolamide, a carbonic anhydrase inhibitor, 1 h after intraventricular injection of 3 U of thrombin resulted in less ventricular enlargement compared with vehicle treatment (16.1 ± 4.2 vs 29.5 ± 5.3 mm^3 in the vehicle-treated group, $p<0.01$) (Fig. 3).

Discussion

In this study, we found intraventricular injection of thrombin caused hydrocephalus and ventricular ependymal wall damage. Acetazolamide, given at 30 mg/kg IP 1 h after thrombin injection, attenuated thrombin-induced hydrocephalus.

Thrombin is a serine protease and an essential component in the coagulation cascade. Experimental investigations have indicated that thrombin formation plays a major role in ICH-induced injury [9, 11, 16]. Thrombin is responsible for early brain edema formation after ICH, and that edema results partly from a direct opening of the blood-brain barrier (BBB). We have demonstrated that intraventricular injection of thrombin can cause significant ventricular dilatation and periventricular parenchyma injury [6]. At present, the mechanisms associated with thrombin-induced ventricular dilatation are unknown. Ependymal injury such as reduced cilia and abnormal of organelle structure were observed in

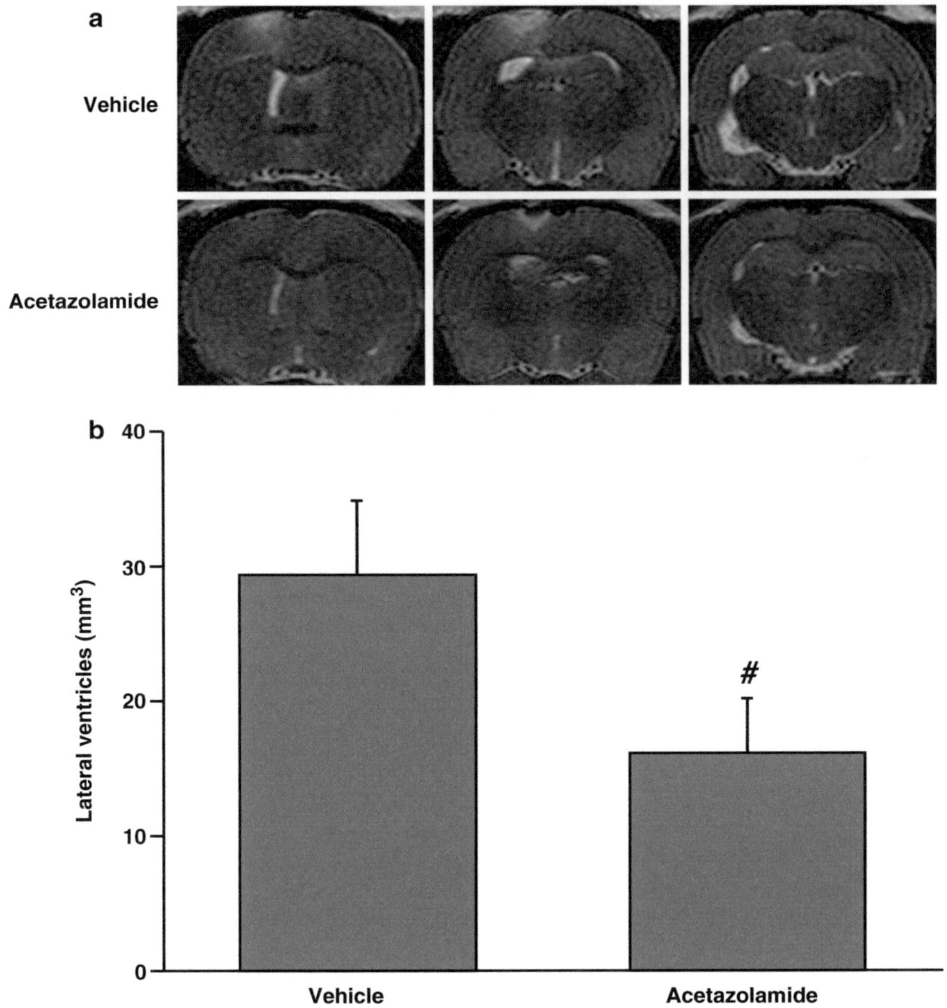

Fig. 3 T2-weighted MRI images (**a**) and lateral ventricular volumes (**b**) 24 h after injection of thrombin (3 U). Rats were treated systemically (IP) with vehicle or acetazolamide 1 h after the thrombin was injected. Values are means ± SD, $n = 6$, # $p < 0.01$ vs vehicle-treated group

thrombin-injected rats [6]. Ependymal damage may lead to increased periventricular brain injury and to hydrocephalus [4, 14]. Activities of normal ependymal cilia are thought to direct cerebrospinal fluid (CSF) current toward the ventricular outlets. Previous study showed absent or functionally defective ependymal cell motile cilia may be a cause of hydrocephalus in a mouse model [1]. Therefore, ependymal damage and abnormal ependymal cilia may play a role in hydrocephalus induced by thrombin.

Acetazolamide, a carbonic anhydrase inhibitor, decreases CSF production in animal models [5, 10, 17]. Acetazolamide has a rapid onset of action. Treatment with 10 mg/kg of acetazolamide resulted in a significant decrease in CSF production and absorption within 3 h of ingestion in dogs [17]. Acetazolamide is also used in both children and adults to treat hydrocephalus and pseudotumor cerebri [6, 7]. We have shown that co-injection of acetazolamide reduced ICH-induced brain injury [7]. In the present study, acetazolamide treatment significantly reduced thrombin-induced hydrocephalus, most likely by reducing CSF production.

Conclusions

Intraventricular injection of thrombin caused ventricular wall damage and hydrocephalus in rats. Inhibition of carbonic anhydrase by acetazolamide effectively reduced thrombin-induced hydrocephalus. The results suggest that thrombin-induced hydrocephalus may result from reduced absorption and/or increased production of CSF.

Acknowledgment This study was supported by grants NS-073959, NS079157, and NS084049 from the National Institutes of Health (NIH), 973 Program-2014CB541600, and grant NSFC 81471168 from National Natural Science Foundation of China.

References

1. Banizs B, Pike MM, Millican CL, Ferguson WB, Komlosi P, Sheetz J, Bell PD, Schwiebert EM, Yoder BK (2005) Dysfunctional cilia lead to altered ependyma and choroid plexus function, and result in the formation of hydrocephalus. Development 132:5329–5339
2. Bhattathiri PS, Gregson B, Prasad KS, Mendelow AD (2006) Intraventricular hemorrhage and hydrocephalus after spontaneous intracerebral hemorrhage: results from the STICH trial. Acta Neurochir Suppl 96:65–68
3. Carrion E, Hertzog JH, Medlock MD, Hauser GJ, Dalton HJ (2001) Use of acetazolamide to decrease cerebrospinal fluid production in chronically ventilated patients with ventriculopleural shunts. Arch Dis Child 84:68–71
4. Chen Z, Gao C, Hua Y, Keep RF, Muraszko K, Xi G (2011) Role of iron in brain injury after intraventricular hemorrhage. Stroke J Cereb Circ 42:465–470
5. Cheng Y, Xi G, Jin H, Keep RF, Feng J, Hua Y (2014) Thrombin-induced cerebral hemorrhage: role of protease-activated receptor-1. Transl Stroke Res 5:472–475
6. Gao F, Liu F, Chen Z, Hua Y, Keep RF, Xi G (2014) Hydrocephalus after intraventricular hemorrhage: the role of thrombin. J Cereb Blood Flow Metab 34:489–494
7. Guo F, Hua Y, Wang J, Keep RF, Xi G (2012) Inhibition of carbonic anhydrase reduces brain injury after intracerebral hemorrhage. Transl Stroke Res 3:130–137
8. Hanley DF (2009) Intraventricular hemorrhage: severity factor and treatment target in spontaneous intracerebral hemorrhage. Stroke J Cereb Circ 40:1533–1538
9. Hua Y, Keep RF, Hoff JT, Xi G (2007) Brain injury after intracerebral hemorrhage: the role of thrombin and iron. Stroke J Cereb Circ 38:759–762
10. Jin H, Xi G, Keep RF, Wu J, Hua Y (2013) DARPP-32 to quantify intracerebral hemorrhage-induced neuronal death in basal ganglia. Transl Stroke Res 4:130–134
11. Keep RF, Hua Y, Xi G (2012) Intracerebral haemorrhage: mechanisms of injury and therapeutic targets. Lancet Neurol 11: 720–731
12. Okauchi M, Hua Y, Keep RF, Morgenstern LB, Xi G (2009) Effects of deferoxamine on intracerebral hemorrhage-induced brain injury in aged rats. Stroke J Cereb Circ 40:1858–1863
13. Okubo S, Strahle J, Keep RF, Hua Y, Xi G (2013) Subarachnoid hemorrhage-induced hydrocephalus in rats. Stroke J Cereb Circ 44:547–550
14. Pang D, Sclabassi RJ, Horton JA (1986) Lysis of intraventricular blood clot with urokinase in a canine model: part 3. Effects of intraventricular urokinase on clot lysis and posthemorrhagic hydrocephalus. Neurosurgery 19:553–572
15. Rosen DS, Macdonald RL, Huo D, Goldenberg FD, Novakovic RL, Frank JI, Rosengart AJ (2007) Intraventricular hemorrhage from ruptured aneurysm: clinical characteristics, complications, and outcomes in a large, prospective, multicenter study population. J Neurosurg 107:261–265
16. Xi G, Keep RF, Hoff JT (2006) Mechanisms of brain injury after intracerebral haemorrhage. Lancet Neurol 5:53–63
17. Zhao J, Chen Z, Xi G, Keep RF, Hua Y (2014) Deferoxamine attenuates acute hydrocephalus after traumatic brain injury in rats. Transl Stroke Res 5:586–594

Effects of Aerobic Capacity on Thrombin-Induced Hydrocephalus and White Matter Injury

Wei Ni, Feng Gao, Mingzhe Zheng, Lauren G. Koch, Steven L. Britton, Richard F. Keep, Guohua Xi, and Ya Hua

Introduction

Low exercise capacity is a risk factor for stroke as well as other forms of cardiovascular disease [11, 13]. Using rats bred for low and high aerobic capacity (low capacity runners, LCRs; high capacity runners, HCRs), our previous study also revealed that low exercise capacity was associated with enhanced brain injury after intracerebral hemorrhage (ICH) [5]. The mechanisms underlying this difference have not been fully elucidated. However, one important component of brain injury after ICH is linked to thrombin. Thus, thrombin can induce blood-brain barrier (BBB) disruption and early brain edema formation after ICH [6, 8, 24]. The effects of thrombin are not limited to ICH; evidence also shows a role in brain injury after intraventricular hemorrhage (IVH). IVH may be caused by hemorrhagic extension after ICH or subarachnoid hemorrhage (SAH). About 67 % of IVH patients develop hydrocephalus, and this is an independent predictor of poor outcome [14]. Data indicate that intraventricular thrombin can induce hydrocephalus and that thrombin contributes to hydrocephalus development after IVH [3, 26].

In this study, therefore, we investigated the effects of exercise capacity on hydrocephalus and periventricular white matter induced by intraventricular thrombin using LCR and HCR rats. We also examined white matter expression of heat shock protein-32, a sensitive marker for brain stress, and microglia activation [18, 19].

W. Ni • M. Zheng
Department of Neurosurgery, University of Michigan, R5018 Biomedical Science Research Building, 109 Zina Pitcher Place, Ann Arbor, MI 48109-2200, USA

Department of Neurosurgery, Huashan Hospital, Fudan University, Shanghai, China

F. Gao
Department of Neurology, the 2nd Affiliate Hospital, Zhejiang University, Zhejiang, China

Department of Neurosurgery, University of Michigan, R5018 Biomedical Science Research Building, 109 Zina Pitcher Place, Ann Arbor, MI 48109-2200, USA

L.G. Koch • S.L. Britton
Department of Anesthesiology, University of Michigan, Ann Arbor, MI, USA

R.F. Keep, PhD • G. Xi, MD • Y. Hua, MD (✉)
Department of Neurosurgery, University of Michigan, R5018 Biomedical Science Research Building, 109 Zina Pitcher Place, Ann Arbor, MI 48109-2200, USA
e-mail: yahua@umich.edu

Materials and Methods

Animal Preparation and Intraventricular Injection

Animal use protocols were approved by the University of Michigan Committee on the Use and Care of Animals. Animals were anesthetized with pentobarbital (50 mg/kg intraperitoneally (IP)) and the right femoral artery was catheterized to monitor arterial blood pressure, blood pH, PaO_2, $PaCO_2$, hematocrit, and glucose levels. Core body temperature was maintained at 37.5 °C with a feedback-controlled heating pad. Rats were then positioned in a stereotaxic frame (Kopf Instruments). A cranial burr hole (1 mm) was drilled and a 26-gauge needle was inserted stereotaxically into the right lateral ventricle (coordinates: 0.6 mm posterior, 4.5 mm ventral, and 1.6 mm lateral to the bregma). Thrombin was infused over 15 min using a microinfusion pump (World Precision Instruments). The needle was removed after injection, the burr hole was filled with bone wax, and the skin incision sutured closed.

Experimental Groups

A previous report provides a detailed description on the development of the rat models for aerobic exercise capacity

R.L. Applegate et al. (eds.), *Brain Edema XVI: Translate Basic Science into Clinical Practice*, Acta Neurochirurgica Supplement, Vol. 121, DOI 10.1007/978-3-319-18497-5_65, © Springer International Publishing Switzerland 2016

[21]. A total of 13 mid-aged (13-month-old) female LCR and 12 mid-aged female HCR rats (Koch/Britton Laboratory, University of Michigan) were used in this study. Rats received an injection of 3 U thrombin in saline (50 μl) and were divided into two groups ($n=10$ for LCR group and $n=12$ for HCR group). LCR control animals received intraventricular saline (50 μl) injection ($n=3$). All rats were euthanized at 1 day after magnetic resonance imaging (MRI) and the brains were used for Western blotting ($n=3$ for each) or histological analysis ($n=5$ for LCR and $n=5$ for HCR).

MRI Scanning and Measurement of Ventricle and White Matter Damage

Rats were anesthetized with 2 % isoflurane throughout MRI examination. MRI scanning was performed in a 7.0-T Varian MR scanner (Varian Inc., Polo Alto, CA) with a T2 fast spin-echo sequence using a view field of 35×35 mm and 25 coronal slices [27]. Ventricular and white matter damage volumes were calculated as described before [1, 15, 16]. Bilateral ventricles and white matter damage were outlined and the areas were measured. Ventricle and white matter damage volumes were calculated by the areas over all slices and multiplying by section thickness. All image analysis was performed using the ImageJ program by a blinded observer.

Immunohistochemistry

Rats were anesthetized with pentobarbital (100 mg/kg IP) and perfused with 4 % paraformaldehyde in 0.1 mol/l phosphate-buffered saline (PBS, pH 7.4). The brains were removed and kept in 4 % paraformaldehyde for 24 h and then immersed in 30 % sucrose for 2–3 days at 4 °C. The brains were embedded in optimal cutting temperature compound and 18-μm-thick slices were cut using a cryostat. Immunohistochemical studies were performed using the avidin-biotin complex technique as previously described [7, 22]. The primary antibodies were rabbit anti-HSP-32 (1:400 dilution; Abcam, Cambridge, MA) and mouse anti-rat OX-6 (1:400 dilution; AbD Serotec, Raleigh, NC).

Western Blot Analysis

Western blot analysis was performed as previously described [25]. Briefly, brain tissue was immersed in Western sample buffer and sonicated. Protein concentration was determined by the Bio-Rad protein assay kit and 50 μg protein from each sample was separated by sodium dodecyl sulfate-polyacrylamide gel electrophoresis and transferred to a Hybond-C pure nitrocellulose membrane. Membranes were probed with the following primary antibodies: rabbit anti-HSP-32 (1:2000 dilution; Abcam, Cambridge, MA) and mouse anti-rat OX-6 (1:2,000 dilution; AbD Serotec, Raleigh, NC). Antigen-antibody complexes were visualized with the ECL chemiluminescence system and exposed to a Kodak X-OMAT film. The relative densities of bands were analyzed with NIH ImageJ.

Statistical Analysis

Values are means ± standard deviation (SD). Student's *t*-test was used to analyze the data. Differences were considered significant at $p<0.05$.

Results

Physiological parameters, including mean arterial blood pressure, blood gases, pH, hematocrit, and glucose, were in the normal ranges. Mortality was not significantly different in LCRs (2 of 10 rats) and HCRs (4 of 12 ras) after intraventricular injection of thrombin (3 U).

In LCR rats, intraventricular injection of thrombin resulted in ventricular enlargement (lateral ventricular volumes: 23.0±2.3 vs12.8±1.9 mm^3 in saline group, $p<0.01$) and periventricular white matter damage (damage volume: 9.3±7.6 vs 0.6±0.5 mm^3 vs in saline group, $p<0.05$; Fig. 1). Compared with LCR rats, HCR rats had less lateral ventricular enlargement (17.3±3.9 vs 23.0±2.3 mm^3 in LCR rats, $p<0.01$, Fig. 1) and white matter injury (2.6±1.2 vs 9.3±7.6 mm^3 in LCR rats, $p<0.05$, Fig. 1) after thrombin injection.

The number of HSP-32-positive cells in the periventricular white matter area was greater in LCR compared with HCR rats (Fig. 2a). This was confirmed by Western blot where HSP-32 protein levels in periventricular white matter were significantly higher in the LCR rats (HSP-32/β-actin ratio: 3.69±0.42 vs 1.83±0.63 in HCR rats, $p<0.01$, Fig. 2b). Similarly, there were more activated microglial, OX-6-positive cells in the periventricular white matter area of LCR than in HCR rats (Fig. 3a). Western blot showed OX-6 protein levels in the periventricular white matter area

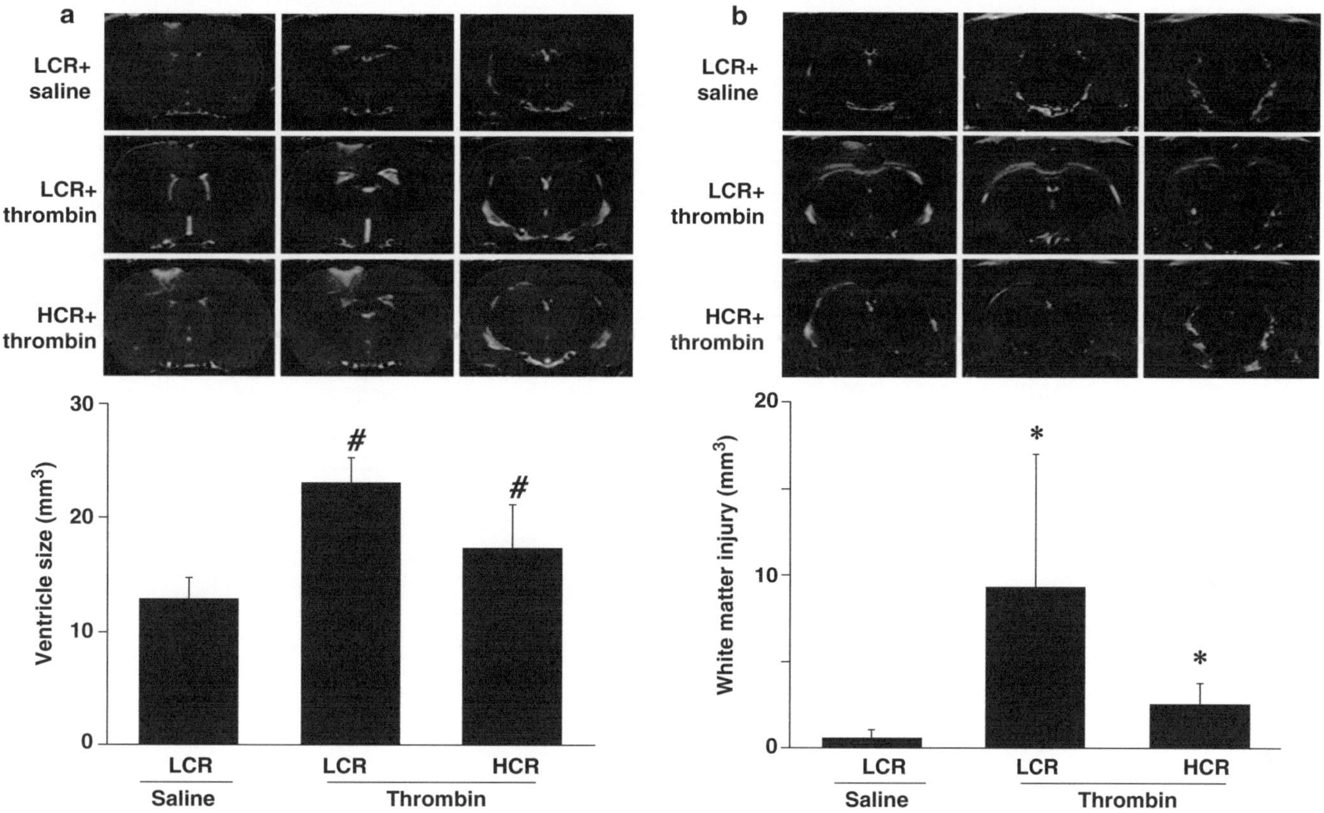

Fig. 1 T2-weighted MRI scans showing lateral ventricles (**a**) and periventricular white matter damage (**b**) at 24 h after thrombin (3 U) or saline (50 μl) injection into the right lateral ventricle in LCR and HCR rats. The *bar graphs* show quantification of the MRIs. Values are expressed as the means ± SD, $n = 3$ in LCR saline group, $n = 8$ in LCR/HCR thrombin group.

were higher in LCR rats (OX-6/β-actin: 0.96 ± 0.09 vs 0.58 ± 0.12 in HCR rats, $p < 0.05$, Fig. 3b).

Discussion

The present study demonstrates that thrombin injection causes more severe hydrocephalus and periventricular white matter damage in LCR rats compared with HCR rats. This was associated with greater HSP-32 expression and microglia activation. These results demonstrate a significant influence of exercise capacity on the initial impact of thrombin.

The LCR–HCR model system was developed based upon the aerobic hypothesis and provides polygenic-based experimental substrate for exploring both diagnostic and prescriptive translational clues that underlie disease risk factors. Low exercise capacity is a risk factor for stroke as well as other forms of cardiovascular disease [11, 13]. Thus, the LCR rats have diminished longevity [10], metabolic syndrome [21], hepatic steatosis [20], and a disordered capacity to oxidize lipids [17]. Thrombin is an essential component of the coagulation cascade and produced immediately in the brain after IVH. Our previous study has shown thrombin formation can contribute to the development of hydrocephalus after IVH [3]. In the present study, we found mid-aged LCR rats developed greater hydrocephalus than HCR rats. This result demonstrated a significant influence of exercise capacity in the initial impact of thrombin.

Hydrocephalus is often accompanied by periventricular white matter damage. Accumulating evidence implicates periventricular white matter damage as the major mechanism underlying poor behavioral outcomes [2]. In the present study, periventricular white matter damage was detected by MRI after intraventricular thrombin injection, and that damage was greater in LCR than HCR rats. The exact mechanisms of white matter damage induced by hydrocephalus are still unclear. It may be related to BBB damage, inflammation, and hypoxia-ischemia [3, 12].

That there is greater white matter damage in LCR compared with HCR rats was supported by the finding of greater

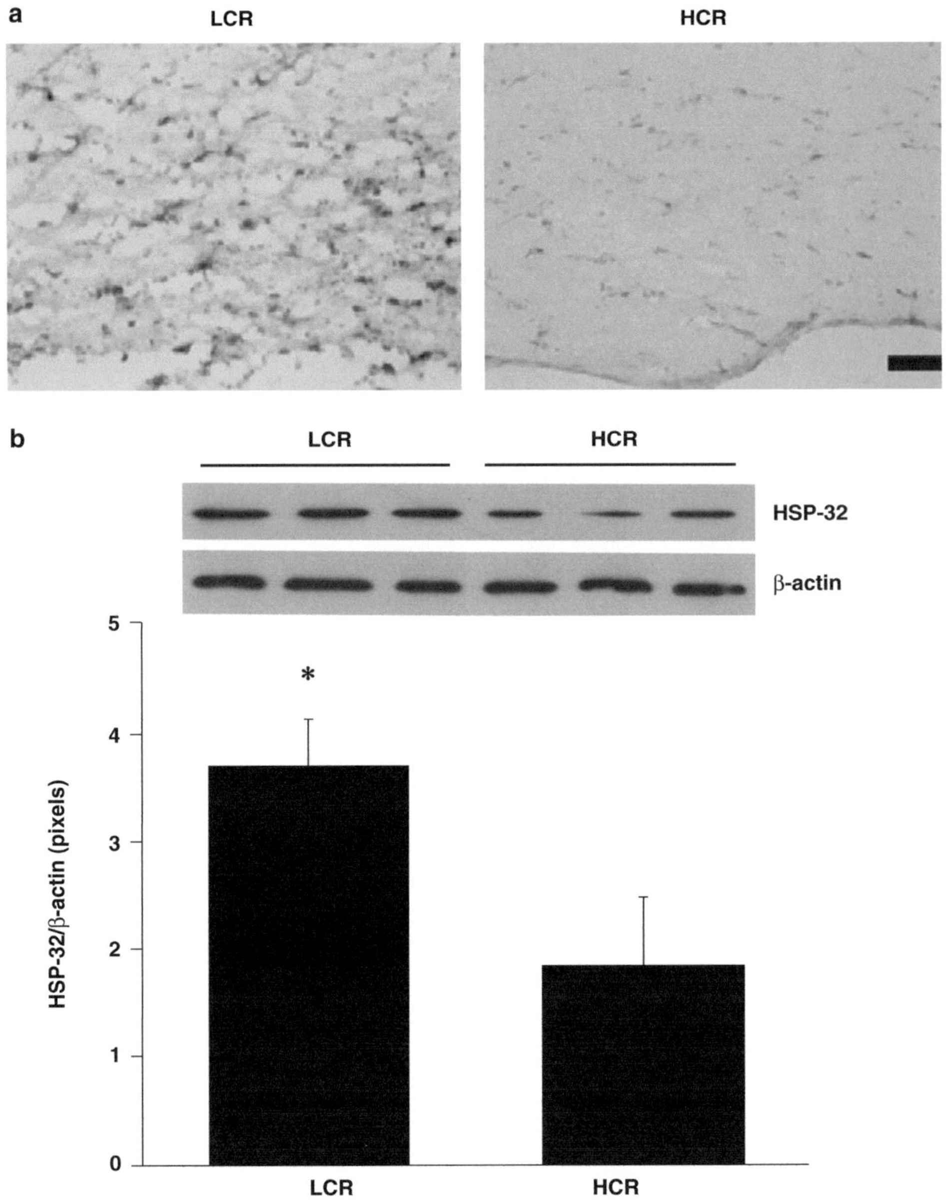

Fig. 2 (**a**) HSP-32 immunoreactivity in the periventricular white matter 24 h after intraventricular thrombin (3 U) injection in LCR and HCR rats. Scale bar = 50 μm. Representative example of $n=5$. Note the increased expression of HSP-32 in the LCR rats. (**b**) HSP-32 protein levels in the periventricular white matter area at 24 h after intraventricular thrombin injection in LCR and HCR rats. Values are expressed as the means ± SD, $n=3$, $^*p<0.05$

HSP-32 expression, a stress marker, and more microglial activation in LCR rats. A question arises as to whether the changes in HSP-32 and microglial activation may participate in causing the greater injury. HSP-32, also called hemeoxygenase-1, is an enzyme involved in the breakdown of heme and the release of iron [4]. There is evidence in ICH that HSP-32 participates in brain injury [6, 8, 24]. Similarly, there is evidence that microglial activation may exacerbate ICH-induced brain injury [23] and that it is also associated with the development of white matter damage [9]. Thus, the changes in HSP-32 and microglia activation may participate in the greater periventricular white matter injury in LCR rats.

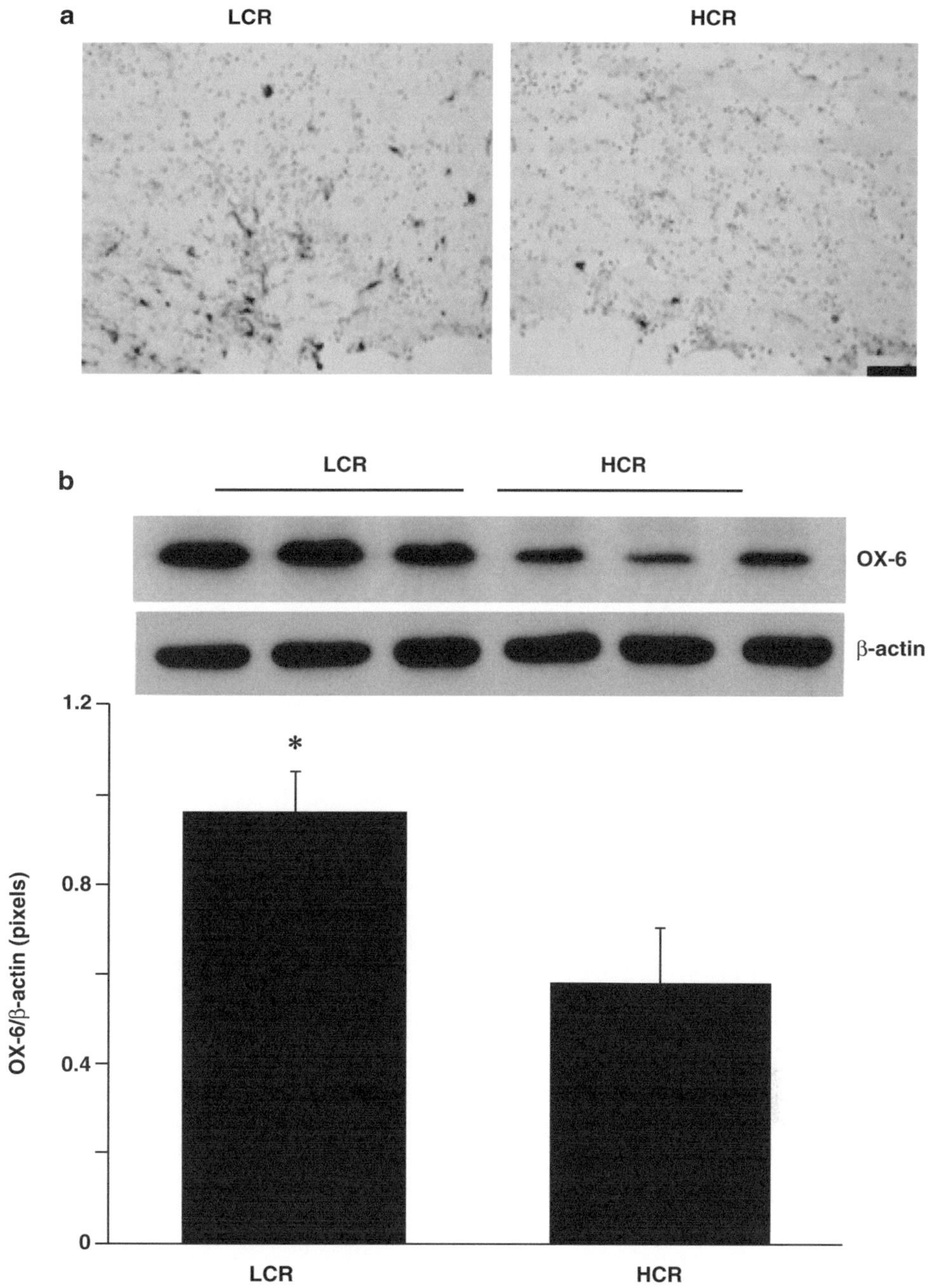

Fig. 3 (**a**) OX-46 immunoreactivity (marker of activated microglia) in the periventricular white matter 24 h after intraventricular thrombin (3 U) injection in LCR and HCR rats. Scale bar = 50 μm. Representative example of $n = 5$. Note the increased expression of HSP-32 in the LCR rats. (**b**) Ox-6 protein levels in the periventricular white matter area at 24 h after intraventricular thrombin injection in LCR and HCR rats. Values are expressed as the means ± SD, $n = 3$, $*p < 0.05$

Conclusion

In summary, thrombin induced more severe hydrocephalus and periventricular white matter damage in the rats with low aerobic capacity. Differences in thrombin-induced injury may contribute to greater brain injury following cerebral hemorrhage in rats with low aerobic capacity.

Acknowledgments This study was supported by grants NS-073959, NS079157, and NS-084049 from the National Institutes of Health (NIH) and 973 Program-2014CB541600. The LCR-HCR rat model system was funded by the Office of Research Infrastructure Programs/OD grant R24OD010950 and by grant R01DK099034 (to LGK and SLB) from the National Institutes of Health. SLB was also supported by National Institutes of Health grants R01DK077200 and R01GM104194. We acknowledge the expert care of the rat colony provided by Molly Kalahar and Lori Heckenkamp. Contact LGK (lgkoch@med.umich.edu) or SLB (brittons@umich.edu) for information on the LCR and HCR rats: these rat models are maintained as an international resource with support from the Department of Anesthesiology at the University of Michigan, Ann Arbor, Michigan.

References

1. Chen Z, Gao C, Hua Y, Keep RF, Muraszko K, Xi G (2011) Role of iron in brain injury after intraventricular hemorrhage. Stroke J Cereb Circ 42:465–470

2. Del Bigio MR, Wilson MJ, Enno T (2003) Chronic hydrocephalus in rats and humans: white matter loss and behavior changes. Ann Neurol 53:337–346
3. Gao F, Liu F, Chen Z, Hua Y, Keep RF, Xi G (2013) Hydrocephalus after intraventricular hemorrhage: the role of thrombin. J Cereb Blood Flow Metab Off J Int Soc Cereb Blood Flow Metab 34(3):489–494
4. Gong Y, Tian H, Xi G, Keep RF, Hoff JT, Hua Y (2006) Systemic zinc protoporphyrin administration reduces intracerebral hemorrhage-induced brain injury. Acta Neurochir Suppl 96:232–236
5. He Y, Liu W, Koch LG, Britton SL, Keep RF, Xi G, Hua Y (2012) Susceptibility to intracerebral hemorrhage-induced brain injury segregates with low aerobic capacity in rats. Neurobiol Dis 49C: 22–28
6. Hua Y, Keep RF, Hoff JT, Xi G (2007) Brain injury after intracerebral hemorrhage: the role of thrombin and iron. Stroke J Cereb Circ 38:759–762
7. Jin H, Xi G, Keep RF, Wu J, Hua Y (2013) DARPP-32 to quantify intracerebral hemorrhage-induced neuronal death in basal Ganglia. Transl Stroke Res 4:130–134
8. Keep RF, Hua Y, Xi G (2012) Intracerebral haemorrhage: mechanisms of injury and therapeutic targets. Lancet Neurol 11: 720–731
9. Koch LG, Britton SL (2001) Artificial selection for intrinsic aerobic endurance running capacity in rats. Physiol Genomics 5: 45–52
10. Koch LG, Kemi OJ, Qi N, Leng SX, Bijma P, Gilligan LJ, Wilkinson JE, Wisloff H, Hoydal MA, Rolim N, Abadir PM, van Grevenhof EM, Smith GL, Burant CF, Ellingsen O, Britton SL, Wisloff U (2011) Intrinsic aerobic capacity sets a divide for aging and longevity. Circ Res 109:1162–1172
11. Kurl S, Sivenius J, Makikallio TH, Rauramaa R, Laukkanen JA (2009) Exercise workload, cardiovascular risk factor evaluation and the risk of stroke in middle-aged men. J Intern Med 265: 229–237
12. Liu DZ, Ander BP, Xu H, Shen Y, Kaur P, Deng W, Sharp FR (2010) Blood-brain barrier breakdown and repair by Src after thrombin-induced injury. Ann Neurol 67:526–533
13. Myers J, Prakash M, Froelicher V, Do D, Partington S, Atwood JE (2002) Exercise capacity and mortality among men referred for exercise testing. N Engl J Med 346:793–801
14. Nieuwkamp DJ, de Gans K, Rinkel GJ, Algra A (2000) Treatment and outcome of severe intraventricular extension in patients with subarachnoid or intracerebral hemorrhage: a systematic review of the literature. J Neurol 247:117–121
15. Okauchi M, Hua Y, Keep RF, Morgenstern LB, Xi G (2009) Effects of deferoxamine on intracerebral hemorrhage-induced brain injury in aged rats. Stroke J Cereb Circ 40:1858–1863
16. Okubo S, Strahle J, Keep RF, Hua Y, Xi G (2013) Subarachnoid hemorrhage-induced hydrocephalus in rats. Stroke J Cereb Circ 44:547–550
17. Rivas DA, Lessard SJ, Saito M, Friedhuber AM, Koch LG, Britton SL, Yaspelkis BB 3rd, Hawley JA (2011) Low intrinsic running capacity is associated with reduced skeletal muscle substrate oxidation and lower mitochondrial content in white skeletal muscle. Am J Physiol Regulat Integr Compar Physiol 300:R835–R843
18. Sharp FR (1995) Stress proteins are sensitive indicators of injury in the brain produced by ischemia and toxins. J Toxicol Sci 20: 450–453
19. Sharp FR, Zhan X, Liu DZ (2013) Heat shock proteins in the brain: role of Hsp70, Hsp 27, and HO-1 (Hsp32) and their therapeutic potential. Transl Stroke Res 4:685–692
20. Thyfault JP, Rector RS, Uptergrove GM, Borengasser SJ, Morris EM, Wei Y, Laye MJ, Burant CF, Qi NR, Ridenhour SE, Koch LG, Britton SL, Ibdah JA (2009) Rats selectively bred for low aerobic capacity have reduced hepatic mitochondrial oxidative capacity and susceptibility to hepatic steatosis and injury. J Physiol 587: 1805–1816
21. Wisloff U, Najjar SM, Ellingsen O, Haram PM, Swoap S, Al-Share Q, Fernstrom M, Rezaei K, Lee SJ, Koch LG, Britton SL (2005) Cardiovascular risk factors emerge after artificial selection for low aerobic capacity. Science 307:418–420
22. Wu J, Hua Y, Keep RF, Nakamura T, Hoff JT, Xi G (2003) Iron and iron-handling proteins in the brain after intracerebral hemorrhage. Stroke J Cereb Circ 34:2964–2969
23. Wu J, Yang S, Xi G, Song S, Fu G, Keep RF, Hua Y (2008) Microglial activation and brain injury after intracerebral hemorrhage. Acta Neurochir Suppl 105:59–65
24. Xi G, Keep RF, Hoff JT (2006) Mechanisms of brain injury after intracerebral haemorrhage. Lancet Neurol 5:53–63
25. Xi G, Keep RF, Hua Y, Xiang J, Hoff JT (1999) Attenuation of thrombin-induced brain edema by cerebral thrombin preconditioning. Stroke J Cereb Circ 30:1247–1255
26. Xi G, Wagner KR, Keep RF, Hua Y, de Courten-Myers GM, Broderick JP, Brott TG, Hoff JT (1998) Role of blood clot formation on early edema development after experimental intracerebral hemorrhage. Stroke J Cereb Circ 29:2580–2586
27. Zhao J, Chen Z, Xi G, Keep RF, Hua Y (2014) Deferoxamine attenuates acute hydrocephalus after traumatic brain injury in rats. Transl Stroke Res 5:586–594

Author Index

R.L. Applegate et al. (eds.), *Brain Edema XVI: Translate Basic Science into Clinical Practice*, Acta Neurochirurgica Supplement, Vol. 121,
DOI 10.1007/978-3-319-18497-5, © Springer International Publishing Switzerland 2016

Subject Index

R.L. Applegate et al. (eds.), *Brain Edema XVI: Translate Basic Science into Clinical Practice*, Acta Neurochirurgica Supplement, Vol. 121,
DOI 10.1007/978-3-319-18497-5,

J

K

T

V

MIX
Papier aus verantwortungsvollen Quellen
Paper from responsible sources
FSC® C105338

If you have any concerns about our products,
you can contact us on
ProductSafety@springernature.com

In case Publisher is established outside the EU,
the EU authorized representative is:
Springer Nature Customer Service Center GmbH
Europaplatz 3, 69115 Heidelberg, Germany

Printed by Libri Plureos GmbH
in Hamburg, Germany